P9-DUC-555

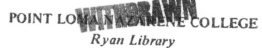

Child, Adolescent, and Family Psychiatric Nursing

Child, Adolescent, and Family Psychiatric Nursing

Barbara Schoen Johnson, PhD, RN, CS
Assistant Professor
School of Nursing
The University of Texas at Arlington
Arlington, Texas

and

Clinical and Research Consultant
Waco Center for Youth
Texas Department of Mental Health
and Mental Retardation
Waco, Texas

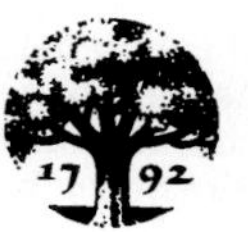

J.B. LIPPINCOTT COMPANY
Philadelphia

Acquiring Editor: Margaret Belcher RN, BSN
Sponsoring Editor: Ellen Campbell
Coordinating Editorial Assistant: Kimberly Oaks
Project Editor: Sandra Cherrey
Indexer: Lynne E. Mahan
Design Coordinator: Melissa Olson
Interior Designer: William T. Donnelly
Cover Designer: Tom Jackson
Production Manager: Helen Ewan
Production Coordinator: Kathryn Rule
Compositor: The Composing Room of Michigan, Inc.
Printer/Binder: Courier Book Company/Westford

6 5 4 3 2 1

Library of Congress Cataloging-in-Publication Data

Child, adolescent, and family psychiatric nursing / [edited by]
Barbara Schoen Johnson ; with 30 contributors.
p. cm.
Includes bibliographical references and index.
ISBN 0-397-54832-X
1. Child psychiatric nursing. 2. Adolescent psychiatric nursing.
3. Family nursing. I. Johnson, Barbara Schoen.
[DNLM: 1. Psychiatric Nursing—in infancy & childhood.
2. Psychiatric Nursing—in adolescence. 3. Mental Disorders—
nursing. 4. Family. WY 160 C5355 1995]
RJ502.3.C475 1995
610.73′68—dc20
DNLM/DLC
for Library of Congress 93-46905
CIP

Any procedure or practice described in this book should be applied by the health-care practitioner under appropriate supervision in accordance with professional standards of care used with regard to the unique circumstances that apply in each practice situation. Care has been taken to confirm the accuracy of information presented and to describe generally accepted practices. However, the authors, editors, and publisher cannot accept any responsibility for errors or omissions or for any consequences from application of the information in this book and make no warranty express or implied, with respect to the contents of the book.

Every effort has been made to ensure drug selections and dosages are in accordance with current recommendations and practice. Because of ongoing research, changes in government regulations and the constant flow of information on drug therapy, reactions and interactions, the reader is cautioned to check the package insert for each drug for indications, dosages, warnings and precautions, particularly if the drug is new or infrequently used.

Miracles, miracles
That's what life's about
Most of you must agree
If you thought it out

I can see and I can hear
I can tell you why
I can think and I can feel
I can even cry

I can walk and I can run
I can swim the sea
We have made [two babies]
And [they] look like me

Miracles, miracles
That's what life's about
Most of you must agree
If you thought it out

"Miracles"
Written by Roger Cook

To Eric and Jessica,
the miracles in our life

CONTRIBUTORS

Jane M. Baggett, MSN, RN, CNS, LCDC, CADAC
Clinical Instructor
Trinity Valley Community College
Executive Director
Day Treatment Center of Dallas
Dallas, Texas

N. Margaret Brunett, MS, RN
Director of Nursing Services
Waco Center for Youth
Texas Department of Mental Health and Mental Retardation
Waco, Texas

John F. Conley, MS, RN
Pathways Program Coordinator
Austin Wilderness Counseling Services
Austin, Texas

Deane L. Critchley, PHD, RN, CS, FAAN
Private Practice and Consultation
Children, Adolescents, and Individuals
Albuquerque, New Mexico

Sue E. Cutbirth, BSN, RN,C
Nurse–Coordinator, Specialized Treatment Unit
Waco Center for Youth
Texas Department of Mental Health and Mental Retardation
Waco, Texas

Alice S. Demi, MSN, BSN, RN, DNS, FAAN
Professor
Georgia State University
School of Nursing
Atlanta, Georgia

Lynn M. Drost, BSN, RN
Clinical Director
Child Psychiatric Unit
The Children's Hospital
Denver, Colorado

Linda M. Finke, PHD, RN
Professor and Associate Dean for Graduate Programs
Indiana University School of Nursing
Indianapolis, Indiana

Sally Francis, MS, MA
Missoula, Montana
Formerly
Assistant Professor
Department of Pediatrics
Children's Medical Center of Dallas
University of Texas Southwestern Medical Center
Dallas, Texas

Anne DuVal Frost, PHD, RN
Psychotherapist, Private Practice
Associate Professor
College of New Rochelle
New Rochelle, New York

Charlotte M. Gilbert, PHD, RN, CS
Assistant Professor
University of South Florida College of Nursing
Tampa, Florida

Judith A. Greene, PHD, RN, CS
Adjunct Faculty Southern College of Seventh Day Adventists
Collegedale, Tennessee
Nursing Coordinator
Westcott Center
Hamilton Medical Center
Dalton, Georgia

Doris S. Greiner, PHD, RN, CS
Associate Professor
University of Alabama School of Nursing
University of Alabama at Birmingham
Birmingham, Alabama

Deborah Ann Gross, DNSc, RN, FAAN
Associate Professor and Practitioner/Teacher
Rush-Presbyterian-St. Luke's Medical Center
Chicago, Illinois

Celeste M. Johnson, MSN, RN
Nursing Director/Psychiatry
Children's Medical Center of Dallas
Dallas, Texas

Maureen R. Killeen, PHD, RN
Associate Professor
Mental Health-Psychiatric Nursing
Medical College of Georgia
Athens, Georgia

Maureen T. McSwiggan-Hardin, MS, RN, CS
Assistant Professor
Medical College of Georgia
Department of Psychiatry
Section of Child, Adolescent, and Family Psychiatry
Augusta, Georgia

Jacqueline M. Melonas, JD, MS, RN
Director of Risk Services
Campania Management Co., Inc.
Vienna, Virginia

Geraldine S. Pearson, MSN, RN, CS
Assistant Clinical Professor
Yale University School of Nursing
New Haven, Connecticut
Clinical Nurse Specialist
Riverview Hospital for Children and Youth
Middletown, Connecticut

Rebecca Personett, MS, RN
Doctoral Candidate
Texas Woman's University
Assistant Vice President of Nursing Practice
Osteopathic Medical Center of Texas
Fort Worth, Texas

Nicki Warren Potts, PHD, RN
Instructor in Clinical Nursing
University of Texas at Austin
Austin, Texas

Lisa Samenfeld Ross, MSN, RN
Manager of Children's Services
West Pines Hospital
Wheat Ridge, Colorado

Alean Royes, MSN, RN, ANP
Adjunct Faculty, School of Nursing
University of Texas at Arlington
Arlington, Texas

Sarah R. Stanley, MS, RN, CNA, CS
Senior Policy Analyst
American Nurses Association
Washington, D.C.

Joyce A. Swegle, PHD, RN
Vice President
Osteopathic Medical Center of Texas
Ft. Worth, Texas

Cheryl Taylor, PHD, RN
Associate Professor
Medical School of Nursing
Louisiana State University
New Orleans, Louisiana

Brenda Wagner, PHD, RN
Licensed Psychologist
Affiliated Counseling Services
Smyrna, Georgia

Susan Mace Weeks, MS, RN
Nurse Psychotherapist, Private Practice
Weeks, Kirkham & Roaten, L.L.P.
Fort Worth, Texas

Sandra J. Weiss, PHD, DNSc, FAAN
Professor and Director
Center for Family Health Studies
University of California
San Francisco School of Nursing
San Francisco, California

Valerie A. Woodard, MSN, RN
Gainesville, Florida
Formerly
Charter Springs Hospital
Ocala, Florida

PREFACE

Child, Adolescent, and Family Psychiatric Nursing is about mental disorders of children, adolescents, and families. It is a shame it has to be written. Most of us would prefer not to read or write or think about these topics. We wish that every child in our nation were protected and happy. We wish that every family were healthy and nurturing. Unfortunately, the reality is often very different from our wishes.

Children and adolescents are abused. They live in poverty. They are depressed. They commit violent crimes. They have mental illnesses as serious and severe as adults. They live with neglectful parenting. They face serious health threats. Families suffer discrimination. They live with unemployment. They have no health care. They feel hopeless.

But there is an up side here, for this book is also about the mental health of children and families. It is about what mental health is and how to encourage it. It is about hope, and wellness, and joy. It is about the means to healthier parenting, relief from sadness, and freedom from fear.

Child-adolescent-family psychiatric and mental-health nursing is the field of work dearest to my heart. I would rather work with and write and teach about children than pursue any other aspect of nursing. And, quite frankly, when Lippincott offered me the opportunity to write and edit this book, I almost panicked. Where would I start such an important work? How could I face this major task? The solution? To begin with the best and brightest child and adolescent psychiatric nurse–authors I could find. And find them I did.

The 30 authors of these chapters are the star throwers of our age (see Acknowledgments). From all areas of the country they bring to their content material the latest scientific knowledge and their considerable experience. The topics are relevant—Problems in Parenting, Homeless Families, Children of the Mentally Ill, Trends in Mental Health Care. The topics are significant—Mood Disorders, Chemical Dependency, Bereavement, Conduct Disorders. Some topics are controversial—Personality Disorders, Law and Ethics, Psychopharmacology.

Together with the authors, my goal was to produce a comprehensive text that addresses the specialized knowledge and skill of child-adolescent-family psychiatric and mental-health nurses. We recognized that our readers already possess a basic familiarity with psychiatric nursing, but we wanted to develop or refine their focused skills in working with children, adolescents, and families. We set about exploring the critical mental health issues of today's youth and their families.

In the introduction the text discusses the mental health of and application of the nursing process to children, adolescents, and families, and important problems in parenting. Theories of attachment, family systems, behavior, and cognition are explored to lay a foundation for nursing approaches. Populations of children, adolescents, and families at risk for mental disorders and addictions—including children of the mentally ill; bereaved youth; victimized youth; children and adolescents with disabilities, chronic illness, and mental retardation; and homeless families—are presented with the goals of both defining the problems or issues and searching for solutions.

The book then examines disorders of anxiety, attention, conduct, personality, and mood; pervasive developmental and tic disorders; eating disorders; and chemical dependency in children, adolescents, and their families. Treatment modalities focus on those most often used with youth and families—play, individual, family, and group therapies; information processing approaches; behavior management; psychopharmacology; and therapeutic environments. Legal issues are examined and trends in psychiatric and mental health care of children, adolescents, and families are forecasted. Research, clinical examples, and the newest approaches to families, such as in-home care and school-based treatment, are integrated throughout the book.

I believe that the authors and I have brought forth a significant and needed work, a stellar contribution to psychiatric-mental health nursing of children and families. I commend them and I commend you. You who work with troubled children, adolescents, and families are making a significant difference in their lives every day. If this book helps you, the psychiatric and mental-health nursing care providers of the nation, then our time, effort, and energy were well worth it.

Barbara Schoen Johnson, PHD, RN, CS

ACKNOWLEDGMENTS

In *The Unexpected Universe,* the naturalist Loren Eiseley related his experience with depression. He tried to fight his despair by taking a long vacation at the seashore. Whenever he awakened before dawn and was unable to return to sleep, he would walk along the beach, hopefully to lift his spirits. Instead of finding solace on these walks, however, he became disturbed by the frenzy of professional shell collectors who raced along the beach, picked up any form of sea life lying there, and stuffed them into bags. Later, the shell collectors would boil the tiny animals out of their shells, dry the starfish in the sun, and sell the shells to tourists. Eiseley said to himself, "Thus the strong exploit the weak."

One morning Eiseley walked farther than usual along the beach, far beyond the shell collectors. There, he spotted someone all alone—a person who crouched beside a shallow pool. Eiseley approached and quietly stood and watched. A starfish arched stiffly in the water, trying to keep its tiny pores from getting clogged with sand. The person picked up the starfish and flung it far out into the sea. Then he continued to move along the shore, search for living starfish, and throw each one out into the sea. Eiseley stared for awhile, then walked on; he thought, "The star thrower is mad! These actions are foolish and a waste of time."

But every morning Eiseley returned to watch the star thrower moving about, hurling stranded starfish into the sea. He was fascinated with the star thrower, who symbolized hope in a discouraging, even hopeless, world. The star thrower's morning ritual restored and revived Eiseley's depressed spirit.

A star thrower acts to affirm life when others may become apathetic or despondent. The authors of this book—those who care and advocate for, teach and teach about, and write about children, adolescents, and families with troubles—are the star throwers of our age. I am proud to know and to have learned from each of them. I thank them for their exquisite dedication and contribution to psychiatric-mental health nursing.

You, the readers, who have chosen child, adolescent, and family psychiatric-mental health nursing, are star throwers, too. I commend you as you face the daily challenges of making a difference in the lives of your clients and pray that this book assists you in your very important work.

The friends who have helped me in so many ways during the years of this work and countless other years are also star throwers. They support, encourage, and keep me on the straight path. And so I thank all of you—Juanita Zapata Flint, Barbara Burke, Sondra George Flemming, Fela Alfaro, Dana Stahl, Diane Snow, Margaret Brunett, Kathy Lee Dunham, Barbara Vernon, Susan Wegman, Bethann Scratchard, Andi Smith, Marjorie Schuchat, Wissa Winslow, and the rest of you who will forgive my not calling you by name.

One of the best discoveries I've made while working on this book has been that of a ready-made group of compadres, soul mates really, in the Association of Child and Adolescent Psychiatric Nurses (ACAPN). Many of the authors are members and officers in this national nursing group that is devoted to the specialty of child and adolescent psychiatric-mental health nursing. They are a membership of colleagues whose warmth and nurturance demonstrate that they've selected the right nursing specialty. Finding them has been like coming home.

The University of Texas at Arlington School of Nursing has welcomed me into its fold and given me an opportunity to work with wonderful psychiatric nurse–role models—Diane Snow, Pat Gordon, Rosalyn Tolbert, and Kathy Lee Dunham. The support of Dean Myrna Pickard, Associate Dean Mary Ellen Wyers, and Assistant Deans Mary Lou Bond and Susan Grove has been a positive force during this endeavor.

For its part, Lippincott has continued to offer me its best in Ellen Campbell, editor, confidante, "commiserator," ally, and friend. As this project winds down, our professional collaboration is ending, but I expect our friendship will continue.

Through my life, my parents Roy and Marie Schoen have set an example of star throwing; they have encouraged, praised, and nurtured me while expecting nothing less than my best. I appreciate the continuing support of my sisters, brother, sisters-in-law, and brothers-in-law—Bobi and Fred Ravagnani, Mary Ellen and Don Makkos, Jeff and Angela Schoen, Bonnie and John Weseloh, and Bryan and Dee Johnson.

I started my nursing career in 1967 in a state hospital in Ohio, working with children and adolescents. At that early age, I saw so many severely disturbed and disabled children that I began to wonder: Was it possible to rear healthy, happy children? What about sane, stable children? How do parents juggle the environmental, genetic, temperamental, and emotional factors just so, to produce and rear thriving children? And I wondered, could we, in the words of Bettelheim, be "good enough parents?" Well, we (Barry and I) surely have tried and continue to work at it. I think that nothing is harder than rearing children well.

Our children have grown up with their mother writing, among other things. It could not, at times, have been easy for them. But they have come through like the champs they are. Eric Schoen Johnson and Jessica Schoen Johnson are 16 and 13 years old. They are born and bred Texans. They are kind, enthusiastic, happy, fun, motivated, unique, and all-around terrific! They are the center of our universe. The sun (that great Texas sun) rises and sets on these two teens. I thank them for their smiles and hugs and, mostly, for being who they are, wonderful people.

Which brings me now to the person I always acknowledge last, maybe because I don't know where to start (or end). My husband Barry should have contributed a chapter to this book, "How to be the World's Best Father." He is patient, strong, kind, and loving. He can coach softball and tutor advanced algebra simultaneously, in good humor, and without missing a beat. He is funny, gentle, goodhearted, and truly sees the glass half-full. He is the ultimate star thrower. I love you, Barry, and thank you for these 25 shining years of laughter, romance, and love.

CONTENTS

Child, Adolescent, and Family Psychiatric Nursing

UNIT I

Introduction

Nobody made a greater mistake than he who did nothing because he could only do a little. —EDMUND BURKE

CHAPTER

1

Mental Health of Children, Adolescents, and Families

Barbara Schoen Johnson

The mental health problems of children, adolescents, and families are monumental. Services to children and families often are fragmented and poorly coordinated. It is conceivable that any psychiatric care provider would feel overwhelmed by the enormity of the issue and wonder if he or she is able to make an impact on it. This introductory chapter overviews the scope of child mental health problems, risk groups, preventive programs, and interventions that address child and adolescent disorders. More importantly, however, this chapter and the following chapters present ways that nurses and other child mental health professionals can, and do, make a difference in the lives of our nation's youth and families.

Child Psychiatric Nursing

Child, adolescent, and family psychiatric nurses are familiar with the consequences of inadequate parenting, non-nurturing environments, poor physical care, and minimal family and community resources. Nurses know what happens when parents do not or cannot effectively parent their children, when they have no one to turn to for help with their children's needs, or when they cannot provide the living environment their children need. Nurses recognize that the latest findings of brain research have determined biochemical and genetic causation of serious brain illnesses, such as bipolar disorder and schizophrenia.

No one denies the difficulty of rearing children today or the compounded difficulty of finding that needed support and resources for a child with a mental illness are lacking.

Child and adolescent psychiatric and mental health nursing is a specialty within the field of psychiatric nursing, which focuses on the developmental and emotional needs of youth and their families. It deals with the mental disorders of children and adolescents from primary, secondary, and tertiary prevention perspectives. The American Nurses Association's Council on Psychiatric and Mental Health Nursing developed Standards of Child and Adolescent Psychiatric and Mental Health Nursing in 1985 (Box 1-1). These 1985 ANA Standards have been superseded by A Statement of Psychiatric-Mental Health Clinical Nursing Practice and Standards of Psychiatric-Mental Health Clinical Nursing Practice, which were published in 1994 by the ANA and are summarized in the Appendix.

Scope of Mental Disorder in Children

In 1983 the American Academy of Child Psychiatry estimated that 11.8% of the children in the United States, that is, more than 7 million children, suffer an emotional disorder. Of these children and youth

BOX 1–1 • STANDARDS OF CHILD AND ADOLESCENT PSYCHIATRIC AND MENTAL HEALTH NURSING PRACTICE (1985)

STANDARD I. THEORY
The nurse applies appropriate, scientifically sound theory as a basis for nursing practice decisions.

STANDARD II. ASSESSMENT
The nurse systematically collects, records, and analyzes data that are comprehensive and accurate.

STANDARD III. DIAGNOSIS
The nurse, in expressing conclusions supported by recorded assessment data and current scientific premises, uses nursing diagnoses or standard classifications of mental disorders for childhood and adolescence.

STANDARD IV. PLANNING
The nurse develops a nursing care plan with specific goals and interventions delineating nursing actions unique to the needs of each child or adolescent, as well as those of the family and other relevant interactive social systems.

STANDARD V. INTERVENTION
The nurse intervenes as guided by the nursing care plan to implement nursing actions that promote, maintain, or restore physical and mental health, prevent illness, effect rehabilitation in childhood and adolescence, and restore developmental progression.

STANDARD V-A. INTERVENTION: THERAPEUTIC ENVIRONMENT
The nurse provides, structures, and maintains a therapeutic environment in collaboration with the child or adolescent, the family, and other health care providers.

STANDARD V-B. INTERVENTION: ACTIVITIES OF DAILY LIVING
The nurse uses the activities of daily living in a goal-directed way to foster the physical and mental well-being of the child or adolescent and family.

STANDARD V-C. INTERVENTION: PSYCHOTHERAPEUTIC INTERVENTIONS
The nurse uses psychotherapeutic interventions to assist children or adolescents and families to develop, improve, or regain their adaptive functioning; promote health; prevent illness; and facilitate rehabilitation.

STANDARD V-D. INTERVENTION: PSYCHOTHERAPY
The child and adolescent psychiatric and mental health specialist uses advanced clinical expertise to function as a psychotherapist for the child or adolescent and family and accepts professional accountability for nursing practice.

STANDARD V-E. INTERVENTION: HEALTH TEACHING AND ANTICIPATORY GUIDANCE
The nurse assists the child or adolescent and family to achieve more satisfying and productive patterns of living through health teaching and anticipatory guidance.

STANDARD V-F. INTERVENTION: SOMATIC THERAPIES
The nurse uses knowledge of somatic therapies with the child or adolescent and family to enhance therapeutic interventions.

STANDARD VI. EVALUATION
The nurse evaluates the response of the child or adolescent and family to nursing actions to revise the data base, nursing diagnoses, and nursing care plan.

STANDARD VII. QUALITY ASSURANCE
The nurse participates in peer review and other means of evaluation to assure quality nursing care provided for children and adolescents and their families.

STANDARD VIII. CONTINUING EDUCATION
The nurse assumes responsibility for continuing education and professional development and contributes to the professional growth of others studying children's and adolescents' mental health.

STANDARD IX. INTERDISCIPLINARY COLLABORATION
The nurse collaborates with other health care providers in assessing, planning, implementing, and evaluating programs and other activities related to child and adolescent psychiatric and mental health nursing.

STANDARD X. USE OF COMMUNITY HEALTH SYSTEMS
The nurse participates with other members of the community in assessing, planning, implementing, and evaluating mental health services and community systems that attend to primary, secondary, and tertiary prevention of mental disorders in children and adolescents.

STANDARD XI. RESEARCH
The nurse contributes to nursing and the child and adolescent psychiatric and mental health field through innovations in theory and practice and participation in research and communicates these contributions.

(From American Nurses Association, Council on Psychiatric and Mental Health Nursing. [1985]. *Standards of Child and Adolescent Psychiatric and Mental Health Nursing Practice.* Kansas City, MO: Author.)

needing mental health treatment, only 7% of them receive any form of help. According to the Joint Commission on Mental Health of Children (1969), 80% of the mental disorders of children were related to "surface conflicts" and "faulty life experiences," such as inadequate or abusive parenting or loss of a parent through death, divorce, or desertion. Fifteen percent of these disorders were due to deeper conflicts or responses to more serious physical illness or disabilities. The remaining 5% of children's mental disorders constituted severe problems, such as autism and pervasive developmental disorder (Pothier, Norbeck, & Laliberte, 1985).

In 1986 the U.S. Congress, Office of Technology Assessment estimated that 12% to 15% of all children in the United States younger than age 18 (that is, approximately 7.5 to 9.5 million children and youth) need some level of psychiatric and mental health service. Again, it was estimated that only 7% of these children, usually the most disordered children, receive the help they need. The maldistribution of services between urban and rural areas continues to compound the inadequate availability of mental health services for children (de Leon Siantz, 1990).

Using multimethod case-finding, Brandenburg, Friedman, and Silver noted in 1990 that estimates of psychiatric disorder in children and adolescents fall in the range of 14% to 20%, reflecting moderate to severe degrees of disorder. Severe disorder seems to be present in approximately 7% of the population. The U.S. Department of Health and Human Services (1990) reported that recent studies suggest that as many as 17% to 22% (or 11 to 14 million) children suffer some type of diagnosable mental disorder.

EFFECTS OF CHILD DISORDER

The effects of childhood mental disorder are staggering. The U.S. Office of Technology Assessment (1986) noted that the many untreated youth will develop into seriously mentally ill adults who are unlikely to become contributing members of society. Almost half of the children with conduct disorder become antisocial adults. Untreated depression in children and young adolescents often results in chronic depression in later adolescence and, especially in girls, the chronic depression continues into adulthood (U.S. Department of Health and Human Services, 1990).

Costs of childhood mental illness to families may include that a potential wage earner must stay home with a particularly disturbed child. The burden to families—in the form of guilt, shame, unrealized hopes—and to siblings whose needs often go unmet is profound (U.S. Department of Health and Human Services, 1990).

These and other costs of child and adolescent mental illness are estimates at best. The financial burdens include the direct cost of mental health treatment and the indirect costs of special education, physical health services, child welfare, and juvenile justice systems. Insurance benefits may not cover the costs of extended treatment; many families are uninsured or underinsured. More than 12 million children in the United States have limited or no access to health care because they lack health insurance (Children's Defense Fund, 1990).

CHILDREN AT RISK

Studying groups at risk for a particular psychiatric disorder requires that the investigators recognize that there is no single causal agent. Rather, etiology of mental disorder is multifactorially determined (Rutter, 1988). However, whether or not a risk variable ultimately leads to a psychiatric disorder depends on what happens with time; at some point, a particular situation may activate the person's vulnerability produced by the risk factor, which results in the psychopathology (Rutter, 1988).

The U.S. Congress, Office of Technology Assessment (1986) and mental health professionals have identified specific groups of children and youth at high risk for emotional and mental disorder.

CHILDREN OF POVERTY. Children are the poorest group of citizens in U.S. society. One out of four to five children is born into poverty; 22 million of these children are younger than the age of 6 years (National Center for Children in Poverty, 1990). The major factor in the rising rate of poor women and children is divorce (Opie, 1990).

Poverty denies children adequate housing, medical care, nutrition, schools, and safe play environments. Parents who live in poverty live under chronic stress. The presence of poverty in a person's life increases the likelihood that other risk factors will exist concurrently; for example, low-income mothers are twice as likely to have a low-birth-weight baby, more likely to lack social support, less likely to be married, and if married, more likely to experience a high level of marital conflict. Low-income parents are three times more likely than other parents to begin childrearing in adolescence. Children of poverty suffer the direct physical effects of deprivation, the indirect effects of additional stress on the parent–child relationship, and the continual effects of having a lowered status in society (Halpern, 1990).

CHILDREN OF MENTALLY ILL AND SUBSTANCE-ABUSING PARENTS. Recent research indicates that in 1991, 375,000 babies were born exposed to drugs prenatally. Eighty percent of these were exposed to cocaine (National Association for Perinatal Addiction Research and Education, 1988).

A recent international review of the literature has discussed the effects of parental alcoholism on children and adolescents. Plant, Orford, and Grant (1989) found that parental alcoholism markedly increases health risks to children and adolescents, such as decreased intellectual ability, and maladaptive and behavioral disorders. The long-term effects of having a parent who drinks excessively also include psychoactive substance abuse, criminality, depression, suicide, personality disorders, and other psychologic and behavioral disorders (Plant, et al., 1989).

Children of mentally ill parents often undergo multiple separations from their parents throughout childhood. They are primarily at risk because their parents suffer a biologically or biochemically caused brain illness. In addition, children born to these parents are poorly stimulated during their infancy. Gross (1989a) notes that although it is unclear exactly how or why, children of mentally ill parents are at greater than normal risk for psychiatric and developmental disorders. These children are a highly vulnerable group who fear becoming ill themselves. Gross (1989a) found that the severity and chronicity of the parent's illness, rather than the parent's specific diagnosis of schizophrenia, bipolar disorder, and so forth, are critical factors in predicting the child's level of functioning. In addition, the risk to the child is greater when the mentally ill parent is the mother, rather than the father.

CHILDREN WHO ARE ABUSED. Each year 675,000 children are abused or neglected (Children's Defense Fund, 1990). Children suffer significantly from the effects of physical and emotional abuse and neglect and sexual and ritualized abuse. Sexually abused children are at higher risk for both short- and long-term mental disorders, including post-traumatic stress and dissociative disorders (Opie, 1990).

Morris and Bihan (1991) found a cluster of behaviors, including sexual acting-out, physical aggression, excessive masturbation, emotional withdrawal, low self-esteem, frequent physical complaints, drop in school performance, and sleep disturbance, in a population of child psychiatric inpatients with a history of sexual abuse. Escalating violence in our homes, schools, neighborhoods, and cities is producing grave physical and psychological consequences for all family members.

CHILDREN OF MINORITY ETHNIC STATUS. One of five people in the United States is a member of an ethnic minority group. African-Americans make up 11.5% of the total population, with one in three African-Americans living in poverty (U.S. Department of Health and Human Services, 1985). One in 12 Americans is Hispanic, with children comprising one third of the Hispanic population. Nearly half of all African-American children and more than 40% of Hispanic children live in poverty (National Center for Children in Poverty, 1990). Children in the Native-American and Alaskan-Native populations have a high rate of disorders, particularly high incidences of substance abuse and adolescent suicide (de Leon Siantz, 1990). Between 1970 and 1980, the population of Asian Americans and Pacific Islanders grew 120%, comprising about 1.6% of the American population. The combination of factors such as ethnicity, poverty, and racial discrimination influence a child or adolescent's developmental progress and mental health.

CHILDREN OF TEENAGE PARENTS. There were 500,000 births to adolescents in 1983. Every year more than 1 million teenagers become pregnant (Johnson, 1991). Teen parents are more likely to have premature infants, infants with low birth weight, and children with health problems. Teen parents are less likely to have the physical, mental, and emotional maturity to deal constructively with the stressors that children add to one's life.

CHILDREN IN FAMILIES WITH PARENTAL CONFLICT OR DIVORCE. Fifty-nine percent of children in the United States will live, at some point, in a single-parent home. More than 15 million children and 54% of young poor children are living in a home with one parent (National Center for Children in Poverty, 1990). Loss of a parent by divorce, death, or desertion is significant. The impact and importance of losses to a child often are overlooked or denied by the remaining, and often grief-stricken, parent (Opie, 1990). The experience of divorce to a child, says Wallerstein (1983), can be compared to the loss of a parent through death or to the losses a community suffers following a natural disaster, that is, a period of acute, time-limited crisis, followed by an extended period of disequilibrium that can last years past the precipitating event.

CHILDREN WITH CHRONIC ILLNESS AND DISABILITY. A child with epilepsy is five times more likely to have psychologic problems than a child without a chronic illness. A child with cerebral palsy, a speech impairment, or other handicapping condition also has a higher risk of emotional problems (Bishop, 1990; de Leon Siantz, 1990). The previously and widely held belief that individuals with mental retardation were "untroubled" emotionally is now known to be untrue; in fact, they are more likely to have psychologic difficulties (Varley & Furukawa, 1990).

Lipsky's writing (1985) has pointed to some of the unusual and positive aspects for the family living with a child with a disability. The family of a disabled child is not dysfunctional, Lipsky has stated, but simply runs out of energy—physically, emotionally, and financially—as they try to do all that is expected of them. The stress in the child's home is not due to psychologic disturbance, but to the lack of a sympathetic social or economic support system (Lipsky, 1985). The disability and rehabilitation literature historically has focused on the family's "chronic sorrow" (Olshansky, 1962) and the stressors facing the disabled child and family. Rarely does the literature speak to the child and family's coping, resilience, and other strengths.

Johnson (1988) has identified "parental straddling," the concept that parents of children with disabilities straddle, or balance precariously, between opposing positions as they try to maximize their children's development. Parents of a disabled child straddle between living in the past (preoccupied with the child's birth, diagnosis, and developmental milestones) and the present, facing often harsh day-to-day realities; dealing with their own and with the child's feelings and issues; and striving for an ideal position of viewing and treating the child as "normal" and helping the child see himself or herself as "normal" when the child is clearly not "normal" (Johnson, 1988). Even with adequate and available resources, the balancing act requires the parents to draw on extraordinary coping skills; in reality, most parents of children with disabilities have neither adequate nor available resources.

ACQUIRED IMMUNODEFICIENCY SYNDROME AND HOMELESSNESS. In addition to these risk groups, the Institute of Medicine (1989) has identified acquired immunodeficiency syndrome (AIDS) and homelessness as two health threats having serious mental health consequences for children. Runaway children, says Opie (1990), often come from homes with a high degree of conflict. The impact of AIDS on the lives of all Americans is steadily growing; this topic is discussed more fully in the chapter on children with chronic illness and disability (Chapter 11).

Gap Between Need and Available Resources

The number of children at risk for, or already demonstrating, mental health problems is growing. The number of available child psychiatric care specialists is inadequate.

Every commission and panel convened to examine the issue of child mental health has arrived at the same conclusion—mental health services to children and adolescents are inadequate, fragmented, and often inappropriate. Of America's 7.5 to 9.5 million children who need help, 70% to 80% either do not receive it or receive inappropriate or inadequate care (Garrison, 1989). The percentage of children receiving inadequate or no help may actually be 90% or higher (U.S. Congress, Office of Technology Assessment, 1986).

The shortage of professionals to work with children, adolescents, and their families continues to increase. In 1980 the American Academy of Child Psychiatry announced that the 3000 child psychiatrists in the United States at that time were not going to be sufficient to meet the needs by 1990. The Academy then urged child psychiatrists to shift their focus away from less severe or complex mental health problems and concentrate instead on children with physiologic involvement or severe psychiatric disorders (Pothier, et al., 1985).

An available source of professional service providers to help meet these needs can be found in graduate child and adolescent psychiatric nurses. The number of child and adolescent psychiatric nursing graduate programs in the United States, however, is small. Many other graduate-level child and adolescent psychiatric nurses have completed a generic Masters program in psychiatric nursing and specialized their didactic and clinical experiences with children, adolescents, and families.

The 1980 statement of the American Academy of Child Psychiatry never referred to the nursing body of care providers as professionals who could step in to help fill the gap between need and resources. The Pothier et al. 1985 study of the educational preparation and practice setting of graduate child and adolescent psychiatric nurses found that these nurses were adequately prepared to diagnose and treat children's emotional disorders. In direct and indirect practice, the nurses were not being used optimally, sometimes because of difficulty finding appropriate positions where they could concentrate their attention on the care of children and adolescents. In addition, Pothier et al. (1985) found that most of the nurses in independent practice spent less than half their time in direct work with children and that the poorest served group of children were the youngest children.

The study concluded that child and adolescent psychiatric nurse specialists are underused and lack professional recognition. Two difficult issues for this group were how to gain access to this underserved population and how to advocate for adequate funding to support mental health services for children (Pothier et al., 1985). The national organization of child and adolescent psychiatric nurses, the Association of Child and Adolescent Psychiatric Nurses, with chapters in many regions of the United States, is an important advocacy resource, which is described more fully in Chapter 32, Trends in Mental Health Care of Children, Adolescents, and Families.

There are estimated to be about 10,000 child psychiatric nurse specialists with Masters or Doctoral degrees in the United States (Bishop, 1989). However, within this group, ethnic minorities are underrepresented at a time when services to children of ethnic minority groups are critically needed (de Leon Siantz, 1990, 1993).

What Is Needed

Education, research, and prevention are needed to reduce the incidence and severity of mental disorders in children, adolescents, and families.

EDUCATION IN CHILD PSYCHIATRIC NURSING

Education in the specialty of child psychiatric nursing is difficult for a prospective student to locate. Only a handful (10 to 15) of these Masters programs exist in the United States, and none are located in the central, southern, or southwestern regions of the country. Higher education for nurses in the specialty of child, adolescent, and family psychiatric-mental health nursing would prepare the nurse specialists and practitioners needed to serve the youth of the nation.

RESEARCH

The need for child mental health and psychiatric research is great. Developmental perspectives, child- and family-focused approaches, and preventive and interventive measures are a few of the critical issues for study in the fields of child psychiatric care.

Research is needed, for example, to identify and treat children at high risk for dysfunctional behavior. Bishop (1990) asks how the various biologic, psychologic, and sociocultural factors interact to produce risk and what the protective factors in the environment that reduce risk are. Children and youth who experience situational and maturational crises, physical and sexual abuse, teenage pregnancy, behavioral problems, substance abuse, poverty, ethnic minority status, or significant losses clearly fall into groups at risk for emotional and behavioral problems. Risk factors rarely occur in isolation, and more often in combinations. Inner-city children, for example, are more likely to encounter several risk factors for mental disorder (e.g., violence, exposure to substance abuse, poverty, and chaotic family life-styles) (Opie, 1990).

Child and adolescent psychiatric nurses need to be poised to participate fully in the national research effort to increase knowledge and understanding of child mental health and disorder. In 1990 the National Advisory Mental Health Council submitted a report, *National Plan for Research on Child and Adolescent Mental Health Disorders,* as requested by the U.S. Congress. One of the goals of this document, produced by the National Institute of Mental Health, was to "stimulate a rapid expansion of scientific knowledge about these disorders" that afflict young people (U.S. Department of Health and Human Services, 1990).

Stanley (1990) identifies the strengths of the report as an overview of child psychiatry research status, a formalized plan for increase in funding, multidisciplinary incentives, a longitudinal focus, attention to child rights and ethical issues of research, and research funding and traineeships for career development tracts. The research plan recommends study of children and substance use and abuse, cultural and minority group response to child psychiatric disorders, communication of preventive aspects of child mental health disorders, alternate family structures, community-level child mental health delivery systems, study of children of chronically mentally ill parents, and case management (Stanley, 1990).

PREVENTION

The research evidence is clear; according to Pothier (1988), "early identification and intervention can prevent more serious mental illness" in children and adolescents. A preventive focus, however, has not yet been a national mental health priority. The American Nurses Association's (1991) *Nursing's Agenda for Health Care Reform* along with President Clinton urge that the nation's system of costly treatment of illness should be replaced with a primary health care system that promotes, restores, and maintains health.

Prevention does not equate to serving children and adolescents already identified as needing mental health services. It means intervening in schools and preschools, play groups, families, and prospective families, so that disorder does not develop. Examples include helping children who have suffered losses to work through their grief, educating children and adolescents on the consequences of drug abuse and establishing rewards with their peer group for not drinking or taking drugs, and assisting families under stress to prevent them from abusing their members.

In planning a continuum of care for children and adolescents, Herrick, Goodykoontz, Herrick, and Hackett (1991) compiled the components of a primary level of care, such as education of health care professionals and the public about mental health concepts, information about resources, identification of high-risk groups, and appropriate referrals.

Community mental health centers can play a critical role in primary preventive efforts. Some examples of prevention programs with at-risk infants are identification and early treatment of depression in mothers with infants and teaching mothers how to stimulate sensory modalities of their temperamentally or developmentally different infants. Prevention with school-age children includes avenues to involve parents in their children's learning in school, such as keeping close contact with teachers and monitoring academic progress. Adolescent disorder may be prevented through support groups and awareness of the need for counseling after a move away from the peer group (Berlin, 1990).

PREVENTING FAMILY ABUSE. Witnessing family violence has been found to affect the adult behavior of male and female children. Preventive approaches are possible through education regarding the intergenerational effects of violence (Bullock, Sandella, & McFarlane, 1989), respite care, and parental nurturing, role modeling, and support. Diminishing societal approval for violent behavior and attitudes is a first step toward changing the society in which violence and abuse thrive.

INFANT MENTAL HEALTH. Nurses are in ideal positions to help prevent, detect, and intervene in developmental delays and mental disorders of infants and toddlers. In this approach to the mental and emotional well-being of the infant and toddler, the client is the "bonding unit," because that relationship is the most important determinant of early emotional health (Hartsfield, 1991). Examples of early educative intervention with parents in the perinatal period include information about parenting, attachment and separation, family systems, and emotional development.

PARENTING SUPPORT. Parents must learn methods to maximize their parenting competence. Some parents need to learn to "ease up" or not hurry their child prematurely into adult situations (Elkind, 1988). Other parents need to realize that they should not try to be a perfect parent rearing a perfect child but a "good enough" parent who tries to rear his or her child as well as possible (Bettelheim, 1987). Importantly, Caplan and Hall-McCorquodale (1985) call for an end to the scapegoating of mothers.

Intervention

STRENGTHENING FAMILIES

Intervention programs to enhance parenting effectiveness must be tailored to the target population. The primary role of the parent, Lipsky (1985) reminds us, is to parent. That means including, not excluding, parents from important decisions about their child. Questions must be asked, such as: What is needed in a particular family? Is it information; parental nurtuance; role modeling; help adjusting to the changing developmental needs and issues of growing children; respite care; assistance in dealing with community agencies, such as schools and health care systems; individual work with a child; or family education and consultation? (Bishop, 1990). Mental health care professionals must recognize the family's responsibility as the primary unit for delivering services to most children (Box 1-2). Services for youth must support family involvement and preservation (Halvorson, 1992).

TARGETING RISK GROUPS

CHILDREN OF THE MENTALLY ILL. Among the target population composed of the children of the mentally ill, specific interventions can be identified to diminish their distress. Early and intensive treatment of mentally ill parents, assistance to the well parent to maximize his or her parenting effectiveness, and support to hold together and strengthen the family relationship are areas of intervention that will reduce the damage suffered by children due to their parents' mental illness (Gross, 1989a).

To reach this population, nurses must provide early intervention through initial assessments of all adults admitted to inpatient treatment to identify parenting problems and abilities, promotion of parent–child contact during the parent's hospitalizations, and discharge plans that include the child and his or her parenting needs (Gross, 1989a). The presence of stable attachment figures in the child's

BOX 1–2 • FAMILY SUPPORT AND SELF-HELP

The National Alliance for the Mentally Ill (NAMI) has formed a Children's and Adolescents' Network, known as NAMI-CAN, whose goal is early detection of and intervention into mental illnesses of children and adolescents.

NAMI believes that parents, educators, and even mental health professionals have difficulty identifying mental illness in children. In addition, stigma is as serious, or more serious, of a problem for children and adolescents than for adults. According to Ron Norris, President of NAMI-CAN and a Board Member of NAMI, it is difficult for people to believe that a child's mental illness can be caused by a biologic brain disease. Rather, lay and professional people tend to attribute children's emotional and behavioral problems to bad parenting or rebelliousness. At least half of NAMI members indicate that their mentally ill family member became ill before age 18. According to NAMI figures, only one in five young people receives appropriate treatment.

Families often faced with an alarming change in their child or adolescent and looking for answers may not know what questions to ask. Referring families to NAMI-CAN may help them with guidance, advocacy, and peer support.

Families also may find help in books, such as *Children and Adolescents with Mental Illness: A Parents Guide,* edited by Evelyn McElroy, PhD. The contributors to this down-to-earth guide, many of whom have mentally ill children of their own, have provided technical information for parents and skills needed for daily management of their child's symptoms. McElroy helps parents with such issues as medications, long-term care and planning, school services, various treatment modalities, and a directory of many state and national resources.

As an example of its far-reaching advocacy efforts, NAMI has recommended that Congress increase research funding on children and adolescent mental illness from $92.3 million in 1991 to $283.3 million in 1995.

REFERENCES

Eisler, L. (1991). Children's network grows in numbers and awareness. *NAMI Advocate, 12*(1), 4.

McElroy, E. (1987). *Children and Adolescents with Mental Illness: A Parents Guide.* Kensington, MD: Woodbine House.

Peschel, E. (1991). Early intervention is NAMI-CAN goal. *NAMI Advocate, 12*(5), 5.

life can help to offset the disruption of multiple separations experienced by children whose parent is repeatedly readmitted to treatment facilities.

ABUSED CHILDREN. Working through the aftermath of physical, emotional, and sexual abuse in children has been increasingly documented in the literature. Stanisz (1990) described a heterogeneous support group, called the safe group, for abused adolescents on an inpatient unit. The foci of the group was the adolescents' expression of feelings about past abuse, keeping themselves safe in the present, and other safety issues. Gilbert (1988) used art in group interventions with children living in women's shelters to help the children learn that they were not alone in their experience with family violence; and through art to express and discuss their experiences (Gilbert, 1988). Identification and treatment of child victims of abuse would decrease long-term psychological suffering (Hall, Sachs, Rayens, & Lutenbacher, 1993).

TEENAGE PARENTS. Marshall et al. (1991) evaluated a teen-parent intervention program designed to strengthen teen-parent families by improving parents' self-esteem and parenting skills and by increasing their knowledge of child development. Goals of the program also included reducing child abuse and neglect and increasing community support for teen families (Marshall, Buckner, & Powell, 1991).

BEREAVED YOUTH. A study of adolescents after the death of a parent conducted by Kuntz (1991) found that adolescents grieve differently than children and adults and even that younger adolescents grieve differently than older adolescents. Because death is a crisis situation for the survivors, Kuntz recommends that nurses offer supportive, educational counseling to all bereaved children through individual, group, or family intervention or make appropriate referrals (1991).

CHILDREN WITH CHRONIC ILLNESS AND DISABILITY. Although her work was the study of adaptation of children with epilepsy and their family resources, Austin's (1988) valuable recommendations were applicable to children with other illnesses and disabilities. Included in these recommendations were the following: consider the child at risk for, and assess for, psychosocial adaptation problems; educate the child about his or her condition; use group interventions to enhance self-esteem and promote positive adaptation; encourage regular school assessment of academic and behavioral performance; complete a comprehensive assessment of family adaptation; and support and educate families.

COMMUNITY-BASED SERVICES

Mental health services must be moved out of traditional settings, such as hospitals and clinics, and into places where children are, that is, the schools, neighborhoods, day care settings, and juvenile justice system (Opie, 1990). Instead of children being expected to fit into existing, available service systems, community-based service systems must be designed to adapt to their individual and family needs (England & Cole, 1992). An array of appropriate services would encourage individualization of care for children and families.

An often-mentioned deficiency in our system of mental health treatment is the overuse of inpatient care, rather than initially using the treatment that is least restrictive. Appropriateness of placement can be determined through interagency coordination. Some placements, such as out-of-state placements and placements of children on adult psychiatric units, should be prohibited. In the school system, the mandates of *PL 94-142,* the Education of All Handicapped Children Act, have not been fully implemented (Garrison, 1989).

Fishel (1990) reported on a multidisciplinary, multiagency pilot project that attempts to provide a continuum of services for children and adolescents and trained mental health professionals to work with youth through community-based services. These services include crisis assessment and intervention and ongoing treatment through individual therapy, respite care, and psychologic testing, evaluation, and treatment. One of the most innovative roles for nurses in this project is that of in-home family therapy and education, an example of the holistic perspective of nursing and recognition that the family as a whole is the unit of care (Fishel, 1990).

POLICY SETTING

Nurses must collaborate with other child mental health professionals in service planning, research, and advocating for social policy that fosters child and family mental health. Nurses should monitor existing practices and policies and ask whether children are being exploited or served by these. De Leon Siantz (1990) urges nurses to analyze what they do, communicate it to other mental health professionals, and recommit themselves to learn about and influence policies affecting child and family mental health.

ADVOCACY

Psychiatric nurses and other child mental health professionals have a dual advocacy role—for the child and for the family (de Leon Siantz, 1988). Children are an inarticulate and vulnerable population and lack the power to speak for themselves (Petr & Poertner, 1989).

The word advocate is both a noun and a verb. An advocate is one who pleads for or in behalf of another. The verb, to advocate, means to plead in favor of or support. Psychiatric nurses are familiar with this role of pleading for and supporting clients and families, especially in the private or institutional arena. Nurses need to become more comfortable speaking publicly on behalf of children, adolescents, and families.

ADVOCATING FOR CHILDREN. The child's rights (Box 1-3), as well as the parent's rights and responsibilities, are safeguarded through the nurse's ethical approach to treatment issues. According to the principle of respect for people, the child is recognized as having human dignity and rights, including rights of which he or she is unaware. The principle of nonmaleficence directs us to do no harm to the child and family; the principle of beneficence directs us to do good and prevent harm to the child and family, such as supporting parental rights to make decisions in the child's best interests. Justice tells us to treat every child and family fairly (de Leon Siantz, 1988).

To advocate for children, nurses must possess comprehensive knowledge of child development. This knowledge drives advocacy behavior and movements. Children are not, for example, evil creatures who have to be saved from themselves.

BOX 1–3 • CHILDREN'S RIGHTS

Traditionally, "children's rights" has been a term meaning special protections accorded to children. Historically, the idea of childhood as a distinct and vulnerable period of life developed during and extended from the 16th through the 19th centuries. John Locke compared the bonds of subjection to the father's authority over his child to swaddling clothes, which support a weak infant but loosen as the child grows in age and reason (Ross, 1982). By the second half of the 19th century, adults were largely being freed from legal authorities' overseeing their daily lives, but children's freedom was increasingly restricted. Today we realize that minors are entitled to certain rights but also need adult care and protection. We seek to balance the special needs of children, the state's interest in ensuring those needs are met, and the perquisites of parental authority with children's rights of citizenship (Ross, 1982).

We want our nation to become responsive to the needs of children. We want to eliminate abuse of children. We want capricious decision making about children to end, and we want services of at least minimal quality for all children (Knitzer, 1982). The litigation involving children in nonfamilial contexts has had a dramatic impact, as reflected in *PL 94-142,* the Education for All Handicapped Children Act. The law requires due process safeguards for children and their parents. *PL 94-142* addresses the responsibility of the services; it states specifically what opportunities for redress clients will have if these requirements are not met (Knitzer, 1982).

REFERENCES

Ross, C. J. (1982). Of children and liberty: An historian's view. *American Journal of Orthopsychiatry, 52*(3), 470–480.

Knitzer, J. (1982). Children's rights in the family and society: Dilemmas and realities. *American Journal of Orthopsychiatry, 52*(3), 481–495.

Children are not miniature adults; they neither think nor perceive as adults do. Not long ago in history, however, these were common, accepted beliefs about children (Cherry & Carty, 1986).

Nurses must assume leadership roles in keeping society aware of the vulnerability of children and the need for social policies that enhance their development (Cherry & Carty, 1986). The goals of child health advocacy are not just to reduce childhood mortality and morbidity, but to enhance the full developmental potential of all children. These goals have been limited by available human and environmental resources and inadequate funding and child development research. The elements of advocacy on behalf of the mental health of children, adolescents, and families include providing information, protection, action, and influence on policy-making. It requires that nurses stand up, demand, and work for change. It means that nurses set an example as pillars of interdisciplinary cooperation and collaboration.

Nurses must become leaders in our communities and take on cooperative, collaborative roles with those who are interested in child mental health—educators, psychologists, social workers, researchers, and parents (Cherry & Carty, 1986). Nurses and other mental health professionals must invite parents to join them as advocates for children.

ADVOCATING FOR FAMILIES. "Advocating for children" are empty words unless we also examine whether or not we are advocating for families and the empowerment of families. Bishop (1988) reminds us that a limited goal of child psychiatric nurses is to engage the family in supporting or assisting the developing child, but an expanded goal would be to help the family increase their abilities to nurture and develop all their members (i.e., to "strengthen the autonomy and competency of families"). The role of nurses then clearly becomes as an advocate of the child and family. Families and mental health professionals need not be adversaries; rather, they need to be partners in the emotional growth of children.

In 1989 Preston J. Garrison, the National Executive Director of the National Mental Health Association, addressed all advocates of child and family mental health with the following words:

> We must begin to preserve families, to create self-sufficiency rather than dependence, and to

meet the needs of our children with the least possible intrusion into their lives, and into the lives of their families (Garrison, 1989).

Summary

The alarming incidence of child and adolescent mental disorders alerts child and family psychiatric nurses and other care providers to take action to ensure the availability of supportive services for families. Services for children and adolescents and their families are notoriously inadequate, fragmented, inappropriate, and poorly coordinated. The identification of groups of children at risk for mental disorders will, hopefully, lead to the planning and implementation of effective prevention and early intervention programs. As Stanley (1990) noted, "Children are this country's best opportunity for illness prevention and wellness promotion."

Research in child mental disorders has proven that prevention is more effective and less costly than treating an actual psychiatric illness. Shifts in focus are required to individualize care of children through an interdisciplinary orientation that places parents and families in primary roles. Advocacy is the responsibility of everyone concerned with children's needs. Ways to advocate for children and families are possible but demand educated, prepared professionals, such as child and adolescent psychiatric-mental health nurses, to come forward and work to affect policies and philosophies of care.

REFERENCES

American Nurses Association. (1991). *Nursing's agenda for health care reform.* Washington, DC: American Nurses Association.

Austin, J. K. (1988). Childhood epilepsy: Child adaptation and family resources. *Journal of Child and Adolescent Psychiatric and Mental Health Nursing, 1*(1), 18–24.

Berlin, I. N. (1990). The role of the community mental health center in prevention of infant, child and adolecent disorders: Retrospect and prospect. *Community Mental Health Journal, 26*(1), 89–106.

Bettelheim, B. (1987). *A good enough parent: A book on childrearing.* New York: Vintage Books.

Bishop, S. M. (1989). Barriers to child psychiatric nursing research: Issues and opportunities to advance the field. *Journal of Child and Adolescent Psychiatric and Mental Health Nursing, 2*(4), 131–133.

Bishop, S. M. (1988). Editorial: The primacy of the family in child psychiatric and mental health nursing. *Journal of Child and Adolescent Psychiatric and Mental Health Nursing, 1*(2), 45.

Bishop, S. M. (1990). Educating for parenthood in the 1990s: Preventive intervention for high-risk youth. *Journal of Child and Adolescent Psychiatric and Mental Health Nursing, 3*(1), 1–2.

Brandenburg, N. A., Friedman, R. M., & Silver, S. E. (1990). The epidemiology of childhood psychiatric disorders: Prevalence findings from recent studies. *Journal of the American Academy of Child and Adolescent Psychiatry, 29*(1), 76–83.

Bullock, L. F. C., Sandella, J. A., & McFarlane, J. (1989). Breaking the cycle of abuse: How nurses can intervene. *Journal of Psychosocial Nursing, 27*(8), 11–13.

Caplan, P. J., & Hall-McCorquodale, I. (1985). The scapegoating of mothers: A call for change. *American Journal of Orthopsychiatry, 55*(4), 610–613.

Cherry, B. S., & Carty, R. M. (1986). Changing concepts of childhood in society. *Pediatric Nursing, 12*(6), 421–424.

Children's Defense Fund. (1990). *Children 1990: Report care, briefing book, and action primer.* Washington, DC: Author.

de Leon Siantz, M. L. (1988). Children's rights and parental rights: A historical and legal/ethical analysis. *Journal of Child and Adolescent Psychiatric and Mental Health Nursing, 1*(1), 14–17.

de Leon Siantz, M. L. (1993). Child and family minority research: How are we doing? *Journal of Child and Adolescent Psychiatric and Mental Health Nursing, 6*(4), 6–9.

de Leon Siantz, M. L. (1990). Issues facing child psychiatric nursing in the 1990's: Issues and recommendations. *Journal of Child and Adolescent Psychiatric and Mental Health Nursing, 3*(2), 65–68.

Elkind, D. (1988). *The hurried child: Growing up too fast too soon.* Menlo Park, CA: Addison-Wesley.

England, M. J. & Cole, R. F. (1992). Building systems of care for youth with serious mental illness. *Hospital and Community Psychiatry, 43*(6), 630–633.

Fishel, A. H. (1990). A community-based program for emotionally disturbed children and youth. *Journal of Child and Adolescent Psychiatric and Mental Health Nursing, 3*(4), 128–133.

Garrison, P. J. (1989). Commentary. America's invisible children need visible services: An executive view. *Journal of Child and Adolescent Psychiatric and Mental Health Nursing, 2*(3), 97–99.

Gilbert, C. M. (1988). Children in women's shelters: A group intervnetion using art. *Journal of Child and Adolescent Psychiatric and Mental Health Nursing, 1*(1), 7–13.

Gross, D. (1989a). At risk: Children of the Mentally Ill. *Journal of Psychosocial Nursing, 27*(8), 14–19.

Hall, L. A., Sachs, B., Rayens, M. K. & Lutenbacher, M. (1993). Childhood physical and sexual abuse: Their relationship with depressive symptoms in adulthood. *Image: Journal of Nursing Scholarship, 25*(4), 317–323.

Halpern, R. (1990). Poverty and early childhood parenting: Toward a framework for intervention. *American Journal of Orthopsychiatry, 60*(1), 6–8.

Halvorson, V. M. (1992). A home-based family intervention program. *Hospital and Community Psychiatry, 43*(4), 395–397.

Hartsfield, B. (1991). Commentary. Infant-toddler mental health an emerging concern. *Journal of Child and Adolescent Psychiatric and Mental Health Nursing, 4*(3), 116–118.

Herrick, C. A., Goodykoontz, L., Herrick, R. H., & Hackett, B. (1991). Planning a continuum of care in child psychiatric nursing: A collaborative effort. *Journal of Child and Adolescent Psychiatric and Mental Health Nursing, 4*(2), 41–48.

Institute of Medicine (1989). *Research on children and adolescents with mental, behavioral, and developmental disorders.* (Research Rep. No. IOM-89-07). Washington, DC: National Academy Press.

Johnson, B. H. (1991). A call to action in behalf of children and families. *Children's Health Care, 20*(3), 185–188.

Johnson, B. S. (1988). *Parenting children with disabilities.* Unpublished doctoral dissertation, Texas Woman's University. Denton, Texas.

Johnson, B. S. (1989). The emotionally disturbed child. In B. S. Johnson (Ed.), *Psychiatric-mental health nursing: Adaptation and growth* (2nd ed.). (pp. 519–549). Philadelphia: J.B. Lippincott.

Kuntz, B. (1991). Exploring the grief of adolescents after the death of a parent. *Journal of Child and Adolescent Psychiatric and Mental Health Nursing, 4*(3), 105–109.

Lipsky, D. K. (1985). A parental perspective on stress and coping. *American Journal of Orthopsychiatry, 55*(4), 614–617.

Marshall, E., Buckner, E., & Powell, K. (1991). Evaluation of a teen parent program designed to reduce child abuse and neglect and strengthen families. *Journal of Child and Adolescent Psychiatric and Mental Health Nursing, 4*(3), 96–100.

McElroy, E. (1987). *Children and adolescents with mental illness: A parent's guide.* Woodbine House.

Morris, P. A., & Bihan, S. M. (1991). The prevalence of children with a history of sexual abuse hospitalized in the psychiatric setting. *Journal of Child and Adolescent Psychiatric and Mental Health Nursing, 4*(2), 49–54.

National Association for Perinatal Addiction Research and Education. (1988). *A first: National hospital incidence survey. Update.*

National Center for Children in Poverty. (1990). *Five million children: A statistical profile of our poorest young citizens.* New York: Author.

Olshansky, S. (1962). Chronic sorrow: A response to having a mentally defective child. *Social Casework, 43,* 190–192.

Opie, N. D. (1990). Issues facing child psychiatric nursing in the 1990's: Response and recommendations. *Journal of Child and Adolescent Psychiatric and Mental Health Nursing, 3*(2), 68–71.

Petr, C., & Poertner, J. (1989). Protection and advocacy for the mentally ill: New hope for emotionally disturbed children? *Community Mental Health Journal, 25*(2), 156–163.

Plant, M. A., Orford, J., & Grant, M. (1989). The effects on children and adolescents of parents' excessive drinking: An international review. *Public Health Reports, 104*(5), 433–442.

Pothier, P. C. (1988). Child mental health problems and policy. *Archives of Psychiatric Nursing, 2*(3), 165–169.

Pothier, P. C., Norbeck, J. S., & Laliberte, M. (1985). Child psychiatric nursing: The gap between need and utilization. *Journal of Psychosocial Nursing, 23*(7), 18–23.

Rutter, M. (Ed.). (1988). *Studies of psychosocial risk: The power of longitudinal data.* Cambridge: Cambridge University Press.

Stanisz, M. M. (1990). A support group for inpatient abused adolescents. *Journal of Child and Adolescent Psychiatric and Mental Health Nursing, 3*(1), 14–17.

Stanley, S. R. (1990). Review of the institute of medicine report on children and adolescents. *Journal of Child and Adolescent Psychiatric and Mental Health Nursing, 3*(2), 62–64.

U.S. Congress, Office of Technology Assessment. (1986). *Children's mental health: Problems and services*—a background paper (Report No.OTA-BP-H-33). Washington, DC: U.S. Government Printing Office.

U.S. Department of Health and Human Services. (1993). *Child Mental Health in the 1990's.* Rockville, MD: U.S. Government Printing Office.

U.S. Department of Health and Human Services. (1990). *National plan for research on child and adolescent mental disorders.* Rockville, MD: National Institute of Mental Health.

U.S. Department of Health and Human Services. (1985). *Report of the secretary's task force on black and minority health.* (Vol. VI). Washington, DC: U.S. Government Printing Office.

Varley, C. K., & Furukawa, M. J. (1990). Psychopathology in young children with developmental disabilities. *Children's Health Care, 19*(2), 86–92.

Wallerstein, J. S. (1983). Children of divorce: The psychological tasks of the child. *American Journal of Orthopsychiatry, 53*(2), 230–243.

If there is anything we wish to change in the child, we should first examine it and see whether it is not something that could be better changed in ourselves. —C.G. JUNG

CHAPTER

2

Applying the Nursing Process to Children, Adolescents, and Families

Barbara Schoen Johnson and Jane M. Baggett

The nursing process is fundamentally a problem-solving method that nurses use to carry out the business of nursing. Applied to children, adolescents, and families in need of psychiatric and mental health intervention, the nursing process directs nurses through five steps to assess and diagnose clients' problems and to plan, implement, and evaluate care.

When a child or adolescent presents for mental health treatment, the "identified client" cannot be isolated from the family. Similarly, when the family unit is the client seeking treatment, family needs cannot be separated from those of individual youth members of the family. Because of their immaturity and dependence, children and adolescents require the continuing involvement of their parents and other family members. In this chapter, however, the nursing process is discussed first in its application to children and adolescents and then to families. References to "parents" in this chapter also are meant to encompass any caregiver, such as a grandparent, who may be responsible for rearing the child.

Assessment of Children and Adolescents

The assessment of a child or adolescent brought for treatment sets the tone for the rest of the interaction and intervention with him or her and the family. It provides an opportunity to deal with the parents' fears and misinformation, support their desire to be "good parents," and teach them to actively participate in their child's care. It should not be a time of exclusively one-sided interaction, that is, parents and child or adolescent answering questions and giving information to the psychiatric-mental health nurse, but rather a time of sharing between the nurse and the child–family unit. The nurse should answer the child's and family's questions and offer them information and options with empathy and honesty. This assessment period will form the foundation of future therapeutic relationships.

Nursing skill at assessing and diagnosing children's and adolescents' mental health problems is based on cognitive and affective abilities that allow the nurse to make high-level inferences about psychiatric and psychosocial problems (Bumbalo & Siemon, 1983). It will be more difficult for some youth to participate openly with the examiner in the assessment process. For example, children of families with an alcoholic member may not volunteer information about their home situation because they have learned from their families to follow certain "rules" of behavior: "Don't talk, don't trust, and don't feel" (Rowe, 1989).

MEANS OF COLLECTING DATA

The nurse gathers data from which nursing diagnoses will be generated by means of therapeutic use of self, information from child and family, and use of specific techniques or tools (Bumbalo & Siemon, 1983). Therapeutic use of self encompasses communication skills, empathy, and establishment of rapport. The child's or adolescent's drawings, games, doll and puppet play, and standardized tests provide important assessment data. As with other assessment techniques, standardized tests should add to the data collection process, not stand alone as a source of information.

Means of collecting assessment data about the child or adolescent client include the interview with the parents about the child; the interview with the child; behavior rating scales completed by parents, teachers, or significant adults in the child's life; physical examination, including neurologic assessment; and laboratory studies and psychologic tests (Box 2-1) (Cantwell, 1988). Data produced from multiple assessment methods are more reliable than those from a single source.

INITIAL DATA COLLECTION

In the initial contact with the client, nurses and other mental health professionals often prefer to meet with the entire family, rather than with the "identified" child or adolescent client. This family meeting gives the message that everyone in the family is involved in the problem and eases some of the pressure placed on the child, particularly if the child functions as the family scapegoat. The child or adolescent seeking treatment may have been referred by parents, school personnel, the juvenile justice system, or other health care providers; rarely is a child self-referred. The nurse must ask why the child has been brought for treatment and what goals or expectations the child and family have formulated. The child may not know why he or she is being brought for treatment; the adolescent may assert that the problem is his family's, not his or hers. Often a crisis event, such as the loss of a loved one, an acute illness of a family member, or a school failure, leads the problem behavior to escalate and precipitates the decision to seek help. If the client goals seem unrealistic and unattainable, the nurse must elicit the child's and family's participation in realistic goal setting.

Assessment data should be gathered, if possible, from multiple sources, including members of the nuclear and extended family, teachers, other health care professionals, and of course, the child or adolescent. Agreement or consistency of information among the sources should be assessed. Although the nurse will learn what the client and family identify as the "problem," an open mind must prevail. An assessment must be broad to prevent preconceived notions about a certain problem or disorder from leading to a premature focus on a particular area and to the exclusion of other relevant information (Bumbalo & Siemon, 1983). In the inpatient setting and in many outpatient settings, the multidisciplinary team collaboratively assesses, diagnoses, and plans treatment with the child–family unit.

DIRECT OBSERVATION

Unlike adults and their mental health problems, most children present inconsistent problems, which they may not recognize as problems, and have short histories marked by rapid change (Reid, Baldwin, Patterson, & Dishion, 1988). Direct observation permits the precise description of minute-by-minute child behavior. These observational data may be gathered from parents and teachers. Because children often act differently in the clinical setting than they do in their home, direct observations in natural settings are preferred. The nurse will find, for example, that a visit to the child's home provides a greater depth of information about family relationships, privacy, openness, community involvement, and so forth than can be determined in a clinical, and thus artificial, environment. Behavior reported to the nurse may include the client's temperament, activity level, habits, school performance, self-care, peer relationships, self-abusive behavior, and interaction with extended family members.

Although adolescents are capable of expressing themselves verbally, children's verbal ability is limited. The assessment of children, therefore, is conducted primarily through the medium of play. The nurse facilitates the child's natural method of expression through play by providing play materials, such as dolls, puppets, art materials (paper, pencils, crayons, paints), movement toys (cars, trucks, planes), age-appropriate games, punching bag, toy telephone, and doll house and furniture (Critchley, 1979).

CONTENT OF DATA COLLECTION

Throughout the assessment interview, the nurse gathers information about the nature of the child's or adolescent's problem; its onset, severity, duration, and impact; perceptions (and misperceptions)

BOX 2–1 • ASSESSMENT TOOLS FOR CHILDREN AND ADOLESCENTS

CHILD BEHAVIOR CHECKLISTS AND RATING SCALES

Numerous child behavior checklists and rating scales exist. They require that the informant share with the investigator a common understanding of the behavior to be rated. Some of the advantages to the use of behavior checklists and rating scales are that they draw information from adults with years of experience with the child across different settings, allow extremely infrequent behavior to be rated, are inexpensive and efficient, incorporate the opinion of significant people in the child's life, and tease out the enduring qualities or characteristics of a child (Barkley, 1988). Behavior checklists and rating scales have not been useful in assessing specific aspects of disturbance or behavior changes due to treatment or developmental effects.

STRUCTURED PSYCHIATRIC INTERVIEWS FOR CHILDREN

Face-to-face interviews have the advantages of establishing rapport, maintaining interest, clarifying misunderstandings, and validating the problems of the child and family. Although mental health professionals still rely heavily on information from adult informants, child interviews provide self-report data from children, such as their own feelings, perceptions, and behaviors.

Structured child psychiatric interviews are relatively new compared with other child assessment tools, and most interview schedules have not developed to the stage of clinical research. All structured interview schedules for children offer a list of target symptoms, behaviors, and events to be discussed, plus guidelines for conducting the interview and recording responses (Edelbrock & Costello, 1988). Interview schedules differ, however, in the information they yield and the degree of structure they impose on the interviewer.

Some examples of structured interview schedules for children are the Kiddie-Schedule for Affective Disorders and Schizophrenia (also known as Kiddie-SADS and K-SADS), 1978; the Child Screening Inventory, 1976; the Diagnostic Interview for Children and Adolescents, 1982; the Interview Schedule for Children, 1982; the Child Assessment Schedule, 1982; and the Diagnostic Interview Schedule for Children, 1982. All of the currently available interview schedules need further testing to verify their validity and reliability. No interview schedule is superior for all purposes, and all have strengths and weaknesses. Structured interviews seem to be less reliable than other assessment methods, such as observation, psychologic testing, and behavioral ratings (Edelbrock & Costello, 1988).

REFERENCES

Barkley, R. A. (1988). Child behavior rating scales and checklists. In M. Rutter, A. H. Tuma, & I. S. Lann (Eds.), *Assessment and diagnosis in child psychopathology* (pp. 113–155). New York: The Guilford Press.

Edelbrock, C. & Costello, A. J. (1988). Structured psychiatric interviews for children. In M. Rutter, A. H. Tuma, and I. S. Lann (Eds.), *Assessment and diagnosis in child psychopathology* (pp. 87–112). New York: The Guilford Press.

of the problem; and any significant events occurring concurrently. The nurse also collects information about the child's developmental stage, temperament, developmental stressors, sociocultural influences, relationships with family and peers, patterns of behavior, strengths and weaknesses, experiences of traumatic events, and school performance. The assessment of adolescents also demands that the nurse collect data about the youth's sense of identity, independence, self-image, impulsiveness, drug and alcohol use, and sexuality (Box 2-2) (McElvain, 1989).

The assessment period is a time of communication with parents. Nurses should ask parents to discuss their perceptions and expectations of the child or adolescent, the level of functioning they believe the child should demonstrate, their goals for the child, and their hopes for his or her future (Johnson, 1989). Answering the parents' spoken and unspoken fears about their child (if they did "something wrong," if their child is OK), the nurse can significantly affect the parents' comfort with their decision to seek treatment. Discussing the multiplicity of etiologic factors in a child and adolescent disorder provides information and reassurance to parents.

DEVELOPMENTAL HISTORY

The developmental history includes an assessment of developmental milestones and the quality of the skill attainment, that is, not just that the child "talked" at age 2 years, but how clearly and how many words the child used. The history also focuses on prenatal, perinatal, postnatal, and environmental risk factors associated with developmental delays such as medication use during pregnancy, precipitous delivery, low birth weight, or poverty (Steele, 1988).

A developmental history should include information about allergies, medical problems, medica-

(text continues on page 20)

BOX 2–2 • ASSESSMENT GUIDE FOR CHILDREN AND ADOLESCENTS

DEMOGRAPHIC DATA:
Name ________ Age ________ Birthdate ________ Sex ________
School ________ Grade ________

SOCIOCULTURAL INFORMATION:
Parents' occupations ________
Parents' education ________
Cultural beliefs and practices ________
____

REFERRAL SOURCE:
Presenting problems: Onset, severity, duration, effects
____
____
____
Concurrent significant events ________
____

PRECIPITATING EVENTS:
____
____

EXPECTATIONS OF TREATMENT:
Client's ________
Parents' ________

GOALS FOR THE CLIENT:
Client's ________
Parents' ________

PSYCHIATRIC HISTORY:
Client's and family's ________
____
____
Drug and alcohol use ________
____
____
Traumatic experiences ________
____
Abuse ________
____
Organic mental disorders in family ________
____
Self-harm ________
____

DEVELOPMENTAL HISTORY:
Milestones achieved ________
____
Level of skill attainment ________
____
Developmental stage ________
____
Developmental stressors ________
____

(*continued*)

BOX 2–2 • ASSESSMENT GUIDE FOR CHILDREN AND ADOLESCENTS (*Continued*)

HEALTH STATUS:
Allergies ____________________
Health history ____________________
____
Current health problems ____________________
____
Eating habits ____________________
Nutritional status ____________________
Vision ____________________
Speech ____________________
Hearing ____________________
Findings of physical examination ____________________
Medications taken ____________________

BEHAVIOR OBSERVED:
Clinical setting ____________________
____
Natural setting (home, school) ____________________
____
Play activity ____________________

BEHAVIOR REPORTED:
Temperament ____________________
____
Activity level ____________________
Patterns of behavior ____________________
____
Habits ____________________
Self-care ____________________
Self-abuse ____________________
School performance ____________________
____

RELATIONSHIPS: FAMILY
With parents ____________________
____
With siblings ____________________
____
With extended family ____________________
____

RELATIONSHIPS: PEERS
____
____
Social skills ____________________
____

SENSE OF SELF:
Identity ____________________
Impulsivity ____________________
Independence ____________________
Self-image ____________________
Sexuality ____________________
Strengths ____________________
____

(*continued*)

BOX 2–2 • ASSESSMENT GUIDE FOR CHILDREN AND ADOLESCENTS *(Continued)*

Weaknesses ______________________________

____

Hobbies/interests ______________________________

____

MENTAL STATUS EXAMINATION:

Appearance ______________________________

Mood ______________________________

Manner of relating to examiner ______________________________

Thinking/intellectual skills ______________________________

Play and fantasy ______________________________

Sensorimotor development ______________________________

DRAWINGS:

Self-portrait

Kinetic family drawing (KFD)

House-tree-person

(Attach client's drawings with descriptions in client's words.)

tions, special education, pregnancy and birth history, developmental course, and adjustment to school entry. Scahill and Sipple (1990) found that although child psychiatric nurses agreed that developmental data were essential in planning treatment for a child and that nurses should collect these data, half of the nurses in their study expressed uncertainty about how to conduct a developmental interview. The results of the study suggest that developmental data are likely to be inconsistent and incomplete when a systematic method of data collection is not used (Scahill & Sipple, 1990).

Children with developmental delays often exhibit scattered performance, that is, different levels of functioning in the domains of physical, language, self-help, and personal or social development. Parents can provide valuable information to the developmental assessment by describing the child's current level of functioning compared to what the parent knows about the development of other children (Steele, 1988). For example, does the 15-month-old child function like other 15-month-olds the parent has known, or does he function more like a 6-month-old? Ongoing or longitudinal assessments are needed to provide information about the child's or adolescent's developmental progress.

PSYCHIATRIC HISTORY

To compile the psychiatric history, the nurse gathers data about the occurrence of mental and emotional disorders, psychiatric symptomatology, drug and alcohol dependence, and organic mental disorders in the client and family members. In addition, the histories of the presenting problem, abuse, and traumatic experiences are explored.

SELF-HARM

Assessing suicidal risk for children and adolescents is an important method of preventing suicide. Because children's and adolescents' suicidal behavior is multidetermined, the assessment must be multilevel and involve follow-up interactions. The purposes of assessing suicidal risk are to diminish the possibility of immediate self-harm and defuse the crisis situation. The nurse clinician should openly discuss with the youth his or her self-harmful behaviors, thoughts, and tendencies to obtain a comprehensive suicidal assessment (Pfeffer, 1989).

Certain trends have influenced suicidal risk factors among children and adolescents, specifically an increased use of guns as a suicide method and an increased use of alcohol prior to suicide. In the assessment of the potentially suicidal child or adolescent, the nurse clinician must determine the availability of lethal methods, such as guns, and a thorough history of substance use. Pfeffer (1989) also recommends that the clinician ask whether the youth has been exposed to suicidal individuals and evaluate the potential for imitative suicidal actions.

In addition to the availability of lethal methods, substance, (particularly alcohol) abuse, and exposure to suicidal people, other risk factors for youth suicide include depression, history of family members who committed suicide, suicidal ideation and specificity of plan, previous suicidal behavior, impaired family relations, poor impulse control, and environmental stress. Other signs of impending suicidal behavior, such as vegetative signs of depression, reticence, noncommunicativeness, and secretiveness, warrant continued assessment (Pfeffer, 1989).

MENTAL STATUS EXAMINATION

A structured mental status examination includes assessment of the following:

- Appearance—dress, gestures, posture, tics
- Mood—predominant feelings, lability, fluctuations, appropriateness, ease or constriction in displaying feelings
- Manner of relating to the examiner—child's perceptions of the reasons
- Modes of thinking and intellectual skills—child's mental development
- Capacity for play and fantasy—amount and kind of involvement in play, use of play materials, themes of play, spontaneity of play, use of examiner in play
- Sensorimotor development—fine and gross motor activities, symmetry of movement, eye–hand coordination, right-left discrimination (Critchley, 1979).

During psychiatric emergencies, the nurse conducts a focused mental status examination to evaluate judgment, impulsiveness, signs of psychosis, organicity, intoxication, and suicidal tendencies.

HEALTH HISTORY

The child's or adolescent's health history includes data about allergies, childhood illnesses, past medical problems, surgeries, current health problems, and previous and current medications. A thorough physical examination, including neurologic examination, is essential in a comprehensive assessment. Health information and assessment must include the child's vision, speech, hearing, eating habits, and nutritional status. Certain chronic illnesses seem to predispose children to mental illness. In her study of adolescents with developmental disabilities, Myers (1987) found that those with epilepsy were significantly more likely to have a major psychiatric disorder, such as schizophrenia or bipolar disorder. (Chapter 11, Disability and Chronic Illness, provides more information about the population of children and adolescents with long-term conditions.)

COMMUNICATION

Children with speech and language disorders are at greater risk for emotional and behavioral problems. Scahill's (1990) retrospective study of referrals of child psychiatric inpatients for speech evaluation found that although speech pathologists made specific recommendations, these were seldom entered into the child's written treatment plan. Undetected communication disorders, existing either comorbidly or as related conditions to the psychiatric disorder, are significant barriers to the treatment of a child's emotional problems (Scahill, 1989).

STRENGTHS AND WEAKNESSES

Identification of a child's or adolescent's strengths gives the nurse and other health care providers areas of functioning to reinforce. Examples of strengths may include social skills, physical health, relationship skills, stability and supportiveness of family, ability to communicate, motivation, intelligence, school success, and cooperation.

ENVIRONMENT

An assessment of the child's or adolescent's environment will reveal supportive or harmful elements affecting all areas of functioning. For example, a supportive environment in the form of social support for the child, adolescent, or family reduces the impact of stress on an individual's psychologic stability. A nonsupportive environment, due to poverty or lack of health care or adequate nutrition, adds to the negative impact of stress on mental health.

RISK GROUPS

The U.S. Congress, Office of Technology Assessment (1986) has identified specific groups of children and youth at high risk for emotional and mental disorder. These risk groups encompass children of poverty, children of mentally ill and substance-abusing parents, children of teenage parents, children of minority ethnic status, children with chronic illness and disability, children who are abused, and children in homes with intense marital conflict or divorce. The Institute of Medicine (1989) has added acquired immunodeficiency syndrome and homelessness to these risk groups as two health threats having serious effects on the mental health of children. In addition, children undergoing maturational and situational crises are at greater risk for emotional disturbance than those in periods of less turmoil.

CHILDREN OF ALCOHOLICS. More often than they realize, nurses may assess a child from an alcoholic or other substance-abusing family. The family life of these children usually hinders, rather than promotes, their healthy development (Rowe, 1989). Keeping the "family secret," for example, that one member is an alcoholic, occupies the members' attention and energy. Although the roles of family members in an alcoholic home, such as mascot, hero, placater, lost child, and so forth, aptly describe what many clinicians observe, they have not been validated by clinical research. When children present with behavior problems, whether or not the nurse recognizes that the child comes from an alcoholic family, the nurse must pose this question: "What purpose does this behavior serve for the family?" (Rowe, 1989).

When assessing children of substance-abusing parents, nurses must be alert for academic difficulties; emotional and social behaviors, such as distrust, defensiveness, social isolation, and low self-esteem; anxiety and panic disorders; attention-deficit hyperactivity disorder; depression; child maltreatment and abuse; and increased risk of alcoholism (Rowe, 1989).

VALIDATING ASSESSMENT DATA

The validity of a nursing diagnosis and resultant plan and intervention depends on the accuracy of the assessment information from which it was derived. As a final step in the assessment process, the nurse must verify the accuracy of assessment data. Bumbalo and Siemon (1983) recommend the following methods to validate data:

- Making observations of the child in more than one setting, that is, sampling behavior
- Reviewing previous health and school records
- Using standardized tests or assessment tools
- Verifying validity of observations of child with parents and teachers
- Using a second observer
- Sharing observations and impressions with the child (if appropriate to age) and family
- Videotaping the child in natural settings of home, school, and neighborhood

A comprehensive assessment of children and adolescents with emotional and mental disorders requires that nurses collect and validate data from multiple sources. The assessment forms the foundation from which the remaining steps of the nursing process are developed.

Nursing Diagnosis

The purpose of assessment is to determine a nursing diagnosis that specifies treatment interventions. Child and adolescent psychiatric nurses must communicate clearly what types of problems they diagnose and treat (Bumbalo & Siemon, 1983). The diagnostic process in child psychiatric treatment requires collecting information from multiple sources, weighing its significance, and making a diagnostic formulation. When interview data are compared, some disorders of children are situation specific, that is the disorders are largely confined to home or school and therefore are identified by parents or teachers (Cantwell, 1988).

To formulate a nursing diagnosis, the nurse synthesizes data and reaches conclusions about the child's or adolescent's problems, strengths, coping abilities, adaptiveness of the symptoms, and inferences about the etiology of the disorder. The critical nature of the developmental process must be recognized. Nursing diagnoses of the child's condition must reflect the child's problems and deficits in functioning and his or her normal, healthy functioning. For example, there are conditions that are normal at one period of life, such as bed-wetting, and abnormal at another period of life. School refusal in 5-, 6-, and 7-year-olds often indicates separation anxiety, but school refusal for the first time in high school students may be related to the early stages of schizophrenia or major depression (Cantwell, 1988).

The nursing diagnosis response statements of Impaired Social Interaction, Ineffective Individual Coping, Self-Esteem Disturbance, Anxiety, and High Risk for Violence: Directed at Others may be supported by data such as poor judgment and impulse control, school failure, and hyperactivity in children with attention-deficit disorder. The nursing diagnosis response statements of Altered Nutrition: Less than Body Requirements, Fluid Volume Deficit, and Body Image Disturbance may be supported by data such as severe weight loss, dehydration, preoccupation with food, and fear of gaining weight, which are seen in adolescents with anorexia nervosa (Townsend, 1991).

The etiology ("related to") statements should list factors that nursing has some ability to alter or treat. Thus, in the first example, possible etiology statements could be "feelings of isolation from other children," "limited repertoire of coping skills," "sense of failure in peer interactions," and "unmet needs." In the latter example, the etiology statements could be "excess physical exertion," "abnormal fluid loss due to self-induced vomiting," and "misperception of being overweight." The response statements of nursing diagnoses direct the establishment of client goals; the etiology statements of nursing diagnoses direct nursing interventions.

There is some controversy about the appropriateness of using nursing diagnoses. In light of increasing economic constraints affecting admission and length of stay in inpatient child psychiatric care, Scahill (1991) has underscored the need for more efficient and effective treatment. Comparing nursing diagnosis to goal-oriented treatment planning, Scahill (1991) asserts that the major disadvantage in using nursing diagnoses is the creation of a parallel system of assessment and intervention, which separates nursing from the rest of the multidisciplinary team and which may cause conflicting plans and interventions. This argument proposes that nurses can ensure holistic care by communicating in language that is meaningful to all treatment disciplines.

PLANNING

Planning should be a collaborative process with the parents and child or adolescent. Involvement of adolescents is crucial because of their sensitivity to being heard, understood, and accepted (McElvain, 1989).

The skillful matching of appropriate interventions with a child's problems, states Looney (1984), is as important as accurately assessing or skillfully applying a treatment modality. The confounding variable in defining the optimal form of treatment is that children's mental health problems are almost always multidetermined. Therefore, it is difficult, but critical, to decide which problems to treat and how they should be treated.

GOALS

General child or adolescent client goals include the following:

- The adolescent will experience fewer and less intense symptoms of the mental disorder.
- The child will exhibit developmental progress.
- The adolescent will display greater autonomy and self-esteem.
- The child will interact appropriately with peers in school and the neighborhood.
- Family members will experience less distress and improve their problem-solving ability.

CLIENT OUTCOMES

Client outcomes are more specific than goals; their specificity helps nurses evaluate whether they have been met. Client outcomes, also called behavioral outcomes, should be measurable, attainable, realistic, specific, time-limited, and client-focused. The following are examples of client outcomes:

- The child will have no temper outbursts during the school hours of 9 AM to noon within 1 week of beginning treatment with methylphenidate hydrochloride (Ritalin) treatment.
- The adolescent will list two positive attributes about himself or herself by (date).
- The child will report that he or she is sleeping soundly and without nightmares by (date).
- The adolescent will gain 1 lb per week until the weight of 95 lb is attained.
- The family will plan and carry out one "fun" activity in which all members participate every 2 weeks.

DISCHARGE PLANNING

The planning for the hospitalized child or adolescent begins at the time of admission to the treatment facility. It involves reaching decisions about placement (if the child or adolescent is not to return home), self-management of symptoms, readjustment to the school and community, carryover of the benefits of inpatient treatment to home life, and follow-up with aftercare services (McElvain, 1989).

Intervention

PRIMARY PREVENTION

Primary prevention takes place in schools, homes, and communities. Nurses interact with children and families in a variety of environments and are in an advantageous position to determine whether a comprehensive assessment of a child is warranted. They are also in ideal positions to educate and support parents and youth, for example, helping teenage parents learn to care for infants and toddlers so that a childhood disorder does not develop in their offspring. Children and adolescents in crises are an important population for prevention-focused child and adolescent mental health nurses to reach.

Nurses working with children who may be from alcoholic and other substance-abusing homes must provide screening programs to identify them and their needs. These needs include education to learn about alcoholism as a family illness and opportunities to share with other children about their common experiences and problems. Learning that they are not alone in their feelings and fears helps reduce the children's sense of isolation (Rowe, 1989).

To help protect against child or adolescent suicide, the family and mental health caregiver should encourage social supports and quality coping skills. According to Pfeffer (1989), one of the best means to prevent suicide is methodic and precise evaluation of suicidal risk that involves multiple assessments within a short period of time.

PROVIDING INFORMATION

Rawlins, Rawlins, and Horner (1990) found that parents of chronically ill children identified information as their major health care need. They also reported that they needed easier access to health care and increased availability of special services. In orchestrating optimal care for children with mental or behavioral disorders, parents likewise need information, access to health care, and special services. Thus, giving information and advocating for improved access to and availability of health care and special services become nursing interventions of primary importance to parents and children.

THERAPIES

The eight chapters of Section V, Treatment Modalities, discuss play therapy, individual therapy, family therapy, group therapy, information processing approaches, behavior management, psychopharmacology, and therapeutic environments in great detail. Treatment approaches to the psychiatric and mental health problems of children and adolescents are often multimodal.

The clinical nurse specialist may function as the therapist in play, individual, group, family, and information processing therapies and may set up behavioral programs for parents to use at home. The nurse providing direct care is instrumental in managing the behavioral programs of inpatient care of children and adolescents and the therapeutic milieu. Nurses also discuss with parents the environmental adaptations that might assist their child's or adolescent's daily routine at home. All nurses must be knowledgeable about the medications, including psychotropic, anticonvulsant, and so forth, that children and adolescents are taking. Parents and youth desperately need the kinds of medication education that nurses are particularly well equipped to carry out.

COLLABORATION WITH OTHER MENTAL HEALTH PROFESSIONALS

Working with members of interdisciplinary teams, child and adolescent psychiatric nurses must communicate clearly what types of problems they diagnose and treat. They must be able to speak the languages of psychiatrists, psychologists, social workers, educators, pharmacists, speech and hearing therapists, music and art therapists, and direct care staff. They must be able to articulate what domains are the responsibility of nursing, while cooperating and collaborating so that the best possible treatment may be available to each client and family.

COORDINATION OF CARE

Often psychiatric-mental health nurses assume the role of coordinator of care. This position places them in an ideal place to advocate for the best interests of the child or adolescent and family and to interpret for them the coordinated and collaborative goals of treatment.

EVALUATION

When client outcomes have been stated in behavioral, specific, measurable, attainable, realistic, time-limited, and client-centered terms in the planning step of the nursing process, the evaluation of these outcomes is relatively simple and straightforward. If the child or adolescent and family have reached the outcomes, they can move on to set other, more advanced outcomes and goals. If the outcomes are not attained, the nurse, in collaboration with the multidisciplinary team, needs to evaluate the appropriateness and importance of the outcomes selected and perhaps devise other treatment strategies to achieve the desired goals.

Families

The very nature of the family is in transition with the explosive increase in stepfamily households and the growth of other nontraditional families; single-parent families now outnumber two-parent families. The changing definition of the family makes it a challenge for the nurse to assess and intervene effectively in the family unit.

Some startling statistics surfaced from the last census. The divorce rate doubled since 1965, and demographers project that half of all first marriages of today end in divorce. Six of 10 second marriages will probably collapse. One third of all children born in the past 10 years will probably live in a stepfamily before they reach 18. One of every four children today is being raised by a single parent. Two thirds of all mothers are in the workplace. Approximately 22% of today's children were born out of wedlock; of those, approximately one third were born to teenage mothers. One out of every four or five children lives in poverty; this rate is twice as high among African-Americans and Hispanics.

What is a family? The census bureau defines a family as "two or more persons related by birth, marriage, or adoption who reside in the same household." A definition put forth by the New York Supreme Court lists four standards that identify a family: 1) the "exclusivity and longevity of a relationship"; 2) the "level of emotional and financial commitment"; 3) how the couple "conducted their everyday lives and held themselves out for society"; and 4) the "reliance placed upon one another for daily service." The state of California decided a family could be measured by the things it should do for its members, which it termed "functions": maintain the physical health and safety of its members; help shape a belief system of goals and values; teach social skills; and create a place for recuperation from external stresses.

Family assessment requires the nurse to be flexible. The nurse cannot measure the family's functioning against his or her own experience. In fact, the nurse's own experience may interfere with the ability to be objective in the assessment. To determine what is a normal family, it is suggested that the nurse look at functions: Are the needs of family members being met? Is the family equipped with the skills to accomplish tasks needed for survival (to feed, clothe, and shelter)? The nurse can then plan interventions that help improve family functioning.

ASSESSMENT

Family assessment involves the nurse changing perspectives. The family is the client, rather than the individuals in the family. The emphasis during the assessment is on process—how do people interact and join together to do what families do? This emphasis on process is the challenge in applying the nursing process to the family.

The diagnostic process begins with the collection of information in keeping with the concept of the client, in this case, the family unit. A system is a whole that consists of more than the sum of its parts. Human beings are complex organisms who respond, grow, and change in the context of relationships with others and in response to the environment. The family system's perspective supports the existence of whole family patterns. These family patterns are thought to be integrative and either enhancing or change-resistant. The objective of the assessment portion of the nursing process is to draw conclusions related to the functional status of the family patterns that will provide the basis for determining interventions.

What is a healthy family? The nurse must be aware of any preconceived ideas that might influence conclusions. It is important to view the family as a functioning system. Interventions are aimed at improving this functioning (by the family's request) or at helping the family to mobilize existing strengths or resources (potential for growth). The nurse facilitates the family's problem-solving ability to determine its own solutions.

Beavers (1977) describes eight variables that are critical for producing competent people. Optimal families have an *open system orientation.* The basic assumptions in an open system are that people need other people for self-definition, behaviors are multidetermined, cause and effect are interchangeable, and there is an appreciation of human limitations.

Healthy families have *permeable boundaries.* The family sees the outside world positively, uses input from society and the environment to enrich members' lives, and discards input that it does not value. The boundaries between subsystems within the family, such as the parental subsystem or the parent–child subsystem, permit privacy and aloneness but allow for the inclusion of others. In contrast are those families who keep secrets from each other and from the caregiver and insist on "taking care of everything themselves." These closed families frequently find themselves "cut off" from outside support networks, resulting in intensified emotional reactions when problems do arise.

The healthy family experiences *contextual clarity,* which means that verbal and nonverbal communications are congruent and clear. There is a strong parental hierarchy and clear intergenerational boundaries; that is, the adults work together to take care of the children. These adults provide a structure that provides for basic needs and encourages growth into independent, autonomous people. In dysfunctional families, children are frequently expected to meet the needs of the adults. Single-parent families are at particular risk for this phenomenon because of the absence of another adult with whom to interact. This reversal of roles has unhealthy consequences.

Power in healthy families is shared and flows from the parental couple. The parental pair have an egalitarian partnership that consists of complementary role behaviors. Roles are not shared but complement one another. Difference is valued in the couple relationship. Sex does not define overt power in optimal families. Children do not assume parental responsibilities, and parents use authoritarian approaches, if needed.

Autonomy is encouraged in healthy families. The parents consciously believe that children are being prepared to leave the family and live independently. Each member's views are respected and each member accepts responsibility for, and communicates clearly, his or her thoughts, feelings, and actions. Children raised in these families possess a high degree of initiative and performance.

The *affective tone* in healthy families is caring, warm, empathetic, and hopeful. Members ask about and attend to feelings; they are involved with each other. Conflict is dealt with and resolved. Anger is expressed at the behavior and not at the person. Because conflict is resolved, anger is not frightening and actually strengthens family members' relationships and increases their confidence in the relationships. A respect for subjective reality exists. Members trust in the caring of each other and do not interpret the behaviors of others in a personalized manner. *Negotiation and task performance* are accomplished with input from all members and attention to the developmental capabilities of children.

The healthy family has *transcendent values;* that is, the family has a belief system that tolerates and transcends the pain of loss and change. This belief system may be in part based on conventional religious beliefs but is usually an intrinsic belief that love is a worthwhile risk even though the loved one may be lost.

The assessment guide provides a structure for gathering family systems data (Box 2-3). The nurse must remember to look at the whole family and not the behavior of one individual. Data are gathered through interview and direct observation of family interactions. The genogram, an elaboration of the family tree, can serve as an assessment tool and as an appropriate intervention strategy. It is a clinical method of taking, storing, and processing information and can be a pictorial way to examine family patterns. It is important to include all family members in the assessment process because each member's perceptions are important and may hold the key to effective intervention.

NURSING DIAGNOSIS

After gathering assessment data from the family, the nurse analyzes the data to formulate nursing diagnoses, which will guide nursing interventions. "Diagnosis is the step in the nursing process that links the observation of phenomenon to the implementation of an activity" (Donnelly, 1990).

Within the NANDA taxonomy, seven approved diagnostic categories address family situations:

- Family Coping: Potential for Growth
- Family Coping: Compromised
- Family Coping: Disabling
- Altered Family Processes
- Altered Parenting
- Parental Role Conflict

Incorporating family diagnoses is appropriate during the application of the nursing process for any client exhibiting emotional or behavioral problems.

PLANNING

Planning with parents and child is a collaborative effort. During the planning stage, the nurse reviews with the family the results of the assessment findings. By clarifying the problem, the family often is able to generate solutions of their own. The nurse is in a position to encourage and reinforce their problem-solving efforts.

During this stage, however, dysfunctional (or helpless) families may ask the nurse to tell them what to do to fix their problem. The nurse may then end up in a position of helplessness when the solutions do not work or are sabotaged by the family. "We did what *you* said and it didn't work," the

BOX 2–3 • FAMILY ASSESSMENT GUIDE*

Date: ______________

Family Composition:

	Name	Age	Relationship
(present)	____________	______	____________
	____________	______	____________
	____________	______	____________
	____________	______	____________
	____________	______	____________
	____________	______	____________
(not present)	____________	______	____________
	____________	______	____________
	____________	______	____________

Significant others: (List any person, related or not related, who resides in the home or has regular contact with this family. Examples: grandparents who provide child care, family-owned businesses, live-in babysitter, boarder)

____________	______	____________
____________	______	____________
____________	______	____________

What is the problem? If you could change one thing to make it better, what would it be? (Ask each member.)

Define context of problem. (Where does it occur? Who is involved? Describe in detail the process from beginning to end. What is the final result? Example: If the child has temper tantrum prior to parents leaving, do parents go out or do parents stay home?)

Developmental stage: (Example: couple without children, couple with young child, couple with school-age children or with teenagers)

Appearance and general behavior: (Where do people sit? Who sits next to whom? Who talks and who listens? Is there a family spokesperson? Are differing ideas allowed?)

Mood: (Angry? Depressed? Range of affect; ie, are all emotions expressed or are their limitations? Are there victims? Do parents attempt to control by inducing guilt?)

*Adapted from a traditional mental status examination.

(*continued*)

BOX 2–3 • FAMILY ASSESSMENT GUIDE (*Continued*)

Thought process: (Is the family goal directed? Are they able to complete tasks? Is there confusion? Who is the leader?)

____

____

____

FAMILY VARIABLES

Boundaries: (Is the family unit clearly defined? Do individual members have their own identities? Are differing thoughts and ideas allowed?)

____

____

____

Roles: (Are they clearly defined? Is there strong parental hierarchy and clear intergenerational boundaries?)

____

____

____

Flexibility in structure: (Can family members change roles as the need arises? Examples: Can dad cook; can mom do the yard; can older children pitch in to get the house clean? Does family fall apart when one member is gone?)

____

____

____

Resolvable conflict? (Do problems get worked out, or do they get buried and resurrected with every encounter? Examples: You never do what I ask. He is always late. Take note of words like "always," "never," and "but.")

____

____

____

Awareness that family self-destructs: (Is family able to let go? How is separation dealt with? Have parents separated from their own parents?)

____

____

____

(*continued*)

family can assert. Responsibility for change would then be shifted from the client to the nurse. This is an ineffective position for the therapist.

DETERMINING CLIENT GOALS

Some of the goals and outcomes of family mental health treatment follow:

- The family will support and encourage healthy growth along the developmental continuum.
- Improved ability to express personal thoughts and feelings will increase the possibility of need fulfillment for each family member.
- The family will be able to function with fewer symptoms of disorder and distress.
- Knowledge of the disorder or illness will help the family plan in an organized way the best strategy for coping.
- The family will access community support networks as needed.

INTERVENTION

The approach for family intervention is selected based on the needs and problems of the child and the family. Treatment interventions may include education, psychotherapy (individual or group), play therapy, family therapy, or a combination of therapies.

Family therapy is based on the idea that the behavior of an individual within the family cannot be understood or changed without understanding and effecting change within the entire family system. All behavior has meaning and through joint effort at understanding the behavior, more functional means of communicating can be developed. The family therapist joins with the family in this quest

BOX 2–3 • FAMILY ASSESSMENT GUIDE (*Continued*)

FAMILY GENOGRAM

GENOGRAM SYMBOLS

Symbol	Meaning	Symbol	Meaning
□	Male (age)	/\/\/\/\	Conflictual relationship
○	Female (age)	———	Close relationship
□ m. ○	Marriage (include date)	. . . .	Distant relationship
□ m. d. ○	Divorce (include date)		

GENOGRAM INFORMATION

Demographic	Critical Events/Losses
For each person list:	Successes/accomplishments
Age	Losses
Occupation	Crises
School level	Previous experience with current problem
Health problems	

for understanding. The therapist must take care to remain nonjudgmental and ally with the family instead of taking sides with an individual member. It is helpful to remember that one person's behavior cannot continue without the behavior of the other person. (For example, in an abusive relationship there is an abuser and an abused. If either party changes his or her role, the system cannot continue.)

Specific strategies of family therapy are discussed in Chapter 25.

EVALUATION

The outcome of family intervention is determined by a variety of factors. Does the family report subjective relief of their presenting symptoms? Does the family verbalize confidence in its ability to manage the behaviors that occur in the child? Is communication more open and spontaneous? Is the family interacting and receiving support from an outside community resource? These and other questions can provide feedback to the nurse about the effectiveness of the interventions. If the situation continues to escalate, the assessment may have missed an important clue. The nurse should share with the family the responsibility of searching for solutions. A driving force in systems theory is toward homeostasis (sameness or stability); therefore, change requires overcoming this natural force. Positively urging and reinforcing the efforts toward change will help the family get through the awkwardness involved in modifying well-practiced patterns of behavior.

The accompanying Clinical Example illustrates the application of the nursing process to a family in conflict.

CLINICAL EXAMPLE

Joey is a 6-year-old white boy referred for an evaluation of his oppositional/defiant behavior as reported by his mother and stepfather. The parents report severe problems getting Joey to cooperate around the home. He is aggressive with younger siblings (a newborn and a 1-year-old brother) and very demanding of his mother's attention. He has few peer relationships because his mother "can't trust him out of her sight." He is in first grade; his teacher reports that although he was immature at the beginning of the year, he was able to adjust to the structure and is now functioning well within the academic and behavioral expectations.

DEVELOPMENTAL HISTORY

Joey's parents were never married but were involved in a rocky relationship over a 10-year period. His father was an alcoholic and a drug addict. His mother reports that she also experimented with drugs and alcohol but denies use during pregnancy. Her pregnancy was not planned; the pregnancy and delivery were normal. Joey was very active as an infant and continues to be so. He met normal developmental milestones without difficulty.

FAMILY HISTORY

Joey's maternal grandfather is an alcoholic and is addicted to prescription drugs. His maternal grandmother had a "breakdown" after a medical illness last year; she is reported to be agoraphobic and depressed. She also had postpartum psychosis after the birth of her youngest child.

Joey's mother reports that her own childhood was dysfunctional. Both parents were in the military, so the family moved frequently. Her father drank heavily; her parents fought continuously and separated several times. The mother's father was abusive to her older siblings but overprotective of her. Her parents divorced when she was 10; the children stayed with their mother. While her mother worked to support them, she was cared for by an older sister. When visiting her father, he would make sexual advances toward her, so she stopped visiting him. She describes her adolescence as rebellious; she shunned authority, experimented with drugs, and generally had a "bad attitude." Nevertheless she graduated from high school and college. Her involvement with Joey's father occurred after college. She left him when Joey was 2, because she knew their living situation was not healthy for a young child, and returned to her family.

Joey's mother met and married her present husband when Joey was 4 years old. Two children have resulted from the marriage. His stepfather views Joey as a problem, but "just like his mother"; he also resents the mother's dependent attachment to her parents.

ASSESSMENT

Ms. S. is overwhelmed with the care of three children. She is able to meet the care needs of the two babies but is totally unprepared for mothering a school-age child. Her own parenting was deficient, and her expectations of Joey are unrealistic; she believes that once a child starts school, he should be able to take care of himself. She resents Joey's demands on her. Joey's behavior serves the function of keeping the family involved with him; however, because they are always angry with him, Joey is frightened that they will send him away or not pick him up from school. The boundaries become very confused when the stepfather is away because his mother allows Joey to sleep with her; Joey is displaced when the father is home.

The family system is one in which none of the members' needs are met. The marital relationship is conflicted because the mother spends too much time with the children. The parent–child relationship with Joey is conflicted because he isn't "cooperative" (i.e., won't take care of himself). Mother expects that her needs will be met by the children and uses the children to keep her husband involved with her. These unmet needs produce angry, depressed people.

NURSING DIAGNOSIS

The following nursing diagnoses are appropriate for this family:

Ineffective Family Coping: related to lack of knowledge of parenting skills, chronic stress in the home, and instability of the family unit

Altered Role Performance: deficit in parenting, related to lack of knowledge of child development and mother's own dysfunctional parenting

Altered Self-Concept: disturbance in self-esteem, related to repeated negative experiences, inadequate peer relationships, and conflicted family relationships.

PLANNING

After completing the assessment, it is decided that interventions will include intensive family therapy and play therapy for Joey. The family work begins with education about a child's normal growth and development and parental interventions at various ages. Mother is quite insecure about her ability to "care for" a child who can verbalize and disagree with her. She lacks skills in dealing with conflict. The situation is reframed so that Joey is giving her the opportunity

(continued)

CLINICAL EXAMPLE (*Continued*)

to learn new skills that she had not learned while growing up. While educating the parents, efforts will be geared toward strengthening the parental dyad and marital relationship. If mother can have her intimacy needs met by her husband, she will be less likely to expect the children to meet them. She also will have more motivation and energy to interact with Joey in an appropriate mother–child manner. The parents are helped to set up a reasonable behavioral plan for Joey with appropriate rewards and consequences.

OUTCOME CRITERIA

1. Parents will not argue about Joey in his presence. They will talk to each other about their concerns and present a consistent approach to Joey.
2. Parents will be able to verbalize their feelings to each other and learn to meet their needs without acting out.
3. Communication between parent–parent, parent–child, and child–parent will be clearer.
4. Joey will not be told he is "just like his father" to stop the negative scripting.

INTERVENTION

See Family Therapy Chapter 25 for a discussion of specific interventions.

EVALUATION

As parents are better able to meet their own needs, the family will experience fewer crises. The presenting symptoms of depression and acting out should be diminished.

REFERENCES

Beavers, W. (1977). *Psychotherapy and growth: A family systems perspective.* New York: Brunner/Mazel.

Bumbalo, J. A., & Siemon, M. K. (1983). Nursing assessment and diagnosis: Mental health problems of children. *Topics in Clinical Nursing, 5*(1), 41–54.

Cantwell, D. P. (1988). DSM-III studies. In M. Rutter, A. H. Tuma, & I. S. Lann (Eds.), *Assessment and diagnosis in child psychopathology* (pp. 3–36). New York: The Guilford Press.

Critchley, D. L. (1979). Mental status examinations with children and adolescents. *Nursing Clinics of North America, 14,* 429–441.

Donnelly, E. (1990). Health promotion, families and the diagnostic process. *Family and Community Health, 12*(4), 12–20.

Ferguson, H. B., & Bawden, H. N. (1988). Psychobiological measures. In M. Rutter, A. H. Tuma, & I. S. Lann (Eds.), *Assessment and diagnosis in child psychopathology* (pp. 232–263). New York: The Guilford Press.

Herth, K. A. (1989). The root of it all: Genograms as a nursing assessment tool. *Journal of Gerontological Nursing, 15*(12), 32–37.

Hogarth, C. R. (1989). Families and family therapy. In B. S. Johnson (Ed.), *Psychiatric-mental health nursing: Adaptation and growth* (pp. 222–247). Philadelphia: J.B. Lippincott.

Institute of Medicine. (1989). Research on children and adolescents with mental, behavioral, and developmental disorders. (Research Rep. No. IOM-89-07). Washington, DC: National Academy Press.

Johnson, B. S. (1989). The emotionally disturbed child. In B. S. Johnson (Ed.), *Psychiatric-mental health nursing: Adaptation and growth* (pp. 519–549). Philadelphia: J.B. Lippincott.

Looney, J. G. (1984). Treatment planning in child psychiatry. *Journal of the American Academy of Child Psychiatry, 23*(5), 529–536.

McElvain, M. S. (1989). The emotionally disturbed adolescent. In B. S. Johnson (Ed.), *Psychiatric-mental health nursing: Adaptation and growth* (pp. 550–574). Philadelphia: J.B. Lippincott.

Minuchin, S. (1974). *Families and family therapy.* Cambridge: Harvard University Press.

Myers, B. A. (1987). Psychiatric problems in adolescents with developmental disabilities. *Journal of the American Academy of Child and Adolescent Psychiatry, 26*(1), 74–79.

Pfeffer, C. R. (1989). Assessment of suicidal children and adolescents. *Psychiatric Clinics of North America, 12*(4), 861–872.

Rawlins, P. S., Rawlins, T. D., & Horner, M. (1990). Development of the family needs assessment tool. *Western Journal of Nursing Research, 12*(2), 201–214.

Reid, J. B., Baldwin, D. V., Patterson, G. R., & Dishion, T. J. (1988). Observations in the assessment of childhood disorders. In M. Rutter, A. H. Tuma, & I. S. Lann (Eds.), *Assessment and Diagnosis in Child Psychopathology* (pp. 156–195). New York: The Guilford Press.

Rowe, J. (1989). Nursing assessment of children of alcoholics. *Journal of Pediatric Nursing, 4*(4), 248–254.

Scahill, L. (1990). A method of screening for communication disorders in child psychiatric inpatients. *Journal of Child and Adolescent Psychiatric and Mental Health Nursing, 3*(3), 98–102.

Scahill, L. (1991). Nursing diagnosis vs goal-oriented treatment planning in inpatient child psychiatry. *Image: The Journal of Nursing Scholarship, 23*(2), 95–98.

Scahill, L., & Sipple, B. (1990). Developmental history collection on a child psychiatric inpatient service. *Journal of Child and Adolescent Psychiatric and Mental Health Nursing, 3*(2), 52–56.

Steele, S. M. (1988). Assessing developmental delays in preschool children. *Journal of Pediatric Health Care, 2*(3), 141–145.

Townsend, M. C. (1991). *Nursing diagnoses in psychiatric nursing: A pocket guide for care plan construction* (2nd ed.). Philadelphia: F.A. Davis.

U.S. Congress, Office of Technology Assessment. (1986). Children's mental health: Problems and services—a background paper. (Report No. OTA-BP-H-33). Washington, DC: U.S. Government Printing Office.

Vander Meer, J. M. & Gabert, H. (1993). A psychiatric nursing admission assessment tool for children and adolescents. *Journal of Child and Adolescent Psychiatric and Mental Health Nursing, 6*(3), 34–40.

Whitley, G. G., & Kachel, J. M. (1991). Altered parenting and the reconstituted family. *Journal of Child and Adolescent Psychiatric and Mental Health Nursing, 4*(2), 72–77.

CHAPTER

3

Problems in Parenting*

Maureen R. Killeen

Parent–Child Relations: An Overview

The influence of parent–child relations on the well-being of family members has been studied by nurse researchers in both physical and mental health (Whall & Fawcett, 1991). Researchers in parent–child nursing (Barnard, 1978) and child psychiatric nursing (Austin, 1988; Killeen, 1992) often share a developmental psychopathology perspective of parenting, focusing on patterns of adaptation of family members over time (Sroufe & Rutter, 1984).

Parenting is a relatively new concept. For many generations, childrearing was considered successful if children survived long enough to become contributing members of their families and society. Socialization attempts stressed survival skills, and social skills linked to survival. *How* children were raised was a private matter, with children considered as property (Siantz, 1988).

Historians trace our focus on childrearing to the early 19th century, when a new spirit of empathy in family relationships emerged (Hiestand, 1991; Sears, 1975). Although punitiveness was discouraged, parenting advice continued to sound quite hostile to children. The primary goals of socialization were to produce adults with respect for authority and a deep sense of responsibility. Willful behavior was not allowed. The only real change advocated by early parenting advisors was in discipline: Witholding love was viewed as more effective than physical punishment.

NATURE AND NURTURE

As interest in children increased, disagreements about the nature of childhood emerged. Contemporary theorists are closely aligned with one of three philosophers who published during the 17th and 18th centuries (Shaffer, 1989). The first, Hobbes, suggested that children are inherently selfish and egotistic and must be controlled and disciplined. Conversely, Rousseau believed that children are born with an innate sense of right and wrong and should be allowed to follow their own best inclinations. The third philosopher, Locke, greatly influenced theories of child development in the United States. Locke believed that children come into the world as a *tabula rasa* or blank slate with no inborn tendencies. He believed that children were the products of their environments, while Rousseau proposed that children were active participants in choosing their own experiences.

Similar disagreements existed about the causes

*Preparation of this chapter was supported in part by a grant from the National Institute of Mental Health, K07 MH 00764-04.

of mental illness. For most of the 19th century, mental illness was viewed as the result of constitutional and hereditary factors alone (Chess, 1988). With the publication of Freud's theories of personality development (1927), parental behavior gained attention. Children were still seen as untamed and in need of socialization (Hobbes' view), but parenting took on new importance. Either cold, inconsistent, nonresponsive mothering, or excessive attention during critical developmental periods were thought to underlie the symptoms of neurosis (Blum, 1953).

The pendulum swung to the point where all childhood dysfunctions were viewed as resulting from faulty parent–child interactions (Bruch, 1954). The constitutional theory of mental illness was replaced by the psychoanalytic view, in which parents' behaviors during critical developmental periods were thought to fundamentally influence personality development and lead to later mental disorders. This view was widely held and led to the widespread blame of parents (especially mothers) for their children's difficulties (Chess, 1988). The most noxious result of this "mal de mere" ideology (Chess, 1964) was the concept of the schizophrenogenic mother (Fromm-Reichmann, 1948).

Behaviorists (following Locke) also focused on the environment as the cause of children's difficulties. Faulty patterns of reward and punishment were deemed responsible for behavior problems (Skinner, 1971). The father of behaviorism, Watson, held the radical view that he could take any set of infants and train them to be anything he chose. "There is no such thing as an inheritance of capacity, talent, temperament, mental constitution, and behavioral characteristics" (Watson, 1925).

Although contemporary theorists are less prone to identify parental behavior as the sole cause of childhood dysfunction, most research has focused on the ways in which parents behave toward their children and has viewed parental behavior as a primary influence on their children's mental health. A popular example is the recent attention to adults and children with an alcoholic parent (Killeen, 1988; Scavnicky-Mylant, 1991). Research on socialization within the family also has focused primarily on the unidirectional influence of parents on children (Maccoby & Martin, 1983). In the past 20 years, however, an impressive body of research has pointed to the bidirectional nature of influence in parent–child dyads (Bell, 1968; Bell & Harper, 1977) and the larger family context (Belsky, 1984). Parents do influence their children profoundly, but the behaviors of parents that are most influential may be responses to their children's behavior, rather than causes of it. Additional evidence is accumulating from research in behavioral genetics (Scarr & Kidd, 1983) and the neurologic bases of behavior (Kagan, Reznick, & Snidman, 1987), which shows that nature does leave its handprint on development. However, the outcome for individuals is by no means programmed by nature alone. The effects of nurturing experiences are profound and long-lasting.

MODELS OF PARENT–CHILD RELATIONS

There are several ways to conceptualize the family and the challenges surrounding childrearing. One way is to trace the development of families as their composition and life circumstances change (Duvall, 1977). Another way is to look at the relative contributions to child outcomes from transactions between children's characteristics and their parents' characteristics (Sameroff & Chandler, 1975) A third way is to invoke a broader contextual and intergenerational process view of parenting (Belsky, Steinberg, & Draper, 1991). Each of these models has been applied to the prediction of health outcomes for individual family members.

FAMILY DEVELOPMENT MODELS. Duvall (1977) chose a life-span developmental framework to study families. Her *eight-stage family life cycle* used information about the presence and ages of children in the home to determine family life cycle stages. For each stage she described family developmental tasks that must be accomplished successfully to ensure the continuation of the family as a unit. These stages and tasks are based on the events surrounding the oldest child's individual development, regardless of the number or ages of younger children. Unfortunately, Duvall's description of family life will not fit the majority of children born in the 1980s or 1990s, who will spend at least part of their childhood in a single-parent home (U.S. Congress, 1986). Nevertheless, Duvall's stages provide a heuristic device for examining problems in parenting throughout the childrearing years.

TRANSACTIONAL MODELS OF PARENT–CHILD RELATIONS. Nurses are familiar with the notion of the family as a system in which all family members influence each other and are affected by each other (Whall, 1991). Studies of the complex multidirectional influences operating in families and their effects on children generally are designed within the theoretical framework of *transactional models* of parent–child relations.

Transactional models were first discussed in relation to infants and children who were vulnerable because of prenatal and early postnatal risk factors, but who nonetheless defied predictions of adverse outcomes. In a classic paper, Sameroff and Chandler (1975) articulated their transactional view:

> Successful prediction regarding long-range developmental outcomes cannot be made on the basis of a continuum of reproductive casualty alone. An equally important continuum of caretaking casualty exists to moderate or perpetuate earlier developmental difficulties (Sameroff & Chandler, 1975).

Sameroff and Chandler critiqued then current models for predicting maladaptive outcomes for children. They criticized main-effects models and interactional models as being too simplistic and static. Transactional models take into account the dynamic nature of individuals and environments. They assume interdependence and mutual influence, leading to changes in children and parents with time. Sameroff and Chandler also stressed the self-righting and integrative tendencies of children as they adapt to environmental change. They viewed deviant development as resulting from *continuous* malfunction in the organism–environment transaction with time (Sameroff & Chandler, 1975). This malfunction can result from a profound insult to the individual's integrative capacities, a serious neurologic deficit, or adverse environmental influences present throughout development. How individuals develop depends on the interplay between these constitutional vulnerabilities and environmental risks (Rose & Killian, 1983). The plasticity of the individual, coupled with the severity and chronicity of adverse environmental forces, ultimately determines whether or not the outcome is adaptive (Garmezy, 1987; Sameroff, Seifer, & Zax, 1982).

Belsky (1984) used the literature on transactional models and deviant parenting to propose a process model of competent parental functioning. He suggested that three domains of determinants lead to individual differences in parental functioning: personal psychologic resources of the parents, characteristics of the child, and contextual sources of stress and support. Each may either enhance parental functioning or constitute an additional source of stress. Belsky further proposed that when two of these determinants are at risk, the most competent parenting occurs when parents have sufficient personal resources to be sensitive caretakers. Conversely, competent parenting is least likely when only the child's characteristics produce sensitive parenting. In his view, when dysfunction exists somewhere in the system, optimal parenting and competent children will result most readily when the personal psychologic resources of the parents remain intact.

Although the empirical literature generally supports Belsky's model (Belsky et al., 1991), a body of literature also points to the buffering role that children's characteristics and contextual support can play in the absence of parental psychologic well-being. Studies of resilent children (Garmezy, 1987; Werner & Smith, 1982), those who do well in spite of serious family dysfunction or adversity, have shown that the abilities to seek and find support from an adult outside the family, to engage in positive peer relations, and to develop a sense of self independent of parental functioning are characteristics that protect the child.

In summary most contemporary researchers in parenting have abandoned the nature–nurture debate in favor of discovering *how* each influences development and how adverse outcomes can be prevented. Increasingly, theorists are espousing a transactional view that children and their parents are shaped by their biologic endowments and their social experiences with each other, with contextual sources of stress and support. Each is seen as bringing certain competencies and risks to their interactions, and the outcome is viewed as the culmination of chronic and pervasive influences throughout their lives. Throughout this chapter, this transactional model permeates the discussion of problems in parenting. The discussion focuses on the competencies and risks of parents and children and the developmental sequelae of different patterns of parent–child relations. The chapter addresses the role of the nurse in assessment and intervention in problems with parenting.

Becoming Parents: The Transition to Parenthood

Reviews of research on parent–child relations from infancy through adolescence (Belsky, 1981; 1990; Maccoby & Martin, 1983) have several conclusions in common. The first conclusion is that the characteristics of the parents as individuals and as a dyad influence their ability to engage in competent parenting. The general mental health of the parents and the quality of the marriage influence their interactions with their children.

The effects of children and parents on each other begin before birth. It is well known that parents may influence their children by their health habits during pregnancy. Prenatal assessments of psychologic variables, such as attitudes toward pregnancy and motherhood, maternal confidence, and the mother–father relationship also have been correlated with responsive mothering and infant competence and development (Maccoby & Martin, 1983).

The marital relationship continues to affect the quality of parenting during the infant's first year. Both mothers and fathers may affect their infants directly and indirectly through the spouse's relationship with the child. When fathers hold their wives in high esteem, the competence of the mother is enhanced, while the mother–infant relationship suffers when husbands are generally negative and critical of their wives (Belsky, 1981). Neither parent is likely to be responsive to their infants when marital problems exist, while positive marital relationships are associated with mutual support and more positive parenting behaviors (Shaffer, 1989). This effect of marital relations on parenting is true even when the effects of parents' psychologic adjustment are taken into account (Cox, Owen, Lewis, & Henderson, 1989). While a supportive relationship with a spouse helps to prevent the intergenerational transmission of negative, rejecting, and insensitive maternal care, the relationship is not always straightforward. Recent evidence suggests that mothers may compensate for poor marriages by more positive mothering (Belsky, 1990).

Parenting also can influence marital relations. The transition from married couple to parents involves changes in marital interactions and marital satisfaction. Mothers and fathers may become more traditional in their sex roles and experience more conflict and decreased marital satisfaction, yet the divorce rates in the early years of parenting are much lower than those of childless couples (Cowan & Cowan, 1990). For some families the changes and disruptions in the couple's routine present only minor difficulties and may ultimately be viewed positively (Randell, 1989). In general, adjustment to parenthood is easier when parents are older, have been married longer, and conceive after marriage and when infants are less demanding (Belsky, 1981). Parents of infants with health problems or who are more demanding experience more difficulty. The reaction to infants who are demanding is not a simple infant-to-caregiver effect, however. The quality of the marriage before birth influences the degree of marital disruption following the birth of a child with special needs (Belsky, 1981).

Infant–Toddler Period

CHARACTERISTICS OF PARENTS

During the infant–toddler period, the task of parents is to encourage the development of the child's interpersonal trust and budding autonomy (Duvall, 1977; Erikson, 1963). What are the characteristics of parents that are related to optimal child outcomes? Numerous studies have shown that sensitive, responsive, and nurturing caregiving by the mother is related to healthy intellectual and social-emotional development (Belsky, 1981; 1990).

Belsky (1984) suggests that mature, psychologically healthy adults are most likely to provide this developmentally flexible and growth-promoting care. Research on the effects of age support this view. Maternal age is positively associated with being responsive and gaining satisfaction from interactions with the infant (Ragozin, Basham, Crnic, Greenberg, & Robinson, 1982). Teenage mothers often express less desirable childrearing attitudes and have less realistic expectations for infants than do older mothers, and they tend to be less responsive and engage in less verbal interaction with their newborns. Negative early environments also affect subsequent parenting in a similar fashion. Children raised in homes characterized by marital conflict, unstable parent personalities, and unaffectionate, harsh, rejecting parenting often continue those parenting practices as adults. The effects of growing up in such stressful, rejecting families may persist for several generations (Belsky et al., 1991).

CHARACTERISTICS OF CHILDREN

Children's characteristics also influence the ways that others, especially parents, relate to them. Even newborns initiate a great deal of their interactions with parents by signaling their need for nourishment or their discomfort. Crying is one characteristic on which infants differ and which may be aversive to parents (Frodi & Lamb, 1978). Physical attractiveness also has consequences for caregiving. Mothers of physically attractive infants hold them closer when feeding, are more sensitive in feeding interactions, and rate their interactions more positively. Parents' expectations, as well as the infants' actual behaviors, are thought to influence parent–child interactions (Maccoby & Martin, 1983).

During infancy parents accomplish their main socialization task, fostering trust, by responding to the infant's cues, alleviating distress, and providing growth-fostering opportunities (Barnard, 1978). For a mother to provide sensitive and responsive care, she must comprehend the signals that her infant is sending. The task of the infant is to produce clear cues and respond to the caregiver. Infant characteristics may interfere with these tasks. For example, infants born prematurely with developmental delays or disorders or sensory defects may be unable to respond appropriately to parents' attempts to alleviate distress or provide stimulation. Other infants may simply lack the energy or ability to communicate clearly whether they wish to engage or disengage from stimulation.

INFANT TEMPERAMENT. The child characteristics that have received the most research attention in relation to parenting are those subsumed under the construct of temperament. Temperament has been described as a person's style of behavior, the *how* rather than the *what* (ability) or *why* (motivation) of behavior (Chess & Thomas, 1984). In general, temperament is considered to be a set of relatively stable biologically based traits that may or may not be inherited (Buss & Plomin, 1984).

Temperament is important to those interested in parent–child relations because aspects of the infant's style of behaving may influence parents' caretaking behavior. Temperament researchers have identified several dimensions of temperament that are associated with the ease or difficulty of caring for a child. Difficult temperament is associated with negative mood, high intensity of reactions, and low rhythmicity. Parents' reports of infant difficultness have been validated by studies of infant cries, assessments of the cries by other mothers, and home-based observations (Matheney, Wilson, & Nuss, 1984). It is easy to imagine that a fussy, irritable infant who is difficult to soothe and has irregular habits for eating and sleeping presents a different set of challenges to parents than does a cheerful, engaging infant who sleeps and eats at regular times and who clearly provides cues to his or her distress. How the caregiver responds to such challenges, the "goodness of fit" between infant and caregiver characteristics, may determine the ultimate outcome. One study suggests that parents may become worn down by a difficult infant. Martin and Gray (Barnard, 1978) found that mothers of relatively unresponsive premature infants persist in their efforts to stimulate their babies for a while but eventually give up being sensitive and responsive.

Although Chess and Thomas assert that infants with difficult temperaments are at greater risk for later behavioral problems (Goldsmith et al., 1987), others have found measures of temperament to be only weakly related to later psychopathology (Garrison & Earls, 1987). Consistent with a transactional view of developmental psychopathology, the effect of temperament variables must be considered in combination with family interactions and contextual sources of stress and support.

FAMILY CONTEXT

The context in which parent–child relations take place also influences the competence of the caretaking and the response of the child. Ample evidence shows that persistent poverty and inadequate social support are adverse conditions that lead to poor outcomes for children and families (Schorr, 1988). Children whose parents divorce or suffer from mental disorders or addictions also are at risk for problems in mental health (U.S. Congress, 1986). Most studies have found a cumulative effect of family stressors on child outcomes. Shaw and Emery (1987) found that children who experienced a greater number of chronic family stressors were more likely to have clinically elevated scores on behavior problems and below-average IQ scores. Further, they found that specific stressors predicted specific child outcomes. Maternal depression, parental conflict, and family income predicted behavior problems for children, while overcrowding predicted IQ.

It has been suggested that stressful life experiences affect children through changes in their mother's behavior toward them. Stressful financial circumstances, single parenting, large numbers of children, and young maternal age at first birth have been associated with mothers' affective behaviors toward their children (Conger, McCarty, Yang, Lahey, & Kropp, 1984). Consistent with a transactional model, the effect of stressful life conditions on the affective behavior of mothers was partially mediated by the mothers' psychologic characteristics. Similarly, high levels of life changes experienced by mothers have been found to have a negative impact on their children's language, IQ scores, and behavior but only if the mothers lacked coping resources or adequate social support (Bee, Hammond, Eyres, Barnard, & Snyder, 1986). Like stress, life changes are thought to affect children directly and indirectly through changes in parent–child interactions. Parents who can cope and who have adequate support are better able to buffer their children from the direct and indirect effects of life changes.

QUALITY OF PARENT–CHILD RELATIONS: SECURITY OF ATTACHMENT

The emotional bond that develops between the infant and caregiver is recognized as an extremely important precursor for mental health. This social bond has been studied extensively in the last 20 years from the perspectives of the infant's attachment to the caregiver. Children demonstrate an attachment relationship by engaging in certain security-seeking behaviors when stressed (Bowlby, 1982). Typically, children seek to be near the attachment figure and show distress when separated and relief when reunited. Infants usually display attachment behaviors toward specific people beginning in the second half of the first year (Bretherton & Waters, 1985). Attachment relationships have been used to examine the precursors of mental health and the effects of maternal behaviors and environmental change on infants. The development of an infant–caregiver attachment relationship is closely related to the developmental tasks of establishing trust and autonomy.

INDIVIDUAL DIFFERENCES IN ATTACHMENT. Ainsworth and colleagues (Ainsworth, Blehar, Waters, & Wall, 1978) developed a laboratory procedure for assessing differences among children in the quality of their attachment relationships with their caregivers. They used a "strange situation" to assess children's reactions to separation from the mother, the presence of a stranger, and reunion with the mother and identified three patterns of reaction to separation distress. *Securely attached* children use their mother as a safe haven and explore when alone with her, are distressed at separation, and welcome physical contact with the mother when she returns. Insecurely attached infants behave quite differently. Two types of anxious attachments were described. *Resistant* children are anxious in the presence of the mother and explore little. When separated from the mother, they become very distressed but resist contact with her when she returns. These infants are wary of strangers, even in the presence of their mothers. Like resistant infants, *avoidant* infants explore little in the presence of their mothers; however, they show little distress when separated from her and avoid contact with the mother at reunion. Although these infants are not wary of strangers, they tend to avoid them.

These different patterns of attachment security have been replicated in numerous studies and have been found to have predictive validity for a variety of later behaviors, including confidence and persistence in problem solving (Bretherton, 1985) and later social competence. Children who are securely attached as infants have been rated higher on positive affect, empathy, and compliance by preschool teachers and higher in self-esteem than children who were anxiously attached infants. Both resistant and avoidant children have poor social skills and more behavior problems in preschool. Resistant children are more inept with peers, dependent, helpless, and fearful with preschool teachers, while avoidant children have demonstrated hostile or distant behaviors with peers and do not seek teachers when injured or stressed (Bretherton, 1985; Erickson, Sroufe, & Egeland, 1985).

In addition to the sequelae of these attachment patterns, numerous studies have explored their precursors. Consistent with a transactional model of parent–child relations, contributors to the attachment relationship include maternal factors, child factors, and contextual factors. The quality of mothering appears to be central to the development of secure attachment relationships (Bretherton, 1985). In a longitudinal study of parent, child, and contextual factors related to attachment in high-risk families, Egeland and Farber (1984) found that maternal characteristics and caretaking skills, *not* infant characteristics, were the predominant influence in *anxious–avoidant* attachment relationships. These mothers lacked confidence, were tense and irritable, had poor caretaking skills, avoided physical contact, and evidenced little responsivity or effectiveness with crying. In contrast, the mothers of securely attached infants were sensitive, encouraged reciprocity, and were more confidant, skilled, and affectionate. For *anxious–resistant* attachments, infants' characteristics were important. At birth these infants were less active and alert than other infants and were less socially engaging during feedings. Egeland and Farber suggest that they may have been more difficult to care for and therefore required more sensitive caretaking, but their mothers were neither skilled nor sensitive. Caretaking was more important than affection for secure attachments. Recent reviews (Clarke-Stewart, 1988; Bretherton, 1985) have upheld these conclusions that the most securely attached infants have the most sensitive mothers; avoidant infants are most likely to have insensitive, angry, tense and sometimes aggressive mothers; and resistant infants are more likely to have mothers who have insufficient knowledge, general ability, and sensitivity and are inept, unsupportive, unadaptable, and sometimes neglectful. When infants' characteristics and social conditions are included in the analysis, even better predictability occurs. Difficult infants with insensitive mothers and low social support were most likely to be insecurely attached.

Finally, studies examining attachment and later behavior problems have provided evidence that subsequent mother–child interactions may be more important than early attachment classification. Erikson, Sroufe, & Egeland (1985) found that children who were securely attached as infants but who developed behavior problems in preschool had mothers who were less effective in helping them with subsequent stages of development, were less supportive of their problem-solving efforts, did not provide warmth and encouragement, and did not let their children know what was expected of them. Conversely, mothers of children who were insecurely attached as infants but who did not display behavior problems in preschool were respectful of their child's autonomy; allowed exploration without intrusion; provided structure and firm, consistent limits without hostility; and provided clear instructions and cues to help their child. In both cases in which preschool behavior differed from expectations based on attachment security, there were changes in the quality of care and support.

Preschool Through Adolescence

Erikson (1963) describes the tasks of preschool and school-age children as developing their sense of initiative and industry, respectively. In adolescence, the lessons learned culminate in a sense of identity. The tasks for parents are to adapt to children's changing needs and interests in stimulating, growth-promoting ways; to fit into the school community; and to balance their children's freedom with parental responsibility (Duvall, 1977). Consistent with a transactional model, individual characteristics, patterns of family interactions, and contextual factors influence the success of family members in accomplishing their tasks.

EFFECTIVE PARENTING

During the preschool period, parents consciously begin the task of socialization, teaching children the values and skills needed to function as adults in their society. Invariably, this involves promoting some behaviors while restricting others. The lessons and admonitions of parents will only be effective if they are internalized, if children adhere to them when parents are absent. Competence in problem solving, mature moral development, and adequate self-esteem are precursors to positive adult functioning. In general childrearing variations have been shown to have consistent effects on development in these areas (Maccoby & Martin, 1983).

Early studies described two kinds of discipline: power-assertive (physical punishment, forceful commands, threats, and shouting) and love-oriented techniques (showing disappointment, praise, love withdrawal, contingent affection, and reasoning). Baumrind and Black (1967; Maccoby & Martin, 1983), classified parents based on two related dimensions of childrearing: parental demandingness and parental responsiveness.

Authoritative parents have a balanced approach to the demanding and responsive aspects of childrearing (Maccoby & Martin, 1983). Authoritative parents foster their children's independence and individuality, demand mature, age-appropriate behavior, and set clear standards. They firmly enforce rules and standards, use more positive reinforcement and less punishment, listen to children's points of view, and respond to their children's reasonable demands. Children raised by authoritative parents have higher self-esteem, more mature moral development, competence, and self-control (Baumrind & Black, 1967; Shaffer, 1989).

Authoritarian parenting involves a high level of demandingness and a low level of responsiveness to children's demands. Authoritarian parents tend to use more power-assertive techniques to control children, value obedience and respect for authority, issue demands as edicts rather than discussing rules with children, and discourage verbal give-and-take between parent and child. They tend to punish transgressions and not to encourage independence and individuality. Children raised in this way have less social competence, spontaneity, curiosity, and originality; show less internalization; and have lower self-esteem (Maccoby & Martin, 1983).

Indulgent–permissive parents also lack balance between demandingness and responsiveness. Permissive parents tolerate children's impulses, use little punishment, and avoid asserting authority or imposing controls or restrictions. They make few demands for mature behavior, allow children to regulate their own behavior, and have few rules. Baumrind emphasizes the price children pay for their parents' failure to exercise control and make maturity demands. Negative effects of permissiveness include impulsivity, aggression, difficulty in taking responsibility, lack of independence, and poor self-control (Shaffer, 1989). Children with permissive parents have lower cognitive and social competence during the school years and adolescence (Dornbusch, Ritter, Leiderman, Roberts, & Fraleigh, 1987).

Parents who fit any one of the patterns of childrearing also may vary in parental involvement, the degree to which they are committed to their role as parents (Maccoby & Martin, 1983). *Involved* mothers tend to have children who are compliant, less demanding, and who have higher self-esteem and an internal locus of control; *indifferent–uninvolved* parenting has been associated with disturbances of attachment in infancy (Egeland & Sroufe, 1981) and delinquency in adolescence (Patterson & Stouthamer-Loeber, 1984). Children whose parents are more involved in the school do better than those whose parents are less involved (Stevenson & Baker, 1987). Involvement should not be confused with intrusiveness. Parental involvement is more likely to promote adolescent school success when it occurs in the context of an authoritative home environment (Steinberg, Lamborn, Dornbusch, & Darling, 1992). The optimal level of involvement depends on the child's age and maturity (Maccoby & Martin, 1983).

Why do these differing patterns of childrearing and levels of involvement affect children's competence, self-esteem, and development of conscience? The answer may lie in what each type of childrearing pattern teaches the child. Hess and McDevitt (1984) suggest that domineering parents who use direct control tactics distract the child's attention away from the specific elements of the task and prevent children from actively participating, so they lack the practice required to develop competence in problem solving. In addition, children whose parents help too much may assume that their success is due to their parents' efforts and that they cannot succeed by themselves. Balanced and flexible independence-promoting approaches can teach children *how* to solve problems and that they *can* solve problems. Conversely, harsh discipline may teach children that the world is a hostile place.

Weiss, Dodge, Bates, and Petit (1992) found a consistent relation between harsh discipline and childhood aggression in two cohorts of children. The relation was not due to child or contextual factors, but was mediated by maladaptive social information-processing patterns that developed in response to the harsh discipline. Children are more likely to internalize standards when parents use reasoning and teach children the effects of their actions (Maccoby & Martin, 1983). Power assertive techniques are effective in getting children to obey in the short run, but they do not produce obedience when the parents are absent. Punishment teaches children what not to do but does not teach them appropriate behaviors. Even when appropriate, such as when a dangerous behavior must be suppressed, punishment is more effective if accompanied by explanations about why the behavior is wrong (Hoffman, 1985).

Despite the consistent findings that children's positive behaviors are related to authoritative parenting, another interpretation is possible. Clarke-Stewart (1988) suggested that authoritative parents use reasoning and listen to their children's views because their children respond to that form of discipline. In general mothers of more difficult children engage in more control attempts and engage in more power-assertive interactions (Belsky, 1990; Maccoby & Martin, 1983). Difficult children, in turn, ignore maternal control attempts and persist in misbehavior. As this pattern of interaction progresses, parents may escalate their attempts to control behavior (Patterson, 1982). Evidence consistent with this comes from a study involving children with hyperactivity (Barkley & Cunningham, 1979). Parents whose children were medicated changed their disciplinary tactics so that they were far less negative and authoritarian than control-group parents, despite the fact that they were unaware of whether their children were receiving medication or placebo. Although negative parenting practices decreased when children were medicated, parent training was required to help parents notice and appropriately respond to their children's positive and compliant behaviors.

Clarke-Stewart (1988) concludes that we can no longer make simple generalizations about one-sided effects of parents' discipline on children's behavior or development. Parents' socialization strategies are clearly related to their children's behavior, their knowledge of child development, and their interpretations of children's behavior. Dix (1991) suggests that emotion is at the very heart of parental competence and that the emotion that parents feel and express also is related to their children's behavior, the parents' knowledge of development, and their interpretations and attributions regarding that behavior. Clarke-Stewart asserts that parent training should be made available to all parents to help them to gain knowledge of development and become skilled in using effective, growth-producing discipline methods.

ADOLESCENCE. Erikson (1963) describes the developmental task for adolescents as the development of a sense of identity versus role confusion. This sense of identity includes acceptance of the physical self, maturity, and a potential role in adult society. The task for parents of adolescents is fostering this independence and self-reliance while balancing freedom with responsibility (Duvall, 1977). Independence and autonomy do not imply rejection of parents. Rather, teens who have secure attachments to their parents are more likely to be independent and autonomous and to feel more emotional security with friends, while those who are emotionally detached from their parents may develop a more negative self-concept and feel less worthy of love (Ryan & Lynch, 1989).

The same kinds of parenting attributes that are associated with competence in preschool and school-age children are associated with psychosocial competence in adolescence (Lamborn, Mounts, Steinberg, & Dornbusch, 1991). For example, Dornbusch et al. (1987) found that authoritative parenting was positively related to adolescents' school performance, while authoritarian and permissive parenting were negatively correlated with grades. Steinberg, Elman, & Mounts (1989) replicated and extended this study and found that each component of authoritative parenting—acceptance and warmth, psychologic autonomy, and a high degree of supervision and strictness—contributes to facilitating academic performance of adolescents. Further, they found that the positive impact of authoritative parenting on achievement is mediated by its effects on the development of a sense of autonomy and a healthy psychologic orientation toward work.

Adolescents respond to contextual stress much as younger children do. Economic hardship has been found to produce distress in adolescents directly and indirectly through changes in parent–child relations (Lempers, Clark-Lempers, & Simons, 1989). Under economic stress, parents often become less nurturing and more rejecting and inconsistent. These hardship-induced changes in parenting have been associated with adverse adolescent outcomes, such as depression and loneliness, delinquency, and drug use. Consistent with a transactional model, Lempers et al. found that inconsistent, rejecting discipline mediated the effects of economic stress on youth.

Another consideration in the relationship between parenting practices and adolescent outcomes concerns the role of culture. Darling and Steinberg (1993) reviewed evidence that the effectiveness of authoritative parenting differs among ethnic groups. Authoritative parenting was found to be most effective in influencing academic achievement among European-American adolescents and least effective among Asian and African-American youth. They suggest that researchers must consider the differing conditions under which different parenting practices may influence children's development.

Problems in Parenting and Children's Mental Health

The serious problems that bring families to professionals for advice and treatment often present in a context of disordered parent–child relations. Studies of families in which one child is aggressive or has a conduct disorder have found consistent patterns of interactions among family members that contribute to the continuation of discipline problems. Patterson (1982) calls these *coercive home environments* and has described the kinds of interactions that typify them. Families who engage in coercive interactions do not use social reinforcers, such as attention or approval, to reward others for appropriate behavior. Rather, they become entangled in hostile interactions that start with noncompliant or irritating behaviors and escalate until the family is out of control and the child or adolescent is punished. Parents of deviant children differ in the behaviors that are tolerated and in their manner of discipline. They are more likely to nag but are inept and inconsistent in enforcing rules, and their environments are more likely to be characterized by family conflict (Hetherington & Martin, 1986).

Effective parents use a number of family-management techniques that distinguish them from the parents of deviant and delinquent children. Effective parents monitor their children's behavior, reinforce positive behaviors, consistently and effectively discipline inappropriate or deviant behaviors, and engage in problem-solving activities with their children. A lack of monitoring of children's friends and activities and decreased discipline by parents are related to delinquency and recidivism, while positive reinforcement and problem solving are related to positive behaviors (Patterson & Stouthamer-Loeber, 1984). The consistent application of effective punishment, such as time out or loss of privileges, is necessary for significant long-term reduction in rates of antisocial behavior (Patterson, 1982).

Patterson's (1982) program for treating out-of-control, defiant children includes the entire family. After observing family interactions and reinforcement patterns, he describes the nature of the problem to the parents and teaches them how to use positive reinforcement and punishment effectively. Parents are taught how to set rules and consequences for breaking the rules. Consistency and effective consequences are stressed. Parents and siblings are taught to negotiate and to make behavioral contracts that specify acceptable and unacceptable behaviors and the positive and negative consequences for each (Patterson, 1975). In essence, Patterson's program incorporates the characteristics that have been associated with effective parenting: balance between demandingness and responsivity and involvement. His program fosters agreement between parents and provides all family members with practice in using effective interpersonal skills. The program has been effective with a wide variety of family problems, seemingly because it takes into account the multidirectional and transactional nature of family problems (Shaffer, 1989).

The Nurse's Role in Parent–Child Problems

Nurses have traditionally focused on the health and well-being of families and individuals within families. Leahey and Wright (1987) distinguish between family therapy and family nursing. In family therapy the family is seen as the patient, with interventions aimed at changing dysfunctional interaction patterns within the family. Family nursing focuses on the individual's illness in a family context. Family nursing traditionally recognized that an individual's illness is shaped by the family's reaction to it, and the family context was considered when planning interventions, but the target of interventions was the individual. However, with new awareness of the transactional nature of family interactions and individuals' mental health, a systems-oriented approach to family nursing has evolved, in which the family is viewed as the unit of care (Leahey & Wright, 1987).

In psychiatric nursing, a focus on the effects of mental disorders and behavior problems on the family as a whole, and particularly on the caregivers of spouses, children, and parents with mental disorders, has emerged. This focus complements the more traditional view that families influence the course of individual problems, and recognizes that individuals may have mental health problems that impact negatively on the rest of the family. Nurses may choose either a family therapy approach or a systems-oriented family nursing approach when intervening with families. Although family therapy is an intervention used only by psychiatric clinical nurse specialists and others with advanced clinical training, all nurses have a role in interventions for families with problems in parenting.

NURSING PROCESS AND PARENT–CHILD RELATIONS

ASSESSMENT. A number of assessment models are available for nurses to use with families. The Nursing Child Assessment Scales (NCAS) (Barnard, 1978) are particularly useful for assessing parent–child interactions for families with children 3 years old and younger. Other models (Friedman, 1986; Leahey & Wright, 1987) use family interviews to identify sources of strength and stress, assess developmental status, and assess family roles and functioning.

Barnard's (1978) NCAS is used to assess the competence of the mother–child dyad from birth through age 3. These observation scales have been used in a variety of studies to examine the contributions of parents, children, and environment to child outcome and as a clinical teaching tool for use with high-risk mothers. The NCAS includes a sleep and activity record, observational checklists for assessment of the parent–child dyads during a feeding session and a teaching task, and the Home Observation for Measurement of the Environment (HOME) (Bradley & Caldwell, 1976). The feeding and teaching observations tap the infant's ability to produce clear cues and respond to the caregiver, and the caregiver's ability to respond to the infant's cues, alleviate distress, and provide experiences that foster cognitive and social-emotional growth. The HOME assesses the degree to which the child's home environment provides adequate social, emotional, and cognitive support. The sleep and activity scales assess rhythmicity and regularity of infants, an indicator of the child's contribution to the parenting task.

For families with parenting problems, it is extremely important to assess each family member's view of the difficulties. It also is important to determine whether family members are experiencing difficulties outside the home, at work, or at school. Parents' marital satisfaction and agreement on childrearing practices should be assessed. Peer relations are an important indicator of children's social skills and should be discussed. Academic progress and teacher reports of classroom interactions are further sources of information on behavior of children and adolescents.

NURSING DIAGNOSES. Several nursing diagnoses may be used for families with the kinds of difficulties described in this chapter. Altered Parenting, High Risk for Altered Parenting, and Altered Family processes; Family Coping: Ineffective; Family Coping: Potential for Growth; and Knowledge Deficit (Doenges, Townsend, & Moorhouse, 1989) are particularly appropriate. In addition, other nursing diagnoses that focus on difficulties of the individuals may be necessary to include in the plan of care.

NURSING INTERVENTIONS AND EVALUATION. Doenges et al. (1989) identified four nursing priorities for promoting effective parenting: (1) promoting positive feelings about parenting abilities; (2) involving parents in problem solving; (3) helping families develop the skills to deal with their current situation; and (4) facilitating learning of new parenting skills. In addition, nursing interventions should focus on promoting communication and problem-solving skills for all family members, including the children. When behavioral approaches, such as Patterson's (1982), are used, interventions can be evaluated easily by determining whether target behaviors have changed in frequency, intensity, or duration in the predicted direction.

Parent training has been suggested as one way to enhance parents' sensitivity to infants' needs and thereby influence the security of attachment (Clarke-Stewart, 1988). A visiting nurse program (Booth, Mitchell, Barnard, Spieker, & Magyary, 1987), which provided either therapy or information and instruction during pregnancy and for 1 year after birth for high-risk mothers, revealed that mothers who improved in social skills were more likely to have securely attached infants, as were mothers who were shown how to interact with their infants in positive and developmentally appropriate ways (Lyons-Ruth, Zoll, Connell, & Odom, 1987).

However, Schorr (1988) warns that parent training is not a panacea. Families who are living in poverty, with multiple problems and few supports, cannot be expected to overcome the stresses in their lives just because they participated in a parent-training program. For the most needy families, parents must not only be taught how to respond to their children, but also must be given adequate support so that they are able to produce optimal responses. For some parents, access to health care, to child-care programs, and job-training or other economic assistance may be necessary before they can use the information provided in parent-training programs.

Summary

This chapter begins with a discussion of the evolution of transactional models of parent–child relations. These models assert that the outcomes for family members derive from the chronic and pervasive influences that operate within the family, the individual, and between the family and its environment. Research evidence supports this view, suggesting that children can survive trauma, if the consistent influences in their lives are positive, but also that they are impervious to "one-shot" interventions that do not change existing chronic and pervasive adverse conditions.

It is clear from the studies on parenting, that we know what to do to raise competent children. The hallmarks of effective parenting, a balance between responding to children's demands and exercising control over them, involvement, consistent discipline, and encouragement of age-appropriate independence, are associated with competent children because they allow children to learn by doing and experiencing in a context of acceptance and safety. Helping parents develop effective parenting skills requires similar strategies. Admonitions to parents to use authoritative family management practices are naive if they do not take into account the characteristics of the children and the family context. Parents need to be supported and provided with help in gaining skill in parenting their children. The most needy families will require the most comprehensive and intensive interventions. Nurses who have access to families in a variety of settings have the opportunity to help parents learn about their children's competencies and special needs and effective parenting strategies. These interventions will be most effective if nurses also reward parents for their efforts, foster independence by helping them to use effective problem-solving skills, and allow parents to learn by doing in a context of acceptance and safety.

REFERENCES

Ainsworth, M. D. S., Blehar, M. C., Waters, E., & Wall, S. (1978). *Patterns of attachment: A psychological study of the strange situation.* Hillsdale, NJ: Erlbaum.

Austin, J. K. (1988). Childhood epilepsy: Child adaptation and family resources. *Journal of Child and Adolescent Psychiatric and Mental Health Nursing, 1,* 18–24.

Barkley, R. A., & Cunningham, C. E. (1979). The effects of methylphenidate on the mother-child interactions of hyperactive children. *Archives of General Psychiatry, 36,* 201–208.

Barnard, K. E. (1978). *The nursing child assessment satellite training series: Learning resource manual.* Seattle: University of Washington.

Baumrind, D., & Black, A. E. (1967). Socialization practices associated with dimensions of competence in preschool boys and girls. *Child Development, 38,* 291–327.

Bee, H. L., Hammond, M. A., Eyres, S. J., Barnard, K. E., & Snyder, C. (1986). The impact of parental life change on the early development of children. *Research in Nursing and Health, 9,* 65–74.

Bell, R. Q. (1968). A reinterpretation of the direction of effects in studies of socialization. *Psychological Review, 75,* 81–95.

Bell, R. Q., & Harper, L. V. (1977). *Child effects on adults.* Hillsdale, NJ: Erlbaum.

Belsky, J. (1981). Early human experience: A family perspective. *Developmental Psychology, 17,* 3–23.

Belsky, J. (1984). The determinants of parenting: A process model. *Child Development, 55,* 83–96.

Belsky, J. (1990). Parental and nonparental child care and children's socioemotional development: A decade in review. *Journal of Marriage and the Family, 52,* 885–903.

Belsky, J., Steinberg, L., & Draper, P. (1991). Childhood experience, interpersonal development, & reproductive strategy: An evolutionary theory of socialization. *Child Development, 62,* 647–670.

Blum, G. S. (1953). *Psychoanalytic theories of personality.* New York: McGraw-Hill.

Booth, C. L., Mitchell, S. K., Barnard, K. E., Spicker, S. T., & Magyany, D. (1987, April). *Evaluating intervention with multirisk mothers: Links between social skills improvements and child outcomes.* Paper presented at the meeting of the Society for Research in Child Development, Baltimore.

Bowlby, J. (1982). *Attachment and loss.* (Vol 1). *Attachment* (2nd ed.). New York: Basic.

Bradley, R. H., & Caldwell, B. M. (1976). Early home environment and changes in mental test performance in children from six to 36 months. *Developmental Psychology, 12,* 93–97.

Bretherton, I. (1985). Attachment theory: Retrospect and prospect. In I. Bretherton & E. Waters (Eds.), Growing points of attachment theory and research. *Monographs of the Society for Research in Child Development, 50* (1–2, Serial No. 209), 3–35.

Bretherton, I., & Waters, E. (Eds.). (1985). Growing points of attachment theory and research. *Monographs of the Society for Research in Child Development, 50,* (1–2, Serial No. 209).

Bruch, H. (1954). Parent education or the illusion of omnipotence. *American Journal of Orthopsychiatry, 24,* 723–732.

Buss, A. H., & Plomin, R. (1984). Early developing personality traits. Hillsdale, NJ: Lawrence Erlbaum.

Chess, S. (1964). Mal de mere. *American Journal of Orthopsychiatry, 34,* 613–614.

Chess, S., & Thomas, A. (1984). *Origins and evolution of behavior disorders.* New York: Brunner/Mazel.

Chess, S. (1988). Child and adolescent psychiatry comes of age: A fifty year perspective. *Journal of the American Academy of Child and Adolescent Psychiatry, 27,* 1–7.

Clarke-Stewart, K. A. (1988). Parents' effects on children's development: A decade of progress? *Journal of Applied Developmental Psychology, 9,* 41–84.

Conger, R. D., McCarty, J. A., Yang, R. K., Lahey, B. B., & Kropp, J. P. (1984). Perception of child, child-rearing values, and emotional distress as mediating links between environmental stressors and observed maternal behavior. *Child Development, 55,* 2234–2247.

Cowan, P. A., & Cowan, C. P. (1990). Becoming a family: Research and intervention. In I. E. Sigel & G. H. Brody (Eds.), *Methods of family research: Biographies of research projects.* (Vol. I). *Normal families.* Hillsdale, NJ: Erlbaum.

Cox, M. J., Owen, M. T., Lewis, J. M., & Henderson, V. K. (1989). Marriage, adult adjustment, and early parenting. *Child Development, 60,* 1015–1024.

Darling, N. & Steinberg, L. (1993). Parenting style as context: An integrative model. *Psychological Bulletin, 113,* 487–496.

Dix, T. (1991). The affective organization of parenting: Adaptive and maladaptive processes. *Psychological Bulletin, 110,* 3–25.

Doenges, M. E., Townsend, M. C., & Moorhouse, M. F. (1989). *Psychiatric care plans: Guidelines for client care.* Philadelphia: F.A. Davis.

Dornbusch, S., Ritter, P., Liederman, P., Roberts, D., & Fraleigh, M. (1987). The relation of parenting style to adolescent school performance. *Child Development, 58,* 1244–1257.

Duvall, E. M. (1977). *Marriage and family development.* Philadelphia: J.B. Lippincott.

Egeland, B., & Farber, E. A. (1984). Infant-mother attachment: Factors related to its development and changes over time. *Child Development, 55,* 740–752.

Egeland, B. S., & Sroufe, L. A. (1981). Developmental sequellae of maltreatment in infancy. In R. Rizlet & D. Cicchetti (Eds.), *Developmental perspectives in child maltreatment* (pp. 77–92). San Francisco: Jossey-Bass.

Erikson, E. H. (1963). *Childhood and society* (2nd ed.). New York: Norton.

Erikson, M. F., Sroufe, L. A., & Egeland, B. (1985). The relationship between quality of attachment and behavior problems in preschool in a high-risk sample. In I. Bretherton & E. Waters (Eds.), Growing points of attachment theory and research. *Monographs of the Society for Research in Child Development, 50*(1–2, Serial No. 209).

Freud, S. (1927). *The ego and the id.* London: Hogarth Press.

Friedman, M. M. (1986). *Family nursing: Theory and assessment* (2nd ed.). Norwalk, CT: Appleton-Century-Crofts.

Frodi, A. M., & Lamb, M. (1978). Sex differences in responsiveness to infants: A developmental study of psychophysiological and behavioral responses. *Child Development, 49,* 1182–1188.

Fromm-Reichmann, F. (1948). Notes on the development of treatment of schizophrenia in psychoanalytic psychotherapy. *Psychiatry, 11,* 263–273.

Garmezy, N. (1987). Stress, competence, and development: Continuities in the study of schizophrenic adults, children vulnerable to psychopathology, and the search for stress resistant children. *American Journal of Orthopsychiatry, 57,* 159–174.

Garrison, W. T. & Earls, F. J. (1987). *Temperament and child psychology.* Newbury Park, CA: Sage.

Goldberg, S. (1983). Parent-infant bonding: Another look. *Child Development, 54,* 1355–1382.

Goldsmith, J., Buss, A. H., Plomin, R., Rothbart, M., Thomas, A., Chess, S., Hinde, R., & McCall, R. (1987). Roundtable: What is temperament? *Child Development, 58,* 505–529.

Hess, R. D., & McDevitt, T. M. (1984). Some cognitive consequences of maternal intervention techniques: A longitudinal study. *Child Development, 55,* 2017–2030.

Hetherington, E. M., & Martin, B. (1986). Family factors and psychopathology in children. In H. C. Quay & J. S. Werry (Eds.), *Psychopathological disorders of childhood* (pp. 332–390). New York: John Wiley and Sons.

Hiestand, W. C. (1991). Nursing, the family, and the "new" social history. In A. Whall & J. Fawcett (Eds.), *Family theory development in nursing: State of the science and art* (pp. 93–106). Philadelphia: F.A. Davis.

Hobbs, D. (1965). Parenthood as a crisis: A third study. *Journal of Marriage and the Family, 27*, 677–689.

Hoffman, M. L. (1985). Moral development. In M. H. Bornstein & M. E. Lamb (Eds.), *Developmental psychology: An advanced textbook.* Hillsdale, NJ: Erlbaum.

Kagan, J., Reznick, J. S., & Snidman, N. (1987). The physiology and psychology of behavioral inhibition. *Child Development, 58*, 1459–1473.

Killeen, M. R. (1988). Self-concept of children of alcoholics: Part I: Family influences. *Journal of Child and Adolescent Psychiatric and Mental Health Nursing, 1*, 25–29.

Killeen, M. R. (1992). *A transactional model of self-esteem.* Paper presented at the Third State of the Art and Science of Psychiatric Nursing Conference, Bethesda, MD.

Lamborn, S. D., Mounts, N. S., Steinberg, L., & Dornbusch, S. M. (1991). Patterns of competence and adjustment among adolescents from authoritative, authoritarian, indulgent, and neglectful families. *Child Development, 62*, 1049–1065.

Leahy, M., & Wright, L. M. (1987). *Families and psychosocial problems.* Springhouse, PA: Springhouse.

Lempers, J. D., Clark-Lempers, D., & Simons, R. L. (1989). Economic hardship, parenting, and distress in adolescence. *Child Development, 60*, 25–39.

Lyons-Ruth, K., Zoll, D., Connell, D. B., & Odum, R. (1987, April). *Maternal depression as mediator of the effects of home-based intervention services.* Paper presented at the meetings of the Society for Research in Child Development, Baltimore.

Maccoby, E. E. & Martin, J. A. (1983). Socialization in the context of the family: Parent-child interaction. In E. M. Hetherington (Ed.), *Handbook of child psychology* (Vol. 4). New York: John Wiley and Sons.

Matheney, A. P., Wilson, R. S., & Nuss, S. N. (1984). Toddler temperament: Stability across settings and overages. *Child Development, 55*, 1200–1211.

Patterson, G. R. (1975). *Families: Applications of social learning to family life* (rev. ed.). Champaign, IL: Research Press.

Patterson, G. R. (1982). *Coercive family process.* Eugene, OR: Castalia.

Patterson, G. R., & Southamer-Loeber, M. (1984). The correlation of family management practices and delinquency. *Child Development, 55*, 1299–1307.

Ragozin, A. S., Basham, R. B., Crnic, K. A., Greenberg, M. T., & Robinson, N. M. (1982). Effects of maternal age on parenting role. *Developmental Psychology, 18*, 627–634.

Randell, B. (1989). Childbearing and its effect on marital quality. In C. L. Gilliss, B. L. Highley, B. M. Roberts, & I. M. Martinson (Eds.), *Toward a science of family nursing.* Menlo Park, CA: Addison-Wesley.

Rose, M. H., & Killian, M. (1983). Risk and vulnerability: A case for differentiation. *Advances in Nursing Science, 5*(3), 60–73.

Ryan, R. M., & Lynch, J. H. (1989). Emotional autonomy versus detachment: Revisiting the vicissitudes of adolescence and young adulthood. *Child Development, 60*, 340–356.

Sameroff, A. J., & Chandler, M. J. (1975). Reproductive risk and the continuum of caretaking casualty. In F. D. Horowitz, E. M. Hetherington, S. Scarr-Salapatek, & G. Siegel (Eds.), *Review of child development research* (Vol. 4). Chicago: University of Chicago Press.

Sameroff, A. J., Seifer, R., & Zax, M. (1982). Early development of children at risk for emotional disorder. *Monographs of the Society for Research in Child Development, 47* (Serial No. 7).

Scarr, S., & Kidd, K. K. (1983). Developmental behavioral genetics. In M. M. Haith & J. J. Campos (Eds.), *Handbook of child psychology* (Vol. 2). *Infancy and developmental psychobiology* (pp. 345–420). New York: John Wiley and Sons.

Scavnicky-Mylant, M. L. (1991). Children of alcoholics. In E. G. Bennett & D. Woolf (Eds.), *Substance abuse: Pharmacologic, developmental, and clinical perspectives* (2nd ed.). (pp. 127–141). Albany, NY: Delmar.

Schorr, L. B. (1988). *Within our reach: Breaking the cycle of disadvantage.* New York: Doubleday.

Sears, R. R. (1975). Your ancients revisited: A history of child development. In E. M. Hetherington, J. W. Hagen, R. Kron, & A. H. Stein (Eds.), *Review of child development research* (Vol. 5). Chicago: University of Chicago Press.

Shaffer, D. R. (1989). *Developmental psychology: Childhood and adolescence* (2nd ed.). Pacific Grove, CA: Brooks/Cole.

Shaw, D. S., & Emery, R. E. (1988). Chronic family adversity and school-age children's adjustment. *Journal of the American Academy of Child and Adolescent Psychiatry, 27*, 200–206.

Siantz, M. L. (1988). Children's rights and parental rights: A historical and legal/ethical analysis. *Journal of Child and Adolescent Psychiatric and Mental Health Nursing, 1*, 14–17.

Skinner, B. F. (1971). *Beyond freedom and dignity.* New York: Knopf.

Sroufe, L. A., & Rutter, M. (1984). The domain of developmental psychology. *Child Development, 55*, 17–29.

Steinberg, L., Elmen, J. D., & Mounts, N. S. (1989). Authoritative parenting, psychosocial maturity, and academic success among adolescents. *Child Development, 60*, 1424–1436.

Steinberg, L., Lamborn, S. D., Dornbusch, S. M., & Darling, N. (1992). Impact of parenting practices on adolescent acheivement: Authoritative parenting, school involvement, and encouragement to succeed. *Child Development, 63*, 1266–1281.

Stevenson, D. L., & Baker, D. P. (1987). The family-school relation and the child's school performance. *Child Development, 58*, 1348–1357.

U.S. Congress, Office of Technology Assessment. (1986). *Children's mental health: Problems and services—A background paper.* Washington, DC: U.S. Government Printing Office.

Watson, J. B. (1925). *Behaviorism.* New York: Norton.

Weiss, B., Dodge, K. A., Bates, J. E., & Petit, G. S. (1992). Some consequences of early harsh discipline: Child aggression and a maladaptive social information processing style. *Child Development, 63*, 1321–1335.

Werner, E. E, & Smith, R. S. (1982). *Vulnerable but invincible: A longitudinal study of resilient children and youth.* New York: McGraw-Hill.

Whall, A. L. (1991). Family system theory: Relationship to nursing conceptual models. In A. Whall & J. Fawcett (Eds.), *Family theory development in nursing: State of the science and art.* (pp. 317–342). Philadelphia: F.A. Davis.

Whall, A., & Fawcett, J. (Eds.). (1991). *Family theory development in nursing: State of the science and art.* Philadelphia: F.A. Davis.

Wright, L. M., & Leahey, M. (1984). *Nurses and families: A guide to family assessment and intervention.* Philadelphia: F.A. Davis.

UNIT

II

Theoretical Bases Underlying Nursing Approaches

CHAPTER

4

Attachment Theory

Sandra J. Weiss

During the last 2 decades, an increasing interest has developed in the attachment relationship between infant and parent. Growing clinical concern with attachment stems to a great extent from research that suggests that disturbance of initial attachment relationships can predict later psychopathology. If there have been secure attachments, the child will be more likely to approach the environment as responsive and helpful versus viewing the world as comfortless and unpredictable, perceptions that may result in social withdrawal or hostility.

Secure attachments have been shown to predict later social competencies, such as effectiveness in peer friendships, ability to empathize with others, assertion, and cooperativeness (Erickson, Egeland, & Sroufe, 1985; Pastor, 1981; Waters & Sroufe, 1983). Security also has been related to development of the self, which influences ego strength and resiliency, self-esteem, self-reliance, and internalized self-control (Arend, Gove, & Sroufe, 1979; Lewis, 1987; Sroufe, 1983; Sroufe & Fleeson, 1986).

This chapter provides an overview of attachment theory, including a discussion of the influence of family environment and infant temperament on patterns of attachment. Applications of the theory to clinical practice will then be described, with relevance for mental health promotion and prevention and treatment of mental disorder.

The Concepts of Attachment Theory

Attachment theory was initially described by John Bowlby (1969; 1973; 1982) and later extended by Mary Ainsworth (1979; Ainsworth, Blehar, Waters, & Walls, 1978) and others (Main, Kaplan, & Cassidy, 1985; Sroufe & Fleeson, 1986). It integrates aspects of psychodynamic, ethologic, and interactional approaches to understanding mental health. The concepts of the attachment behavioral system and internal working models are central to the theory.

THE ATTACHMENT BEHAVIORAL SYSTEM

Attachment refers to the socioemotional tie or bond of the infant with an individual who is perceived as stronger or more powerful in the world and to whom the infant can turn for protection and support in situations of perceived danger or adversity. Attachment behaviors are specific proximity or contact-promoting behaviors by children in interactions with parental (or other) attachment figures under conditions of uncertainty, novelty, fatigue, sickness, fear, or other potential stressors that they may experience. Bowlby suggested that

Barbara Schoen Johnson: CHILD, ADOLESCENT AND FAMILY PSYCHIATRIC NURSING, © 1994 J.B. Lippincott Company

infants appraise or evaluate environmental conditions and internal feeling states to determine how much proximity or contact they need to feel secure. This appraisal is seen to be the result of an adaptive behavioral system that all infants possess as part of their biologic makeup (Fig. 4-1). From an evolutionary perspective, the purpose of this control system was to help infants survive in adverse conditions.

The attachment behavioral system actively monitors and processes information taken in by sensory systems, including cues to physical and psychologic danger, accessibility of the attachment figure, and the child's own ability to handle independently the perceived danger. Comparison of the degree of needed proximity with existing proximity will then determine whether the infant activates behaviors such as vocalizing, approaching, or clinging.

WORKING MODELS OF ATTACHMENT

The unique nature of each person's behavioral system is determined by the working model of attachment that that individual gradually builds during childhood. This model is a psychologic frame of reference that guides an individual's evaluation of his or her own capacity to handle stress and of the expected responses of his or her attachment figures when they are turned to in times of need. Internal models of attachment are not necessarily an objective picture of specific events but the integration of various experiences with time that become generalized into expectations for current and future experience. They develop from the infant's actual experiences with attachment figures whereby these figures are seen as accessible and loving or as inaccessible and unloving. Accompanying representations of one's self may come to be viewed as worthy and lovable or the opposite. It is these psychologic models that organize and influence an individual's pattern of behavior with the interpersonal environment when experiencing stress. From initial relations with attachment figures are formed the prototypes influencing the quality of subsequent socioemotional relationships in life, including the nature of relationships that are sought and the responses elicited from others. Thus, patterns of attachment behavior have significant implications for later social support networks, intimate relations, and parenting.

Three different types of internal working models (or patterns of attachment) were initially identified through research (Ainsworth, et al., 1978): secure, insecure-avoidant, and insecure-resistant. More recently, another pattern has been discovered in which the child shows disorganized or disoriented attachment behavior in response to stress (Main & Solomon, 1986).

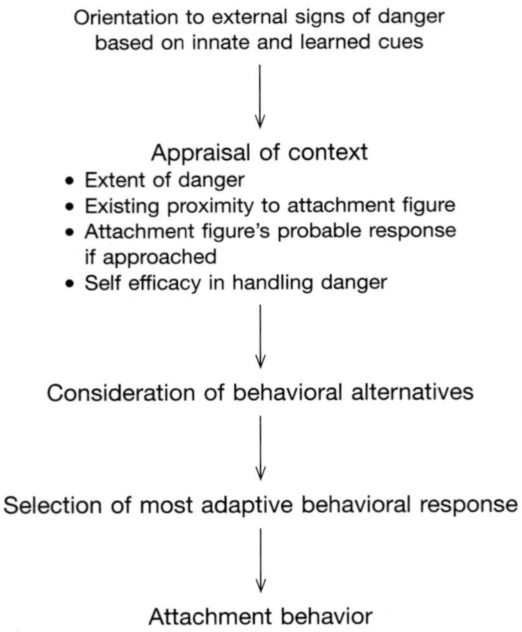

Orientation to external signs of danger based on innate and learned cues

↓

Appraisal of context
- Extent of danger
- Existing proximity to attachment figure
- Attachment figure's probable response if approached
- Self efficacy in handling danger

↓

Consideration of behavioral alternatives

↓

Selection of most adaptive behavioral response

↓

Attachment behavior

FIGURE 4–1 • Simplified model of processes in the attachment behavioral system

SECURE MODEL. According to Bowlby, the infant with an internal model of the attachment figure that is available and responsive will view the caregiver as protecting, soothing, comforting, and helping under conditions of perceived stress. Thus, the child will seek security through proximity and contact. The pull of the attachment figure will be less when the environment is perceived as nonthreatening, but during these times, the child will closely monitor the parent's whereabouts because her or his responsiveness can be counted on if the need arises.

Ainsworth and colleagues (1978) identified the existence of certain attachment behaviors that were common to securely attached infants and consistent with Bowlby's theory. Secure infants tend to seek proximity to and contact with attachment figures when reunited after a period of separation. They also show clear preferences for the attachment figure over a stranger. Four subgroups of secure infants also have been described, each with its own unique style of behavior. For instance, one subgroup relies more on distant modes of interaction with parents rather than physical proximity but shows delighted vocalizations and smiling when reunited with the parent. Another subgroup conspicuously seeks proximity and physical contact with their attachment figures when distressed but is easily soothed when this goal is accomplished. Regardless of the distinctions of the various subgroups, all infants use the attachment figures as a secure base. They are constantly alerted to the need to increase proximity in strange environments or in the face of separation, show signs of missing the parent when separated, and are able to return to exploration and play when confident that the parent is available.

INSECURE MODELS. Ainsworth's research identified two groups of infants whose behaviors did not seem to fit the criteria for being securely attached. Insecure-avoidant infants appear indifferent to stress and uncertainty, including separation from the parent. They ignore and actively avoid their attachment figure when reunited after separation, focusing instead on toys and other aspects of the environment. They fail to cling when held and treat a stranger the same or sometimes better than the attachment figure. Some of these infants show strong, clear cut avoidance of the parent and no distress on being left completely alone. Others are more moderately avoidant, with some distress when alone but easily soothed by a stranger's presence.

A second insecurely attached group of infants has been called insecure-resistant (also referred to as insecure-ambivalent); they tend to resist interaction and contact with the attachment figure when it is available yet manifest contact and proximity-seeking behavior when it is not. They vacillate between seeking and rejecting the parent, for example, by demanding attention but hitting or pushing the parent away when he or she approaches. They seem to excessively monitor the whereabouts of the attachment figure even in situations of low stress. This focus on the parent inhibits their exploration of and learning about the environment. They are very distressed during separation and cannot be settled or soothed when the parent returns. After being separated from the parent, some of these infants combine marked proximity and contact-seeking with conspicuously angry, resistant behavior, while others show less aggressive, almost passive behavior and some resistance to being held.

Both of the insecure patterns of attachment are presumed to reflect internal working models, or expectations, that responsive care in time of need will be unavailable, unpredictable, or disrupted in some way. Such models yield distrust and anxiety concerning the relationship. Main (1981; Main & Weston, 1982) has proposed that infants with the avoidant attachment pattern may be trying to divert their attention away from anxiety-producing cues. The infant seems to be ignoring stress or uncertainty. This pattern may largely reflect defensive attempts to deactivate attachment cues and thus better cope with the experience by denying their existence. In contrast, the insecure-resistant infant appears to be exhibiting extreme dependence on the attachment figure. Through a heightened display of emotion and dependence, the infant may believe he or she can successfully attract the attention of the parent to meet attachment needs yet convince the parent of the need to be more attentive in the future through angry responses of displeasure toward the parent.

THE DISORGANIZED OR DISORIENTED MODEL. Disorganized or disoriented infants are thought to be lacking any coherent internal model to guide their attachment behavior. These infants exhibit the following responses to stress or uncertainty:

- Unexplainable behavior, such as greeting the parent with raised arms then freezing with a frightened expression
- Contradictory behavior, such as smiling while forcefully striking the parent's face or reaching out to touch the parent and then quickly withdrawing the hand
- Stereotypical behavior, such as extended rocking or ear pulling
- Direct indices of confusion and apprehension, such as disorganized wandering or dashing away from the parent with a hunched or tucked head
- Behavioral stilling or freezing

These infants act as though they are experiencing fear or distress that cannot be deactivated or denied, as in the avoidant working model, nor ameliorated through approaching or calling to the attachment figure, as in other working models (Main & Hesse, 19). They seem to have no organized pattern of response to guide their behavior during stress.

Factors Influencing the Development of Attachment Patterns

The exact etiology underlying each working model of attachment is not fully understood. However, research suggests that specific characteristics of parent interaction and the infant's own biologically determined characteristics may influence the resulting pattern of attachment.

PARENTAL RESPONSE TO THE INFANT

The parental behaviors associated with different models of attachment are shown in Table 4-1. Most research to date has studied the mother's behavior as the primary attachment figure. However, it is believed that similar behavioral approaches would be found for any attachment figure. More studies of adoptive parents and fathers will be needed to establish the validity of these assumptions.

BEHAVIOR ASSOCIATED WITH A SECURE MODEL. Parent sensitivity to the infant's cues during feeding, face-to-face play, and physical contact has been a major predictor of the child's security of attachment (Ainsworth et al., 1978). Sensitivity involves noticing cues, accurately interpreting them, and promptly responding to signals. Mothers whose infants show secure attachment also have been found to be more affectionate, tender, and careful in their use of close bodily contact (Egeland & Farber, 1984). They are more accepting of the infant's behavior; that is, they are more willing to respect the baby's interests or needs by allowing him or her to remain involved in activities with which he or she seems interested or by using gentle persuasion, instead of aggressive control, if redirection is needed. They also are more accessible to the infant than are mothers of insecure infants, even when faced with other demands.

Main and Goldwyn (1984) have described parents of securely attached infants as "autonomous" in their own working models of attachment. These parents can easily recall their early experiences as children and are self-reliant and realistic about their relationships with their own attachment figures. In general, they have positive memories of being cared for and responded to in situations of distress. If they have painful memories, they are able to acknowledge them and have developed some insight about how their past experiences have influenced their current relationships.

BEHAVIOR ASSOCIATED WITH AN AVOIDANT MODEL. Mothers of avoidant infants have been found to be insensitive to their infant's signals and rejecting of the infant as shown in abruptness, irritation, and scolding. They may appear resentful and use angry, threatening approaches with the infant. They also may appear emotionally unavailable (detached, uninvolved, or affectless), being unresponsive to the infant's needs, interests, or crying. Many of these mothers show aversion to physical contact, and refuse to hold the child when he or she signals the desire or need to be held (Main, 1990; Main & Stadtman, 1981). There also is growing evidence that mothers who physically abuse their children are likely to have infants who use avoidance as an attachment strategy (Egeland & Sroufe, 1981; George & Main, 1979).

Parents of children with avoidant attachment have been described as frequently detached from their own early attachments or devaluing the importance and influence of attachments on their lives (Main et al., 1985). They recall little of their childhood and tend to idealize any memories they may have of their parents. However, the details that are recollected suggest parental neglect or rejection in spite of their interpretation of the parent as ideal.

TABLE 4–1 Parental Behaviors Associated with Different Models of Attachment

	Models of Attachment			
Parent Behavior	***Secure***	***Avoidant***	***Resistant***	***Disorganized***
Sensitive	High	Low	Low	Low
Rejecting	Low	High	Moderate	High
Interfering	Low	High	High	Unpredictable
Accessible	High	Moderate	Unpredictable	Low
Tender and gentle physical contact	High	Low	Low	Low
Flexible	High	Low	Low	Unpredictable
Role-reversing	Low	Low	Moderate	High
Frightening	Low	Moderate	Low	High

BEHAVIOR ASSOCIATED WITH A RESISTANT MODEL. Mothers who are likely to have infants with a resistant model of attachment also have been identified as unresponsive to their infant's crying and somewhat abrupt and interfering but less so than mothers of avoidant babies. In contrast to mothers of avoidant children who are overtly rejecting, mothers of resistant babies appear unpredictable in their accessibility. Primarily, they are inept in their care of the infant, that is, less adaptable, hesitant, inflexible, and occupied with routines rather than being focused on providing tender, sensitive care (Main & Weston, 1982; Weber, Levitt, & Clark, 1986). Other studies also suggest that while physical abuse may be related to avoidant attachment patterns, physical neglect by parents is more often related to a resistant pattern of attachment (Egeland & Sroufe, 1981; George & Main, 1979).

Parents of children with resistant patterns of attachment tend to be preoccupied with their own early attachments or enmeshed with their family of origin (Main et al., 1985). They are flooded with intense negative memories that elicit anger and dependency. They seem overinvolved with the parents and have difficulty separating from them; they still feel a need to please the parent but never feel as if they do.

BEHAVIOR ASSOCIATED WITH A DISORGANIZED OR DISORIENTED MODEL. Because the attachment classification of disorganized or disoriented has only recently been identified, little research is available concerning the characteristics of parents whose infants show this pattern. However, Main and Hesse (19) have found that some of these parents appear to reverse roles with the infant, seeming "timid, solicitous, or deferential" toward the child. Other parents behave in frightening or threatening ways toward the infant, using ominous gestures and tones or sudden, unpredictable movements. At 6 years of age, children who had disorganized attachment behavior in infancy tend to reverse roles with the parent, often telling the parent what to do or acting in a caretaking way with the parent. Their drawings also depict their families in ominous, irrational ways (Kaplan & Main, 1985; Main & Cassidy, 1988).

Parents of disorganized infants seem to have suffered unusual trauma in their own attachment histories, such as death of the attachment figure or abuse (Main & Hesse, 19). Their recollections of childhood reflect a lack of resolution of mourning for the parent and a substantial degree of incoherence regarding the meaning of the trauma in their lives.

THE ROLE OF THE INFANT IN ATTACHMENT

Studies offer evidence of the role played by constitutional factors, specifically temperamental attributes of the infant. These attributes may be the result of either perinatal health problems (e.g., low birth weight) or genetic variables. For instance, infants who are more capable of focusing their attention on and responding to the parent and who have less irritability as neonates are more likely to be securely attached later in life (Grossman, Grossman, Spangler, Suess, & Unzner, 1985). In contrast, most studies suggest that infants who show difficult temperaments early in life are likely to develop resistant patterns of attachment as they grow. As neonates, they cry significantly more than secure infants, are less able to focus their attention, react to the environment more rapidly and intensely, are more prone to sleep problems, and are described as more difficult to manage. In general they show less central nervous system integrity as newborns (Belsky & Rovine, 1987; Crockenberg, 1981; Miyake, Chen, & Campos, 1985). In addition, in the second half of their first year, infants who later develop resistant patterns of attachment show more fear of strangers and greater behavioral inhibition in uncertain situations (Schneider-Rosen, Braunwald, Carlson, & Cicchetti, 1985). They appear to have a very low threshold for uncertainty, become distressed easily, and are difficult to soothe.

In contrast, infants who later develop an avoidant attachment pattern do not appear to be distressed by new experiences or uncertain situations as infants. From early in life, it takes a lot to upset them, and they can easily recover if they do become distressed (Kagan, 1974; 1987).

Based on these findings, it has been proposed that attachment patterns may in part reflect individual differences in susceptibility to stress. Avoidant babies may act nonchalant and detached when separated from their parents because they are not distressed by being alone and thus do not experience the insecurity that initiates attachment behavior. If distressed, their self-regulatory processes may function more effectively, dampening their distress without seeking the attachment figure. Resistant babies may cry intensely under these same conditions because they feel more distress. Such infants may find even sensitive and responsive parents inadequate in helping them to overcome their distress.

In light of such research, Sroufe (1985) has proposed that avoidant attachment results when a robust infant (i.e., low reactive, easy temperament, alert, and responsive) encounters insensitive parental care. The infant's reliance on his or her own self-efficacy may, by necessity, be strengthened in the infant's attempt to cope with his or her interpersonal environment. Resistant attachment may result when a less optimally functioning infant encounters insensitive care. For this type of infant, the lack of perceived self-efficacy increases every time distress is felt and left unresolved. From the opposite vantage point, sensitive parenting may help to determine whether infants with more difficult temperaments and less central nervous system integrity develop a sense of self-efficacy and whether robust infants can come to value the interpersonal world as providing support or comfort superior to their own self-comforting.

Although little research exists concerning predictors of disorganized attachment behavior, it may be that underlying neurologic abnormalities in the infant create a greater vulnerability to the development of disorganized attachment and are exacerbated by the responses of an insensitive attachment figure. Such a proposal remains to be supported by research.

Thomas and Chess (1984) argue that it is the poorness of fit or dissonance between the environment and the capacities or needs of the child that leads to psychopathology. The onus of achieving a good fit is clearly on the caregiver during the early months of life. Whether a parent appreciates the nature of an infant's independence, fearfulness, or other unique qualities and can adjust his or her behavior to these qualities will determine the degree of fit (Table 4-2). If a mismatch in temperaments exists between parent and infant or the parent is lacking in the competencies associated with sensitivity, accessibility, or flexibility, the child will likely experience more distress. In turn, distress may cause him or her to use avoidant or resistant strategies to feel more secure. The repetitive experience of distress and its lack of effective resolution through interpersonal support may then yield the development of an insecure working model of attachment or the absence of any organized working model as in the disorganized or disoriented pattern.

TABLE 4–2 The Relationship Between Parent Attachment History Classifications and the Attachment Classifications of Their Children

Parent Attachment History Classifications*	Child Attachment Classifications
Secure/autonomous	Secure
Dismissing of attachment/detached	Avoidant
Preoccupied/entangled in past attachments	Resistant
Unresolved attachment traumas	Disorganized/disoriented

*Main & Goldwyn (1990). Adult attachment rating and classification system. In M. Main (Ed). *A typology of human attachment. Organization: Assessed in discourse, drawings and interviews.* New York: Cambridge University Press.

Implications for Clinical Practice

The clinical nurse specialist (CNS) can apply knowledge derived from attachment theory in three primary spheres of the health care continuum: 1) promotion of secure attachment patterns for children, 2) prevention of child mental illness through early assessment of risk for attachment disorders, and 3) treatment of attachment disorders. The grid shown in Figure 4-2 summarizes the major areas for emphasis by the CNS across each dimension of the nursing process.

PROMOTION OF SECURE ATTACHMENT PATTERNS

As a psychiatric liaison to prenatal clinics and hospital nurseries, the CNS can play a major role in promoting child mental health through psychoeducational interventions with parents. The goal for nursing care in this area is to engender cognitive and emotional states within the parent that will enhance the child's potential for a secure attachment.

ASSESSMENT AND DIAGNOSIS. With regard to mental health promotion, there are four important areas for assessment: the parents' values and beliefs about parenting, their own attachment histories, their capacity for empathy and emotional availability, and their knowledge of infant temperament and communication. Main and Goldwyn's (1990) Attachment History Interview, Rohner, Savedra, and Granum's (1979) Acceptance–Rejection Questionnaire, and Wilson's (1991) Pictures of Adult–Infant Relations Test are a few of many useful assessments that are available.

Assessment of these areas may result in a number of nursing diagnoses.* For instance, a parent

*All diagnoses described in this chapter are based on the ANA classification of human responses of concern for Psychiatric-Mental Health Nursing Practice (Loomis, M., O'Toole, M., Brown, P., Pothier, P., West, P., & Wilson, H. Copyright, 1986).

may be identified as having a Knowledge Deficit in regard to the accuracy of his or her expectations about infants, the understanding of infant temperament and communication, or skills in caregiver empathy or availability. Based on the assessment, the CNS may determine that if knowledge were available to the parent, he or she would be able to more effectively parent the infant after birth. On the other hand, assessment may indicate that lack of knowledge is not a problem, but emotional processes may prevent optimal parent–infant interaction. A diagnosis of Distorted Memory may be appropriate, for instance, if assessment of the parent's attachment history suggests that defensive processes, such as idealization, are operating in regard to memories of his or her own childhood experience. Similarly, the parent's attachment history or beliefs about parenting may suggest diagnoses of Altered Feeling Patterns or Undeveloped Emotional Responses. If the parent is bringing substantial anger or unresolved grief into the parenting experience from his or her own attachment history, the potential to be emotionally available with the infant can be severely compromised. Likewise, if the parent is detached from his or her own attachment needs, the capacity for full emotional responsiveness to the infant may be impeded.

PLANNING AND INTERVENTION. The diagnosis made by the CNS will guide the specific objectives for care, such as increased knowledge of infant communication, resolution of grief and mourning, or development of realistic expectations for parenting. The major mode of intervention for any of these objectives will be psychoeducation. Psychoeducation may be defined as the provision of informational content, with recognition of its interconnectedness to the psychodynamic processes of the individual receiving the content.

Attitudes, beliefs, knowledge, and feelings about parenting are all intimately related to the parent's own experiences as a child. Thus, psychoeducation will raise important psychologic issues that the CNS must be prepared to address. Strong feelings may emerge as parents become familiar with ways of assessing infant cues and their meaning or are exposed to alternate beliefs about optimal parenting. They may experience a deep sense of loss based on increased awareness of their own deprivation during childhood or resist the validity of any new information as a result of the pain caused by its consideration. For most parents, these responses will require supportive intervention and cognitive reframing to assist their growing awareness and change in attitudes or feelings. However, for some parents, any necessary change in cognitive or affective processes may require substantial therapeutic work. Depending on the identified role and educational preparation of the CNS, he or she may work directly with a parent to address the psychodynamic issues related to informational content or refer the parent for more intensive, longer term therapy by another mental health professional.

Psychoeducation can occur within the context of a dyadic relationship with one parent, a triadic relationship involving both parents, or a parent group. If the assessment suggests that a parent needs individualized attention to address deeper problems, group approaches are less appropriate. Instead, individual or couple counseling may be the method of choice. However, for most parents, the group context is extremely useful because they can learn a great deal from one another while acquiring mutual support. Parent groups are also a more effective use of resources because the CNS can reach a larger pool with less extensive commitment of time. Media resources, such as books and videotapes on parenting, also can be used with great success in parent groups. Discussion of their content facilitates exploration of common and unique parental concerns and questions.

For some parents the socioeconomic conditions in which they are living can be a major influence on their capacity for effective parenting. If necessities such as food or housing are lacking in their lives, the CNS should refer them to social services for assistance. The nurse's help in coordinating these aspects of care may make the critical difference for a parent in creating an emotional reservoir from which to pull when faced with the substantial needs of a new infant.

RISK IDENTIFICATION AND EARLY PREVENTIVE INTERVENTION

Another major role for the CNS involves risk factor identification and early prevention efforts with parents and infants. These activities occur primarily through liaison work with hospital nurseries and pediatric clinics where agency personnel may identify the potential for interactive problems and refer the parents for further assessment. The goal of the CNS in this arena of child mental health is to enhance the use of sensitivity, acceptance, cooperation, and accessibility by parents when interacting with their child. As described previously, attachment research has shown that these behavioral approaches or their absence in the parents' interaction with the infant predict the pattern of attachment in the child.

(text continues on page 56)

Dimensions of the Nursing Process	Spheres of the Mental Health Continuum		
	Promotion of secure attachment patterns	***Risk identification and early preventive intervention***	***Treatment of attachment disorders***
Goals for nursing care	• Engender cognitive and emotional states within the parent that will enhance the child's potential for secure attachment.	→	→
		• Increase the use of sensitivity, acceptance, cooperation, and accessibility by parents when they interact with their child.	→
			• Increase the child's ability to elicit and maintain desired amounts of proximity and support from attachment figures. • Increase an appropriate balance of attachment and exploration/initiative in the child's social interactions.
Areas for assessment	• Parent values and beliefs about parenting • Parent attachment history • Parent knowledge of infant temperament and communication • Parent capacity for sensitivity	→	→
		• Infant behavior with parent • Parent behavior with infant • Infant temperament	→
			• Child's response pattern during stress or uncertainty • Child's social interactions

Potential nursing diagnosis	• Parent response patterns - Knowledge deficit - Distorted memory - Altered feeling patterns - Undeveloped emotional responses	→	→
		• Parent response patterns - Altered communication processes - Dysfunctional behaviors - Altered parenting role performance • Infant response patterns - High risk for altered emotional processes - High risk for altered interpersonal processes - Undeveloped perception processes - High risk for altered perception processes	→
			• Child response patterns - Altered feeling patterns - Undeveloped emotional processes - Altered communication processes - Dysfunctional behaviors - Altered social interaction - Altered self-concept
Modes of intervention	• Psychoeducation with parents • Referral for intensive therapy • Referral for social service aid	→	→
		• Cognitive-behavioral counseling with parents	→
			• Child counseling • Family counseling
Evaluation	• Evidence of change related to goals and specific nursing diagnoses	→	→

FIGURE 4–2 • Nursing care of attachment problems across the continuum of health care

ASSESSMENT AND DIAGNOSIS. As indicated by the grid in Figure 4-2, early assessment of risk must first consider those areas of assessment relevant to the promotion of secure attachment patterns. Parental values and beliefs, attachment history, capacity for sensitivity toward the infant, and knowledge of infant temperament and communication should all be assessed. The actual interaction between parent and infant needs to be examined so that any problematic behaviors of parent and infant can be identified for intervention. The infant's temperament also should be assessed so that parents can be assisted in appropriately responding to the particular disposition of their infant.

There are many useful methods of assessing parent behavior toward the infant, including a rating scale devised by Ainsworth et al. (1978), the Home Observation for Measurement of the Environment (Bradley & Caldwell, 1988), and the Feeding and Teaching Scales developed by Barnard, Hammond, Booth, Bee, Mitchell, & Spieker (1989) as part of the Nursing Child Assessment Project.

The infant's temperament is particularly important to assess because interactional problems may stem from a parent's difficulty relating to an infant whose signals or cues are confusing or who is not responsive to a parent even when he or she tries to provide positive experiences. The CNS can assess the infant's temperament with a variety of well-accepted methods. For very early assessments, the Neonatal Perception Inventory (Broussard & Hartner, 1971) and the Neonatal Behavioral Assessment Scale (Brazelton, 1984; Brazelton, Nugent, & Lester, 1987) can be used. For later infancy, many temperament assessments are available. Some of the most widely used are the Revised Infant Temperament Questionnaire (Carey & McDevitt, 1978), the Infant Behavior Questionnaire (Rothbart, 1981; 1986), and the Infant Characteristics Questionnaire (Bates, Freeland, & Lounsbury, 1979).

A number of diagnoses may be pertinent to the nurse's risk assessment. These may include diagnoses related to parent response patterns and those related to the infant's response patterns. Parent response patterns may suggest one of three diagnoses: Altered Communication Processes, Dysfunctional Behavior, or Altered Parenting. For instance, Altered Communication Processes may be indicated by the observation that the parent does not show any facial affect when interacting with the infant, increasing the likelihood that the infant may not understand how the parent feels about the infant or their interaction. Dysfunctional Behavior may be indicated by the parent's tendency to interfere with the infant's activities or attempt to continually modify the infant's behavioral state rather than accepting it as valid. There may be direct evidence of rejecting behavior based on constant criticism, harsh vocal tones, or rough and even abusive handling of the infant. A diagnosis of Altered Parenting would reflect a constellation of both Altered Communication and Dysfunctional Behavior, which appeared to influence the parent's ability to respond appropriately to the infant's distress signals or to foster the infant's cognitive or socioemotional growth.

In regard to the infant's response patterns, diagnoses such as the Potential for Altered Emotional Processes, Altered Interpersonal Processes, Undeveloped Perception Processes, or the Potential for Altered Perception Processes may be appropriate. Diagnoses related to perception processes would be called for if assessment suggested that the infant might have a genetic diathesis for hyperreactivity to environmental stimulation or that physical health problems (e.g., resulting from intrauterine exposure to alcohol or other drugs) had left the infant's nervous system excessively vulnerable to stimulation. Undeveloped or altered perceptual processes due to such factors can leave the infant extremely vulnerable to overstimulation by the parents, with implications for the infant's perceived security in a world that is experienced as overly arousing. A diagnosis of the Potential for Altered Interpersonal Processes might be indicated if the assessment showed, for instance, that an infant had difficulty providing clear cues to the parent regarding his or her needs or did not respond to the parent's attempts to please or soothe him or her when distressed. A diagnosis of the Potential for Altered Emotional Processes might be suggested if temperament assessments portrayed an infant who either cried intensely and frequently and was extremely difficult to console or showed no affective response, being "poker faced" and unresponsive a great deal of the time. At this stage of early risk identification, most infant diagnoses reflect the *potential* for certain problems rather than the actual problems. Early intervention may prevent their development into attachment problems.

PLANNING AND INTERVENTION. Objectives for nursing care will be determined by the specific diagnosis. For example, the diagnosis may reflect a need for a decreased use of interfering behaviors by parents or an increased ability of the parents to modify their stimulation of the infant based on cues of infant distress. Regardless of the objectives, cognitive–behavioral counseling with parents represents an effective mode of early intervention. Cognitive–behavioral interventions focus on changing specific behaviors while also changing the beliefs that influence these behaviors (Epstein, Schlesinger, & Dryden, 1988).

If the diagnosis reflects parent response patterns, the CNS will need to determine the degree to which the problem can be influenced by directly working with a certain type of behavior. If problematic behaviors seem too deeply rooted in a parent's altered feeling patterns, distorted memory, or undeveloped emotional responses, then more intensive therapeutic work with the parent to resolve these underlying distortions or defensive processes is necessary. The goal of this work would be to help parents gradually reorganize their own internal models of attachment and open themselves to ways of relating with their infant that they may not have experienced in their own childhood. If it seems apparent that the behavior of a primary attachment figure cannot be modified until substantial change occurs in his or her own internal model of attachment, the CNS should attempt to involve another attachment figure (e.g., father, grandmother) in the infant's care. The CNS may need to help the primary figure continue to feel central in the infant's life and not in any way negated by the support of an additional attachment figure.

If the assessment and diagnosis suggest that parental change is likely without intensive individual therapy, the CNS can work with the parent to modify his or her behavior toward the infant and the cognitions influencing the behavior. One very effective intervention is to videotape parent–infant interaction during a typical aspect of caregiving, such as feeding, bathing, or teaching the infant a new skill. These videotapes can then serve as an excellent focus for discussion with parents regarding how they view the infant's behavior and its meaning and how they interpret their own behavior in response to the infant. The CNS can use specific interactions within the videotape to help parents become more aware of their interactional process, to understand the effects of varied approaches on the infant, and to identify optimal behaviors in response to specific infant signals or cues. For instance, the nurse may identify certain types of touch to which the infant seems sensitive and help the parents learn how to use their touch differently to reduce infant distress.

When both parents are involved in the counseling, they can help one another with suggestions and support. Specific "homework" can be given to parents to spend time attending to the infant's facial and body language and together discussing what it means. They also can be asked to experiment with different approaches to situations, for instance, allowing the child to cuddle with them when distressed rather than preventing physical access and expecting the baby to calm down on his or her own. The CNS can then ask them to bring to subsequent sessions their thoughts and feelings about new approaches with the infant and how a new approach affected the child's response. A focus on concrete behavior is essential in helping parents modify problematic interactions.

The interactions that occur between parent and infant when the CNS is present also provide important learning opportunities. There can be immediate discussion about what the CNS observes, how the parents feel, their rationale for responding as they do, and what they might do differently next time. The CNS also can use every opportunity to model sensitive, accepting, and accessible approaches with the infant. It is essential to describe the reasons for using certain approaches through use of minilectures that will help the parents integrate new ways of thinking about parenting. Such modeling can be followed by encouragement for the parent to try the approach while the CNS is present to give support and feedback.

TREATMENT OF ATTACHMENT DISORDERS

The third sphere of health care in which the CNS can influence the attachment behavior of children is when they are referred for treatment of attachment disorders. Identification of attachment-related problems will normally occur during the preschool years; however, some children may be referred at later stages, especially children who have experienced the loss of an attachment figure or have had multiple out-of-home placements throughout their childhood. In most cases, work with the child will occur in the context of a mental health clinic, day care center, or psychiatric unit of a hospital. The CNS also may function as a resource to preschools or child care centers where agency personnel have identified attachment-related problems. In all cases, the goals for nursing care in the treatment of attachment disorders are twofold: (1) to increase the child's ability to elicit and maintain desired amounts of proximity and support from attachment figures, and (2) to increase an appropriate balance in the child's social interactions between attachment behavior and exploratory self-initiative.

ASSESSMENT. To understand fully the factors contributing to an attachment disorder, the CNS should conduct a complete assessment, including the areas related to promotion of secure attachment patterns and early risk identification (see Fig. 4-2). These are essential for determining parental contributions to the attachment problem and factors in the child's temperament that could influence his or her attachment behavior. In addition, two other areas are important to assess when an attachment disorder has been established: the child's response pattern during stressful or uncertain situations and the child's social interactions with significant others and strangers.

Observational periods can be set up during which the child's behavior is watched in different contexts, with peers, parents, and other adults. If the child has markedly disturbed social relations, he or she may fail to initiate or respond to most social interactions on a persistent basis; display indiscriminate sociability, engaging all adults (including strangers) with hugs, kisses, and clinging behavior; or approach all peers as if they were close friends. Other children with attachment problems may have less extreme behavior, but in contrast to children with secure attachments, they will show more difficulty in peer relations. Children with avoidant attachment patterns are more likely to be hostile toward others and more impulsive in their behavior, and they frequently try to victimize other children. They also show a high degree of anger and noncompliance with adult requests or expectations. Children with resistant attachment patterns often are more socially isolated: withdrawing from other children, being targets for victimization, or acting fearful and helpless in many situations. They tend to seek more nurturance from all adults, to show more immature behavior, and to be excessively dependent and clinging.

Observations also provide information about the child's degree of balance between attachment behavior and independent exploration. Lieberman and Pawl (1988) have identified three patterns of distortion in this balance. In the first, the child shows excessive danger seeking in play and exploration. The authors associate this pattern with insufficient maternal protection or the mother's tendency to discount the child's security-seeking behavior. In the second pattern, the child has excessive fear of danger when this does not appear warranted. These children also exhibit more restricted affective expression, show greater vigilance and withdrawal if unfamiliar people are present, and tend to have minimal exploratory behavior. Such behaviors have been associated with parents who are unpredictable and punitive; the child sees the parent as a source of danger rather than a secure haven from danger. The third distorted pattern of attachment exploration has been labeled precocious competence or hypercompetence. The child typically shows overconcern for the mother and caretaking behaviors toward her, consoling her and being solicitous of her welfare rather than seeking her out for security in times of distress. This pattern is found in children whose mothers may be depressed or for some other reason incapable of providing a child with optimal caretaking.

Aside from direct observations of the child's interactions with others, assessments of the child's view of the social world through play dynamics and drawings provide very useful information. In particular, doll families and family drawings (Boxes 4-1 and 4-2) nicely elicit the child's projections related to attachment situations. With either assessment strategy, children can be given no directives or the CNS can guide the play and drawings with a structure of relevant situations. The rapidity with which a more directive, guided approach can be introduced will depend on the child's level of trust and apparent resistance to dealing with content that may frighten or overwhelm him or her.

BOX 4–1 • AN EXAMPLE OF DIRECTED DOLL PLAY TO ASSESS ATTACHMENT ISSUES

Begin the doll play by introducing and defining the roles of the characters in the doll family and setting the context for the child. Provide a period of free play with the dolls, reflecting observations and using gentle questions to help clarify how the child views the situations he or she creates. After the child appears somewhat comfortable, take the role of the mother doll. At first follow the child's lead, not forcing any interaction into the play. Then, when the child appears to accept your involvement, have the mother doll say that she has to leave the house and the child for a while to go out, that some scary noise or stranger is outside the house, or any other uncertain or stressful event. The choice of situations presented will be most useful if based on the presenting symptoms of the child.

Each child may respond more freely to the use of drawings or doll play as a technique for assessment. The use of whichever modality the child prefers will enhance his or her expressiveness and the usefulness of the assessment. This becomes especially important for avoidant children because their internal working models will yield a detachment from their attachment feelings and make it difficult to express attachment behaviors even in fantasy play.

Some specific assessment procedures also have been developed as a direct measure of attachment patterns. For instance, a story completion procedure with dolls has been developed (Bretherton, Ridgeway, & Cassidy, 19), as well as a bear family story completion (Silver, 1990). The "strange situation" is a videotaped assessment of a child's internal model of attachment through rating of child behavior during structured separations and reunions with the parent (Ainsworth et al., 1978).

Because attachment problems usually are identified as a focus for treatment in early childhood, the above assessments are useful primarily for preschool and early school-age children. However, observation of interactional patterns, family drawings, and age-appropriate story completion tasks can be used with school-age children and adolescents. In addition, attachment history interviews (Main & Goldwyn, 1990) can be an effective means of identifying internal working models of attachment with adolescents.

Two schools of family assessment have particular relevance for older children and adolescents: transgenerational and structural family theories. Transgenerational family assessment focuses on how a parent's past relationships with his or her attachment figures may influence current parent–child behavior. A clinical interview and accompanying observation of family interaction are used with the entire family to acquire information about significant life events in the family's history, the nature of the relationships among all family members, and their relationships with extended families. A Family of Origin Scale has been developed (Hovestadt, Anderson, Piercy, Cochran, & Fine, 1985) to assess some of the key areas of early experiences for various family members. Williamson (1982) and Bowen (1978) provide further details on assessment using a transgenerational approach.

Structural family assessment focuses primarily on boundary issues present in family subsystems using a continuum from extreme enmeshment to extreme disengagement. In enmeshed relations, togetherness or belongingness are pursued to the detriment of individuation. Family members speak for one another, interrupt and interfere with one another, and view the need for privacy or personal autonomy as being equated with disloyalty to the family. Enmeshment is akin to the process observed in families in which the child has developed a resistant attachment pattern, and the attachment figure appears to be entangled in or preoccupied with past relationships. In contrast, disengagement

BOX 4–2 • AN EXAMPLE OF DIRECTED DRAWING TO ASSESS ATTACHMENT ISSUES

Ask the child to draw a picture of his or her family. Then ask him or her to describe who is in the picture and what they are doing. More directive comments also can be used, if the child seems ready, to get at the specific features of the drawings. For instance, if the child in the picture is clinging to the mother or is very distant from her with other family members between them, you might reflect the observation that "the boy is very far away from the mother. I wonder how come?" or "The boy is holding onto his mother very tightly. I wonder what he is feeling. What do you think he is feeling?"

The drawings can be used in an even more focused way to get at attachment behavior. For instance, after you have given the child an opportunity to draw a few pictures of the family without any guidelines, then you might say, "I've got an idea. Let's pretend that the boy [or girl depending on the sex of the child] is very upset because he hurt himself. Can you draw a picture of the boy and his family just after he has been hurt and is very upset?" Another focus for the drawing might be the following: "Let's draw one more picture. In this one, the boy has accidentally broken something. Can you draw the boy and his family right after the parents find out that something has been broken?"

in families supports a low degree of interpersonal contact and an alienated version of individuality. Family members may act as if they have no common bond, showing little reciprocal support, mutual consolation, or nurturance. Family disengagement is closely related to the avoidant pattern of attachment in children. Refer to Minuchin (1974) for a more thorough discussion of structural assessment and its interrelatedness with treatment.

DIAGNOSIS. The child being assessed may have already been diagnosed with a DSM-IV classification of reactive attachment disorder of infancy or early childhood (Box 4-3) or possibly separation anxiety (Box 4-4). However, children may have other psychiatric diagnoses with attachment-related etiology, such as disruptive behavior disorders (especially conduct disorders of the solitary aggressive type) or depression (related to separation, loss, rejection, or abuse). Some of the children may have no established psychiatric diagnosis. Regardless, the nursing diagnosis will specify response patterns of the child at which intervention should be aimed or provide essential data for further referral if deemed appropriate.

Two relevant nursing diagnoses involve response patterns in emotional processes: Altered Feeling Patterns and Undeveloped Emotional Processes. The altered feelings may relate to underlying anger, anxiety, or sadness associated with unmet attachment needs. Undeveloped emotions may be more specific to the case of children who have avoidant attachment patterns. Their detachment from feelings of distress or fear in uncertain or stressful situations most likely evolved as a coping response within their first year of life. Thus, the child may have never fully developed the ability to experience such emotions. A restricted emotional repertoire could have significant implications for the ability to express emotions accurately and meet needs effectively in future relationships.

Two other potential nursing diagnoses involve response patterns in interpersonal processes: Altered Communication Processes and Dysfunctional Behaviors. Altered Communication Processes relate primarily to the child's difficulty providing verbal and nonverbal cues to a parent regarding the need for proximity and contact. It also could reflect difficulties communicating attachment needs to teachers or other adult figures. A diagnosis of Dysfunctional Behaviors reflects age-inappropriate responses, such as precocious competence and role reversal with the caregiver, immature behavior involving excessive clinging and dependence, or excessively vigilant behavior. It also could apply to situations in which the child shows disorganized responses, such as stereotypies or freezing when approached by an attachment figure.

A diagnosis of Altered Social Interaction may be appropriate as well. It would be relevant if the child's interaction with others demonstrates intrusiveness, as seen in the child who tends to victi-

BOX 4–3 • Diagnostic Criteria For 313.89 Reactive Attachment Disorder of Infancy or Early Childhood

A. Markedly disturbed and developmentally inappropriate social relatedness in most contexts, beginning before age 5, as evidenced by either 1 or 2.
   1. Persistent failure to initiate or respond in a developmentally appropriate fashion to most social interactions, as manifest by excessively inhibited, hypervigilant, or highly ambivalent and contradictory responses (e.g., the child may respond to caregivers with a mixture of approach, avoidance, and resistance to comforting, or may exhibit frozen watchfulness)
   2. Diffuse attachments as manifest by indiscriminate sociability with marked inability to exhibit appropriate selective attachments (e.g., excessive familiarity with relative strangers or lack of selectivity in choice of attachment figures)

B. The disturbance in criterion A is not accounted for solely by developmental delay (as in mental retardation) and does not meet criteria for a pervasive developmental disorder.

C. Pathogenic care as evidenced by at least one of the following:
   1. Persistent disregard of the child's basic emotional needs for comfort, stimulation, and affection
   2. Persistent disregard of the child's basic physical needs
   3. Repeated changes of the primary caregiver that prevent formation of stable attachments (e.g., frequent changes in foster care)

D. There is a presumption that the care in criterion C is responsible for the disturbed behavior in criterion A (e.g., the disturbances in criterion A began following the pathogenic care in criterion C).

BOX 4–4 • Diagnostic Criteria For 309.21 Separation Anxiety Disorder

A. Developmentally inappropriate and excessive anxiety concerning separation from home or from those to whom the individual is attached, as evidenced by three (or more) of the following:
   1. Recurrent excessive distress when separation from home or major attachment figures occurs or is anticipated
   2. Persistent and excessive worry about losing, or about possible harm befalling, major attachment figures
   3. Persistent and excessive worry that an untoward event will lead to separation from a major attachment figure (e.g., getting lost or being kidnapped)
   4. Persistent reluctance or refusal to go to school or elsewhere because of fear of separation
   5. Persistently and excessively fearful or reluctant to be alone or without major attachment figures at home or without significant adults in other settings
   6. Persistent reluctance or refusal to go to sleep without being near a major attachment figure or to sleep away from home
   7. Repeated nightmares involving theme of separation
   8. Repeated complaints of physical symptoms (such as headaches, stomachaches, nausea, or vomiting) when separation from major attachment figures occurs or is anticipated

B. The duration of the disturbance is at least 4 weeks.

C. The onset is before age 18.

D. The disturbance causes clinically significant distress or impairment in social, academic (occupational), or other important areas of functioning.

E. The disturbance does not occur exclusively during the course of a pervasive developmental disorder, schizophrenia, or other psychotic disorder and, in adolescents and adults, is not better accounted for by panic disorder with agoraphobia.

Specify if:

Early Onset: If onset occurs before age 6.

mize other children or shows excessive familiarity and affection with strangers. It also would be relevant if the child were socially isolated or withdrawn.

A diagnosis of Altered Self-Concept may be fitting for many children with attachment problems. Feelings of rejection or neglect associated with attachment needs may have a substantial impact on their inner confidence, efficacy, and self-worth.

PLANNING. Depending on the diagnosis, specific objectives for care may be to resolve the child's underlying anger at the attachment figure, to reduce anxiety experienced when separated from the attachment figure, or to enhance the child's ability to communicate distress appropriately. In general, all objectives seek to decrease the child's reliance on avoidant, resistant, or disorganized patterns of attachment during stress or uncertainty, and to enhance age-appropriate attachment behaviors with adults and peers.

INTERVENTION. Modes of intervention to achieve treatment goals will ideally include a combination of individual child counseling and family counseling, with approaches selected as appropriate to the child's developmental status.

For *preschool and early school-age children,* individual play therapy can be used in conjunction with conjoint work involving parents and the child. At the beginning of the working relationship, individual counseling sessions with the child can use fantasy play as a way for the child to achieve catharsis through acting out attachment issues in his or her play. Reflective comments and support as the child encounters negative emotions will help children to attend better to what they are feeling and to realize that feelings of distress are not necessarily rejected and unsupported. The child can then begin to learn new styles of relating by building on a transference with the CNS and gradually testing out new behaviors within the context of a trusting relationship.

Focused or structured play can be very effective once the child has developed an initial level of comfort with the CNS. In this approach, the playroom is set up with family toys of many kinds, and play themes are created that will elicit attachment-related conflicts. The CNS can gradually assume a more influential role in creating stress themes in the play situations and responses of attachment figures and the child using doll or bear families. In taking the role of the mother or father, the CNS can begin to respond sensitively and with emotional availability toward the child. Similarly, he or she can model responses through the doll children that show how a child could more directly ask for comfort and support during stressful situations, exposing the child to other possibilities for response patterns. Initially, the child may react to such interventions with traditional attachment patterns of avoidance or resistance, along with signs of accompanying anxiety, anger, or other forms of distress. The reflections and interpretations of the CNS during these reactions can help the child identify his or her feelings and their relationship to certain events in his or her life. In addition, the child's beginning attempt to change the play interactions to achieve more satisfying outcomes can serve as a corrective emotional experience that can build hope and comfort. See Chapter 23, Play Therapy; Slavson and Schiffer (1981); or Schaefer and O'Connor (1983) for further discussion of play therapy techniques.

For *older school-age children and adolescents,* individual work is initially preferable to group treatment because children at this age have difficulty acknowledging and discussing their attachment needs with peers. They often bring deeply held beliefs that they should have outgrown such needs and feel embarrassed dealing with them. However, the CNS may decide that group work is an important sequel to individual counseling, especially if the diagnosis indicates Altered Social Interaction with other children, including intrusiveness or social withdrawal.

Cognitive–behavioral approaches can be an especially effective means to address attachment issues in the older child and adolescent. These approaches aim to influence behavior and feelings by changing thinking patterns. The child's internal model of attachment and its accompanying attachment patterns are the target for change. Techniques include active discussion by the CNS of alternative ways to meet attachment needs or to view the responses of an attachment figure; self-instruction exercises for the child, such as teaching the child to say "It's OK for me to feel upset and tell mom about it"; and challenging maladaptive beliefs held by the child.

Effectively combined with these more cognitive approaches are behavioral exercises, such as role-playing different attachment behaviors and modeling procedures. Videotapes or films of other same-age children in attachment situations can be very useful. The child in the video can show both ineffective and effective strategies for eliciting support and proximity with parents that can then serve as a source of discussion. Active confrontation of the child's existing beliefs and role playing of anxiety-producing situations can be difficult for the child and may increase his or her distress. Therefore, careful timing of interventions and a supportive climate of trust are critical if any change is to occur (DiGiuseppe, 1981; Epstein et al., 1988; and Hersen & Van Hasselt, 1987).

Unless parents are unable or unwilling to be involved in the child's treatment, they should be viewed as an integral aspect of the therapeutic process. The child cannot be expected to make any lasting changes in attachment behavior if he or she lives in an environment where change is actively resisted or at best, not reinforced. Family counseling enables the parents to learn and experiment with new behaviors along with the child. Although the younger preschool child may not directly understand the content of the family sessions, his or her presence enables the CNS to work directly with actual behaviors that emerge in the course of interaction, helping parents talk about their responses to the child and try out different approaches with support and feedback. Older children and adolescents will benefit as much as their parents from family discussions, the modeling of empathy, and emotional availability by the CNS.

As indicated under the previous discussion of assessment, transgenerational and structural family therapies are particularly relevant to attachment concerns. In transgenerational family counseling, the resolution of old attachments is central to the approach. The primary goal is to reduce the influence of past relationships with attachment figures on the present behavior of family members. Primary techniques to accomplish this goal are interpretation (calling attention to unconscious factors in a given behavior) and education (asking strategic questions, modeling, minilectures, and readings). Through these techniques, the CNS can reduce family projection (i.e., the process whereby current relationships are used as stand-ins for the past) and help parents and children more effectively experience their relationships in the realities of the present (Bowen, 1978; Brown & Christensen, 1986; Levant, 1984).

Through structural family therapy, techniques can be used to modify dysfunctional patterns of disengagement or enmeshment in the family. Among the many available techniques within the structural approach, enactment and reframing are especially useful. Enactment involves the activation of dysfunctional patterns related to attachment behavior during family sessions and then helping the family to discuss these patterns and alternative ways of handling attachment situations.

The technique of reframing involves helping the

family to see a different reality in the situation by highlighting aspects of the child's behavior that could reflect a request for proximity and support, aspects of the parent's behavior that encourage the child to avoid or resist support and nurturance, and potential reasons for any difficulties family members may have in expressing what they really think and feel. Like transgenerational therapy, the structural approach also includes a strong educational component in which the CNS assists the family in understanding their interactions and trying out new ones in a safe environment (Brown & Christensen, 1986; Minuchin & Fishman, 1981; & Tavantzis, 1984).

Whether the CNS conducts these family counseling sessions or refers the family to another mental health professional should depend on the degree to which the CNS has received educational preparation and training in family therapies. More harm than good can be done if a CNS encourages the family to confront deeply engrained attitudes and interactions yet does not have the skill to work effectively through issues with families to achieve some level of resolution.

CLINICAL EVALUATION

Regardless of the specific therapeutic approaches selected by the CNS, their usefulness and efficacy with each child and family must be evaluated as part of the nursing process. Evaluation needs to first address the major goals for nursing care as they relate to attachment. Has the care engendered cognitive and emotional states within the parents that will enhance the child's potential for a secure attachment? Has the care increased the use of sensitivity, acceptance, cooperation, and accessibility by parents when interacting with their child? Has the care increased the child's ability to elicit and maintain desired amounts of proximity and support from attachment figures? Has the care increased an appropriate balance between attachment and exploration or initiative in the child's social interactions?

In addition to evaluation of these overall attachment goals, specific criteria must be established for each child and family that are pertinent to the nursing diagnoses. For example, does a parent show evidence of increased knowledge regarding the potential meaning of his or her infant's behavior (Knowledge Deficit)? Does a parent show increased use of consistent and sensitive caregiving behavior with the child rather than interference and criticism (Dysfunctional Behaviors)? Does a child show an increased ability to express his or her needs for support and nurturance rather than hiding them behind behaviors of withdrawal or aggression (Altered Social Interaction)?

If the answers to such questions are negative, then clearly the approaches to care need reconsideration and potential modification. It is possible, however, that the care plan is appropriate, but more time is needed before the effects are visible. It also is possible that the approaches need to be intensified in frequency or in the degree to which they overtly confront the problem areas being addressed. On the other hand, the entire care plan may need reconceptualization, based on continued assessment and modification in light of new information being acquired.

Through this evaluation, the CNS can help to assure that his or her interventions are accurately addressing the attachment issues of a particular child and family. In addition, evaluation can raise important questions for future research, which can contribute to the expansion and refinement of existing attachment theory.

REFERENCES

Ainsworth, M. D. S. (1979). Attachment as related to mother-infant interaction. In J. S. Rosenblatt, R. A. Hinde, C. Beer, & M. Busnel (Eds.), *Advances in the study of behavior* (Vol. 9). New York: Academic Press.

Ainsworth, M., Blehar, M., Waters, E., & Walls, S. (1978). *Patterns of attachment.* Hillsdale, NJ: Lawrence Erlbaum.

Arend, R., Gove, F., & Sroufe, I. A. (1979). Continuity of individual adaptation from infancy to kindergarten: A prospective study of egoresilience and curiosity in preschoolers. *Child Development, 50,* 950–959.

Barnard, K., Hammond, M., Booth, C., Bee, H., Mitchell, S., & Spieker, S. (1989). Measurement and meaning of parent-child interaction. In F. Morrison, C. Lord, & K. Deating (Eds.), *Applied developmental psychology.* (Vol. III). New York: Academic Press.

Bates, J., Freeland, C., & Lounsbury, M. (1979). Measurement of infant difficultness. *Child Development, 50,* 794–803.

Belsky, J., & Rovine, M. (1987). Temperament and attachment security in the strange situation: An empirical rapproachment. *Child Development, 58,* 787–795.

Bowen, M. (1978). *Family therapy in clinical practice.* New York: Aronson.

Bowlby, J. (1969). *Attachment and loss.* (Vol. I). *Attachment* (2nd ed.). New York: Basic Books.

Bowlby, J. (1973). *Attachment and loss.* (Vol. II). *Separation.* New York: Basic Books.

Bowlby, J. (1982). Attachment and loss: Retrospect and prospect. *American Journal of Orthopsychiatry, 52,* 664–678.

Bradley, R., & Caldwell, B. (1988). Using the home inventory to assess the family environment. *Pediatric Nursing, 14*(2), 97–102.

Brazelton, T. B. (1984). *Neonatal behavioral assessment scale* (2nd ed.). Philadelphia: J.B. Lippincott.

Brazelton, T. B., Nugent, J. K., & Lester, B. (1987). Neonatal behavioral assessment scale. In J. Osofsky (Ed.), *Handbook of infant development* (pp. 780–817). New York: John Wiley & Sons.

Bretherton, I., Ridgeway, D., & Cassidy, J. (1990). Assessing internal working models of the attachment relationship. In M. Greenberg, D. Cicchetti, & M. Cummings (Eds.), *Attachment in the preschool years: Theory, research and intervention* (pp. 273–308). Chicago: University of Chicago Press.

Broussard, E., & Hartner, M. (1971). Further considerations regarding maternal perceptions of the first born. In J. Hellmuth (Ed.), *The exception infant: Studies in abnormalities.* New York: Brunner/Mazel.

Brown, J., & Christensen, D. (1986). *Family therapy: Theory and practice* (pp. 51–82). Monterey, CA: Brooks/Cole.

Brown, J., & Christensen, D. (1986). *Family therapy: Theory and practice* (pp. 115–139). Monterey, CA: Brooks/Cole.

Carey, W., & McDevitt, S. (1978). Revision of the infant temperament questionnaire. *Pediatrics, 61,* 735–739.

Crockenberg, S. (1981). Infant irritability, mother responsiveness, and social support influences on the security of mother-infant attachment. *Child Development, 52,* 857–865.

DiGiuseppe, R. (1981). Cognitive therapy with children. In G. Emery, S. Hollon, & R. Bedrosian (Eds.), *New directions in cognitive therapy* (pp 50–67). New York: Guilford Press.

Egeland, B., & Farber, E. (1984). Infant-mother attachment: Factors related to its development and changes over time. *Child Development, 5,* 753–771.

Egeland, B., & Sroufe, L. A. (1981). Developmental sequelae of maltreatment in infancy. In R. Rizley & D. Cicchetti (Eds.), *Developmental perspectives in child maltreatment* (pp. 77–92). San Francisco: Jossey-Bass.

Epstein, N., Schlesinger, S., & Dryden, W. (1988). *Cognitive-behavioral therapy with families.* New York: Brunner/Mazel.

Erickson, M., Egeland, B., & Sroufe, L. A. (1985). The relationship between quality of attachment and behavior problems in preschool in a high risk sample. In I. Bretherton & E Waters (Eds.), Growing points in attachment theory and research. *Monographs of the Society for Research in Child Development, 50*(1–2, Ser. No. 209), 147–186.

George, C., & Main, M. (1979). Social interactions of young abused children: Approach, avoidance, and aggression. *Child Development, 50,* 306–318.

Grossman, K., Grossman, K. E., Spangler, G., Suess, G., & Unzner, L. (1985). Maternal sensitivity and newborn's orientation responses as related to quality of attachment in Northern Germany. In I. Brazelton & E. Waters (Eds.), Growing points of attachment theory and research. *Monographs of the Society for Research in Child Development, 50* (1–2, Serial No. 209).

Hersen, M., & Van Hasselt, V. (1987). *Behavior therapy with children and adolescents.* New York: John Wiley and Sons.

Hovestadt, A., Anderson, W., Piercy, F., Cochran, S., & Fine, M. (1985). A family of origin scale. *Journal of Marital and Family Therapy, 11*(3), 287–297.

Kagan, J. (1974). Discrepancy, temperament and infant distress. In M. Lewis & L. Rosenblum (Eds.), *The origins of fear.* New York: John Wiley and Sons.

Kagan, J. (1987). Perspectives on infancy. In J. Osofsky (Ed.), *Handbook of infant development* (pp. 1150–1198). New York: John Wiley and Sons.

Kaplan, N., & Main, M. (1985). Internal representations of attachment at six years as indicated by family drawings and verbal responses to imagined separations. In M. Main (Ed.), *Attachment: A move to the level of representation.* Symposium conducted at the meeting of the Society for Research in Child Development, Toronto.

Levant, R. (1984). *Family therapy: A comprehensive overview.* (pp. 86–121). Englewood Cliffs, NJ: Prentice-Hall.

Lewis, M. (1987). Social development in infancy and early childhood. In J. Osofsky (Ed.), *Handbook of infant development* (pp. 419–493). New York: John Wiley and Sons.

Lieberman, A., & Pawl, J. (1988). Clinical applications of attachment. In J. Belsky & T. Nezwarski (Eds.), *Clinical implications of attachment* (pp. 327–351). New York: Erlbaum.

Main, M. (1981). Avoidance in the service of attachment. A working paper. In K. Immelmann, G. Barlow, L. Petrinovich, & M. Main (Eds.), *Behavioral development* (pp. 651–693). Cambridge: Cambridge University Press.

Main, M. (1990). Parental aversion to infant-initiated contact is correlated with the parent's own rejection during childhood: The effects of experience on signals of security with respect to attachment. In K. Barnard & T. B. Brazelton (Eds.), *Touch: The foundation of experience* (pp. 461–495). Madison, CT: International Universities Press.

Main, M., & Cassidy, J. (1988). Categories of response to reunion with the parent at age six: Predictable from infant attachment classification and stable over a one-month period. *Developmental Psychology, 24*(3), 415–426.

Main, M., & Hesse, E. (1990). Parents' unresolved traumatic experiences are related to infant disorganized attachment status. In M. Greenberg, D. Cicchetti, & M. Cummings (Eds.), *Attachment in the preschool years: Theory, research and intervention* (pp. 161–182). Chicago: University of Chicago Press.

Main, M., & Goldwyn, R. (1990). Adult attachment rating and classification system. In M. Main (Ed). *A typology of human attachment. Organization: Assessed in discourse, drawings and interviews.* New York: Cambridge University Press.

Main, M., Kaplan, N., & Cassidy, J. (1985). Security in infancy, childhood and adulthood: A move to the level of representation. In I. Bretherton & E. Waters (Eds.), Growing points in attachment theory and research. *Monographs of the Society for Research in Child Development, 50*(Whole No. 209), 66–104.

Main, M., & Goldwyn, R. (1984). Predicting rejection of her infant from mothers representation of her own experience: Implications for the abused-abusing intergenerational cycle. *Child Abuse & Neglect, 8,* 203–217.

Main, M., & Solomon, J. (1986). Discovery of an insecure-disorganized/disoriented attachment pattern. In T. B. Brazelton & M. Yogman (Eds.), *Affective development in infancy.* Norwood, NJ: Ablex Publishers.

Main, M., & Stadtman, J. (1981). Infant response to rejection of physical contact by the mother: Aggression, avoidance, and conflict. *Journal of the American Academy of Child Psychology, 202,* 292–307.

Main, M., & Weston, D. (1982). Security of attachment to mother and father: Related to conflict behavior and the readiness to establish new relationships. *Child Development, 52,* 932–940.

Minuchin, S. (1974). *Families and family therapy.* Cambridge, MA: Harvard University Press.

Minuchin, S., & Fishman, H. (1981). *Family therapy techniques.* Cambridge, MA: Harvard University Press.

Miyake, K., Chen, S., & Campos, J. J. (1985). Infant temperament, mother's mode of interaction, and attachment in Japan: An interim report. In I. Bretherton & E. Waters (Eds.), Growing points in attachment theory and research. *Monographs of the Society for Research in Child Development, 56*(1–2).

Pastor, D. (1981). The quality of mother-infant attachment and its relationship to toddler's initial sociability with peers. *Developmental Psychology, 17*(3), 326–335.
Rohner, R., Savedra, J., & Granum, E. (1979). Parental acceptance-rejection questionnaire: Test manual. Washington, DC: American Psychological Association.
Rothbart, M. (1981). Measurement of temperament in infancy. *Child Development, 52,* 569–578.
Rothbart, M. (1986). Longitudinal observation of infant temperament. *Developmental Psychology, 22*(3), 356–365.
Schaefer, C., & O'Connor, K. (1983) *Handbook of play therapy.* New York: John Wiley Publications.
Schneider-Rosen, K., Braunwald, K. G., Carlson, V., & Cicchetti, D. (1985). Current perspectives in attachment theory: Illustration from the study of maltreated infants. In I. Bretherton & E. Waters (Eds.), Growing points of attachment theory and research. *Monographs of the Society of Research in Child Development, 50* (1–2, Serial No. 209).
Silver, D. H. (1990). Representation of attachment and social behavior in preschool children. Unpublished manuscript, Department of Psychology, University of California, Berkeley.
Slavson, S., & Schiffer, M. (1981). *Group psychotherapies for children.* New York: International Universities Press.
Sroufe, L. A. & Fleeson, J. (1986). Attachment and the construction of relationships. In W. Hartup & Z. Rubin (Eds.), *Relationships and development.* Hillsdale, NJ: Lawrence Erlbaum Associates.
Sroufe, L. A. (1983). Infant-caregiver attachment and patterns of adaptation in preschool: The roots of maladaptation and competence. In M. Perlmutter (Ed.), *Minnesota symposia in child psychology* (Vol. 16). (pp. 41–83). Hillsdale, NJ: Erlbaum.
Sroufe, L. A. (1985). Attachment classification from the perspective of infant-caregiver relationships and infant temperament. *Child Development, 56,* 1–14.
Tavantzis, T. (1984). Family therapy: An introduction to a structural perspective. In J. Gumaer (Ed.), *Counseling and therapy for children,* (pp. 287–314). New York: Free Press.
Thomas, A., & Chess, S. (1984). Genesis and evolution of behavioral disorder: From infancy to early adult life. *American Journal of Psychiatry, 141,* 1–9.
Waters, E., & Sroufe, L. A. (1983). A developmental perspective on competence. *Developmental Review, 3,* 79–97.
Weber, R. A., Levitt, M. J., & Clark, M. C. (1986). Individual variation in attachment security and strange situation behavior: The role of maternal and infant temperament. *Child Development, 57,* 56–65.
Williamson, D. (1982). Personal authority via termination of the intergenerational hierarchical boundary: Part II. The consultation process and the therapeutic method. *Journal of Marital and Family Therapy, 8*(2), 23–28.
Wilson, P. (1991). Pictures of adult-infant relations test. Unpublished doctoral dissertation. School of Nursing, University of California, San Francisco.

CHAPTER

5

Family Systems Theory

Judith A. Greene

Children are born into families and remain dependent on them until they achieve sufficient maturity to leave home. During infancy, childhood, and even adolescence, human beings do not hold positions of leadership, authority, or power in their families. Thus, children have little responsibility for the decisions their families make. In many ways children are virtually at the mercy of their parents and other significant adults during their formative years. The child's survival and emotional health are thus contingent on the effective functioning of his or her parents and other important adults in his or her life. For these reasons, therapeutic intervention needs to be conducted with the responsible adults (usually parents) when children exhibit emotional or behavioral problems.

Bowen Family Systems Theory and Therapy and Research Foundations

HISTORIC AND RESEARCH FOUNDATIONS OF THE THEORY AND THERAPY

Bowen family systems theory and therapy were developed by the late Murray Bowen and his associates over 30 years. Murray Bowen and two of his associates, Michael Kerr and Daniel V. Papero, have described the historic origins of this theory and therapy in several writings. Readers interested in the history of Bowen's work are referred to those sources (Bowen, 1978; Kerr & Bowen, 1988; Kerr, 1981; Papero, 1990).

BOWEN FAMILY SYSTEMS THEORY

Bowen family systems theory and associated therapy provide a practical guide for clinicians faced with decisions regarding how to help emotionally or behaviorally disordered children. Therapy based on this theory provides direction to parents in a way that promotes their own emotional maturity. Helping parents through this therapy assists their children to function with increased emotional control. Stated more simply, parents in possession of increased emotional control are more helpful, effective parents. Children, in turn, reflect their parents' improvement by behaving more effectively.

Bowen family systems theory consists of eight interrelated concepts. These concepts serve to describe and explain processes that govern human behavior. Underlying these concepts are some important assumptions about human development, human relationships, and behavior.

Assumptions

The following assumptions underlie the concepts of Bowen family systems theory.

- *The occurrence of a symptom reflects an acute or chronic disturbance in the balance of emotional forces in the affected person's relationship system, especially the family system* (Bowen, 1978; Kerr & Bowen, 1988; Kerr, 1981).

Barbara Schoen Johnson: CHILD, ADOLESCENT AND FAMILY PSYCHIATRIC NURSING, © 1994 J.B. Lippincott Company

- *The individual on whom other family members rely for their own successful emotional functioning is generally the person most vulnerable to symptom formation* (Kerr, 1981). In some families this individual may be a parent. In others, however, this individual is a child.
- *Central to this theory is the assumption that two counterbalancing life forces operate in all natural systems.* These life forces also operate in the natural system known as the human family.

  These two forces consist of a force toward togetherness (the herd instinct) and a force toward individuality. The togetherness force, or need for others, stems from an instinctual need for connectedness to a group or another person. It also is expressed as pressure for conformity and assurance that mutual needs will be met in the relationship. The force toward individuality, on the other hand, stems from an instinctual need for independence, self-reliance, and self-containment (Kerr, 1981).

  Another part of this assumption is that these two forces are in a dynamic, ever-changing state. Individuals in a relationship carefully monitor and respond to fluctuations in these two forces. To illustrate, a feeling of too much togetherness may be associated with a sense of loss of self. This loss triggers efforts to achieve an increased sense of individuality. In a similar way, a feeling of too much independence or too little togetherness prompts a drive toward increased togetherness (Bowen, 1978; Kerr, 1981).
- *Anxiety plays a major part in the automatic or reflex-like operation of these counterbalancing forces.* For example, when anxiety increases, a human family, like other mammals, tends toward increased togetherness. This increased drive toward togetherness fosters increased cohesion, which in turn is associated with family members feeling and behaving as though they were responsible for each other's welfare and behavior (Bowen, 1978; Kerr, 1981).

  If anxiety continues to increase, the togetherness drive and the concomitant loss of individuality increases. This high anxiety situation can be positive or negative (Papero, 1990). In negative family relationships, rebellion against or overcompliance with family expectations is common. Both of these reactions stem from family pressure for cohesion, conformity, and sameness. If anxiety remains chronically high in a family, the life course of its members tends to be directed largely by various emotional reactions (Kerr, 1981; Papero, 1990).
- *Although human behavior is largely governed by emotions, humans also have the capacity for intellectually determined behavior.* Intellectually based behavior derives from the intellectual system, and emotionally based behavior derives from the emotional system. As long as the two systems can stay functionally separate, the individual can choose whether to act out of the intellectual or emotional systems (Kerr, 1981; Papero, 1990).

  When these two systems are not functionally separate, the emotional system tends to dominate, resulting in emotionally based behavior. The lack of emotional separateness between the intellectual and emotional systems is referred to as fusion (Kerr, 1991). The fusion of these two systems occurs and increases when the individual's anxiety increases.

  During periods of emotional calm, the individual can keep the emotional and intellectual systems fairly separate. This permits the person to think more clearly and objectively. Stormy, intense emotional periods, however, lead to fusion of these two systems and increased subjectivity and irrationality. In such situations the intellect functions in the service of emotion rather than as a counterbalancing force (Kerr, 1981; Papero, 1990). Examples of the intellect functioning in the service of emotion include the defense mechanisms of intellectualization, rationalization, and projection. The individual in these circumstances loses the capacity to choose between acting out of emotionality or intellectuality.
- *The extent to which people are apt to succumb to fusion of these two systems is variable.* Some people can sustain intense stress and emotionality before separateness of the intellectual system is lost. Other individuals, however, experience fusion of their emotion and intellectual systems even under mild to moderate stress and anxiety. This variability in the ability to maintain separateness of the emotional and intellectual systems tends to be related to what is referrred to as basic differentiation between the two systems (Kerr, 1981). To illustrate, people who maintain considerable separation of the intellectual and emotional systems in a variety of circumstances, especially emotionally charged ones, are thought to have a higher degree of basic differentiation. Individuals lacking such flexibility are thought to have a lesser degree of basic differentiation.

  Individuals with a lesser degree of differentiation between their intellectual and emotional systems are influenced more by their emotions. If the emotional system dominates, the individual's functioning is more affected by his or her togetherness life force (Kerr, 1981).

The dominant influence of the togetherness life force is exhibited in several ways. People whose thinking, feeling, and behavior are dependent on, or influenced by, the emotionality of others demonstrate dominance of the emotional system and the drive toward togetherness. Additionally, this oversensitivity to the emotionality of others is revealed in approval-seeking or people-pleasing, conforming behaviors and anxiety about and emotional reactivity to what other people say and do. In some cases this oversensitivity and emotional reactivity are expressed in diametrically opposite behaviors, such as rebelling against the perceived wishes of others in an effort to gain social disapproval. These rebelling cases, however, do not differ from the people-pleasing, conforming cases, because both are produced in reaction to the emotionality of others (Bowen, 1978; Kerr, 1981).

- *The emotional reactivity of people to each other is what produces the social pressure people feel from each other to think, feel, and act in certain ways* (Kerr, 1981; Papero, 1990). The capacity to exert pressure on one hand and be vulnerable to it on the other are opposite sides of the same emotional coin. In other words, these capabilities can be considered emotional equivalents (Kerr, 1981).
- *The degree to which the individual's (emotional and intellectual) systems are fused reflects the extent to which the individual loses self in relationships.* This loss of self in relationships is called relationship fusion (Kerr, 1981). As stated previously, fusion of intellectual and emotional functioning in the individual leads to dominance of the togetherness force. When this occurs, it is difficult for the individual to maintain a clear sense of self in relationships, hence the development of relationship fusion.
- *People with similar levels of emotional functioning and togetherness needs attract each other in terms of forming long-term relationships, such as marriage.* The greater the togetherness needs of each person in the relationship, the greater and more intense the relationship fusion. The greater and more intense the relationship fusion, the greater the loss of individuality (Kerr, 1981).

  Usually each partner in a relationship fusion acts out the opposing sides of the togetherness force previously described. On the surface, it may appear that one partner is more emotionally mature and independent. On closer analysis, however, both have very similar needs for togetherness.

  To illustrate, couples are commonly composed of one spouse who in the name of peace and harmony surrenders his or her own values, principles, and opinions by way of relationship fusion. This spouse may appear inadequate, vulnerable, and weak. The other spouse, in contrast, may appear independent, competent, and calm. This spouse may experience less felt need for closeness and approval from his or her mate. Additionally, this spouse may overvalue himself or herself while at the same time devaluing his or her mate for being inadequate, dependent, weak, and so forth. The spouse who appears stronger is said to gain self by way of relationship fusion. Conversely, the spouse who appears weak is described as losing self by way of relationship fusion. This twosome, thus, acts out mutually reciprocal roles in the relationship fusion (Bowen, 1978; Kerr, 1981; Papero, 1990).
- *The greater the separation of emotional and intellectual systems within an individual, the greater his or her basic level of differentiation.* The greater the degree of differentiation, the greater the individuality in the person. The greater the individuality force, the greater the tendency toward separation of the emotional and intellectual systems. Individuals with more basic differentiation of self thus experience a lesser degree of relationship fusion. Such relationships tend more toward individuality and are characterized by less emotional intensity and togetherness (Kerr, 1981). Thus, these individuals are freer emotionally to pursue independent activities outside the relationship.
- *Relationship fusion can alleviate and cause anxiety.* Individuals with less differentiation of self experience more anxiety when they feel emotionally isolated or alone. In turn, they seek togetherness in the relationship to reduce anxiety. This increased togetherness, however, increases the emotional intensity of the relationship. Thus, the individuals involved in such relationships need closeness to reduce anxiety associated with emotional isolation and distance to reduce the anxiety associated with closeness. Individuals involved in relationships characterized by intense emotional fusion many times experience great difficulty in balancing this closeness–distance dilemma (Bowen, 1978; Kerr, 1981; Papero, 1990).

  Relationships with a high degree of fusion

often produce so much anxiety and so many problems that neither spouse can escape impairment. In some cases, the spouse who compromised the most or surrendered more of self to the relationship may be the first to become impaired. This spouse may be described as underfunctioning. The spouse who appeared more adequate or healthy may be described as the overfunctioning member of the couple. This overfunctioning spouse can eventually feel compromised and become impaired by the burden of the other's underfunctioning. This relationship process is driven by anxiety, and both spouses are victims of it (Bowen, 1978; Kerr & Bowen, 1988; Kerr, 1981; Papero, 1990).

The preceding assumptions underlying Bowen family systems theory provide the basic foundation for the interlocking concepts of the theory itself.

Interlocking Concepts

TRIANGLES. According to Bowen, a relationship composed of just two people is unstable. The reason for this is that when tension and anxiety increase, one or both of the individuals become anxious. Usually, one feels more anxious than the other. In an effort to gain relief from anxiety or other strong emotion, this individual involves a third person in the relationship. The involvement of a third person tends to reduce the anxiety between the original dyad (Kerr, 1981; Papero, 1990).

The involvement of a third person usually provides the more uncomfortable member of the dyad an opportunity to ventilate his or her emotions and complaints about the other member of the dyad. The other member of the dyad may, for a short time, feel less anxious as a result of the third party's involvement. The reason for this is that the relationship between the original dyad has become less intense (Kerr, 1981). The decreased intensity of the relationship results in their interactions becoming less difficult and emotional.

An example of this kind of transaction in a family might take place in this manner: A husband and wife develop an ongoing conflict about with which of their respective parents they will spend the Thanksgiving holiday. Each partner wants to spend the holiday with his or her own parents. The wife, who in the past has compromised her wishes to preserve harmony in the marriage, becomes increasingly angry and emotional about this issue. As her discomfort mounts, the wife cries and complains about her husband and all their misspent past Thanksgiving holidays to their 12-year-old son. The husband and wife predictably cease arguing about where to celebrate the Thanksgiving holiday. Additionally, their interactions as a couple become more calm and congenial. The husband erroneously believes the conflict has been resolved. Actually what has happened is that the mother and child relationship has intensified. As a result, the father has moved into the outside position, and doing so has afforded him some anxiety relief. At this point in the family triangle, the father has a fairly comfortable position in relation to his wife and son. The mother and son, however, occupy uncomfortable positions in relation to each other.

As the relationship between the mother and son becomes progressively more intense, the son begins to have nightmares about being chased by men with guns. Traditionally, the son and his father, along with paternal uncles and male cousins, have gone deer hunting on Thanksgiving. The mother becomes very anxious about the son's nightmares and eventually finds the situation intolerable. At this point, the mother goes to her husband to express her anxieties about their son. The father then becomes involved with the son in an intense manner in an effort to understand and stop the son's nightmares. The father's doing so thus places the mother in the more comfortable outside position of the triangle.

The son tells the father that his nightmares would probably go away if they did not have to go hunting on Thanksgiving. At this point, the father becomes angry with the son for not fulfilling his expectations about deer hunting on Thanksgiving. The emotional intensity of their interaction results in the mother's intervening. Her intervention takes the form of her criticizing her husband for being "a bad father" who makes his son miserable on Thanksgiving. This turn of events results in increased tension between the parents, with the son returning to the more comfortable outside position.

This example illustrates the fluidity of movement among the triangle positions. When circumstances are calm, individual members of the triangle appear more calm and independent. In less differentiated people, the operation of the triangle is more active and obvious. Additionally, more than one triangle can exist within a nuclear family. Other triangles can emerge involving other offspring in the family. Still other triangles involving the parents' families of origin can be activated.

A system of interlocking triangles can come into play when anxiety cannot be contained within a single triangle. The activation of other triangles usually can be predicted with a fairly high degree of accuracy (Kerr, 1981). For example, it is highly probable that a fourth party may be drawn into the family situation previously described. In this case, the mother appeals to her own father for support by confiding to him about her husband's selfishness and insensitivity regarding his son's emotional difficulties and nightmares. Her father becomes incensed and gives his daughter emotional support by agreeing with her about her husband being "a bad father." Thus, a triangle composed of the mother, her father, and the husband is activated. The wife's father draws yet another person into the struggle, his own wife.

The wife's mother has had a few minor physical problems in the past year and consequently fears that this may be her last Thanksgiving. The wife's mother calls her son-in-law and actively accuses him of being cold and insensitive to his own family and to his in-laws. The wife who has always resented her mother for "being interfering" aligns with her husband against her mother. Thus, another triangle composed of the wife, husband, and wife's mother is activated. The activation of this triangle stabilizes, at least temporarily, the intactness of this nuclear family, the father, mother, and son.

The preceding example describes the automatic manner in which individuals move within interlocking triangles to maintain involvement or noninvolvement with each other and to keep anxiety within themselves and the family at a tolerable level.

NUCLEAR FAMILY EMOTIONAL PROCESS. When a marriage experiences acute or chronic anxiety, The marital pair can cope with or reduce anxiety in four ways (Kerr, 1981; Papero, 1990):

1. Distance themselves emotionally from each other
2. Develop conflict with each other
3. Transfer their own anxiety to one or more children
4. Allow one partner to become dysfunctional either emotionally or physically

Factors influencing which of these options are selected depends on the level of relationship fusion between the marital pair, how they related as children to their own parents, and the degree of chronic anxiety present in their relationship (Kerr, 1981).

Each of these options represents an attempt to preserve an emotional balance within the individuals comprising the family and the family itself. Sometimes, however, the intactness of one person's functioning is undermined to preserve the functioning of the other. The exclusive overuse of one of these options to maintain family balance results in little use of the other options. Thus, some families use one option exclusively, while other families use a mixture of them. Additionally, the greater the relationship fusion of a nuclear family, the greater the chronic anxiety within the family; therefore, the greater the need for using these options. Also, extreme anxiety within a nuclear family generated by external stressors can result in the family's use of these options even though the relationship fusion may be relatively low (Kerr, 1981).

EMOTIONAL DISTANCE. Emotional distance describes what happens when people involved in relationships such as marriage react to the emotional intensity of the relationship by withdrawing from each other. Emotional distancing is a way of reducing the anxiety associated with too much closeness. The closeness in the relationship may be experienced as either positive or negative togetherness (Kerr, 1981). In either case, the participants in the relationship distance from each other as if they were allergic to each other.

In this way, emotional distance differs from the way better differentiated persons function in a relationship. That is, better differentiated people may choose to be separate from each other to pursue their own individual activities. Their distance from each other is by choice, not by a strong need to escape the other (Kerr, 1981; Papero, 1990).

Behaviorally, emotional distance may take several forms. Physical separation due to a job requiring long hours at work or long distance traveling can be a way of achieving emotional distance. Interpersonal mechanisms, such as avoiding specific topics, protracted silence, and not looking at each other for long periods, are other ways of achieving distance.

Because distancing occurs automatically, the marital pair may not be aware of what is happening. This way of relating may become an accepted feature of their marriage, which serves to reduce the tension between the couple. If one spouse is aware of the distance, he or she may try to change the pattern. Attempts to change the pattern by seeking more closeness may produce the opposite effect, even greater distancing. A shift to marital conflict also may result from attempting to change the distancing pattern. This shift can result in the pattern of marital conflict alternating with distancing (Kerr, 1981; Papero, 1990).

Despite the fact that distancing is automatic, it

usually is a dissatisfying relationship pattern. One or both partners may experience discomfort because of it. If one of the spouses becomes too uncomfortable, he or she may become involved with an outside third party in a triangle. This third party may be a lover, a child, a relative, a friend, or an associate. In any case, it is common for spouses involved in emotional distancing to consider the other as "the problem," despite the fact that each contributes equally to the process (Kerr, 1981).

MARITAL CONFLICT. This is a relationship pattern that takes yet another approach to coping with anxiety associated with too much or too little emotional closeness in a marriage. Such a relationship is characterized by intense emotional involvement. Both spouses' emotional reactiveness is focused on the other. Time spent together is used to debate, discuss, and argue. Neither spouse gives in or backs off because both strive to win. When they are apart, they remain focused on the other. Often their thoughts are preoccupied with how they have been unfairly treated by the other. Their protracted periods of intense verbal warfare occasionally alternate with brief periods of positive emotional closeness. These periods are short lived, however, because a mere change in facial expression, voice tone, or a casual remark can set off further conflict (Kerr, 1981).

The effect of intense marital conflict has traditionally been considered harmful to the offspring of such marriages. Contrary to this assumption, Bowen and his associates have found that the more anxiety can be contained between the marital dyad, the less offspring are affected (Kerr, 1981). Their observations also seem to indicate that children are at greater risk when one or both parents become anxious about the effects of their marriage on the child. This kind of anxious involvement often leads to parents banding together and transferring their own anxiety to their children.

TRANSFER OF ANXIETY AND SYMPTOMS TO A CHILD. As described in the section on triangles, parents can avoid fusion-caused difficulties and anxiety by transferring their concerns to one or more children. This takes place when one parent, usually the mother, becomes overly involved with one or more children. The other less involved parent either supports this overinvolvement or distances from it. In doing so, the less involved parent becomes equally involved in this process (Kerr, 1981; Papero, 1990).

The exact way in which parents transfer their anxieties to a child are difficult to discern. Generally, however, it seems that the anxiety in a parent is expressed in sensitivity and emotional reactivity to a child. This emotional reactivity prevents the mother or father from parenting in an effective manner (Kerr, 1981). In some cases the parent may have difficulty setting limits with the child. In other cases the parent may focus on real or imagined problems in the child. In still others the parent may assume an overly loving stance, which promotes idealization of the child and his or her capabilities. Often the parent encourages and undermines the child's becoming independent. The child, unsurprisingly, either responds by behaving in an overly dependent or overly independent way. In both instances the child is impaired by a misperception of his or her true capabilities and limitations (Kerr, 1981). (This process is discussed further in the section on the family projection process.)

IMPAIRED SPOUSE. Marital tension and anxieties can be reduced if one spouse gives in or compromises himself or herself to the other to preserve marital harmony. Pressure to reach such a solution usually arises from both spouses. The spouse who compromises self does so to avoid making decisions. The spouse who appears dominant assumes responsibility for decision making. This willingness to assume responsibility for decision making arises from his or her feeling that he or she knows what is best. Such couples experience little flexibility, as evidenced by their inability to defer to the other's areas of expertise (Kerr, 1981).

As a result of the couple interacting in this manner, one spouse, the dominant decision maker, usually emerges as the overfunctioning spouse. The compromising spouse, on the other hand, presents as the underfunctioning one. This pattern of interaction may work effectively for the couple as long as stress and anxiety remain at manageable levels.

When this overfunctioning–underfunctioning pattern confronts sustained periods of high stress and anxiety, it is common for one spouse to become impaired. The impairment may take the form of physical illness, mental illness, or some type of social acting-out problem, such as gambling or alcohol or drug abuse (Bowen, 1978; Kerr, 1981). The spouse who becomes symptomatic is the one whose sense of self has deteriorated most during the course of the relationship. This deterioration of self can occur either through overfunctioning or underfunctioning.

The basic differentiation of people involved in a marriage characterized by spouse dysfunction is usually low. In such marriages, each partner usually has unrealistic expectations of others and himself or herself. These unrealistic expectations can be revealed in the extent to which one spouse feels personally responsible for the well-being of his or her mate and other family members. For example, one spouse may feel so overly responsible for others that he or she feels that investment in meeting one's own basic survival needs threatens the survival of other family members. This form of feeling overly responsible can occur to a mild degree or can reach psychotic proportions in severe cases (Kerr, 1981). In other cases, feeling unrealistically responsible for the other may lead to one spouse feeling and acting as though he or she knows what is best for the other. This form of over-responsibility can result in one spouse anxiously hovering over the other to ensure that he or she stays on course. This anxious hovering can result in the other spouse becoming impaired in some way (Papero, 1990).

In each case, the spouse who feels over-responsible is matched with the spouse who has equally unrealistic expectations about his or her mate's over-responsible functioning. This marital agreement regarding over-responsible functioning in the marriage is unspoken and unconscious. The more undifferentiated the couple, the more automatic the process of assigning and accepting responsibility becomes (Kerr, 1981).

The effect of such marriages on the child usually is minimal if the couple's undifferentiation or emotional immaturity are largely confined to this type of marital relationship pattern. If the child is affected, it will be to a lesser degree than in the relationship pattern in which symptoms are transferred to the child.

FAMILY PROJECTION PROCESS. This concept describes the way in which parents transfer their own undifferentiation or immaturity to their children. The result is that their children's levels of differentiation usually correspond closely to their own. Because this process does not focus evenly on all the children, it is possible for their children's differentiation levels to vary within a limited range. Some children may be more or less differentiated than their parents, while some may be differentiated to the same extent as their parents (Kerr, 1981; Papero, 1990).

The family projection process operates within the triangles composed of the father, mother, and child. This process is so universal that it exists in all father–mother–child triangles to some extent. The extent to which this process occurs varies from minimal to severe (Kerr, 1981; Papero, 1990).

In all marriages a certain amount of undifferentiation or emotional immaturity must be bound in some way. The use of distancing, marital conflict, spouse dysfunction, or transfer or projection to the child serves to bind parental emotional immaturity. The exclusive use or overuse of projection to the child results in impairment of the child. Most families, however, use all of these options to bind undifferentiation. The more the family shifts emphasis on use of these options, the less likely severe impairment will occur (Kerr, 1981; Papero, 1990).

The family projection process is the process whereby parental emotionality defines who the child becomes. This definition may or may not conform to who the child actually is. In time, however, this definition does determine what the child will be like and who the child becomes. This process serves to stabilize the individual functioning of the spouses and their relationship at the expense of the child (Papero, 1990).

The selection of the child affected by this process is determined by several factors. The process of selection is automatic and usually is influenced primarily by the degree of undifferentiation of the parents (Papero, 1990). Additionally, the degree of parental anxiety at the time of the child's conception, the parents' attitudes toward marriage and children, and the degree of stress impacting on the mother at the time of conception until the child's birth play a great part in determining whether a child will be affected by this process (Kerr, 1981). Examples of frequently selected children include the firstborn, the oldest son or daughter, an only child, or a child who is emotionally special to either or both of the parents. A child born with a physical or mental defect also may be a recipient of this process (Papero, 1990).

While the child may possess a characteristic that plays a part in his or her being singled out as a target of the projection process, this process is the product of parental anxiety, parental emotional reactivity, and parental undifferentiation.

DIFFERENTIATION OF SELF. This concept is the cornerstone of Bowen's family systems theory and describes how people differ in terms of their ability to cope with the daily drives for individuality and togetherness (Bowen, 1978). According to this concept, people can be placed on a continuum referred to as the scale of differentiation. The scale ranges from the lowest to the highest levels of differentiation of self. It is further theorized that humans have probably not evolved to the highest possible levels of differentiation of self (Bowen, 1978).

People at the lower end of the scale are those whose lives are dominated by the togetherness force. These are people whose emotional and intellectual systems are fused, and as a consequence they lead lives guided by emotion rather than reason and intellect. People approaching the upper end of the continuum are those whose lives are in balance with regard to togetherness and individuality forces (Bowen, 1978). This balance permits people to be well defined in their own right while also being effective team members. However, most people probably fall somewhere near the midrange of these two extremes (Kerr, 1981).

People at the lower end of the scale seem to be affected by a large number of human problems. These are people who are less adaptable to stress and more emotionally dependent on others. They seek togetherness and become dysfunctional even under minor stress. Once they succumb to stress, these people require longer to recover (Bowen, 1978).

In contrast, people at the upper end of the scale seem to escape a great many human problems. When they are faced with problems, they cope more effectively. Their effective coping derives from their increased adaptability and independence from the emotionality of others. For these reasons, their lives achieve more order, success, and freedom from problems (Kerr, 1981).

The scale of differentiation of self, however, does not correspond with psychiatric diagnoses. While people at the upper end of the scale may be less vulnerable to symptom formation, people at all points on the scale can develop symptoms if subjected to sufficient stress and anxiety, according to Bowen's theory (Bowen, 1978). Thus, the scale of differentiation of self does not arbitrarily assign what is or is not normal.

MULTIGENERATIONAL TRANSMISSION PROCESS. This concept describes the ways in which the family emotional process affects the generations. This concept expands on the nuclear family process to include multigenerations. In doing so, it becomes possible to view the multigenerational family as an emotional unit (Bowen, 1978).

Viewing the multigenerational family as an emotional unit explains how the family projection process occurs generation after generation. It also explains how in a nuclear family, one or more children escape serious symptom development, such as schizophrenia, and another sibling does not (Kerr, 1981).

Usually in a group of siblings, one child is more involved in the family process than others. This child develops a greater sensitivity to its parents' emotional states. The parents in turn project their own undifferentiation onto this child in the manner previously described in the section on the family projection process. As a consequence, this child emerges from the family with a lower level of differentiation than his or her siblings. The siblings who were minimally or less involved in the family's emotional process emerge with a higher degree of differentiation than their less fortunate sibling (Kerr, 1981).

In the multigenerational transmission process, individuals develop a higher, the same, or a lower level of differentiation than their parents. In the same manner, as descendants evolve from a given family with lower levels of differentiation, dysfunctional symptoms eventually occur. Similarly, descendants with higher levels of differentiation evolve from the family, and in this way the family system remains in balance.

SIBLING POSITION. This concept in Bowen's family system theory is adapted from Walter Toman's book entitled *Family Constellation: A Psychological Game,* published in 1961. Toman describes 10 profiles of different sibling positions. The fact that people born into the same family position in different families share many common personality characteristics illustrates what Bowen refers to as the functioning position in a family system. The emotional forces in a family system determine how individual members will function. A child born into a given family system is molded to a great extent by the family emotional process as it affects his or her functional position in the family (Kerr, 1981).

The functional expectations of the oldest, youngest, oldest son, and so forth are part of family structure across the generations and exceed the wishes, desires, and even control of any one person. These expectations also outweigh the influence of cultural values (Kerr, 1981; Papero, 1990). The following provides a brief description of the personality characteristics associated with each of the ten possible birth positions:

- *The only child* prefers not to have his or her own children, tends to look for a father or mother rather than sibling in his or her spouse, wants to remain a child, has a difficult time getting along with peers, and tends to have difficulty adjusting to marriage.
- *The oldest brother of brother(s)* (OBB) is aggressive, assertive, in control, a leader; gets along well with other males and usually prefers their company over that of women; often dislikes women; tends to undermine authority figures; is a perfectionist; likes neatness; dislikes de-

pendence on others; and seldom seeks advice of others.

- *Youngest brother of brother(s)* (YBB)—capricious, willful, daring, imaginative, is reactive to superiors, is an irregular worker, tends to be artistic, likes scientific endeavors, accepts authority, does not understand women but is soft and tender with them, competes with his children for attention from his wife, has a laissez-faire attitude, is dependent and counts on his needs being met;
- *The oldest brother of sister(s)* is a ladies' man, adores women, just wants to make a living, can accept failure, is a responsible worker, accepts authority as long as it does not interfere with his private affairs, is a good father, male friends are less important, and is less tolerant of exclusively male company than OBB or YBB.
- *The youngest brother of sister(s)* is adored by girls, is the object of female attention, is dependent on women for caretaking, is an irregular worker, is capable of great accomplishments as long as he has a "mother figure" for support, is usually nice to women but takes them for granted, resents a working wife because he wants her around to care for him, competes with his children for his wife's attention and is not necessarily a good father, and does not get along well with male peers as a rule.
- *The oldest sister of sister(s)* is dominant, assertive, and bossy; becomes unhappy, angry, and sullen when in a subordinate position; is a good worker when in a leadership position; only heeds authority of older males; expects submission from other women; tries to boss around men to whom she is attracted; tends to be a proud and protective mother; and deemphasizes her husband's role in the family.
- *The youngest sister of sister(s)* is charming, adventurous, and colorful; likes entertainment and change; is unsettled and can discard friends and relationships easily to start over; remains enthusiastic and youthful; is seductive and traditionally feminine; wins men easily; is variable as a worker; and is willing to have children but does not want to care for them.
- *The oldest sister of brother(s)* is independent, strong, and practical; relates well to men; is a peacemaker at work; will give up her career for a man; views nothing as important as the man in her life; and likes motherhood and childcare.
- *The youngest sister of brother(s)* is very desirable to men; is feminine, friendly, kind, tactful, submissive, a good companion, and a good sport; may be extravagant; usually does not become a professional; usually marries for keeps; and is an ideal employee but does not get along well with other women (Toman, 1970).
- *Others*—If people occupy a mixture of these positions, they will have characteristics of the mixture. Usually, however, there will be a predominance of one position over the others. Siblings who are 5 or more years apart in age may function more like only children (Kerr, 1981).

This concept provides a useful tool to understand how a specific child is selected for involvement in the family projection process. For example, if an oldest child functions more like a youngest child in a family, then this indicates that this child was the one most triangled with the parents (Kerr, 1981; Papero, 1990).

Additionally, this concept is helpful in understanding complementarity patterns in marriages. For example, two oldest children or two youngest children who marry each other would have a rank conflict. While they would identify with each other, they would nevertheless seek and even compete for the same role in the marriage relationship. Another type of marital problem emerges when a brother of brothers and a sister of sisters marry each other. In this pattern, a sex conflict would likely occur because neither spouse would have experienced a sibling peer relationship with the opposite sex (Kerr, 1981). Marriages in which partners hold complementary or partially complementary roles in terms of sibling position (e.g., oldest brother of sisters and youngest sister of brothers) are likely to have less conflictual marriages. The concept of sibling position also can be applied to parent–child relationships. Parents and children with rank or sex conflicts also could be expected to have greater difficulty adjusting to each other than those who have greater complementarity with each other (Kerr, 1981).

According to Toman and Bowen family systems theory, it appears that individuals' sibling positions affect not only their interactional expectations of marital partners, but also their offspring. Thus, it seems that sibling position together with the family projection process determine to a significant degree the nature of individuals' relationships (Kerr, 1981).

EMOTIONAL CUTOFF. The concept of emotional cutoff depicts the way in which individuals commonly cope with their emotional attachment (fusion) to their parents and families of origin (Kerr, 1981; Papero, 1990). To cope with their emotional attachment to their families of origin, individuals may use physical distance to control and reduce the frequency of interactions (Papero, 1990). In other instances, individuals may use internal mechanisms, such as emotional withdrawal or avoidance of emotionally charged topics while in the presence of their families (Kerr, 1981).

According to Bowen, people who use internal mechanisms to emotionally cut off from their families of origin while also remaining in supportive contact with them are more prone to develop symptoms of physical illness or depression (Bowen, 1978). On the other hand, individuals who use physical distance to accomplish emotional cutoff are more prone to develop relationship problems with new acquaintances resembling those they have had with their families of origin (Kerr, 1981). As a result, these individuals may go from relationship to relationship searching for, yet escaping, intense emotional closeness.

Some examples of emotional cutoff include the following:

- Adolescents who have been intensely fused or attached to their parents begin to cut off from their parents by entering into intense relationships with their peers.
- An adult who maintains a marital relationship through the use of internal cutting off mechanisms, such as extramarital affairs or alcohol or drug abuse, is not only emotionally cutting off from the marital partner, but also his or her family of origin.
- An individual leaves home and goes from relationship to relationship seeking need satisfaction, while cutting off from relationships when they get too intense (Kerr, 1981).
- An individual gives up on relationships altogether by maintaining a fixed distance from all other people (Papero, 1990).

EMOTIONAL PROCESS IN SOCIETY. This concept contends that the processes of the nuclear family are similar to those of society at large (Papero, 1990). The forces toward individuality and togetherness operate in society similarly to their operation in the family. Forces toward individuality and togetherness operate to counterbalance each other on a societal level as they do in the family. As in the family, increasing societal anxiety alters the functional balance of these forces by increasing the tendency toward togetherness. This increased tendency toward togetherness gradually erodes individuality and results in lowering society's functional differentiation level. As the togetherness tendency progresses, increasing symptoms and complications arise. Decisions are made on a societal level to reduce societal discomfort. Such decisions, as with the nuclear family, often are made not on the basis of principles and thoughtful deliberation, but rather on the basis of what "feels good" (Kerr, 1981).

The following examples illustrate the similarity between the emotional process in society and in the family:

- A teenager demands certain "rights" from his or her parents. If the parents lack a clear set of guiding principles for decision making concerning such matters, they are apt to react irrationally to the teenager's demands. For example, the parents may tend to placate or appease the teenager, or they may react harshly. In either case, the teenager's demands will probably escalate.
- A group of teenage high school students demand certain "rights" from their high school principal and faculty. If the principal and faculty lack clear principles for dealing with a situation, they may react irrationally to student demands. If they react irrationally, then student demands and problems will probably increase. These two examples illustrate that public officials, like parents, may lack the ability to respond rationally to teenagers with problems.

Other examples of societal emotional process include group-think, scapegoating phenomenon, violence, and government and economic instability (Kerr, 1981). These factors and others are considered symptoms of an intensely anxious society, which in turn affects the emotional process of individual families.

BOWEN FAMILY SYSTEMS THERAPY

Families can present for therapy for several reasons. Universally, however, families come to therapy because anxiety has risen to an uncomfortable and sustained high degree. Additionally, families seeking help tend to have a high degree of emotional reactivity or acting-out behavior. Furthermore, family members are usually having great difficulty maintaining a sense of self in relationship to others and the issues existing between and among themselves.

Given that the preceding examples constitute universal conditions motivating families to seek therapy, the therapist has the following tasks to perform.

THERAPIST TASKS REMAINING OBJECTIVE AND NEUTRAL. The family in therapy has a natural tendency to attempt to involve the therapist in the family's emotional process. The intensity between and among family members, however, will resolve automatically if the therapist can remain in contact with each of them while remaining neutral (Kerr, 1981). Remaining neutral and objective is the equivalent of the therapist keeping himself or herself detriangled from the family's emotional process (Papero, 1990).

Staying detriangled from the family's emotional process, however, is no simple task. It is natural for humans to participate emotionally in relationships (Kerr, 1981). Emotional participation in relationships ranges from covert physiologic responses to overt emotional expressions. The therapist's task is to be aware of and to control this natural inclination (Papero, 1990).

CLARIFYING THE FAMILY'S EMOTIONAL PROCESS BETWEEN AND AMONG ITS MEMBERS. A first step in completing this task is to obtain the history of the family's presenting problem. Questions beginning with who, when, what, where, and how are most helpful in maintaining the focus on the family's emotional process. Questions beginning with "why" need to be avoided because they tend to focus on causes of the problem and blame (Kerr & Bowen, 1988; Kerr, 1981). Causal thinking can lead to the therapist becoming triangled into the family's emotional process (Papero, 1990).

A second step in clarifying the family's emotional process is to obtain the history of the nuclear family. This history begins with when the two parents met, what was happening in their individual lives at the time, the geographic moves before and after their marriage, the birth of their children, and events happening in close proximation to those births. Additionally, information concerning their general health, educational, and vocational background is obtained (Kerr, 1981).

This information is useful in assessing the family's approximate level of differentiation. For example, couples having very short or very long courtships usually have lower levels of differentiation of self. Similarly, couples with lower levels of differentiation are more likely to experience serious problems after having a child or undertaking a geographic relocation. Better differentiated families, on the other hand, usually have fewer and milder symptoms and lead more orderly, organized lives, even when circumstances are stressful (Kerr, 1981).

Clarifying the family's emotional process also involves a third step, obtaining a history of the husband's and wife's extended family systems: information concerning their sibling positions, assessment of the emotional process in their siblings' families, and assessment of past and current functioning of their respective parents. Additionally, basic information regarding their parents' and siblings' health, educational, vocational, and marital backgrounds is needed. Such information reveals the extent to which their extended families are stable and provides the basis for estimating their levels of differentiation of self (Kerr, 1981).

Additionally, information concerning previous residences, geographic proximity to the extended family, and exact dates of significant family events is collected. Such information is important to indicate occurrences of emotional cutoff and to discern correlations of events currently taking place in the nuclear family (Kerr, 1981). Past traumatic events in the family or in the life of one of its members can result in an "anniversary reaction" affecting the entire nuclear family.

As a therapist collects this information, he or she attempts to help the family identify "something" in fairly specific terms that they are willing to address in therapy. While helping the family to do so, the therapist needs to remain differentiated from the family to maintain his or her own objectivity. By remaining objective, the therapist is able to keep the focus off the symptom or symptomatic family member. This way the therapist is in a better position to get the family to focus on their emotional process as a group. Keeping the focus on the family's emotional process enables family members to recognize that they *all* contribute and react to the tension and anxiety in the family. This recognition gradually enables them to begin changing themselves and to stop insisting that the others are to blame, and therefore they must change. It is necessary for only one family member to gain this recognition and to translate it into his or her behavior (to maintain increased emotional control and to follow his or her intellect) to initiate a chain reaction in other family members (Kerr, 1981). Just one family member entering family systems therapy can initiate this process of change in his or her own family. The specific approach used by the family systems therapist varies based on the specific clinical situation. Therapy can be undertaken with the individual couple with the focus on nuclear family relationships. Family systems therapy also can be undertaken with individual family members; the therapeutic focus in these cases is on the family of origin and other family issues.

Summary

While Bowen's family systems theory and therapy apply to a broad range of clinical problems affecting people of all ages, it is especially useful in working with families whose dysfunction is expressed by the symptomatic child or adolescent. The accompanying clinical example provides an illustration of how this therapy and theory apply to a family with a supposedly problem child.

(text continues on page 79)

CLINICAL EXAMPLE

Mrs. T called for an appointment saying that her 4-year-old son had become a discipline problem since she and her husband separated 2 weeks ago. Mrs. T stated that she also has been anxious and has had difficulty coping since the separation. Mrs. T was given an appointment for her and her son. The therapist provided a brief description of family systems therapy and requested that Mrs. T ask her estranged husband to accompany her son and her to the initial session.

On their initial visit, the therapist met with the couple and their child to assess their interactional pattern and the child's physical condition and development. During this visit, the therapist noted that each member of this nuclear family appeared outwardly physically healthy. The couple kept their focus on their son by giving a thorough history of his physical problems since his birth. The boy's physical problems included surgical correction of pyloric stenosis at age 3 weeks, repeated respiratory infections, and Rocky Mountain spotted fever at age 3.

Both parents reported a great deal of anxiety about their son's health despite the fact that he had recovered from all previous illnesses without any residual effects and had been physically healthy for 1 year. During that portion of the interview, both parents kept their eyes fixed on their son for the most part and seldom looked at each other. Their son's activity level was consistent with that of most 4-year-old boys during the interview. The therapist noticed that their son's activity increased when the parents disagreed with each other regarding answers to the therapist's questions.

At that point in the interview, the therapist asked the couple if she could continue the interview with them while their son went to the children's playroom. The father readily agreed to this arrangement while the mother hesitated saying, "but our son is the reason for our being here." The mother agreed to her son going to the playroom after her estranged spouse suggested that perhaps they, as parents, needed to talk with the therapist alone. Once the mother agreed to this interview arrangement, the child readily departed for the playroom.

On continuing the interview without the child present, the couple related that they could not pinpoint exactly when their son's discipline problem began. They stated, however, that it became obvious after Mr. T moved out of the home. The mother described her son's discipline problem as refusing to go to bed at bedtime, refusing to stay in bed when he finally did go to bed, crying for his mother when he was in bed, refusing to eat at regular mealtimes, dawdling before fulfilling requests or instructions about putting away toys, slapping and screaming at his mother, and crying and clinging to his mother every morning when she attempted to leave him at kindergarten.

The father's description of the son's discipline problems was prefaced with this comment, "She's really a good mother and has really devoted herself to our son. They are really close." He went on to describe his son's problems as "not doing what his mother tells him to do." The father denied that their son presented a discipline problem to him. He further elaborated that his estranged wife often accused him of being "too stern" with their son. The father denied that he was "too stern," and the mother was not able to give specific examples of when or how the father had been "too stern." Instead, she asserted that, "It just hurts sometimes to see [the son] jump to do whatever [the father] says." The mother also confided that on many occasions, she had had to enlist the father's assistance to gain control over their son.

At that point in the interview, it was becoming apparent that the nuclear family triangle, consisting of the father, mother, and son, was operating automatically to maintain involvement or noninvolvement with each other and to control their anxiety. The therapist at that time began to collect information about their history as a nuclear family unit.

The couple related that they had decided to live together prior to marriage "to make sure that we were compatible." Originally, they had planned to live together for 1 year and at the end of that time, marry if "we still felt the same way." Despite the wife's use of oral contraceptives, their son was conceived after 3 months of living together. They married 2 months later. At the time of their marriage, they had known each other for 7 months. Both wife and husband described themselves as being "head over heels in love" and as not really considering or thinking about the consequences of their actions. Both the husband and wife denied being upset about the unplanned pregnancy and subsequent marriage. The husband, however, stated that he was unprepared to cope with the responsibility of fathering a child born with fairly serious health problems. He also complained about feeling "left out and overlooked" by his wife. He asserted, however, that he loved his son very much and wanted to be a "good father if she will let me."

The wife expressed anger at her husband for spending too much time with his buddies and leaving her at home with their child. She asserted

(*continued*)

CLINICAL EXAMPLE (*Continued*)

that she had done most of the work in terms of child care and housework for the past year. She admitted that her husband, however, had always been there during their son's previous illnesses.

Both parents confided that they had been preoccupied during the first years of their marriage with the pregnancy, birth of their child, and his subsequent physical health problems and needs. Both parents described being chronically anxious about their child, their marriage, and their adequacy to meet these challenges. With the improvement of their child's physical health, they had expected their situation to improve. Instead, their dissatisfaction with themselves and the marriage increased. Eventually, the tension, conflicts, and intense emotional disagreements about parenting their child and the husband's time away with his buddies reached an intolerable level. The couple described their separation as being as emotionally driven as their original union.

Both parents were able to offer information concerning their families of origin. Interestingly, both were the oldest of same-sex siblings. Both sets of parents were alive, in relatively good health, and lived in close proximity to the couple. Additionally, both sets of parents were still involved in providing and caring for their respective younger siblings.

Neither Mr. nor Mrs. T had informed their respective parents about their separation and current difficulties. Mr. T had refrained from informing his parents because he did not wish to burden them with problems. According to Mr. T, his parents were struggling financially to keep his three younger brothers in college and were having family and marital problems of their own. Mrs. T had not informed her parents of the separation because she was ashamed to do so. Apparently, she had always perceived her parents as being extremely critical of her and her major life choices, including marrying Mr. T. Mrs. T's parents reportedly also were actively involved in keeping her two younger sisters in college and planning a wedding for another. Both Mr. and Mrs. T denied significant relationship difficulties with their parents or siblings.

At the conclusion of the interview, Mr. and Mrs. T continued to assert that their primary problem was their son's discipline problem. Mr. T contended that he did not feel that he was part of this problem and that he should, therefore, be excluded from future therapy sessions. Mrs. T, on the other hand, expressed the opinion that Mr. T should attend future sessions because he *obviously* contributed to their son's problem by being absent from the home. Neither directly expressed a desire to work on their marital relationship. Mrs. T, however, readily agreed to proceed with family therapy sessions for the purpose of improving her interactions with her son.

THERAPIST'S ASSESSMENT OF THE T FAMILY

Both Mr. and Mrs. T appeared to have similarly lower levels of differentiation of self as evidenced by their emotional reactivity to each other and their son's behavior. Their short courtship, emotionally charged union and separation, and chronic anxiety about their child and their own adequacy as parents added further support to this assessment. Their undifferentiation or emotional immaturity was managed primarily through transfer of symptoms to the child, marital conflict, and distancing.

The triangle most obviously in operation consisted of the father, mother, and son. At the outset of their marriage, the parents managed instability and emotional tension between themselves by focusing on the pregnancy and then on the child and his health problems. In doing so, they were able to bind their emotional immaturity and relationship instability to some degree. As the child's physical health improved, however, the emotional intensity between the parents increased. This heightened emotional intensity was handled through the father's distancing himself from the situation by spending large amounts of time with his buddies. His doing so soon led to marital conflict. Their marital conflicts not only centered around the father's absence, but also "inequities" with regard to child care and household tasks. Their conflicts, which can be characterized as sex and rank conflicts, were most likely products of their sibling positions as the oldest of same-sex siblings.

In an attempt to deal with the ever-increasing emotional tenseness in the marriage, the mother began to focus on what she perceived as a behavior problem in their son. The mother's increased attention to, and focus on, the son stabilized the marital relationship for a while. When the intensity between the mother and son reached an intolerable degree, the mother sought the father's assistance to deal with their son's behavior. The mother then assumed the comfortable outside position of the triangle formerly occupied by the father. This attempt to stabilize the family's emotional functioning did not work very long. When the father was "stern" with their son, the mother intervened and once again entered into open conflict with the father regarding child discipline.

(*continued*)

CLINICAL EXAMPLE (*Continued*)

Hence, the family's emotional functioning once again intensified.

Because both parents were emotionally cut off from their families of origin as evidenced by their keeping their problems and separation secret, they had diminished emotional resources to cope with their predicament. Moreover, their cutoff from the previous generation (their respective parents) tended to intensify the emotions within their own nuclear family system. The other primary triangle operative in this nuclear family was the father and his buddies, with his wife and child in the outside position. The father's access to this outside resource probably enabled him to have better control of his emotions and thus in some ways present himself as being more adequate and mature than his wife.

PROVIDING FAMILY SYSTEMS THERAPY

While some family therapists might insist on working with both parents or even insist on including the child in therapy sessions, the family systems therapist in this case was willing to work with the family member most motivated for therapy. In this case, the mother was the one most motivated to do therapeutic work.

The therapist worked with this mother who was able eventually to gain more control of her emotions. This increased emotional control allowed her better access to her intellectual system. The mother was then better able to exercise her principles and beliefs about how to relate to and care for her son.

Within eight sessions, the mother reported that she no longer was having a discipline problem with her son. Mr. and Mrs. T remained separated, but Mr. T had begun to spend more time with his son and Mrs. T. Both had informed their respective parents about their separation and had found them surprisingly supportive, available, and concerned.

Mrs. T expressed her desire to stop therapy at the ninth session, stating that she planned to resume therapy if and when she and Mr. T decided to reunite. At that time, neither of them were pursuing a divorce. Mrs. T simply said, "We're enjoying our son and each other for the first time, and we aren't in any hurry to change things."

The preceding example illustrates how the concepts of Bowen family systems theory interlock and provide a strong tool for assessment and intervention in a nuclear family system. In this case, by remaining neutral and detriangled, the therapist was able to relate effectively with one family member, the mother, to reduce her anxiety sufficiently so that she could be different with her son and estranged husband. The mother's reestablishment of communication with her own family of origin and her estranged husband's following suit also helped defuse the emotional tension within the nuclear family unit. Mr. and Mrs. T's decision to postpone further action regarding their marriage and simply to enjoy each other and their son for a while also demonstrate a change from their usual emotional and impulsive pattern of relating to each other.

Whether this nuclear family unit will survive to evolve toward increased functional differentiation, however, remains to be seen. The application of this theory and therapy, nevertheless, has provided an increased chance for the survival of its members and the nuclear family unit itself.

REFERENCES

Bowen, M. (1961). Family psychotherapy. *American Journal of Orthopsychiatry*, *1*(1), 40–60.

Bowen, M. (1966). The use of family therapy in clinical practice. *Comprehensive Psychiatry*, *7*, 345–374.

Bowen, M. (1971). Family therapy & family group therapy. In H. Kaplan & B. Saddock (Eds.), *Comprehensive group psychotherapy* (pp. 384–421). Baltimore: Williams & Wilkins.

Bowen, M. (1975). Family therapy after twenty years. In S. Areeti (Ed.), *American handbook of psychiatry, 5, treatment* (pp. 367–392). New York: Basic Books.

Bowen, M. (1976). Theory in the practice of psychotherapy. In P. Guerin (Ed.), *Family therapy* (pp. 42–90). New York: Gardner Press.

Bowen, M. (1978). *Family therapy in clinical practice*. New York: Jason Aronson.

Gilbert, R. M. (1991). Extraordinary relationships: A new way of thinking about human interactions. Minneapolis: Chronimed Publications.

Kerr, M. E., & Bowen, M. (1988), *Family evaluation*. New York: W.W. Norton and Company.

Kerr, M. E. (1981). *Family systems theory and therapy*. In A. S. Gurman & David P. Knisken. *Handbook of family therapy*. New York: Brunner-Mazelle.

Papero, D. V. (1990). *Bowen family systems theory*. Boston: Allyn and Bacon.

Toman, W. (1961). *Family constellation: A psychological game*. New York: Springer.

Toman, W. (1970). Birth order rules all. *Psychology Today*, 45–49, 68–69.

CHAPTER

6

Behavioral Theory

Joyce Swegle and Rebecca Personnett

Behavioral methodology has made a significant impact on childhood mental health. The original studies in behaviorism were conducted with children. Ollendick (1986) reported that an exhaustive review of the literature conducted in 1968 found 70 studies related to behavior therapy with children and adolescents. By 1981 a selective literature review found more than 1000 child and adolescent studies using behavioral therapy techniques.

From a theoretical standpoint, behaviorism represented a paradigmatic shift in scientific thinking as depicted by Kuhn (1962). Behaviorism developed out of an experimental tradition and formed the basis of behavior therapy. The underlying principles of behavior therapy reflect a way of knowing about another person that is far removed from the mystical realm of the psychoanalyst. Behaviorism and psychoanalysis can be viewed as dichotomous ways of knowing about human beings. From an existential standpoint, one knows another person as one knows himself or herself. Feelings, attitudes, and intentions are shared through empathy and intuition. The assumption is that another person will behave according to what he or she is.

Juxtaposed to this is the behavioristic view that one knows another person by examining what a person does. This way of knowing is directly observable. Pertinent to this view is the contention that behavior can be explained on the basis of the environment rather than inner states (Skinner, 1978).

Historic Perspective

The methodology and philosophy of behaviorism originated with the work of John Watson. Watson (1924) emphasized the role of experimental technique and the study of behavior and opposed psychoanalysis. His opposition to psychoanalysis was based on the premise that the mind did not exist. As a result of this conjecture, Watson is considered a radical behaviorist.

Watson and Raynor (1920) were heavily influenced by the Pavlovian model of classical conditioning. In this model an unconditioned stimulus (food) elicits an unconditional response (salivation) in a hungry dog. A conditioned stimulus (bell) is paired with the unconditioned stimulus. This process resulted in the elicitation of a conditioned response (salivation) to the conditioned stimulus (bell).

The influence of the Pavlovian model was demonstrated in the work of Watson and Rayner (1920) in which the researchers were able to develop a phobic response in Albert. This response was elicited by pairing a previously neutral stimulus, a rat, with a loud noise. The child subsequently exhibited a conditioned response to the rat's presence unaccompanied by the loud noise.

Jones (1924), a colleague of Watson, reported the ability to treat phobias by pairing the offensive

Barbara Schoen Johnson: CHILD, ADOLESCENT AND FAMILY PSYCHIATRIC NURSING, © 1994 J.B. Lippincott Company

object with a pleasure sensation. This was reported as a study of Peter, whose fear of furry objects was decreased by feeding him in the presence of a rabbit, while gradually bringing the rabbit closer.

Following a few initial studies, behaviorism was relatively dormant until the 1950s. The behavioral movement then began to flourish with the report of treatment successes using operant conditioning and reciprocal inhibition. Since the 1920s, the behavioral movement has undergone significant changes. To some extent, the sharp demarcation in the existential–behavioral dichotomy has softened.

Eysenck (1976) defended the scientific derivation of behavioral therapy. Behavioral therapists advocate for the acceptance of the scientific status of behavioral therapy. Eysenck (1976) characterized the discipline as a progressive paradigmatic shift that replaces the degenerative one of Freud and psychoanalysis.

Eysenck (1976) compared the hypotheticodeductive path of behavioral therapy to the hard and applied sciences. Facts in these sciences are often involved in temporary patching and upsets of empirical findings. It follows that this same scientific progress in behavioral therapy should be viewed not as a sign of weakness, but of strength. Eysenck (1976) challenged the hard sciences to view the behavioral sciences as scientific, acting in the same manner, and willing to change as new knowledge is discovered.

Behavioral theory is a young discipline. To expect unification in such a young discipline, as compared to the hard sciences of physics and chemistry, which fall short as unified theories, is unreasonable (Eysenck, 1976).

Behavioral Theory

Four different schools of thought have developed since the introduction of behaviorism in the early 20th century: neobehavioristic mediational model; applied behavior analysis model; social learning model; and finally the cognitive behavior modification model.

COMMON CHARACTERISTICS

Although there are conceptual differences in the behavior therapy approaches, there also are commonalities in the basic beliefs and assumptions under which behavior therapists function. The two basic characteristics that provide a common core for all forms of behavior therapy were identified by Agras, Kazdin, and Wilson (1979).

First, behavioral therapists use "a psychological model for human behavior that differs fundamentally from the traditional intrapsychic, psychodynamic, or quasi-disease model of mental illness" (Agras, Kazdin, & Wilson, 1979, p. 15). The implications of this psychologic model are numerous. Abnormal behavior that cannot be attributed to some type of brain dysfunction or chemical imbalance is believed to be produced and perpetuated in the same manner as normal behavior. The abnormal behavior is frequently characterized as a "problem of living." As such, abnormal behavior is inseparable from the situation in which it occurs. Breaking the problem of living into smaller component parts provides direction to the therapist for intervention. The treatment is considered successful when the problem of living, or abnormal behavior, is resolved. Because abnormal behavior occurs in a social context, successful intervention may result in a generalization to other behaviors. As a result of this conceptualization of the problem, there is no need to identify or dwell on an etiology.

Second, behavior therapy is characterized by a commitment to the scientific method (Agras et al., 1979). This emphasis on empirical demonstration has provided behavior therapy with one of its greatest strengths—the possibility of research on the effectiveness and outcome of therapy. This is the direct result of the specificity in problem identification and intervention. This characteristic has increased the objectivity and thus allowed the replication of studies.

Much of the work in operant conditioning and neobehavioristic mediational approaches was grounded in learning theory. These models represent an application of learning theory rather than a derivation of learning theorems. The heuristic relationship between these models and learning theory was felt to increase the probability of success because of the antecedent support for similar techniques in learning theory (Erwin, 1978).

Empirical confirmation and the alliance with theories of learning have resulted in the report of single-subject studies. This trend also is influenced by the irreducible nature of behavior and situation.

Neobehavioristic Mediational Model

The neobehavioristic mediational model developed in the 1960s uses concepts of conditioning and counterconditioning as they were described by Watson (1920) and Jones (1924), respectively. The theoretical framework for the neobehavioristic model was constructed along the same lines as learning theory and classical conditioning. The methodologic assumptions of neobehaviorism acknowledge personal observations as the foundation of scientific knowledge. Unlike Watson, who totally rejected the existence of the mind, the neobehaviorists stated methodologic reasons that mental events could not be studied scientifically. The theorists most frequently associated with this school of thought are Eysenck, Wolpe, and Rachman.

RECIPROCAL INHIBITION

Wolpe (1958) devised reciprocal inhibition, a treatment for abnormal behavior based on a classical conditioning paradigm. The principle underlying reciprocal inhibition stated that if a response inhibiting anxiety could be made to occur during the presence of anxiety-evoking stimuli, the bond between the stimuli and the anxiety could be weakened. Reciprocal inhibition was not correlated with anxiety alone, but also could be effective in verbal and conceptual relearning (Wolpe, 1973).

The systematic use of reciprocal inhibition was extended by Wolpe (1958) to include three varieties of responses antagonistic to anxiety: assertive, sexual, and relaxation responses. Assertive responses were targeted against anxieties coming from the client's interactions with others. Sexual responses were appropriate for use when the anxiety responses were conditioned to sexual situations. Relaxation responses were to be useful against anxieties from any source. The principle was that a relaxation response would assist clients in prolonged training in relaxation of all muscles not in use.

SYSTEMATIC DESENSITIZATION

The technique of reciprocal inhibition evolved into the principle of systematic desensitization. A physiologic inhibition of anxiety is prompted by means of muscle relaxation. The client is then exposed to a weak anxiety-producing stimulus. This is repeated several times until the stimulus loses the ability to induce anxiety. The stimuli introduced are then progressively stronger, and the process is repeated until optimal results are obtained (Wolpe, 1973).

AVERSIVE THERAPY

An additional technique of neobehaviorism is aversive therapy. Wolpe (1973) reported that aversive therapy consisted of administering an aversive stimuli to inhibit an unwanted response. This process will thereby decrease habit strength of the unwanted response. In aversive therapy the stimulus and response occur simultaneously rather than the stimulus following the response as in punishment.

Wolpe (1973) advocated that aversive therapy is most useful in obsessions, habits of attraction to inappropriate objects, and compulsions. The aversive stimulus is presented at the same time as the undesirable response. The purpose is that the aversive stimulus inhibits the undesired response. A weakening of the habit is then achieved.

Techniques of aversive therapy may include electric shock, drug therapy, covert sensitization, or anything that is unpleasant. Wolpe (1973) warned that aversive therapy should not be attempted without exploring anxiety bases of the behavior first.

The scope of behavior therapy has been identified as unadaptive habits that are sought to be replaced by adaptive ones. When the habit is based on learning, the learning process provides the key to the needed change. It follows that to unmake the unadaptive habits learned, unlearning is the logical process. When the unlearning is achieved, the symptoms disappear, and there is nothing left to do. If there is no reference to learning of unadaptive behavior, then behavior therapy use is questionable (Wolpe, 1973)

Applied Behavior Analysis Model

This model of behavior therapy is commonly called operant conditioning and is the result of B.F. Skinner's work. Skinner (1953) developed theories of human behavior closely aligned with the early learning theorists. He considered himself a radical behaviorist and renounced the existence of the mind. He conceptualized human behavior as a result of the environment acting on the person. Therefore, therapy based on an operant conditioning paradigm is centered around overt behavior and its consequences. There is no emphasis on mental processes.

Response refers to a movement of an organism. The term is borrowed from the study of reflex action and implies a prior event, called a stimulus. The terms stimulus and response generally are associated with involuntary behavior responses. The paradigm of classical conditioning involves respondent behavior in which an unconditioned stimulus is paired with a previously neutral stimulus to produce a conditioned response (Thomas, 1968).

A second fundamental class of behavior identified by Skinner (1953) is operant behavior. The word operant is used to describe a class of responses that has already occurred and that cannot be predicted or controlled. The prediction is made concerning similar responses that would occur in the future. The term stresses that the behavior operates on the environment, which generates consequences. In operant behavior, a reinforcer is contingent upon a response. The strengthening of behavior resulting from reinforcement is termed conditioning. An operant, then, is strengthening of behavior preceded by a reinforcement, which makes a response more probable.

Operant behavior has further been described as involving voluntary muscles under the client's control. The origin of operant behavior is governed by consequences (Thomas, 1968). Six operant techniques have been identified: positive reinforcement, extinction, differential reinforcement, response shaping, punishment, and negative reinforcement.

POSITIVE REINFORCEMENT

Wolpe (1973) stated that any state of affairs that, following a response, serves to increase the rate of responding is called a reinforcer. Further, when reward is the state of affairs, it is a positive reinforcer, and the future rate of responding is increased.

Reinforcers are further classified as primary, secondary, and generalized secondary. Primary reinforcers function innately to increase the rate of responding. Examples are food, sex, water, approval, and affection. Secondary reinforcers acquire the capacity to increase the rate of responding because of learning history when they have been paired with various conditions or primary reinforcers. Examples of secondary reinforcers are money, domination, and submissiveness. The generalized secondary reinforcers have been learned on the basis of primary reinforcers, and their effectiveness is presumed to be relatively independent of states of deprivation involving primary reinforcers (Thomas, 1968).

EXTINCTION

Extinction is an operant technique of withholding a reinforcer following an operant response that had previously produced that reinforcer. Behavior during extinction is the result of the conditioning that preceded it. Extinction is an effective way of removing an operant from the organism (Skinner, 1953). A problem associated with extinction is that most problem behaviors have been acquired over long periods, and these responses are noted to be resistant to extinction. Therefore, the extinction process should be controlled and monitored carefully (Thomas, 1968).

DIFFERENTIAL REINFORCEMENT

Differential reinforcement is a combination of positive reinforcement and extinction. Positive reinforcement strengthens appropriate responses, and extinction reduces or eliminates problem behavior. The positive reinforcement must be immediate or the precision of the differential effect is counteracted (Skinner, 1953).

RESPONSE SHAPING

Response shaping is a gradual changing of the quality of a response. Initially a simple response would receive reinforcement. After the desired response is performed consistently, the reinforcement is given for more difficult responses. The final product seems to have a special unity and is the result of a continuous shaping process (Skinner, 1953). The pattern continues until the final behavior is achieved, and reinforcement is given only for complex responses.

PUNISHMENT

Punishment is the most common technique of behavior control. A punishment is ideally administered with the intent to inhibit an unwanted response, thereby diminishing its strength. Skinner (1953) discouraged the use of punishment. He noted three effects of punishment. The first was that the stimuli used in punishment is confined to the immediate situation and need not be followed by a change in behavior at a later date. The second effect of punishment is that behavior that has consistently been punished becomes the source of conditioned stimuli, which evokes undesirable behavior. The third effect of punishment is that the behavior that reduces this aversive stimulation will be reinforced, whether it arises from the behavior or from the circumstances. If punishment is discontinued, the unwanted behavior may return in full strength.

Skinner (1953) identified alternatives to punishment. The use of punishment may be avoided by weakening an operant in other ways. One way is to allow time to pass in accordance with a development schedule. Extinction is the most effective alternative to punishment. Positive reinforcement also is an alternative to punishment.

NEGATIVE REINFORCEMENT

Negative reinforcement is an operant conditioning procedure in which a response is followed by the termination of a negative reinforcer. Negative reinforcement is not the same as punishment. Negative reinforcement also may be referred to as time-out from positive reinforcement. The response-strengthening effects involve an increase in the future rate or magnitude of the response (Poling, 1985).

Social Learning Model

The social learning model was introduced in the late 1960s and is primarily the contribution of Albert Bandura. In contrast to other models, this model acknowledges the influence of mental processes and cognition on behavior. Also, social learning model is based on principles of vicarious conditioning rather than operant or respondent conditioning. Human behavior is believed to be developed and maintained through three interacting regulatory systems. These include the pairing of response patterns with external stimuli, external reinforcement, and cognitive mediational processes (Bandura, 1977a).

Modeling is a major component of social learning theory. Terms such as vicarious learning, imitation learning, observational learning, and copying are used interchangeably with modeling. All of these terms are used to describe the same phenomenon (Ollendick & Cerny, 1981).

Bandura (1965) supported a theory of no-trial learning. He suggested that few humans would reach adulthood if the socialization process resulted from trial and error responses typical of operant conditioning. This model recognized the ability to learn rapidly in large, rather than minute, units.

In contrast to the operant model, which stresses performance rather than learning, the social learning model does not require a subject to perform a response before he or she can learn. The social learning model also rejects the notion that learning is suspended until a reinforcer occurs. However, Bandura (1977b) recognized that reinforcement might affect the rate, magnitude, latency, or speed of a performed response. Reinforcement can serve as an antecedent or a consequence. In this context, reinforcement is conceptualized as a regulator rather than a controller of behavior.

Bandura (1971) contended that modeling served three psychologic functions: the transmission of new behavior, the inhibition and disinhibition of unnecessary responses, and the facilitation of already established responses.

Four subprocesses of observational learning have been identified: attentional processes, retention processes, motor reproduction, and reinforcement. Attentional processes include the modeling stimuli and the observer characteristics. Retention processes are either imaginal or verbal and represent a cognitive coding of observed behavior. Motor reproduction is the practice of targeted behaviors. Finally, reinforcement promotes the translation of observation into an actual performance. This process may provide incentive for each of the other subprocesses.

An analysis of research on the social learning model was undertaken by Rachman (1976). He identified four significant findings related to the social learning model. First, symbolic modeling, where the subject observes a real or recorded model but does not actually come in contact with the situation, resulted in some lasting behavior change. Supplementing this process with participant modeling resulted in even longer lasting behavior change. Observational learning was found to be facilitated by a combination of audio and visual presentations, repeated practice, and prolonged exposure to and use of multiple models. Finally, he found that participant modeling facilitated the translation of learning into behavior change.

Cognitive Behavior Modification

The cognitive behavior modification model represents the most current development in behavior therapy. Behavioral procedures have been shown to work through cognitive mechanisms. Systematic rational restructuring has sometimes been paired with behavioral interventions. Rational–emotive therapy (RET) also has been combined with behavioral techniques. Cognitive therapy is an integrated technique with a behavioral approach.

Ellis (1972) described RET. Clients are taught to recondition themselves through insight into their dysfunctional behavior. Acknowledging one's own perpetuation of dysfunctional behavior, addressing one's own irrational beliefs through counterconditioning, and acting against the causes of one's own disordered behavior are the focuses of RET. RET is an integration of attacking problems through cognitive, emotive, and behavioristic techniques. Ellis primarily viewed humans as responding, creative individuals who bring stimuli a kind of receiving apparatus in connection with events they experience.

Goldfried, Decenteceo, and Weinberg (1974) wrote about the systematic rational restructuring. Initially, this technique was seen as an operationalization of Ellis' RET. There are four major components of systematic rational restructuring: presentation of a rationale, overview of assumptions, analysis of the client's problems, and training session for the client to put into practice what is taught.

Cognitive therapy trains individuals to push for a test of particular beliefs. The reliance on hypothesis testing justifies the cognitive behavioral integration in this technique. An alternative construct system may preclude hypothesis testing (Hollon & Beck, 1986)

BOX 6–1 • THE S-O-R-K-C MODEL

S—Internal or external stimulus events thought to be related to the behavior
O—Biologic condition of the organism
R—Observed or reported behaviors
K—Schedules or contingency-related conditions, frequency and timing of response outcomes
C—Environmental or organismic events that follow observed or reported behaviors

(Adapted from Kanfer, F., & Saslow, G. [1969]. Behavioral diagnosis. In C. M. Franks [Ed.], *Behavior therapy: Appraisal and status* [pp. 417–444]. New York: McGraw-Hill.)

Behavioral Assessment of Children

In keeping with the behavioral therapy perspective, assessment is a crucial step in the treatment process. Ollendick and Hersen (1984) describe child behavioral assessment as "an exploratory, hypothesis-testing process in which a range of specific procedures are used in order to understand a given child, group or social ecology and to formulate and evaluate specific intervention strategies" (Table 6-1).

The characteristics of child behavior assessment include a multimethod approach, selection of empirically validated procedures, and sensitivity to developmental processes. While each characteristic is presented separately, it is important to recognize that all three characteristics are interrelated. Choosing a multimethod approach has implications for empirical validity because it may result in compounding of measurement error. Tools used in assessment must take into consideration the developmental process. Obviously, the child's level of development impacts the number and types of possible assessments.

TABLE 6–1 Comparison of Assessment Perspectives

Traditional Perspective	Behavioral Perspective
Search for underlying personality characteristics	Search for antecedent and consequent events of behavior
Personality produces consistency in behavior that is stable and independent of situational variation	Temporal and cross-situational behavior not necessarily expected
Tests on basis of a priori theoretical assumptions about the role of personality variables in behavior	Tests on the basis of stimulus situations associated with behavior
Response viewed as indirect manifestation of underlying personality traits	Response involves sampling approach with a low level of inference

MULTIMETHOD APPROACH

Behavior assessment has traditionally been directed at the identification of target behaviors. However, recent advances have incorporated a broader view of child behavioral assessment, including antecedent and consequent events, physiologic reactions, affective responses, covert cognitions, and distal and proximal events affecting behavior (Ollendick & Hersen, 1984).

An assessment model has been proposed by Kanfer and Saslow (1969), which accommodates a multimethod approach. The S-O-R-K-C model (Box 6-1) allows a wide range of assessment strategies to be used, including interviews, checklists, observations, and self-reports. A functional analysis is then conducted using a six-step process (Box 6-2).

EMPIRICALLY VALIDATED PROCEDURES

A second consideration in behavioral assessment is the validity of the assessment procedures. Choice of a tool or technique may be influenced by the target behavior, characteristics of the child, referral source, assessment setting, social and cultural milieu, and the purpose of the assessment. In addition, the psychometric qualities of all tools should be taken into consideration (Ollendick & Hersen, 1984).

DEVELOPMENTAL PROCESSES

Finally, the behavioral assessment must be sensitive to developmental processes. Edelbrock (1984) outlined common problems in the behavioral assessment of children. Historically, children have been treated as miniature adults without recognition that child behavior is qualitatively different from adult behavior. Failure to identify childhood differences has been compounded by the fact that children rarely refer themselves for treatment, report on their problems, or negotiate interventions. Children are frequently passive responders in the assessment process.

Childhood is characterized by constant change in behavior and attitude. Adults working with children have not consistently taken into consideration the differences existing among children of various ages and age groups.

Significant differences exist between developmental and behavioral perspectives (Table 6-2). Edelbrock (1984) suggested that children could best be served by an assessment synthesized from both perspectives. The synthesis would necessitate the establishment of a normative baseline for behavior, an identification of age difference in the relations among behaviors, and the study of stability and change in behavior over time.

BOX 6–2 • FUNCTIONAL ANALYSIS: SIX-STEP PROCESS

1. Initial analysis of problem situation: behavior excesses, deficits, and assets
2. Clarification of the problem: antecedent and consequent events, consequences of behavior change, determination of how behaviors are functional at the time, consequences of successful and unsuccessful treatment
3. Motivational analysis: determine incentives and aversive conditions operating for the child currently and historically
4. Developmental analysis: biologic, cognitive, and social variables affecting behavior
5. Self-control capacity: analysis of situations in which child can control behavior
6. Analysis of social–cultural–physical environment: analysis of interpersonal relationships that may have affected the development of the target behavior and those that could be a resource in treatment

(Adapted from Kanfer, F., & Saslow, G. [1969]. Behavioral diagnosis. In C. M. Franks [Ed.], *Behavioral therapy: Appraisal and Status* [pp. 417–444]. New York: McGraw-Hill.)

TABLE 6–2 Developmental and Behavioral Assessment

Developmental Approach	Behavioral Approach
Nomothetic	Idiographic
Establish general laws pertaining to groups	Intraindividual changes in behavior
Seeks an identification of patterns	Isolates specific behavior
Emphasizes historic antecedents and developmental precursors to current functioning	Emphasizes role of current environment in shaping and controlling behavior

Nursing Process and Behavioral Therapy

ASSESSMENT

The first step of the nursing process is assessment. The nurse may participate in some or all of the assessment procedures noted previously. The nurse synthesizes information gleaned from other sources with the nursing history to facilitate a complete data base. Because behavior is situationally specific, the nurse may detect conflicting accounts of behavior from different sources or observe behavior that is incongruent with reports.

NURSING DIAGNOSIS

Nursing diagnosis results from a synthesis of assessment data. The treatment of children and adolescents in mental health settings has been optimized through use of a multidisciplinary approach. Nursing diagnosis defines the nursing dimension of the treatment process and nursing's unique contribution to the multidisciplinary team.

Nursing diagnosis has two component parts. Behavioral theory can serve as a theoretical framework from which nursing diagnoses can be derived. In keeping with behavioral theory, the client's response is conceptualized as a directly observable behavioral excess or deficit. The etiology component also is derived from the theoretical framework and reference reinforcers, consequences, perception of self-efficacy, or irrational beliefs.

PLANNING

Team involvement is necessary in planning behavioral intervention. Consistency among staff members is important to reduce the chance reinforcement of maladaptive behavior. The choice of effective reinforcers, a reinforcement schedule, and a precise plan for implementation are needed.

INTERVENTION

Intervention involves the implementation of the treatment plan. Nursing intervention might be a singular technique, such as time out from positive reinforcement, or it might include multiple techniques. For example, interventions directed at impulsive behavior might include time out, positive reinforcement for not demonstrating impulsive behavior for a given time, self-monitoring of behavior, modeling social skills, or possibly self-instruction procedures.

The Council for Children with Behavioral Disorders (1990) has identifed four general strategies for reducing problem behavior in children: modifying the environment; reinforcing alternative behaviors that compete with or are incompatible with the target behavior; withholding, withdrawing, or suspending access to preferred events or stimuli contingent on inappropriate behavior; and administering aversive events contingent on inappropriate behavior. All of these techniques are implemented in home, residential, school, and clinical settings by individuals who espouse and deny affiliation with behavioral methodology.

In general, techniques used with children are derived from either an operant conditioning or social learning model. The use of cognitive approaches has been limited to children developmentally aware enough to understand and follow through with the procedures. Techniques derived from the neo-behavioristic mediational model have been used effectively to reduce fear in children with anxious and withdrawn disorders and pervasive developmental disorders. However, these techniques are rarely implemented with aggressive behaviors (Ollendick, 1986).

The question of the appropriateness of various behavior-reducing techniques has sparked continued controversy. Moral and ethical concerns have surfaced regarding the use of aversive, intrusive, and restrictive techniques. This has been countered by concern for the rights of individuals to access appropriate and effective treatment. Although there is no clear-cut answer to this question, the Council for Children with Behavioral Disorders (1990) has offered recommendations to guide individuals who use behavior reduction techniques (Box 6-3).

BOX 6–3 • GUIDELINES FOR IMPLEMENTATION OF BEHAVIOR-REDUCING TECHNIQUES

1. Practitioners planning to use these behavior-reducing procedures, especially those involving more aversive, intrusive, or restrictive techniques, should obtain prior consent from the child's parents or legal guardians, from administrators, and clearance from human rights committees.
2. Practitioners should carefully analyze potential target behavior(s) and the factors associated with their occurrence before initiating behavior reduction procedures.
3. As a general rule, practitioners should implement and document the use of appropriate, less aversive, intrusive, or restrictive procedures prior to implementing other procedures.
4. Practitioners should develop and follow appropriate guidelines involved in using behavior-reduction strategies.
5. Practitioners should develop and subsequently follow a plan detailing the behavior reduction procedure(s) to be used in a particular case.
6. Once aversive behavior reduction procedures are selected and approved, practitioners should select appropriate procedures for specific situations.
7. People responsible for carrying out behavior-reduction procedures must be appropriately trained.
8. Practitioners should keep data on the efficacy of the behavior-reduction procedures and should communicate these in regularly scheduled staff and parent meetings.

(Data from Council for Children with Behavioral Disorders (1990). *Behavioral Disorders, 15,* 243–260.)

EVALUATION

The objective nature of the behavioral framework makes evaluation comparatively simple. However, the ability to evaluate the results of intervention is directly related to assessment precision and the clarity and measurability of outcomes. Another consideration is whether the interventions were carried out as planned. Finally, the nurse should evaluate whether the interventions modified the identified etiology.

Summary

Behavioral methodology has had a rich tradition in the treatment of childhood mental health problems. Historically, the orignal studies in behaviorism were conducted with child subjects.

Four different models of behavior therapy have been identified; neobehavioristic mediational model; applied behavior analysis model; social learning model; and cognitive behavior modification model. Each model conceptualizes behavior and behavior therapy differently. However, they are all characterized by a psychologic model, rejection of the disease model, use of various behavioral techniques, and a commitment to the scientific method.

Through the nursing process, nurses play a major role in the identification and treatment of childhood and adolescent behavior problems. Behavior theory provides nurses with a theoretical means of deriving nursing diagnosis, thus defining nursing's unique contribution to the mental health care team.

REFERENCES

Agras, W., Kazdin, A., & Wilson, G. (1979). *Behavior therapy: Toward an applied clinical science.* San Francisco: W.H. Freeman.

Bandura, A. (1965). Behavioral modification through modeling procedures. In L. Krasner & L. Ullmann (Eds.), *Research on behavior modification: New developments and implications* (pp. 310–340). New York: Holt, Rinehart, and Winston.

Bandura, A. (1971) *Psychological modeling: Conflicting theories.* Chicago: Aldine-Atherton.

Bandura, A. (1977a). Self efficacy: Toward a unifying theory of behavioral change. *Psychological Review, 84,* 191–215.

Bandura, A. (1977b). *Social learning theory.* Englewood Cliffs, NJ: Prentice-Hall.

Council for Children with Behavioral Disorders (1990). Position paper on use of behavior reduction strategies with children with behavioral disorders. *Behavioral Disorders, 15,* 243–261.

Edelbrock, C. (1984). Developmental considerations. In T. H. Ollendick & M. Hersen (Eds.), *Child behavioral assessment: Principles and procedures* (pp. 20–37). New York: Pergamon Press.

Erwin, E. (1978). *Behavior therapy: Scientific, philosophical and moral foundations.* London: Cambridge University Press.

Ellis, A. (1972). *Humanistic psychotherapy: The rational-emotive approach.* New York: McGraw-Hill.

Eysenck, H. J. (1976). Behaviour therapy-dogma or applied science? In M. P. Feldman & A. Broadhurst (Eds.), *Theoretical and experimental bases of the behaviour therapies* (pp. 333–364). London: John Wiley and Sons.

Goldfried, M. R., Decenteceo, E. T., & Weinberg, L. (1974). Systematic rational restructuring as a self control technique. *Behavior Therapy, 5,* 247–254.

Hollon, S., & Beck, A. (1986). Research on cognitive therapies. In S. L. Garfield & A. E. Bergin (Eds.), *Handbook of psychotherapy and behavior change* (pp. 443–482). New York: John Wiley and Sons.

Jones, M. C. (1924). The elimination of children's fears. *Journal of Experimental Psychology, 7,* 383–390.

Kanfer, F., & Saslow, G. (1969). Behavioral diagnosis. In C. M. Franks (Ed.), *Behavior therapy: Appraisal and status* (pp. 417–444). New York: McGraw-Hill.

Kuhn, T. (1962). *The structure of scientific revolutions.* Chicago: University of Chicago Press.

Ollendick, T. H. (1986). Behavior therapy with children and adolescents. In S. L. Garfield & A. E. Bergin (Eds.), *Handbook of psychotherapy and behavior change* (pp. 525–564). New York: John Wiley and Sons.

Ollendick, T. H., & Cerny, J. (1981). *Clinical behavior therapy with children.* New York: Plenum Press.

Ollendick, T. H., & Hersen, M. (1984). An overview of child behavioral assessment. In T. H. Ollendick & M. Hersen (Eds.), *Child behavioral assessment: Principles and procedures* (pp. 3–19). New York: Pergamon Press

Poling, A. (1985). Punishment. In A. S. Bellack & M. Hersen (Eds.), *Dictionary of behavior therapy techniques* (pp. 176–77). New York: Pergamon Press.

Rachman, S. J. (1976). Observational learning and therapeutic modeling. In M. P. Feldman & A. Broadhurst (Eds.), *Theoretical and experimental bases of the behaviour therapies* (pp. 193–226). London: John Wiley and Sons.

Skinner, B. F. (1953). *Science and human behavior.* New York: Macmillan Co.

Skinner, B. F. (1978). *Reflections on behaviorism and society.* Englewood Cliffs, NJ: Prentice-Hall.

Thomas, E. J. (1968). Selected sociobehavioral techniques and principles: An approach to interpersonal helping. *Social Work, 13,* 12–26.

Watson, J. B. (1924). *Behaviorism.* New York: Norton.

Watson, J. B., & Rayner, R. (1920). Conditioned emotional reactions. *Journal of Experimental Psychology, 3,* 1–14.

Wolpe, J. (1958). *Psychotherapy by reciprocal inhibition.* Stanford: Stanford University Press.

Wolpe, J. (1973). *The practice of behavior therapy* (2nd ed.). New York: Pergamon Press.

CHAPTER

7

Cognitive Theory

Anne DuVal Frost

Information processing in therapy and other psychosocial interventions can be enhanced by metaphors, analogies, anecdotes, axioms, and other concrete cognitive mechanisms. Such mechanisms can facilitate therapeutic goals by simplifying intellectual examination and by providing an easy to remember context for continued examination following sessions or programs. The ability of a client to remember reframing or new information is influenced by cognitive capability, resistance, the level of concrete association, and a triggering device for recall. These criteria are addressed in the cognitive framework of information processing. While this framework is typically recalled for guidance in learning strategies, it is equally applicable for the transformation of perceptions or information related to therapy and other psychosocial interventions.

Information Processing

Information processing is viewed as a serial transformation from old to new information involving three memory components: long-term memory (LTM), short-term memory (STM), and external memory (Newel & Simon, 1972). LTM is a limitless, permanent storage consisting of symbols organized associatively. Associating and storing occurs within a few hundred milliseconds. STM has a limited capacity of five to seven symbols and a requirement of 50 milliseconds for processing. STM is the working division where stimuli are compared to information retrieved from LTM. During the working phase, the encoding from STM may result in an addition to or modification of previously stored information.

External memory consists of the immediate visual field. There is some question as to its exact functioning, but it is accepted as adding to the capacity and stability of STM. External memory may be a part of STM, but empirical studies have not determined whether it is processed into STM for symbolizing or whether the symbols are in external memory and while in view become part of STM without additional processing efforts.

One attends to a stimulus, such as new information, and encodes its meaning in STM after a comparison with prior knowledge in LTM. The mix between new and old information for final storage in LTM is influenced by characteristics of the environment and the total internal state of the individual (Cormier, 1986).

CHUNKING

The characteristics of the functional divisions guide the development of a therapeutic strategy. The limited capacity of STM (Miller, 1965) calls for efficient processing strategies, such as "chunking." This means that information can be consolidated into organizational contexts. There are several types of chunking: one to one, many to one, one to many, and many to many. The most efficient is many to one, in which many new pieces of information can be chunked with one association of prior knowledge (Evans, 1974).

Chunking strategies that are used to assist in the storage of information in LTM or for retrieval of information from LTM are called mnemonics (Hunt, 1982; Norman, 1976). "A mnemonic technique can be defined as any mental strategy that aids the learning of one material by using other, initially extraneous, material as an aid to such learning" (Turnure & Lane, 1987, p. 331). Mnemonic strategies include rules, rhymes, and narratives. A familiar mnemonic rule is "*i* before *e* except after *c*." The following rhyme is often used for remembering the number of days in a month:

> Thirty days has September,
> April, June, and November.
> All the rest have thirty-one
> except February, which has twenty-eight

A rhyme used in a grade school Smurf program for "hyperactive" children was designed as a reminder to practice impulse control: "Smurfs are great; Smurfs can wait!" (Frost, 1984).

Health professionals traditionally use case studies as narratives. Therapists often use metaphors, analogies, anecdotes, axioms, and myths as part of narratives.

In my practice, slogans that incorporate these mechanisms have provided dramatic effectiveness as many to one mnemonics. A single slogan can represent a major therapeutic theme that is easy to recall and that triggers recall of the many associated meanings and applications considered in therapy. Its concrete quality appears to increase understanding, limit distortion, and lower resistance.

IMAGERY

Mnemonics that evoke visual imagery strengthen encoding and retrieval. Research indicates that this is so because there is a verbal (sequential) and imagery (spatial) representational (thought) system in LTM. Horowitz (1970) found that each perceptual experience produces an imagery representation, which during encoding also may be translated into a verbal representation. Pavio's (1972) dual-coding theory states that a word that has an image representation produces two codes that may act together or independent of each other. This means that the word can be retrieved by using either the word code or image code. Hildegard and Bower (1975) also accept the premise that there are two different memory codes. They believe that stimuli such as concrete words, real objects, and pictures produce a sensory image that will activate dual coding. They state, "A large number of learning experiments have now been done indicating that imaginable or pictorial representation of information usually facilitates memory by factors ranging from 1.5 to 3.0 or so" (Hildegard & Bower, 1975, p. 588). The work of Danner and Taylor (1973) supports this conclusion in word pair associations. In the work of Anderson and Kulhavy (1972) and Levin and Divine-Hawkins (1974), imagery also was a key factor in prose learning.

Metaphors and analogies are often powerful imagery-evoking mnemonics that also provide a many to one type of chunking. Arieti (1976), Shibles (1971), and Langer (1951) suggest that metaphors and analogic thinking are a foundation process of human thinking. Folk tales are examples of metaphors that provide concrete transmission of abstract concepts (Bettleheim, 1977; Gardner, 1971; 1972; 1988).

REHEARSAL

STM has rehearsal capability. Klatzky's and Ryan's (Klatzky, 1980) research indicates two kinds of rehearsal: maintenance and integrative. Maintenance is based on rote information and remains only as long as it is given active attention. Integrative rehearsal facilitates association with information in LTM and therefore facilitates permanent storage. There has been controversy over the time factor as a determinant in the effectiveness of rehearsal. However, Klatzky's and Ryan's (1980) research demonstrates that the length of time that information is rehearsed only makes a difference when there is association with information in LTM.

Bower (1970) stresses the ability of mnemonics to engage the subject actively. He believes that this increases the depth of processing and explains why in his studies; adults in the experimental group recall two to seven times more material than those in the control group.

To complement the functions of STM, a therapeutic strategy should be designed to promote integrative rather than rote rehearsal. This might be accomplished through organizational chunking with imagery-evoking mnemonic metaphors, analogies, or anecdotes based on the prior knowledge of the client. Milton Erickson (Haley, 1973) is well recognized for his use of metaphors in adult therapy, while Richard Gardner (1988) supports this approach for children to prevent sterile, unproductive use of abstractions.

NOVELTY

LTM is characterized by an unlimited capacity and a network of symbols or abstract representations of interrelated information in a hierarchic structure (Mandler & Parker, 1976). This taxonomic network reflects developmental and experiential complexity. It functions as a permanent storage for everything that has been experienced and stored. Consequently, it assists in the organization of information and the retrieval and reconstruction of information (Anderson & Bower, 1973).

Encoding for storage in LTM is dependent in part on the relationship of the information to the "typical instance" (Reese, 1977). When information is processed, it is compared with the typical or prototype stored in LTM. As LTM's hierarchic structure is developed, information is divided into categories of stereotypic expectations for people, places, and so forth (Hunt, 1982). These expectations explain why individual interpretation often differs from that which is intended in written and verbal communication.

For atypical or new information to be integrated, a novel or more elaborate generic image must be developed (Gregg, 1986; Cormier, 1986; Luria, 1965). If the sensory stimulus is weak, the information will be absorbed into the typical storage. Therefore, novelty should be designed to challenge or contradict the typical storage. This provocative intent can be achieved through mnemonics that are intellectually clever, humorous, or alarming (Box 7-1).

Reese (1970) suggests that even when change has occurred, repetition or use of the modified image must be ongoing to prevent a return to former memory images. In Renz and Cohen's (1977) parent education programs, they include a component that is a natural adjunct to daily life. This provides environmental replication as a stimulus for recall. In my parent education programs, this example is followed by stories from traditional and contemporary children's literature as intellectual contexts of analogic representation of children's developmental and psychodynamic conflicts. It is suggested to parents that these or similar stories with therapeutic themes be read to support their children and assist in their own recall of the associated parenting principles.

Development of Mnemonic Strategies

Analysis of various learning or processing "styles" reveals that these styles are approaches to the organization of information. Some theorists (Kagan, Moss, & Siegel, 1963; Hunt, 1982) believe that such styles are learned, natural processing strategies. Goldman's (1972) study reported that successful processing was more accurately predicted according to the type of strategy used than to the level of ability. Research has demonstrated positive results for facilitating recall in children with learning disabilities. Mnemonics improved recall and attention (Dawson, Hallahan, Reeve, & Ball, 1980), organizational strategies (Dallago & Maily, 1980), and reading comprehension (Rose, Cundick, & Higbee, 1983).

Gfeller (1986) and Nicholson (1972) found improvement in recall among children with mental retardation by using musical mnemonics. Gfeller hypothesized further improvement when familiar melodies were used with new lyrics.

A Krebs, Snowman, and Smith study (1978) demonstrates the effectiveness of improved prose learning after instruction in the use of mnemonics. There were dramatic differences in results between undergraduate students' usual learning methods and the use of mnemonics. Recall of information units from the first session before instruction consisted of an average of 23% for immediate recall with a range of 15% to 35%. A mean of 13% resulted at the 2-week delayed recall with a range from 6% to 27%. A mean of 10% resulted at the 4-week delayed recall with a range of 6% to 16%.

Using the loci mnemonics, immediate recall was 75% with a range of 48% to 86%. A mean of 83% resulted at the 2-week delayed recall with a range of 59% to 96%. A mean of 84% resulted at the 4-week delayed recall with a range of 55% to 96%.

There was a highly significant difference ($p < 0.001$) between usual study methods and the loci mnemonics for immediate and both delayed recalls. There also was significance ($p < .05$) for recall decay time with the typical study method.

In a 1973 study, Goldman and Hudson compared the learning of student groups representing low, middle, and high grade point averages. The results did not indicate a difference in ability levels but did indicate a difference in processing strategies.

BOX 7–1 • WAYNE'S SLOGAN

In therapy, mnemonic "slogans" provide a ready stimulus for recall. Wayne, age 8, was referred by his mother, Pat, because of difficulty in dealing with the third grade bully and a general reluctance to "stand up for himself." Wayne was the class scapegoat. The daily threats of peers and subsequent loss of clout was creating a vicious cycle of deprecation. "Setting himself up" and accepting the consequences was reportedly also his pattern at home.

Pat described Wayne as unhappy and complacent about making something of himself—much like his father. Wayne's physical similarity with his father seemed proof to his mother of a genetic connection that explained her son's behavioral predisposition. Wayne's younger brother, Tommy, age 4, was the "cute, adorable child" who was given very little discipline. Wayne was punished for defending his "property" or "rights" with his little brother. His mother contributed to Wayne's victim myth by clearly stating that the father had never given as much attention or care to Wayne as he had to Tommy and that Tommy "got away with everything" at Wayne's expense. The mother's self-righteous tone whenever she made these declarations underscored an attempt at aligning herself with Wayne as his protector. During the assessment, Wayne appeared quiet with a blank affect. He waited for directions and seemed intent on trying to please. His drawing portrayed himself as a tiny figure in the center of the large sheet of paper. Wayne's drawings of his mother often featured a moustache, although in reality, facial hair was not apparent.

The goal of the first mnemonic strategy was to transform Wayne's long-term memory store of bullies as powerful. When asked to describe the bully, Wayne said, "He's loud, gets in your face, and shakes his fist." With each description his voice reflected increasing alarm. Wayne seemed astonished at the following novel challenge to his beliefs: "That bully sounds as if he is afraid." He exclaimed, "Afraid?" "Sure, like the lion in The Wizard of Oz." As Wayne was encouraged to recall LTM stores about the Cowardly Lion, he described the concrete image of this mythic character as jumping out from behind a tree, roaring, and shaking his fist. At the last description, Wayne looked excited about the similarities.

The next sessions focused on analyzing examples of risking-taking in The Wizard of Oz and making associations with Wayne's experiences in school and at home. The story's themes acted as a supply of therapeutic affirmations easily recalled because of their rich imagery and analogic applicability. The symbol of the cowardly lion becoming courageous inspired a mnemonic slogan. "We won't take this *li on* down." Wayne's animated response to the humor of this novel, intellectual twist of a familiar idiom was followed by several attempts of appropriate confrontation at school. Wayne's own proclivity for mnemonic strategies was evidenced by his retort to the mythic lion's challenge, "Put 'em up. Put 'em up" with "Yea, so I can put 'em down. Put 'em down."

Dansereau, Atkinson, Long, and McDonald (1974) suggest that a processing strategy should facilitate the selecting, storing, manipulating, managing, and output of information.

Norman (1976) suggests mnemonic techniques as learning or processing strategies. He offers three steps in their development:

1. Arrange the learning material into small, self-contracted sections.
2. Organize the sections so that various parts fit together in a logical self-ordering structure.
3. Establish relationships between the material to be learned and material already learned through such mental activities as imagery or narrative stories (Norman, 1976).

The work of Anderson and Bower (1973) highlights the third step by suggesting that the effectiveness of a mnemonic structure is largely related to its relevance to the type of information being taught. For example, the theme of Harry Chapin's ballad "The Cat in the Cradle" (Furlong, 1982) suggests that adult behaviors are a replication of those modeled by one's parents. Consequently, it was a relevant theme to use in a program on child abuse because of its cyclical nature. The lyrics then become a stimulus for remembering the stored information. The sequential structure of the lyrics also supports Norman's first and second steps.

Although not mentioned in Norman's work, novelty is a key variable in the processing, storing, and accurate recall of new information (Reese, 1977). When new information is compared with prior knowledge, the information must be presented in a way that prevents an easy "fit" and instead promotes modification. Chapin's ballad, for example, provides an intellectually clever context to challenge prior knowledge.

Bower (1970) stresses the ability of mnemonics to engage the learner in an integrative rehearsal of new information. He believes that the more the learner "works" on the association between old and new information, the more deeply the new information will be processed. Chapin's ballad, which is usually associated with entertainment and is culturally compatible with select clients, may seem less academic and less anxiety provoking than a didactic strategy. Easy recall of the familiar lyrics provides a powerful one-to-one mnemonic for consideration of the new information.

A synthesis of elements of the information processing framework previously described suggests criteria for a working strategy, which can be summarized as the mnemonic CRIPRN (pronounced "cry prin") (Frost, 1989):

C—chunking of new information in a context of
R—relevant
I—imagery-provoking
P—prior knowledge, which increases
R—rehearsal with
N—novel associations for new storage

SLOGANS AS MNEMONICS

Slogans can use all of the criteria of CRIPRN and have proven to be a therapeutic strategy that clients are quick to learn. Their ready understanding seems to spark their own creativity and an eagerness to develop new slogans (Box 7-2).

In the author's practice, consultation–education programs are a regular part of community-based psychosocial interventions. Using the CRIPRN framework not only facilitates mnemonic recall, but the use of media related themes limits the "teachy preachy" quality of some health-education programs and associates them with entertainment and pleasure. The following are examples of these programs. (See the chapter on information processing approaches, Chapter 27, for details of clinical application.)

"Family Violence is a 'Thriller?'" Adolescents use Michael Jackson's music video to examine family violence.

"Fun with the Flintstones"—Flintstone cartoons are used to help latency-aged children discuss and accept the imperfections in themselves and others.

"Over the Rainbow"—A case study of Dorothy Gale in *The Wizard of Oz* is used to help young adolescents understand the relationship between their own developmental needs and conflicts and their academic performance in school.

SMURF (Social Maturation Using Recreation and Fantasy)—Smurf characters and cartoons are used to teach latency-aged "hyperactive" children greater inner control by using Smurf behavior.

"The Marlboro Man Speaks with Forked Tongue"—Young adolescents use commercial ads to discuss multilevel family communications.

"The Good Side of Bears, Wolves and Witches"—Parents use children's literature for support of young children's developmental and situational crises.

STORIES AS MNEMONIC

I examined the credibility of a popular program, "The Good Side of Bears, Wolves and Witches." Story contexts were considered for mnemonic effectiveness. An examination of the literature began with Johnson and Mandler (1977), who studied the structure of simple stories, such as folk tales, fables, and myths, for representative structures to facilitate encoding and retrieval.

> The essential structure of a single episode story is that a protagonist is introduced in the setting; there follows an episode in which something happens, causing the protagonist to respond to it, which in turn brings about some event or state of affairs that ends the episode. The simplest story must have at least four propositions, representing a setting, beginning, development, and ending, if it is to be considered a story (Johnson & Mandler, 1977, p. 10).

Rummelhart's (1975) work supports the concept of story schema, which he called story grammars. Thorndyke (1977) advanced Rummelhart's work on a general story structure familiar to many people. The symbol of this story "grammar" consists of SETTING + THEME + PLOT + RESOLUTION. Thorndyke's research demonstrated that a story structure that matched the reader's expectation re-

BOX 7–2 • CHARLIE'S SLOGAN

Charlie, 11 years old, was referred by his mother, Kay, for an obsession with cleanliness. Kay reported that besides frequent handwashing, he insisted on having his sneakers washed whenever he entered his home from the outside. Charlie also expressed disgust for the wash cloths that his parents used in the diaper changes of his baby sister. In addition to these concerns, Charlie often positioned his hands in a "claw-like" half fist, usually when he thought he was not being observed.

During assessment Charlie appeared cognitively gifted but shy. His slight build, frequent squinting, and postured hands reflected the tension compatible with his history of migraine headaches. When asked if he had glasses, Charlie said "Yes," but he didn't like wearing them because people called him a "nerd."

Charlie's history contained a series of recent losses. Abstractly, the birth of his sister represented a loss of "what had been," corroborated by Kay's statement, "Until Susan, Charlie had been my baby." In addition, Charlie's 40-year-old uncle died, resulting in his aunt and two cousins moving into the already crowded, two-family home shared by Charlie, his parents, older brother, baby sister, and grandmother and grandfather. An elderly friend in the neighborhood also died, followed by the death of a cherished dog owned by another neighbor. This series of losses was compounded by the death of Charlie's grandfather with whom he had been very close.

Charlie's grandfather died of emphysema after a long history of smoking. During the final stages of the illness, the grandfather's physician forbade him to smoke anymore, saying that "it would kill him." However, the grandfather had pleaded with Charlie and finally convinced him to buy a pack. Shortly thereafter, his grandfather died. The other remarkable feature of the grandfather's failing health was that he had arthritis, resulting in rigidity of his hands and a "claw-like" position. Charlie's overzealous superego and depleted ego strength predisposed him to excessive guilt and a phobic reaction. The positioning of his hands seemed to reflect an attempt at "holding on" to his grandfather.

The mnemonic that was to act as a philosophic framework for treatment was "Some rules are meant to be broken." This was introduced through the board games during our second session. It was suggested that one of the cards in the game of "Sorry" be modified. Charlie looked shocked at this novel idea and said, "but that would be changing the rule." It was casually suggested that some rules don't make much sense anyway and could be changed. He seemed very disgruntled with this idea and stated that he preferred having "things the way they were." This very phrase seemed to represent his hope for comfort from the painful disruptions he had experienced. A subsequent slogan became "Nobody's perfect," which the therapist used to discount a seemingly poor ability to remember the rules to the new card games that Charlie attempted to teach her.

After 4 weeks, two sessions a week, Charlie began to share examples from school of classmates who "broke rules." This allowed a discussion of whether these were rules meant to be broken. By the sixth week, the therapist gently confronted Charlie about his grandfather. It was explained that his mother had shared information about the grandfather's emphysema and his history of smoking. Charlie said, "Yea, and the doctor wouldn't let him have any more cigarettes because he said it would kill him." To test his readiness for change of his most stringent and antitherapeutic beliefs, his statement was countered with "Isn't that silly!" With shock but great intensity, he remarked, "but you can't smoke if you have emphysema." The reply was, "But Charlie, perhaps that is true for some situations and not for others. Perhaps this is one of those 'Some rules are meant to be broken' situations." With his rapt attention, this theme was continued, "Your grandfather smoked for years. His health was already failing, and he didn't have long to live. Cigarettes were a great source of comfort. Perhaps the doctor had to state the 'usual rule' but needed to give a 'Prescription for comfort' (new mnemonic). Charlie then blurted out "Grandpa made me buy him cigarettes." Seizing the opportunity, the therapist commented, "That was your very thoughtful 'prescription for comfort.'"

Charlie asked many questions about the intellectual context of "prescription for comfort" for the next two sessions. The "mixing" between old and new information was demonstrated by a permanent relaxation of his "claw-like" hands and a report by his mother that he no longer mentioned dirty sneakers. Charlie continued in therapy for 2 more months in which he reported how he was helping some new friends "chill out" about rules.

"Some rules are meant to be broken" provided *chunking* of new information in a *relevant* philosophic theme to "soften" a stringent superego. The concrete axiom is not *imagery* provoking itself, but is associated with the concrete image of the games. It also stimulated use of the metaphor, the "rules of life." The familiarity of the axiom as part of prior knowledge created interest in *rehearsal* because of *novelty* of using it for opposite meaning.

quired minimal processing and a high percentage of recall.

The processing efficiency of a story grammar supports Dyer's (1987) concept of scripts: "a knowledge structure containing a stereotypic sequence of actions." For example, "$ RESTAURANT = ENTER + BE SEATED + WAITRESS COMES + FOOD + EAT + RECEIVE CHECK + LEAVE TIP + PAY BILL + LEAVE" (Dyer, 1981). However, scripts, like stories, have a more effective mnemonic function when intentions are supplied as part of the new information. This is said to limit the distortion with time and a return to typicality.

Supporting the concepts of typicality and the need for inclusion of all aspects of the four propositions of story structure is the study of Owens, Bower, and Black (1979) called, "The Soap Opera Effect in Story Recall." The purpose of the study was to show that when people are learning about the actions of a story's character, one's memory is influenced by assumptions concerning the character's motives. The character's motives become a schema for the actions, the importance of the actions, and the connections between the two.

The control group was given a series of five scripts with stereotypic sequences of action. These were boring vignettes about a character named Nancy or Jack who prepares a cup of coffee, keeps an appointment with a doctor, attends a lecture, goes to a grocery store for shopping, and attends a cocktail party. The "problem" groups read a short description of the character's problem before reading the more neutral scripts.

In determining the results (Owens et al., 1979), scoring reflected the total number of episodes recalled. Those in the "problem" group scored higher with a 4.7 out of 5, compared with a 4.0 for the control group. Next, the recall of the order of the episodes was determined. Again, those in the "problem" group scored higher with 10 recalling the correct order against eight in the control group. Third, correct analysis of the text was scored according to two criteria, the number of correct propositions and the number of false propositions. The two groups did not demonstrate a difference on the correct propositions. However, there was a statistically reliable difference [$t\,(18) = 5.08, p < .001$] for the "intrusions." The majority of intrusions came from the "problem" group who added motives for the primary character (Owens et al., 1979).

The result clearly indicated that providing the subject with a motive and problem for the prime characters promoted accurate recall for the details of the vignettes and the correct order (Owens et al., 1979). In summary, a story that is to function as an effective mnemonic should follow a simple story structure. It also should provide adequate elements to prevent the development of intrusions and subsequent diversion from the association of information to be relevant to the therapeutic or psychosocial goals.

FAIRY TALE AS STORY MNEMONIC

When a simple story structure is chosen to act as a mnemonic, the themes and symbols also should be relevant to the information to be learned. The work of Laughlin and Stephens (Foster & Brandes, 1980) suggests that the symbols used in myths derive from common imagery of visual experiences that the people of a culture share in various stages of consciousness. Because myths are based on primordial imagery and are hermeneutic, there is relevance from childhood to adulthood. Myths have two primary cognitive functions:

> (a) as a system of transformation by which operations upon the myth effectively order (reorder) information both stored in memory and gleaned from immediate and direct experience; and (b) as a system of transposition permitting the reduction of complexity and richness of direct experience and the encoding of that reduced experience for storage as "meaning" within the unconscious (Foster et al., 1980, p. 176).

Bruno Bettleheim (1977) believes that fairy tales are symbolic vehicles that represent the developmental conflicts of childhood. The value of fairy tales is underscored by a statement made by Charles Dickens, "Little Red Riding Hood was my first love. I felt that if I could have married Little Red Riding Hood, I should have perfect bliss." (Bettleheim, 1977, p. 23). The inference is that Little Red Riding Hood became a mnemonic and "many-to-one" chunking symbol that represented the whole of a developmental task.

Goldilocks and the Three Bears as a Media Mnemonic

Media mnemonics (Frost, 1989) were developed to use the principles of information processing while enhancing their ability to entertain and decrease client anxiety and resistance. A media mnemonic is defined as a media-related context or theme that is developmentally and culturally appropriate to the client group and is relevant to the topic. *Goldilocks and the Three Bears* was designed as a fairy tale mnemonic representative of media mnemonics. The story is culturally familiar to most American-born adults, and as such, provides a common base of knowledge between nurse and client to promote a collaborative relationship. The pleasure and innocence often associated with a fairy tale also may decrease the threat of technical and emotionally charged knowledge.

The story also fulfills the criteria of CRIPRN. It provides chunking of new information with a sequence of story events in a relevant analogy of parent–child interactions that represent the developmental thinking and psychosocial stress of children 3 through 5 years of age when there is a new baby in the family. The concrete characters and actions of the fairy tale provide stimuli for imagery representations. The familiarity of *Goldilocks and the Three Bears* provides a context of prior knowledge that may create interest and encourage rehearsal, while encoding with novel associations for storage of new information.

The study used an author-designed developmental questionnaire of 24 questions to test cognitive and psychosocial principles of development for these children. The works of Jean Piaget and Erik Erikson were used as theoretical bases for the questions. Content validity was determined by a panel of five doctorally prepared experts in child development. A Kuder-Richardson reliability coefficient of .66 was obtained for the test as administered in the study.

Three hypotheses were proposed in the study:

1. Greater recall will result from adult learners using a story grammar mnemonic than a didactic format.
2. Greater recall will result from adult learners using a fairy tale mnemonic than a didactic format.
3. Greater recall will result from adult learners using a fairy tale mnemonic than a story grammar mnemonic.

The sample consisted of 102 parents between the ages of 25 and 44 years. They were all white and married. More than half were employed, with the majority in professional positions. Level of education ranged from some amount of college to graduate degrees. Combined family income ranged from $21,000 to $80,000. Place of residence included suburban Virginia and suburban New York. The number of children in each family ranged from one to four.

Data were collected in community settings with random distribution of test packets, each of which contained one of three possible scripts. The first script used the fairy tale mnemonic, the second script used the story grammar mnemonic, and the third used a didactic format. The test data were analyzed using two independent three-factor analyses of variance with repeated measures.

The conclusions in this experimental design with 102 subjects and three treatment groups in community settings follow:

- There was statistical significance for greater adult learner recall using a fairy tale mnemonic than a didactic format.
- There was statistical significance for greater adult learner recall using a fairy tale mnemonic than a story grammar mnemonic.
- There was no statistical significance for greater learner recall using a story grammar mnemonic than a didactic format.

The results suggest that the analogic relevance as well as the imagery and novelty of the fairy tale provide a possible explanation for the unexpected weakness of the story grammar mnemonic.

Mnemonic strategies including media mnemonics are considered in a variety of clinical applications in chapter 27, Information Processing Approaches. The use of mnemonic strategies in psychiatric-mental health nursing is still new but offers promise for time- and cost-efficient interventions that yield effective results.

REFERENCES

Anderson, J. R., & Bower, G. H. (1973). *Human associative memory.* Washington, DC: Winston.

Anderson, R. C., & Kulhavy, R. W. (1972). Imagery and prose learning. *Journal of Educational Psychology, 63,* 242–244.

Arieti, S. (1976). *Creativity: The magic synthesis.* New York: Basic Books.

Bettleheim, B. (1977). *The uses of enchantment.* New York: Vintage Books.

Bower, G. H. (1970). Analysis of a mnemonic device. *American Scientist, 58,* 496–510.

Bower, G. H. (1972). Mental imagery and associative learning. In L. Gregg (Ed.), *Cognition in learning and memory.* New York: John Wiley and Sons.

Cormier, S. (1986). *Basic processes of learning, cognition and motivation.* Hillsdale, NJ: Erlbaum.

Dallago, M., & Maily, B. (1980). Free recall in boys of normal and poor reading levels as a function of task manipulations. *Journal of Experimental Child Psychology, 30,* 62–78.

Danner, F. W., & Taylor, A. M. (1973). Integrated pictures and relational imagery training in children's learning. *Journal of Experimental Child Psychology, 16* (1), 47–54.

Dansereau, D. F., Atkinson, T. R., Long, G. L., & McDonald, B. (1974). Learning Strategies: A review and synthesis of the current literature. *Educational Resources Information Center,* 103–403.

Dawson, M., Hallahan, D., Reeve, R., & Ball, D. (1980) The effect of reinforcement and verbal rehearsal on selective attention in learning disabled children. *Journal of Abnormal Child Psychology 8,* 133–134.

Dyer, M. G. (1981). $ Restaurant revisited or "lunch with Boris." *Proceedings of the Seventh International Joint Con-*

ference on Artificial Intelligence Vancouver, BC, Canada: (pp. 234–236). University of British Columbia. 234–236.

Evans, S. (1974). The structure of instructional knowledges: An operational model. *Instructional Science, 2,* 421–450.

Foster, M. L., & Brandes, S. H. (Eds.). (1980). *Symbol as sense, new approaches to the analysis of meaning.* New York: Academic Press.

Foster M. L. (1984). The use of rock music to assist adolescent sexual identity. *Imprint, 13*(4), 36–42.

Frost, A. (1984). The use of smurfs for increased body control and self-accountability. *Journal of Holistic Nursing, 2,* 38–42.

Frost, A. (1989). Helping teens discuss issues of sexuality. *Imprint, 67,* 68–70.

Furlong, B. (1982). Setting the stage for learning. *American Journal of Nursing, 82,* 300–301.

Gardner, R. A. (1971). *Therapeutic communication with children: The mutual storytelling technique.* Northvale, NJ: Jason Aronson.

Gardner, R. A. (1972). *Dr. Gardner's stories about the real world* (Vol. I). Cresskill, NJ: Creative Therapeutics.

Gardner, R. A. (1988). *Psychotherapy with adolescents.* Cresskill, NJ: Creative Therapeutics.

Gfeller, K. (1986). Musical mnemonics for learning disabled children. *Teaching Exceptional Children, 19,* 28–30.

Goldman, R. D. (1972). Effects of logical versus mnemonic learning strategy on performance in two undergraduate psychology classes. *Journal of Educational Psychology, 63,* 347–352.

Goldman, R. D., & Hudson, D. A. (1973). A multivariate analysis of academic abilities and strategies for successful and unsuccessful college students in different major fields. *Journal of Educational Psychology, 65,* 364–370.

Gregg, V. (1986). *Introduction to human memory.* London: Routledge & Kegan Paul.

Haley, J. (1973), *Uncommon therapy: The psychiatric techniques of Milton H. Erickson, M.D.* New York: W.W. Norton and Co.

Hildegard, E. R., & Bower, G. H. (1975). *Theories of learning.* Englewood Cliffs, NJ: Prentice-Hall.

Horowitz, M. J. (1970). *Image formation and cognition.* New York: Appleton Century-Crofts.

Hunt, M. (1982). *The universe within.* New York: Simon & Simon.

Johnson, N. S., & Mandler, J. M. (1980). A tale of two structures, underlying surface forms in stories. *Poetics, 9,* 51–86.

Kagan, J., Moss, H. A., & Siegel, I. G. (1963). The psychological significance of styles conceptualization. In J.F. Wright & J. Kagan (Eds.), Basic cognition processes in children. *Monographs of the Society for Research in Child Development, 28,* 73–112.

Klatzky, R. L. (1980). *Human memory.* San Francisco: W.H. Freeman.

Krebs, E. W., Snowman, J., & Smith, S. H. (1978). Teaching new dogs old tricks: Facilitating prose learning through mnemonic training. *Journal of Instructional Psychology, 5*(2), 33–39.

Langer, S. K. (1951). *Philosophy in a new key.* New York: The New American Library.

Levin, J. R., & Divine-Hawkins, P. (1974). Visual imagery as a prose learning process. *Journal of Reading Behavior, 6,* 22–30.

Luria, A. R. (1969). The mind of a mnemonist. In L. Solotaroff (Trans.). New York: Avon Books. (Original work published 1965)

Mandler, J. M., & Parker, R. E. (1976). Memory for descriptive and spatial information in complex pictures. *Journal of Experimental Psychology: Human Learning and Memory, 3,* 38–48.

Mastropieri, M. A., & Scruggs, T. E. (1991). *Teaching students ways to remember: Strategies for learning mnemonically.* Cambridge: Brookline Books.

Miller, G. A. (1965). The magical number seven, plus or minus two: Some limits on our capacity for processing information. *Psychological Review, 63,* 81–97.

Newell, A., & Simon, H. A. (1972). *Human problem solving.* Englewood Cliffs, NJ: Prentice-Hall.

Nicholson, D. (1972). Music as an aid to learning. *Dissertation Abstracts International, 33,* 1–352 A. (University Microfilms Number 72-20-653).

Norman, D. H. (1976). *Memory and attention.* San Francisco: W.H. Freeman.

Owens, J., Bower, G. H., & Black, J. B. (1979). The soap opera effect in story recall. *Memory and Cognition, 7*(3), 185–91.

Pavio, A. (1972). A theoretical analysis of the role of imagery in learning and memory. In P. W. Sheehan (Ed.), *The function and nature of imagery.* New York: Academic Press.

Reese, H. W. (1970). Imagery and contextual meaning. In H. W. Reese (Ed.), *Imagery in children's learning: A symposium. Psychological Bulletin, 73,* 404–14.

Reese, H. W. (1977). Toward a cognitive theory of mnemonic imagery. *Journal of Mental Imagery, 2,* 229–244.

Renz, L., & Cohen, M. (1977). Interpersonal skill practice as a component in effective parent training. *Community Mental Health Journal, 13*(1), 54–57.

Rose, M., Cundick, B., & Higbee, K. (1983). Verbal rehearsal and visual imagery: Mnemonic aids for learning-disabled children. *Journal of Learning Disabilities, 16,* 352–354.

Rummelhart, D. E. (1975). Notes on a schema for stories. In D. G. Bobrow & A. Collins (Eds.), *Representation and understanding.* New York: Academic Press.

Shibles, W. A. (1971). *Metaphor: An annotated bibliography and history.* Whitewater, WI: The Language Press.

Thorndyke, P. W. (1977). Cognitive structures in comprehension and memory of narrative discourse. *Cognitive Psychology, 9,* 77–110.

Turnure, J., & Lane, J. (1987). Special educational applications of mnemonics. In M. A. McDaniel & M. Pressley (Eds.), *Imagery and related mnemonic processes* (pp. 329–357). New York: Springer-Verlag.

UNIT

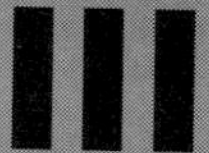

Children, Adolescents, and Family Groups at Risk for Mental Disorders

CHAPTER

8

Children of the Mentally Ill

Deborah Ann Gross

The children of mentally ill parents are more likely to develop psychiatric and psychosocial disorders than are children of well parents. Although the mechanisms for risk remain controversial, longitudinal, cross-sectional, and single case studies have all converged on this finding (Bleuler, 1974; Brockington & Kumar, 1982; Cohler & Musick, 1983; Drake, Racusin, & Murphy, 1990; Gross, 1989; Weissman, Prusoff, Gammon, Merikangas, Leckman, & Kidd, 1984). This chapter reviews some of the documented effects of parental psychiatric illness on children's mental health and selected issues pertaining to the assessment and treatment of this population.

Parental Psychopathology: Maternal Versus Paternal Illness

The majority of research on parental psychopathology and its effects on children has focused on the mentally ill mother rather than the mentally ill father. There are several reasons for this focus. First, in most cultures mothers are the children's primary caregivers. As such, their symptoms are integrally woven into the children's daily lives. For example, paranoid mothers may isolate their children from friends, neighbors, and other family members, thus engendering a fear of social relationships within the children. Depressed mothers may be too preoccupied to feed their infants, change their diapers, or get them out of the crib, leaving them at risk for failure-to-thrive and developmental delay. While the symptoms of paternal mental illness are felt by the children, their influence is considered to be less crucial because fathers tend not to be their children's primary caregivers. This point has been supported by research that has shown a stronger relationship between maternal illness and child dysfunction than paternal illness (Keller, Beardslee, Dorer, Lavori, Samuelson & Klerman, 1986; Kokes, Harder, Fisher, & Strauss, 1980; Welner & Rice, 1988).

Second, when mothers are hospitalized for psychiatric illness, the children's daily caregiving routines are more disrupted than when fathers are hospitalized. In a study of children with hospitalized mentally ill parents, Ekdahl, Rice, and Schmidt (1962) reported that 41% of the children of hospitalized mothers had to be moved out of their homes to live in a variety of surrogate care arrangements, while only 3% of the children of hospitalized fathers were moved out of their homes. This difference is significant on two levels. First, most psychiatric admissions are unplanned, which means that surrogate care needs to be found quickly. As a result, child care often is inadequate, or children may be left at home without adult supervision (Shachnow, 1987).

Third, when children are moved out of their homes, they also may be moved away from their friends and school and the security of their possessions and routines. At a time when the children most need a predictable environment and familiar supports, these resources become unavailable to them.

Finally, more American families are being headed by single or divorced mothers than ever before. According to recent estimates, more than one in five children live in one-parent, female-headed households (Children's Defense Fund Reports, 1989). Of these families, 53.2% live below the poverty line. This demographic trend suggests that the occurrence of maternal psychiatric illness may have an even greater impact on children for two reasons: There may be fewer consistent adult figures with whom the children can develop healthy attachment relationships, and the trend toward lower socioeconomic status in single, female-headed households increases the number of other potentiating risk factors associated with poor child outcomes (i.e., living in violent communities, drug abuse, adolescent pregnancy, low birth weight, and child abuse or neglect). Thus, an assumption underlying much of the research reviewed in this chapter is that the relationship between the mentally ill mother and her children is the most salient one. It is important to note, however, that while this assumption is supported by research, the father's illness does have direct (i.e., through genetic loading and poor quality of father–child interactions) and indirect (i.e., through marital discord and quality of the home environment) effects on child outcomes (Forehand & Brody, 1985; Jouriles, Pfiffner, & O'Leary, 1988). As a result, it is important to acknowledge that parental psychiatric illness is a family matter that extends well beyond the mother–child dyad.

Vulnerability to Disorder: Genetic and Environmental Effects

Until recently, the dominant paradigm underlying psychiatry has been a psychologic–environmental paradigm (Liaschenko, 1989). Child psychiatric nurses have downplayed the significance of genetic and biologic factors in their practice and educational curricula. However, advances in biologic psychiatry and the findings from twin and adoption studies have led to a paradigmatic shift and the realization of the need to integrate the biologic sciences (neurobiology, genetics, and immunology) with the behavioral sciences in psychiatric nursing (McBride, 1990).

For example, in a longitudinal study of 5483 adopted Danish children and a comparison group of biologic children, Kety (1988) and his colleagues reported a statistically significant concentration of schizophrenia spectrum disorders in the biologic relatives of schizophrenic adoptees. In fact, the prevalence of schizophrenic illness in the biologic relatives of schizophrenic adoptees was similar to that in the relatives of nonadopted schizophrenic patients. Similarly, twin studies have consistently demonstrated at least a threefold greater risk for illness in monozygotic twins versus dizygotic twins and a 40- to 60-fold greater risk in monozygotic twins than in the general population (Pardes, Kaufman, Pincus, & West, 1989).

Others who have studied the genetic risk of affective disorder have reported higher rates of illness within families with an affectively ill member than within the general population (Weissman et al., 1984). Bertelsen et al. (1977) found a 79% concordance rate between monozygotic twins with bipolar affective disorder versus a 19% concordance rate between dizygotic twins. Their findings point to the high risk of acquiring bipolar (manic–depressive) illness within families with the same genetic endowment.

However, there is far from a perfect match in the expression of mental illness between twins with the same genetic endowment. It would appear that while the children of mentally ill parents are genetically vulnerable to psychiatric illness, the expression of symptoms is, at least in part, contingent on extensive exposure to disorganized, hostile, or unresponsive environments (Rutter & Quinton, 1984). Thus, having a mentally ill parent can serve as a genetic marker of vulnerability, but its importance lies in its ability to help identify families who may be amenable to pharmacologic and environmentally based interventions.

An assumption underlying this review is that the children of mentally ill parents are vulnerable to psychiatric and psychosocial disorders through a number of pathways. These pathways include those directed by genetic loading for psychiatric illness, the child's temperament and its fit with the parents' temperament (Thomas & Chess, 1984), the manner in which the child selectively perceives his or her environment (Plomin & Daniels, 1987), and the overall quality of the parenting environment.

Parental Psychopathology and Child Outcomes

The literature extensively reports the differences between children of psychiatrically ill and well parents and the risk for disorder. The most dramatic deviations have been demonstrated among the children of affectively disordered parents, beginning as early as 3 months of age.

Field and her colleagues (1988) have shown that infants of depressed mothers interact differently than infants of well mothers. During videotaped structured interaction episodes, Field (1984) found that 3-month-old babies displayed fewer positive facial expressions and more negative facial expressions and produced fewer vocalizations when interacting with their mothers than did the control group. When videotaped with research assistants, the infants continued to show more negative facial expressions and less interactive involvement (Field et al., 1988). Thus, 3-month-old infants of depressed mothers interacted differently than infants of well mothers. According to Field and her colleagues (1988), these infants had already learned a "depressive interactive style," which was exhibited with their mothers and with strangers.

Toddlers of mothers with an affective disorder have more infant–parent attachment disturbances than toddlers of well mothers (Gaensbauer, Harmon, Cytryn, & McKnew, 1984; Radke-Yarrow, Cummings, Kuczynski, & Chapman, 1985). This is an important finding because toddlerhood is the developmental phase during which separation and individuation issues need to be negotiated (Mahler, Pine, & Bergman, 1975). It is hypothesized that the depressed and bipolar mother's blunted affect and preoccupation with herself precludes her ability to be emotionally available to her children. When the attachment figure is emotionally unavailable, children cannot use them as a secure base for exploration. This deficit in the attachment relationship adversely affects the child's social, emotional, and intellectual growth (Bretherton & Waters, 1985).

School-age and adolescent children of depressed parents experience more anxiety and depressive symptoms and have more difficulty learning and getting along with others in school. In a longitudinal study, Billings and Moos (1983; 1985) reported significantly higher rates of dysfunction among the children of depressed parents than among the control children. The depressed families also reported higher levels of family stress and disorganization. In a 1-year follow-up of the same families, 52.2% of the families in which the depressed parent's illness had not remitted had at least one child with marked dysfunction, compared with 9.5% in the control families. Childhood symptoms included depression, anxiety, behavioral problems, academic and disciplinary problems, and high-risk health behaviors. Even among families with a remitted parental depression, child dysfunction remained significantly higher (26.5%) than the control group (9.5%).

During adolescence, when clear psychiatric diagnoses become manifest, the children of mentally ill parents have an increased risk of developing mental illness. Weissman et al. (1984) reported that the risk for psychiatric illness is three times higher when mothers are affectively disordered than in the well population and even higher if both parents are ill. Similarly, Beardslee et al. (1988) found that 30% of children in a sample of affectively disordered parents were depressed, compared with 2% of the children with well parents. Keller et al. (1986) reported that 65% of the children of depressed parents in their study received at least one DSM-III diagnosis, and 46% received two or more diagnoses. In all of these studies, the most common diagnosis among the children of affectively disordered parents was major depression.

Children of schizophrenic mothers also are at risk for developing disorders, although there appears to be less consensus around its specific effects. Marcus, Auerbach, Wilkinson, and Burack (1981) described a subgroup of infants born to schizophrenic parents who repeatedly scored poorly on measures of motor and sensorimotor performance during the first year of life. Their findings support a cluster of other studies suggesting that some children of schizophrenic parents suffer from genetically transmitted neurointegrative deficits (Asarnow, 1988). Such deficits are associated with attentional and information-processing disorders during later childhood (Fox, 1990).

Children of schizophrenic parents are at risk for receiving poor quality of parenting. Goodman and Brumley (1990) reported that in comparison to well and depressed mothers, schizophrenic mothers provided significantly poorer childrearing environments as measured by the HOME Inventory (Bradley & Caldwell, 1977). One methodologic problem with the research examining the children's home environments is that the diagnosis of schizophrenia often is confounded by the severity and chronicity of the parent's illness. For example, the schizophrenic mothers in Goodman and Brumley's study had significantly more hospitalizations and poorer Global Assessment Scale scores (measuring the severity of disturbance) than the depressed and control groups. It has been noted that the chronicity of the parent's illness is more salient to the children's development than the specific diagnosis (Gross, 1983; Sameroff, Seifer, & Zax, 1982), which is discussed in more detail later in this chapter.

The Experience of Having a Mentally Ill Parent

Although children of mentally ill parents are at greater risk for psychopathology, most of these children do not become mentally ill. Approximately 40% to 50% of the children of psychotic parents develop psychosocial or psychiatric disorders (Bleuler, 1978), which means that at least half of the children do not develop diagnosable disorders. However, much of the qualitative data culled from interviews with children point to the profound effects of living with a mentally ill parent. Even among children who do not demonstrate clear maladjustment, a feeling of psychologic vulnerability and loss remains.

For example, children become acutely aware of community reaction to families with a "crazy" member. The social stigma associated with having a mentally ill parent often falls onto the shoulders of children who are too young to understand why their mother or father is not like other parents but who are profoundly aware that this is the case. Children do not know how to explain their parent's bizarre behavior or sudden absence following admission to a psychiatric hospital. They feel different from other children and ultimately fear that they too will become mentally ill. The following are children's statements about growing up in a home with a mentally ill parent. Their comments convey feelings of sadness, fearfulness, and confusion.

> "You cannot believe what it is like to wake up one morning and find your mother talking gibberish" (Anthony, 1985, p. 299).
>
> "My earliest recollection is that my father was different and he was in the hospital and kids would ask, 'where is your father?', and we'd make up stories. We never said he was in a psychiatric hospital. I tended not to socialize much because I didn't know what to say when people asked me those kinds of things. And if I brought friends home, I could never be certain how he would behave; he might talk to himself, or just ignore them" (Canadian Mental Health Association, 1987, p. 4).
>
> "I was sitting at the table just eating my cereal, and as I was pouring out the milk, my hand hit his cup and it went over his lap, and he jumped up and shouted at me and said that I did it on purpose and that I was trying to kill him, and that he knew I hated him. Then he hit me on the head and said I had plans and he knew about them, and he would get me first; and I said it was an accident, but he just wouldn't listen to me. He wasn't so grouchy last year. He has become real mean" (Anthony, 1985, p. 300).
>
> "Mother and I shared a room with twin beds. When Mother was lying down, she would start to moan as if she were talking in her sleep. 'I can't stand that girl. She's evil; she's a bitch. She's just like her father.' I was terrorized, but I dared not move . . . I used to lie in bed, wishing I were dead, believing that I was the worthless girl she was describing" (Lanquetot, 1984, p. 469).
>
> "When you've gone through that you can never really be happy; you can never laugh as others do. You always have to be ashamed of yourself and take care not to break down yourself" (Bleuler, 1974, p. 106).

Buckwalter, Kerfoot, and Stolley (1988) interviewed nine children of parents with an affective disorder about methods they used to cope with having a mentally ill parent. Most of these children had never confided with friends or relatives about their problems and chose not to deal with their feelings about having a psychiatrically ill parent. Their coping strategies included avoiding the parent, ignoring the existence of the family's problems, crying alone, attempting to control their anger, and running away from home.

It is particularly difficult for children to know how to respond to the ill parent's behavior when the well parent denies or minimizes its existence. However, this often is the case in families in which the well parent has become distant from or frightened by the ill spouse. Shachnow (1987) relates the story of Mrs. J, who was admitted after setting fire to her husband's clothing and running outside naked in fear of little men shooting at her. Mr. J, described as a workaholic, denied the impact of his wife's psychotic behavior on his children and assured the interviewer that his children were functioning well. According to the grandmother, however, the children had become aggressive with other children and had begun walking and talking psychotically like their mother.

In a second case, Shachnow (1987) describes two other children who returned home from school one day to see their mother, severely bleeding and delusional, being carried to an ambulance following a suicide attempt. Their father told the children that their mother had accidentally cut herself while carving a turkey. Like the children described by Buckwalter et al., well parents may choose to deny the potent effects of the illness on the family, leaving the children confused and frightened.

Children of mentally ill parents mourn the loss of having a healthy, emotionally available caregiver. As Anthony (1973) pointed out, the loss of a parent to psychiatric illness can be more devastating to the child than losing a parent who has died. When a parent dies, the grieving process ends, and the child can grow and move beyond it. However, when a parent is mentally ill, the child continues to hope that one day that parent will be well and behave normally. Delusional behavior and repeated hospitalizations serve as reminders that their mother or father is different from other parents. Mourning the loss of a mentally ill parent remains incomplete because the children cannot feel certain that there will never be another frightening episode.

> "I felt protective pity for her, but I could not honestly acknowledge loving her. To do that would mean feeling the awful pain of having lost her somehow, and I was sure feeling that pain would probably be strong enough to kill me, so I just skipped it" (Crosby, 1989, p. 508).

Protective Factors

Despite growing up in a family with a mentally ill parent, a portion of children appear to function quite well. It is estimated that 10% of the children with mentally ill parents have been able to distance themselves from the ill parent and have sought to understand their parent's pathology. These children have been referred to as "resilient" (Rutter, 1985) or "invulnerable" (Anthony & Cohler, 1987) children, and they have provided insights into how some children manage to grow from adverse circumstances.

However, the term "protective" does not necessarily mean that the children have emerged from their childhoods unscathed. Rutter (1985) has noted that in distancing themselves from the disturbed parent, some children may have learned to maintain shallow or rigid relationships with people and a self-centeredness about their own needs. Thus, the concept of resilience implies the absence of an expected outcome (i.e., clinical pathology) rather than the quality of being a happy, socially competent individual. This point is not intended to diminish the importance of protective factors in assessing the children's well-being, but rather to place in perspective the relative importance of having a mentally ill parent.

Nonetheless, a number of factors have been associated with favorable outcomes in children at risk for psychiatric illness. These factors include the availability of at least one healthy attachment figure (Rutter, 1985) or several caretakers who take an interest in the child (Werner, 1988); having an easier, more adaptable temperamental style (Rutter & Quinton, 1984); the ability to focus their energies into some area of achievement, such as school, which gives them an inner sense of competence (Rutter, 1985); and not having a chronically mentally ill mother (Gross, 1983; Shachnow, 1987).

In a longitudinal study, Fisher, Kokes, Cole, Perkins, and Wynne (1987) described a profile of some well-functioning children of mentally ill parents. These children tended to have mothers whose disorders were not chronic and that began when the children were older. They also came from families that were still able to provide warm and nurturant relationships despite the parent's illness. That is, in the absence of a warm and responsive mother, a healthy father or grandparent provided the children with support and nurturance. Thus, children who are given the opportunity to develop strong, healthy attachment relationships early in life appear to function well in spite of their parent's illness.

The Impact of Chronic Psychiatric Illness

Many authors have taken the stance that the specific parental diagnosis is less significant in predicting the effects on the child's mental health than is the chronicity of that illness. Indeed, in most of the studies described in this review, having a chronically ill mother is one of the most powerful predictors of their children's vulnerability to disorder.

In a longitudinal study of infants and toddlers with mentally ill mothers, Sameroff et al. (1982) concluded that the chronicity of the mother's illness was the most important factor affecting the children's social–emotional competence. Children with chronically ill mothers had poorer obstetric and neonatal statuses, more difficult temperaments, and lower scores on developmental tests and were less responsive during interactions with their mothers. Similarly, their mothers were observed to be less responsive and more negative when interacting with their children in the home.

In a study of mother–toddler interactions among a group of mentally ill mothers and a matched group of well mothers, Gross (1983) found no significant differences in the mothers' abilities to be sensitive and effective with their children when analyzed by a maternal diagnostic group. However, there was a crucial difference if the mothers had a history of multiple psychiatric hospitalizations. Chronically ill mothers were significantly less sensitive to their children's cues and far less effective in setting limits on their toddler's behavior.

Why is chronicity such a potent factor? By definition, chronic mental illness implies the persistence of disability. The more chronically ill the parent has become, especially if the target parent is the mother, the more likely that her illness and disability will have intruded on every realm of her life, including her children. For example, chronically ill mothers are likely to be hospitalized more frequently, leading to more abrupt separations from the children and more frequent disruptions in their children's daily lives. Moreover, each admission creates a crisis for the children who may not know or understand what has happened to their parent. In Shachnow's (1987) study of the children of psychiatrically hospitalized parents, the most disturbed children interviewed had a chronically ill mother who functioned poorly between episodes of acute illness.

The following Clinical Examples highlight some of the implications of having a chronically mentally ill parent. Two mothers of young children are presented; one suffered from chronic schizophrenia, and the other had a good premorbid history prior to her postpartum psychotic depression. Both mother–child dyads were eventually seen for treatment in a program for psychiatrically ill mothers and their young children (Gross, 1984; Musick, Stott, Cohler, & Dincin, 1981). While she and her husband wanted their daughter to have a better life than they had had, they did not know how to create it for themselves and their child. Both parents had histories of chronic psychiatric illness, childhood abuse, poor academic and social skills, poverty, and social isolation. In addition, their child's difficult temperament taxed what little energy these parents had. Moreover, Lucy's lack of attachment behavior made Martha feel ineffective as a parent. The pervasiveness of this family's illness and disorganization placed Lucy at highest risk for psychiatric and psychosocial disorder. At 16 months, she had already met DSM-III-R criteria for a disorder of attachment. As a result of their mental illnesses, Martha and Judy demonstrated a re-

CLINICAL EXAMPLE

Martha was the child of an alcoholic mother and a sexually abusive stepfather. She remembers very little about her unhappy childhood until the age of 12 when she was placed in foster care after reporting her stepfather for repeatedly molesting her. Martha's first psychiatric hospitalization occurred at 15 years of age for "acting out" behavior. At 16, she dropped out of high school following a history of failing grades and poor peer relationships. By 18, Martha was married, drinking heavily, and experiencing psychotic symptoms. Her husband, Ralph, was physically abusive, alcoholic, and perpetually unemployed. Together, they had four children. Martha recalls that as a parent she was "terrible . . . I did terrible things." One day, during a psychotic episode, Martha threw her youngest child out of a window. All four children were subsequently removed from her care.

Having nothing to tie them together, she and Ralph subsequently divorced. Martha was devastated by the loss of her children and husband and spent the next 8 years in and out of state psychiatric hospitals. One record cites 28 psychiatric hospitalizations.

Martha later married Larry, a chronic schizophrenic whom she met on a psychiatric inpatient unit. He, too, had been abused as a child, and the couple decided to begin a new life together and raise another family. When Martha was 36, she gave birth to Lucy.

Lucy was a colicky baby, and Martha became extremely anxious caring for a seemingly unhappy and unresponsive baby. Larry was unavailable to help with Lucy's care and did not understand that his wife needed his support. Having had no positive parenting experiences from her own childhood and no friends or family with whom she could confide, Martha felt unable to care for her difficult baby. She asked to have Lucy placed in foster care at 3 months of age.

By 16 months, Lucy was back with her parents but had spent most of her life in a series of foster homes. She displayed no attachment behaviors to her parents; was grossly delayed in her cognitive, social, and language skills; and refused to use adults as a source of comfort. She presented herself as a strong-willed, intense child. Neither parent knew how to set clear, predictable limits on her behavior or engage her in a nurturing relationship. Lucy felt no attachment to her parents and therefore did not reward them with hugs, smiles, and the desire to be loved by them.

One year following treatment, Martha and Larry chose to relinquish parental rights to Lucy. Lucy was quickly adopted by another family with whom Lucy eventually developed a strong attachment relationship.

CLINICAL EXAMPLE

Judy was a first-generation American daughter of a close-knit, working-class Asian family. She had been a shy, bright child whom her parents described as "a good girl." She married her husband 2 weeks after graduating from college and became pregnant within 3 months of her marriage. Her husband had strong expectations that his wife remain at home and care for what he hoped would be many children.

For 6 months, Judy refused to talk about her pregnancy. Her family became very concerned about her lack of joy and unwillingness to prepare for a new baby. They refused to seek help, however, feeling that this was a family problem and one that the family would somehow manage.

When their daughter Kim was born, Judy did not want to hold her. She claimed that the new baby was "the devil" and told her mother that she would not touch nor care for "that baby." Kim was a placid child who rarely cried. Since she demanded little attention, the baby spent much of the time in her crib until her father returned home from work.

As Judy's behavior became more erratic, the family became concerned about the infant's safety. Judy's mother eventually took over the daily care of her granddaughter, but by 3 months of age, the family could no longer cope with Judy's increasingly psychotic behavior. Kim did not smile at, nor make eye contact with, her mother. She had a bald spot on the back of her head from laying supine in her crib for long periods of time. Judy was diagnosed and treated for postpartum psychotic depression. Her 3-month-old daughter was significantly delayed in her socioemotional and motor development.

One year following treatment, Judy and Kim were doing well. Judy could not believe that she ever hated her child, while Kim grew into a happy and healthy toddler. Judy's husband eventually agreed to participate in treatment to work out their marital difficulties.

markable lack of connectedness with their young children. They were both so overwhelmed and frightened by their infants that they were unable to care for them. Their husbands maintained distance from their ill wives and had limited participation in the care of their children. According to Musick et al. (1981), this profile is typical of many mentally ill mothers. However, in contrast to Martha's history of chronic psychiatric illness, lack of supportive resources, poor academic experiences, and social pathology, Judy's history appears much more positive. Most noteworthy, Judy had a good premorbid history, close relationships with an extended family, a history of having received positive parenting experiences, and previous experiences in which she felt competent and effective. Martha and Larry, however, had no resources on which to draw to help them through their crises. As a result, Lucy's parenting options consisted of an inadequate foster care system or an overwhelmed, ineffective mother and an uninvolved father.

Both acute and chronic mental illness severely impair a mother's ability to respond to her children's needs. However, the children of chronically mentally ill parents are at greatest risk for poor outcomes. The parent's pervasive pathology and persistent inability to gain access to supportive resources keep them from being able to make a better life for themselves and their children.

Implications for Clinical Practice

This review provides strong evidence that children of mentally ill parents are at high risk for developing psychiatric and psychosocial disorders; many psychiatrically ill parents are unable to provide a healthy environment for their children because of their illness; and children experience a sudden and profound loss when their parent, particularly their mother, is hospitalized for psychiatric illness. While some important efforts have been made to legislate the development of programs for families at risk (Meisels, 1989), no mechanisms have been established within our health care system for identifying and treating the children of mentally ill parents.

It is proposed that using the parent's hospitalization or outpatient treatment as an opportunity to evaluate the children's mental health is a feasible and effective method for identifying children at risk (Gross, 1989; Gross & Semprevivo, 1989). When children have been included in their mentally ill parent's treatment, the results have been remarkable.

For example, Rosenheck and Nathan (1984) describe a program for evaluating and treating children of chronically ill psychiatric patients in a Veterans Administration hospital. The authors reported that their chronically ill adult patients were deeply concerned about their children's well-being but had avoided seeking help because of their distrust of psychiatric settings and of how they would be judged as parents. When the children's treatment was instituted as part of the patient's treatment, the family became extremely receptive to psychiatric help.

Shachnow (1987) interviewed the offspring of 22 hospitalized patients to explore the impact of the parent's mental illness and hospitalization on their children's mental health. Interestingly, simply including the children's evaluation as a part of the parent's treatment yielded a number of positive outcomes outside of the initial research goals. First, the author found that 50% of the children were experiencing psychiatric symptoms severe enough to require treatment. These children were subsequently referred for outpatient care. Second, children received an opportunity to discuss openly their parent's illness and how it had been affecting them. Third, expressing an interest in the children's well-being sensitized the well parent to the effects the illness and hospitalization were having on their children. In subsequent family sessions, well parents paid more attention to their children's concerns and symptomatic behavior. Finally, information gained from the children's interviews added to the treatment team's understanding of the patient as an individual and as a parent with many of the concerns that other parents face in raising their children.

While Shachnow (1987) and Rosenheck and Nathan (1984) demonstrate the feasibility of assessing the parent's capabilities and the children's mental health as part of the treatment program, two recent nursing studies underscore the extent to which this opportunity lies untapped. Rudolph, Larson, Hough, and Arorian (1990) reviewed the charts of 35 hospitalized pregnant psychotic women, most of whom had been hospitalized previously at least five times. Although five patients had been homeless and 25 were receiving some form of government subsidy, few charts contained any documentation regarding access to supportive resources that would enable these mothers to care for their newborns. In addition, prenatal assessments of their ability to retain infant custody were absent in 30 cases. The absence of parenting assessments were of particular concern because 23 women had given birth to other children, but only two were still living with their children.

Similarly, Gross and Semprevivo (1989) reviewed the charts of 21 hospitalized mentally ill mothers of children younger than 6 years of age. The purpose of this review was to describe the parenting issues raised by these mothers during their hospitalizations. None of the records reviewed addressed the mother's ability to care for her children following discharge or the status of the children's mental health. Only one chart contained a note indicating who was caring for the children in the mother's absence. Notes regarding the mother's parenting concerns were evident in nine charts, although the patient's concerns were used to plan treatment and discharge in only one case.

The lack of a plan for assessing the children's mental health is a missed opportunity to identify children at risk and provide treatment for families in crisis. Moreover, having to care for children following discharge from a psychiatric hospital can be a major stressor that might eventually precipitate readmission. For example, in the study by Gross and Semprevivo (1989), most mothers were the primary caregivers for two or more children. Thus, not assessing the mother's ability to manage the stressors inherent in caring for children ignores a potential factor in her recovery following discharge.

The Parenting Interview

When a parent is hospitalized, the psychiatric team should address the following parenting issues as part of the treatment plan:

- Identify parenting problems that affect the children's mental health and the parent's ability to resume their parental role following discharge.
- Help the parent maintain contact with her children during her hospitalization.
- Develop discharge plans that will enable the parent to maintain or develop healthy relationships with her children.

When the parent is admitted, at least one actual or potential problem related to parenting should be added to the care plan. For example, High Risk for Altered Parenting related to illness and hospitalization would signal the treatment team to the need for assessing how the parent's hospitalization and illness have affected the children, their daily care, and the mother's feelings about being a parent. Once sufficient information is obtained, this potential problem can be clarified or resolved.

A treatment goal for parents admitted for psychiatric care might be, "Patient will discuss how she feels about her children, her caretaking ability, and resuming her maternal role following discharge."

Once additional information is obtained, this goal can be more specific to the parent's needs.

Mentally ill parents often are ambivalent about revealing their concerns regarding their children or themselves as parents. They fear that others will consider them poor parents, threaten to take their children away from them, or blame them for any problems their children are experiencing. However, many parents also want to talk about how their illness impairs their ability to care for their children, how difficult it can be to raise children when you do not feel well, and how much they rely on their children for love and affection (Gross & Semprevivo, 1989).

The parenting interview is a guide for nurses to use when interviewing hospitalized mentally ill parents about their children and about themselves as parents (Gross, 1989) (Box 8-1). It is not a validated instrument but a series of pertinent questions culled from the author's clinical experience. The interview gives parents an opportunity to discuss their concerns with a health care professional and identify parenting issues that may require intervention.

> Mrs. J was a 26-year-old mother admitted to the psychiatric unit with a diagnosis of manic depression. Mrs. J described her day with her 16-month-old son as "exhausting." As a result of her depression, Mrs. J had difficulty awakening in the morning and was often unable to get her son dressed and fed until her husband arrived home in the evening. Prior to Mrs. J's discharge, the primary nurse worked out a schedule with Mr. and Mrs. J that included help for Mrs. J in getting her son dressed and fed in the morning. Discharge plans also included a referral to a community-based outpatient program for parents and children. The purpose of the referral was to engage Mrs. J in a program that would provide parenting support, ongoing parent–child assessments, and opportunities for social interaction with other mothers with young children.

The parenting interview guide also includes a question about the parent's plans for maintaining contact with his or her children during the hospitalization. Buckwalter et al. (1988) assert that an important goal during the parent's hospitalization is to keep family relationships intact. Often, parents are fearful of their children's reactions to their impaired state or fear they will be unable to answer their children's questions. It is important for children to know their mother or father is alive and receiving care. Thus, phone calls, pictures, or letters can be reassuring to children when parents feel unable to see their children during the hospitalization. Asking the parents how they will keep contact with their children conveys the message

BOX 8–1 • PARENTING INTERVIEW QUESTIONS

1. Who is caring for your children while you are in the hospital?
2. How do you feel about those child care arrangements?
3. Who usually cares for your children during the day and during the night?
4. Tell me about your children. For example, are they easy going or difficult to handle at home? What kinds of things do they do well? What kinds of things do you wish they did better?
5. What things do you do best as a mother/father?
6. Do you have any concerns about the way your children are getting along in life and in the family? Please explain.
7. Do you have any concerns about how you are raising your children? Please explain.
8. One of the most difficult parts of raising children is disciplining them. What methods do you use to discipline your children when they disobey or do something dangerous?
9. To whom do you go to for support or advice when you need help with your children? How do these people help you?
10. What plans have you made for keeping contact with your children during your hospitalization?
11. Raising children can be a very stressful experience for parents. Is there any way we can help you cope with the stresses of parenting when you return home?

(Adapted from Gross, D. [1989]. At risk: Children of the mentally ill. *Journal of Psychosocial Nursing, 27,* 14–19.)

that their relationships with their children are important and need to be maintained.

> Mrs. P was hospitalized for major depression following a suicide attempt in her home. She expressed concern about her oldest daughter, who was a bright but depressed 9-year-old, "She knows why I am here, but I don't want her to see me like this. So I have told her she cannot come. But I feel terrible. I know she needs me, and she's worried about me. The other day she asked me if I was going to die." Her primary nurse asked Mrs. P what she feared her daughter might think or say if she were to see her. Mrs. P replied "I don't know if I'm not going to die. I still haven't decided if I want to live, but I'm afraid to tell her that." Mrs. P and the nurse discussed the mother's ambivalence about seeing her daughter and possible responses to the questions the little girl might ask should she choose to see her. Other options for reassuring her daughter that she was alright were discussed, including sending a card or picture home.

Assessment of the Children

Because children of mentally ill parents are at risk for developing psychiatric and psychosocial disorders, an assessment of the children is strongly recommended. School-age and adolescent offspring of mentally ill parents should be interviewed to determine how they are feeling about their parent's illness and hospitalization and how they are coping with living with a mentally ill parent. If the child reports academic problems, poor peer relationships, difficulty concentrating, depressive symptoms, suicidal ideation, or other symptoms indicative of poor psychosocial functioning, a more extensive psychiatric assessment is necessary to determine if referral for psychiatric treatment is warranted.

The interview also is an opportunity to provide information and to correct misinformation regarding their parent's illness. Children often feel responsible for their parent's illness or do not understand what is wrong with their parent. Shachnow (1987) reported that some of the children in her sample had assumed they had caused their parent's illness and hospitalization by misbehaving or not doing something they should have done.

Assessing the mental health of infants and preschoolers requires expert observation and interviewing skills specific to the developmental issues that arise during the first 5 years of life. The quality of the parent–infant interaction and the degree to which the child is functioning at his or her developmental level are important indicators of the home environment. Because most child psychiatric nurses do not have expertise assessing infants and preschoolers, consultants may be necessary. For example, many occupational and physical therapists have expertise in conducting developmental assessments of young children. Nurses who have received standardized training in the use of the Nursing Child Assessment Feeding and Teaching Scales (Barnard, 1978) can rate the quality of mother–child interaction following an unobtrusive observation period. Nurses who are experienced in assessing attachment and other childhood emotional disorders should be contacted for consultation.

Important warning signs that young children may be at risk for a psychosocial disorder are listed in Box 8-2. These signs include evidence of inadequate well baby care, evidence of growth failure, atypical or delayed development (as evidenced by failure on a standardized screening test), evidence of attachment disorder, and delay or abnormality in achieving expected emotional milestones (Blackman, 1986).

Although it is not realistic to expect that the health care team can treat the children's psychosocial disorders during the parent's hospitalization, appropriate outpatient programs can be contacted prior to discharge. For example, we have developed a directory of early intervention programs for psychiatrically high-risk parents and young children in the Chicago area for nurses to use when planning discharge. Other organizations, such as The Family Resource Coalition in Chicago, have developed a resource guide that includes support programs throughout the United States (Levine, 1988).

The Parenting Alliance

Because parents may be reluctant for their children to be evaluated or to admit to parenting problems, it is crucial for families to feel that these assessments are intended to be supportive. Raising children, especially young children or adolescents, is a stressful experience for all parents and requires an enormous amount of energy. Thus, in planning the parent's discharge, it is crucial for the psychiatric team to better understand the children and their needs so they can anticipate the types of stressors the parent will face when going home and identify strategies for managing those stressors; assist the parent in addressing some of the concerns their children have about the illness and hospitalization; and identify and initiate contact

BOX 8–2 • SIGNS OF POOR PARENT–CHILD RELATIONSHIPS (AGES BIRTH TO 5 YEARS)

1. Lack of well child care
2. Evidence of growth failure
3. Atypical or delayed cognitive, socioemotional, motor, sensory, or behavioral development as evidenced by failure on a standardized screening or assessment instrument
4. Parent's concern that the child is significantly less competent or happy than other children
5. Evidence of an attachment disorder, such as the following:
   - Persistent failure to initiate or respond to most social interactions
   - Fearfulness and hypervigilence that does not respond to comforting by parent
   - Indiscriminant sociability, such as seeking affection from a stranger or no preference for play and affection displayed by the child between parent and a stranger
6. Delay or abnormality in achieving expected emotional milestones, such as the following:
   - A lack of pleasurable interest in the social world
   - An inability to communicate needs clearly and appropriately for age, either through verbal or nonverbal cues

(Cited from Blackman, J. [1986]. *Warning signals: Basic criteria for tracking at-risk infants and toddlers.* Washington, DC: National Center for Clinical Infant Programs and American Psychiatric Association [1994]. DSM-IV. Washington, DC: Author.)

with appropriate outpatient services for all members of the family.

Parents are exquisitely sensitive to other people's judgments about their children. For example, a nurse who soothes a baby's distress when the infant's mother cannot may no longer be seen as an ally, but a competitor who is more competent than the mother. Thus, nurses must understand the mentally ill parent's view of themselves, their children, and the childrearing culture that guides the parent's behavior and attitudes. Parents must be treated as allies and as the people who are most knowledgeable about their children.

Finally, nurses must enter the assessment process with the assumption that the parents may already have a feeling that something is wrong, although they may not be able to verbalize that feeling to the nurse, and that they ultimately want their children to be healthy. If the health care team approaches the family as collaborators rather than investigators, they are more likely to achieve a working alliance.

Summary

There are two ironies in the literature on the children of mentally ill parents. First, we lament the absence of funding for services that focus on the prevention and early treatment of mental illness but have failed to capitalize on opportunities for early intervention when they arise. Second, "family involvement" in child psychiatry appears to be operationalized as the inclusion of parents, while the same term in adult psychiatry appears to be operationalized as the inclusion of spouses. Because a large number of children of mentally ill parents will develop psychosocial or psychiatric disorders and one day enter the adult psychiatric treatment system, children should be included in the care of their mentally ill parent. To neglect this component of nursing care is a missed opportunity for the assessment and early detection of parenting problems and childhood disorders.

REFERENCES

Anthony, E. J. (1973). Mourning and psychic loss of the parent. In E. J. Anthony & C. Koupernik (Eds.), *The child in his family* (Vol. 2). (pp. 255–264). New York: John Wiley & Sons.

Anthony, E. J. (1985). Psychotic influences on parenting. In E. J. Anthony & G. Pollack (Eds.), *Parental influences: In health and disease* (pp. 259–315). Boston: Little, Brown & Co.

Anthony, E. J., & Cohler, B. (1987). *The invulnerable child.* New York: The Guilford Press.

Asarnow, J. R. (1988). Children at risk for schizophrenia: Converging lines of evidence. *Schizophrenia Bulletin, 14,* 613–631.

Barnard, K. (1978). *Nursing child assessment satellite training project: Learning resource manual.* Seattle: University of Washington School of Nursing.

Bertelsen, A., Harvald, B., & Jauge, M. (1977) A Danish twin study of manic depressive disorders. *British Journal of Psychiatry, 13,* 330–351.

Billings, A., & Moos, R. (1983). Comparisons of children of depressed and nondepressed parents: A social-environmental perspective. *Journal of Abnormal Child Psychology, 11,* 463–485.

Billings, A., & Moos, R. (1985). Children of parents with unipolar depression: A controlled 1-year follow-up. *Journal of Abnormal Children Psychology, 14,* 149–166.

Blackman, J. (1986). *Warning signals: Basic criteria for tracking at-risk infants and toddlers.* Washington, DC: National Center for Clinical Infant Programs.

Bleuler, M. (1974). The offspring of schizophrenics. *Schizophrenia Bulletin, 8,* 93–107.

Bleuler, M. (1978). In S.M. Clemens (Trans.), *The schizophrenic disorders.* New Haven: Yale University Press.

Bradley, R., & Caldwell, B. (1977). Home observation for measurement of the environment: A validation study of screening efficiency. *American Journal of Mental Deficiency, 81,* 417–420.

Bretherton, I., & Waters, E. (1985). Growing points of attachment theory and research. *Monographs of the Society for Research in Child Development, 50,* 1–2, (Serial No. 209).

Brockington, I., & Kumar, R. (1982). *Motherhood and mental illness.* London: Academic Press.

Buckwalter, K., Kerfoot, K., & Stolley, J. (1988). Children of affectively ill parents. *Journal of Psychosocial Nursing, 26,* 8–14.

Canadian Mental Health Association. (1987). *Is anybody listening? Children at risk from the major mental disabilities of their parents.* Toronto, Ontario: Canadian Mental Health Association.

Children's Defense Fund Reports. (1989). *Poverty drops slightly in 1988 but continues to rise for young children and young families* (pp. 1 and 4). Washington, DC: Children's Defense Fund.

Cohler, B., & Musick, J. (1983). Psychopathology of parenthood: Implications for the mental health of children. *Infant Mental Health Journal, 4,* 140–164.

Crosby, D. (1989). First person account: Growing up with a schizophrenic mother. *Schizophrenia Bulletin, 15,* 507–509.

Drake, R., Racusin, R., & Murphy, R. (1990). Suicide among adolescents with mentally ill parents. *Hospital and Community Psychiatry, 41,* 921–922.

Ekdahl, M., Rice, E., & Schmidt, W. (1962). Children of parents hospitalized for mental illness. *American Journal of Public Health, 52,* 428–435.

Field, T. (1984). Early interactions between infants and their postpartum depressed mothers. *Infant Behavior and Development, 7,* 517–522.

Field, T., Healy, B., Goldstein, S., Perry, S., Bendell, D., Schanberg, S., Zimmerman, & Kuhn, C. (1988). Infants of depressed mothers show "depressed" behavior even with nondepressed adults. *Child Development, 59,* 1569–1579.

Fisher, L., Kokes, R., Cole, R., Perkins, P., & Wynne, L. (1987). Competent children at risk: A study of well-functioning offspring of disturbed parents. In E. J. Anthony & B. Cohler (Eds.), *The invulnerable children* (pp. 211–228). New York: Guilford Press.

Forehand, R., & Brody, G. (1985). The association between parental personal marital adjustment and parent-child interactions in a clinic sample. *Behavior Research and Therapy, 23,* 211–212.

Fox, J. M. (1990, November). *Schizophrenia: Perceptual and cognitive deficits.* Paper presented at the State of the Art and Science of Psychiatric Nursing Conference, National Institute of Mental Health, Bethesda, MD.

Gaensbauer, T., Harmon, R., Cytryn, L., & McKnew, D. (1984). Social and affective development in children with manic–depressive parent. *American Journal of Psychiatry, 141,* 223–229.

Goodman, S., & Brumley, H. E. (1990). Schizophrenic and depressed mothers: Relational deficits in parenting. *Developmental Psychology, 26,* 31–39.

Gross, D. (1983). How some dyads "fail": A qualitative analysis with implications for nursing practice. *Infant Mental Health Journal, 4,* 272–286.

Gross, D. (1984). Relationships at risk: Issues and interventions with a disturbed mother-infant dyad. *Perspectives in Psychiatric Care, 22,* 159–164.

Gross, D. (1989). At risk: Children of the mentally ill. *Journal of Psychosocial Nursing, 27,* 14–19.

Gross, D., & Semprevivo, D. (1989). Mentally ill mothers of young children: Analysis of in-patient chart reviews. *Journal of Child and Adolescent Psychiatric Nursing, 2,* 105–109.

Jouriles, E., Pfiffner, L., & O'Leary, S. (1988). Marital conflict, parenting and toddler conduct problems. *Journal of Abnormal Child Psychology, 16,* 197–206.

Keller, M., Beardslee, W., Dorer, D., Lavori, P., Samuelson, H., & Klerman, G. (1986). Impact of severity and chronicity of parental affective illness on adaptive functioning and psychopathology in children. *Archives of General Psychiatry, 43,* 930–937.

Kety, S. (1988). Schizophrenic illness in the families of schizophrenic adoptees: Findings from the Danish national sample. *Schizophrenia Bulletin, 14,* 217–222.

Kokes, R., Harder, D., Fisher, L., & Strauss, J. (1980). Child competence and psychiatric risk: V. Sex of patient parent and dimension of psychopathology. *Journal of Nervous and Mental Disease, 168,* 348–352.

Lanquetot, R. (1984). First person account: Confessions of the daughter of a schizophrenic. *Schizophrenia Bulletin, 10,* 467–471.

Levine, C. (1988). *Programs to strengthen families: A resource guide.* Chicago: Family Resource Coalition.

Liaschenko, J. (1989). Changing paradigms within psychiatry: Implications for nursing research. *Archives of Psychiatric Nursing, 3,* 153–158.

Mahler, M., Pine, F., & Bergman, A. (1975). *The psychological birth of the human infant.* New York: Basic Books.

Marcus, J., Auerbach, J., Wilkinson, L., & Burack, C. (1981). Infants at risk for schizophrenia: The Jerusalen infant development study. *Archives of General Psychiatry, 38,* 703–713.

McBride, A. B. (1990). Psychiatric nursing in the 1990's. *Archives of Psychiatric Nursing, 4,* 21–28.

Meisels, S. (1988). Meeting the mandate of public law 99–457: Early childhood intervention in the nineties. *American Journal of Orthopsychiatry, 59,* 451–460.

Musick, J., Stott, F., Cohler, B., & Dincin, J. (1981). Posthospital treatment for psychotic depressed mothers and their young children. In M. Lansky (Ed.), *Family therapy and major psychopathology* (pp. 91–121). New York: Grune & Stratton.

Pardes, H., Kaufmann, Pincus, H., & West, A. (1989). Genetics and psychiatry: Past discoveries, current dilemmas, and future directions. *American Journal of Psychiatry, 146,* 435–443.

Plomin, R., & Daniels, D. (1987). Why are children in the

same family so different from one another? *Behavioral and Brain Sciences, 10,* 1–60.

Radke-Yarrow, M., Cummings, E., Kuczynski, L., & Chapman, M. (1985). Patterns of attachment in two- and three-year-olds in normal families and families with parental depression. *Child Development, 56,* 884–893.

Rosenheck, R., & Nathan, P. (1984). Treatment of children of volatile psychotic adults in the adult psychiatric setting. *American Journal of Psychiatry, 141,* 1555–1558.

Rudolph, B., Larson, G., Hough, E. E., & Arorian, K. (1990). Hospitalized pregnant psychotic women: Characteristics and treatment issues. *Hospital and Community Psychiatry, 41,* 159–163.

Rutter, M. (1985). Resilience in the face of adversity: Protective factors and resistance of psychiatric disorder. *British Journal of Psychiatry, 147,* 598–611.

Rutter, M., & Quinton, D. (1984). Parental psychiatric disorder: Effects on children. *Psychological Medicine, 14,* 853–880.

Sameroff, A., Seifer, R., & Zax, M. (1982). Early development of children at risk for emotional disorder. *Monographs of the Society for Research in Child Development, 47,* 7. (Serial No. 199).

Shachnow, J. (1987). Preventive intervention with children of hospitalized psychiatric patients. *American Journal of Orthopsychiatry, 57,* 66–77.

Thomas, A., & Chess, S. (1984). Genesis and evolution of behavioral disorders: From infancy to early adult life. *American Journal of Psychiatry, 141,* 1–9.

Weissman, M., Prusoff, B., Gammon, D., Merikangas, K., Leckman, J., & Kidd, K. (1984). Psychopathology in the children (ages 6–18) of depressed and normal parents. *Journal of the American Academy of Child Psychiatry, 23,* 78–84.

Welner, A., & Rice, J. (1988). School-aged children of depressed parents: A blind and controlled study. *Journal of Affective Disorders, 15,* 291–302.

Werner, E. (1988). Individual difference, universal needs: A 30-year study of resilient high risk infants. *Zero to Three, 4,* 1–5.

You cannot prevent the birds of sorrow from flying over your head, but you can prevent them from nesting in your hair. —(CHINESE PROVERB)

CHAPTER

9

Bereavement in Children

Alean Royes

Loss and grief are a natural part of life and are unavoidable. Most people associate grief with death, but we grieve over the loss of anything important. Because of their limited developmental capacities and level of maturity, children are especially vulnerable and experience greater difficulty than adults in resolving and managing losses. Also, the ability to adapt to losses depends "on the relationships that exist between a child and many other individuals in his or her life" (Rosen, 1986, p. 8). Losses are inherently stressful and inevitably bring about changes; tremendous losses become numbing experiences. Children who have experienced and coped with a previous loss may cope more successfully with intense losses, such as a family member through death, divorce, or other separation (Salladay & Royal, 1981).

Children experience grief over the loss of many things, including pets, toys, and friend relationships. This chapter examines the impact of death and divorce on children. These losses increase the risk of problems for children because of the threat they pose to a child's security (Jackson, 1982). In this chapter the nursing process is applied to the problems of children's grief and loss, using interventions to lessen the negative impact on their growth and development.

Death

Various customs related to death and grieving have evolved and changed throughout history. In earlier times death was not a mystery. Medical knowledge with sophisticated technology was limited. Mortality rates were high, and many people died at home; thus, children were exposed to death. People were encouraged to grieve; women wore black clothing, and men black arm bands for 1 year. This period allowed them time to mourn the deceased person's birthday, holidays, and special events. Mourning was normal and necessary, giving the bereaved person time to gradually let go of the emotional energy invested in the lost loved one.

Increased medical knowledge, improved technology, advanced nursing care, and changes in society revolutionized our outlook on death. People began living longer, and death in hospitals became more common than death at home. Children were not exposed to death, and death became a frightening and upsetting experience.

Kubler-Ross (1974) ignited a new interest in death through her work with dying patients and publications on death and dying. Dying patients were encouraged to talk about death, and once again the subject of death became more acceptable. Despite this, and Koocher's (1974) work to help lift barriers on discussing death with children, "the subject remains a taboo topic within the American culture" (Zambelli, Clark, Barile, & de Jong, 1988, p. 43).

Death remains frightening and a topic often avoided with children. Parents, overwhelmed by their own grief, are often unavailable to help their children mourn. Also, most parents want to protect their children from emotional pain and are not aware of the impact that death has on children, their need for honesty, and the need to grieve. Children should be told the truth about death, enabling them to "make sense of their changed circumstances and the reactions of those around them, and to be able to mourn their loss effectively. What to tell will depend on their age and understanding" (Black & Kaplan, 1988, p. 626). When children are not given the truth, they will grieve again when they learn the truth, often manifesting abnormal behavior. Understanding how children of various ages conceptualize death and accepting their feelings and behaviors related to death will help nurses to prepare for the task of helping parents and children grieve and possibly escape long-term emotional scars.

CHILDREN'S CONCEPTS OF DEATH

Most authorities agree that a child's ability to cope with bereavement is closely related to age level and corresponding cognitive development. Nagy's (1948) classic work during war times was one of the first research studies that related to children and death. Analyzing interviews, she developed stages of children's conceptualization of death. Wass and Scott (1978) used Piaget's (1970) framework to describe children's conceptualization of death. They described children's concepts of death as progressing from the preoperational to concrete to formal stages of thought.

Piaget's (1970) framework offers a description of the evolution of learning and adaptation, which remains relevant to nurses working with bereaved children. It provides a tool for assessing a child's cognitive level and helps to identify misconceptions. Piaget's theory is primarily concerned with what and how children learn. Cognitive growth occurs as children pass through definite stages representing a change from one type of behavior or thought to another. Individuals progress from the earliest sensorimotor stage to preoperational, followed by concrete operations and finally formal operations stage at different ages.

Preoperational children generally misunderstand death, and discussions about death should be brief, structured, and honest. Children in the concrete operational stage of development begin to accept the irreversibility of death, and their curiosity arouses questions related to actual facts about death and life after death. At this stage children begin to focus on grief reactions. During the formal operational stage of development, children's understanding of death is more sophisticated, yet their struggle for a new identity and emotionality impacts their grieving (Gaffney, 1988b).

INFANCY TO 2 YEARS

Children younger than 2 years of age have no concept of death. However, they perceive, and are affected by, responses from their caretakers. Therefore, they may react to feelings of separation. For toddlers, the loss of a mother or significant person can cause worry, anger, and withdrawal. Infants are extremely sensitive to maternal communications, including speech, movement, and expressions. Ongoing deficits in these areas may result in cognitive and emotional problems (Goodyer, 1990). At times of separation and loss, infants and toddlers need gentleness, patience, comfort, consistency, and continuation of a regular routine.

2 TO 5 YEARS

Children 2 to 5 years of age see death as temporary and often conceptualize death in "reference to animals, creatures, and nature" (Jozefowski, 1983, p. 277). They will be confronted with death at some time during this age, especially through television where death is artificial, which reinforces their belief that death is completely reversible. They act out death through play, "playing dead" one minute and alive the next. "Preschool children's sense of well being is linked to being able to play"; they must have adequate play time to preserve their emotional health and expedite their grieving process (Royes, 1990, p. 2). Two- to 5-year-olds perceive death through magical thinking, believing that they are somehow responsible for a death and that it is a way of punishing them for a wrongdoing. Children of this age move between fantasy and reality with death, which is confusing for them. It is very painful for them when someone who used to be there for them is no longer there. They recognize that people around them feel sad and frightened and they too become frightened. They are upset by their natural tendency to associate evil and darkness. Nightmares are common; they become afraid of the dark.

Play allows 2- to 5-year-old children to talk and think about the threatening aspects of death. Fantasy and play offer relief from the intense feelings associated with death, allowing children to confront death free of sadness, fear, and hurt. Brief, honest explanations are required to respond to their impressive curiosity. Adults must be realistic without interrupting the child's need for magical thinking.

CLINICAL EXAMPLE

Donny was 18 months old when his mother, Jane, was suddenly killed in an automobile accident. Jane had not worked outside of the home since Donny was born. He was left occasionally with a sitter. He had depended heavily on Jane and had begun to mimic her feelings and actions. When she suddenly disappeared from his life, he changed from a happy, content toddler to one with frequent temper tantrums. He began banging his head, sucking his thumb, and hiding under his bed. Donny's father was overwhelmed with his own grief and was easily frustrated with Donny's actions. By age 4, his behavior had become an established pattern and considered part of his personality. Professional counseling at the age 5 produced noticeable and positive changes in his behavior.

6 TO 9 YEARS

Children at age 6 or 7 still possess magical thinking and may associate death with monsters and witches. Gradually they develop a clearer understanding of death and begin to become aware that they too can die. They start to fear death yet become secretive and reluctant to share their thoughts and feelings. Worries about mutilation or destruction are common. Feeling responsible and guilty, they continue to link thoughts of death with fears of wrongdoing and punishment. At this age boys frequently associate death with violence; girls associate it with life events and nature (Jozefowski, 1983).

Six- to 9-year-old children dealing with death require compassion and nonjudgmental responses. They need an opportunity to say "good bye" and to resolve their relationship with the person who died. Often they have feelings of anger at the person who died and need opportunities to express and ventilate these feelings. Reassurance that they were loved by the person who died, accompanied by acceptance and empathetic listening, helps them deal with their loss. They seek strength from their parents and want to hear their beliefs about death.

10 TO 12 YEARS

Children of this age realize that death is permanent and that everyone dies. They are curious about the biologic aspects of death and ask questions, such as "Was blood everywhere?" They are fascinated by the shock aspects of death, the horrible, terrible, and "gory" aspects. They associate death with evil and sadness. When death occurs in their own family, 10- to 12-year-old children show ambivalent feelings and are greatly affected by the loss. Their separation anxiety increases, along with continued fears of mutilation and suffocation. They may be reluctant to leave home. Children at this age may try to act "tough" to cover for their true feelings, such as feeling ashamed of their tears. Daydreaming, problems concentrating in school, and a drop in school performance are common grief reactions in latency-age children.

Others may bargain with themselves to do everything "perfectly" to make up for the death, especially the death of a sibling. Their performance in school and sports may improve. These children often think that the sibling who died was the parent's favorite, because bereaved parents may idealize the lost child or raise him or her to sainthood as a self-protective mechanism. Emotionally the

CLINICAL EXAMPLE

Janice was 3 years old when her father died from cancer. She asked her mother, "Who shot Daddy?" She believed people died from being shot "just like on T.V." She also asked, "Will he be home tomorrow?"

Amy was 4 when her 8-year-old sister died. Her parents honestly discussed the death with her; however, Amy began having nightmares and screamed in the middle of the night. After exploring issues with her, Amy admitted that she had kicked her sister and thought if she went to sleep, she also would die. She continued to ask when her sister was coming back so they could play together.

When visiting the cemetery, where his baby sister was buried, with his mother, 4-year-old Tommy became upset and concerned that nobody was feeding the baby or changing her diapers.

CLINICAL EXAMPLE

Jonathan, age 10, and his sister, 8-year-old Nancy, were outside playing when Jonathan rode his bike into the street and was struck by a car and killed. Nancy became withdrawn and had frequent episodes of crying and nightmares. She felt angry toward Jonathan for riding his bike in the street and guilty for feeling angry. Her parents, overcome by their own problems and grief, were unavailable to help Nancy or see that she received professional help. Later, at age 30, Nancy continued to feel responsible and guilty about the accident.

children begin to distance themselves from others and need comfort and reassurance from an empathetic listener. They must be allowed to vent their feelings and know that it is acceptable to cry.

ADOLESCENTS

Adolescents view death more abstractly, more similar to adult views. They are striving for independence and may try to break away from parental beliefs about death and formulate their own ideas. Adolescents also think that nothing can happen to them, only to others. However, they feel threatened by death because it involves destruction of life, and they are concerned with their own bodies. Their own mortality is threatened when someone close to them dies; they may withdraw and deny the loss. With unpredictable emotions, they may respond to minor events with much more emotion than when confronted with the death of a loved one.

Adolescents may reject family rituals, such as funerals, yet when a friend dies and other peers mourn, they too may mourn openly in large groups. At such times, they realize that life is fragile. Adolescents need time, understanding, and support from people around them. Compromising is generally the best way to deal with them while they mourn in their own way. It is important to include them in the decision making regarding funerals of loved ones. By viewing the body and attending the funeral, adolescents see firsthand the reality of death, which helps them to confront their own denial used to protect themselves. The loss of the same-sex parent increases an adolescent's risk for prolonged depressive symptoms (Rutter, 1986).

Although concepts of death related to age and cognitive level are useful guidelines when working with children affected by death (Table 9-1), it is important to remember that children do not fit neatly into categories; their individuality must be considered. Furman (1964) believed children ages 2 to 3 could comprehend death. Spinetta and Deasy-Spinetta (1981) observed children with cancer between the ages of 6 and 10 and indicated that these children with life-threatening diseases comprehended the finality of death. "Family, social networks, and cultural norms" are significant factors in determining the impact of loss on children (Rosen, 1986, p. 9). All children need permission to grieve, cry, express their feelings, and hurt (Lester, 1987). The family is the best place to express this permission. Unresolved grief at any age will manifest itself eventually. Children's fears may remain submerged until life situations trigger them, but they will resurface then as physical and psychiatric problems.

Divorce

Since the 1950s the divorce rate has increased alarmingly. There are more than 300,000 divorces in the United States annually, affecting approximately 600,000 children (Wahlstrom, 1983). Social changes within American society contribute to the problem. Children and adolescents are thrown into situations without choices and feel not only the

CLINICAL EXAMPLE

Becky was 12 years old when her beloved grandfather died. She started worrying about her own death. She had extreme outbursts of crying and sorrow, followed by anxiety attacks marked by shortness of breath.

CLINICAL EXAMPLE

Margaret was 15 years old when her 7-year-old brother died of leukemia. She said, "I helped a lot at home and tried to do everything right. My parents had enough to deal with. I didn't want to upset them more. I just pretended it never happened. It doesn't matter how hard I try though, I can't please my parents. My brother was their favorite. I am not good enough for them."

loss of both parents' presence, but also changes in homes, schools, friends, and their sense of security. Rarely are children relieved by their parents' decision to divorce. Children continuously involved in marital disharmony suffer constant losses and have an increased risk of psychiatric problems (Rutter, 1989). The antecedent effects and quality of social disruptions must be considered when determining the impact of loss children suffer. Hetherington (1989) found that circumstances involved in the decision to divorce and postdivorce relations affect children's social and emotional well-being. When the father is absent in divorced families, mother–son relations are tense with ongoing con-

TABLE 9–1 Progression of Age-Related Concepts About Death, Related Behaviors, and Needs

Age	Concept of Death	Common Behaviors Related to Death	Needs
Infancy to 2 years	No concept of death Death means separation	Worry Anger Withdrawal Lots of crying Clinging Upset stomach	Comfort Gentleness Patience Regular routine Caregiver consistency Warmth
2 to 5 years	Death seen as temporary Death only happens to other people Death seen through magical thinking Relate cause to themselves May see death as punishment	Nightmares Fear of the dark Frightened easily followed by anger, regression Inappropriate comments Wants to hear story of death over and over Act out death through play	Honesty Allow to cry Give brief explanations Allow to play act death Avoid punishment Patience Help to be realistic without interrupting need for fantasy
6 to 9 years	Magical thinking still present in 6–7 years of age Begin to develop clearer understanding of death Awareness that they too can die Begin to fear death	Difficulty talking about death Guilt feelings Anger at loved one for dying Uses art to tell story of death Death may be play acted in war and violence Worries about abandonment Concern about loss Sadness Worries about own death—or parent's death Try to reason the meaning of life, heaven, and life after death	Help in expression of anger and guilt Acceptance and empathetic listening Avoid punishment Reassurance that they were loved by the loved one who died Information on parents' beliefs about death

(continued)

TABLE 9–1 Progression of Age-Related Concepts About Death, Related Behaviors, and Needs *(Continued)*

Age	Concept of Death	Common Behaviors Related to Death	Needs
10 to 12 years	Understand that death is permanent May think death is punishment for bad behavior Realize that everyone dies Death is seen as terrible and horrible and associated with evil and sadness	Worries about own death Fear of being buried alive Worries about pain and suffering Separation anxiety Reluctant to leave home Daydreaming Ambivalent Ashamed to cry Drawings contain symbols of lifelessness such as closed eyes and mouth and broken hearts May be embarrassed by death Curious about biological aspects of death	Compassion Avoid punishment Allow to vent feelings Explain that crying is normal and OK Comfort and reassurance
Adolescents	See death abstractly, more like adults May break away from parental concepts (both religious and secular) and try to formulate own ideas	Not predictable Feelings of hopelessness, neglect, and that no one cares Think nothing can happen to them Withdrawal and denial of loss Rejection of funeral custom, with exception of when a classmate dies—then attends funeral in large numbers and mourns openly	Need "room to breathe" and to think No set rule or pattern to follow, but do not exclude Include in decision making Avoid punishment

flict. However, when the father is involved in the son's life and shows concern, the harmony between mother and son improves dramatically (Block, Block, & Gyerde, 1988). If stepfathers enter into the relationship, existing problems increase in intensity (Hetherington, 1988). There are no simple ways to describe how divorce affects children. In addition to family relations before and after the divorce, other factors contributing to a child's response and adjustment include the child's age, cognitive developmental status, and social factors outside of the home. Piaget's (1970) stages of age and cognitive development are useful when assessing specific effects of divorce experienced by children (Table 9-2).

INFANCY

Infants react to feelings of separation, to the stress of their caretakers, and to stress within their environment. Parents experiencing divorce often are depressed and preoccupied and project these feelings onto their infants. Infants may have a disrupted sleeping pattern, spit up more frequently, cry for prolonged periods, cling to caregivers, and generally be more irritable. They need physical care and comfort, caregiver consistency, gentleness, and a regular routine.

> James, an only child, was 11 months old when his father and mother divorced. James' father had always played with him before bedtime, bathed him, and rocked him. Suddenly his routine changed. His mother was tired and irritable at the end of the day. He became likewise irritable and slept poorly at night.

PRESCHOOL AGE

Responses of preschool children to divorce are dominated by attention-seeking behaviors. They exhibit noticeable aggression, sleep disturbances, and acting out behavior (Hetherington, 1988). Pre-

TABLE 9–2 Age-Related Emotions and Behaviors Related to Divorce

Infancy	Preschool	School Age	Adolescents
Behaviors	***Behaviors***	***Behaviors***	***Behaviors***
Increased crying Disruption in sleeping pattern Spitting up Irritability Clinging to caregiver	Increased aggression, especially in boys Acting out Sleep disturbances Nightmares Social withdrawal Fear of abandonment Fighting with peers Regression Impulsive behaviors Difficulty distinguishing reality from dreams and fantasies Intense feelings of loss	Tearfulness Fearfulness Social withdrawal Poor grades Anger usually directed toward peers Boys show more negative behaviors May eat compulsively Idealize parent who left Girls have low self-esteem	Depression Overt anger Blames parent who leaves Poor grades Social difficulties Sexuality Antisocial acting out
Emotions	***Emotions***	***Emotions***	***Emotions***
Separation anxiety	Fear Separation anxiety Anger Guilt Grief	Fear and anxiety Anger Grief	Fear and anxiety Anger Grief

schoolers commonly withdraw socially, cry, and fight with peers. Although their symptoms of disruption improve with time, 2 years after divorce these children remain quantitatively different in their social, cognitive, and emotional well-being as compared with children of nondivorced parents, and they continue to be more impulsive and exhibit more attention-seeking behaviors (Block, Block, & Gyerde, 1988). Some preschool children may not develop significant problems, whereas others become clinically depressed (Wallerstein & Kelly, 1980).

Preschoolers of divorcing parents need reassurance and increased nurturing. Brief, honest explanations about what happened and parental cooperation regarding children's issues help to alleviate their fears and anxieties. They need to be reassured that they are not to blame for the divorce.

> Anna's parents divorced when she was 3 years old. Prior to the divorce, an atmosphere of quarreling and fighting prevailed in the home. Anna was the youngest of four children ranging in ages from 3 to 10 years. She began pinching, biting, and kicking her siblings and playmates, and exhibiting hyperactive behavior. She "wouldn't listen to anyone."

SCHOOL AGE

School-age children commonly respond to divorce through affective symptoms, such as crying, fearfulness, and moodiness. They can cognitively understand the changes occurring in their lives but emotionally have a difficult time (Richards, 1988). Hetherington (1989) found that boys have greater problems in school and evidence educational underachievement, while girls of divorce suffer from low self-esteem. Social withdrawal is a common response. Children often direct their anger at parents toward peers and siblings because they fear further parental loss. Sibling rivalry intensifies during the school-age years.

School-age children need to be accepted and to know that they continue to be loved by both parents. Empathetic listening and consistent limit setting with natural and logical consequences of behavior help to alleviate aggressive behavior. Punishment should be avoided.

CLINICAL EXAMPLE

Maria was 9 years old and the oldest of three children when her parents divorced. She felt responsible for the divorce, thinking that if she had helped more with chores around the house, made better grades in school, and fought less with her brothers and sisters, her dad would not have left. Her parents were involved with their own problems, and Maria felt ignored. She became depressed and cried for prolonged periods. She did not want to go to school and began having night terrors and enuresis.

ADOLESCENTS

The impact of divorce on adolescents is usually noticeable; they are at high risk for depression (Hodges & Bloom, 1984). Overt anger is typically directed toward the parent who left. Parental divorce may bring on adolescents' sexual acting out, leading to an increase in teenage pregnancies and illegitimate births (Richards, 1988). Adolescents become distressed with parents who develop social lives similar to theirs. Runaway behavior, alcohol and drug abuse, and delinquency may be used as coping strategies to deal with their losses.

Immediate effects related to divorce, such as shock, distress, and grief are not always resolved; sometimes they lead to long-term problems, for example, an increased risk for adult relationship difficulties. The behavior patterns developed through adverse social experiences of children of divorce influence their increased risk of divorce as adults (Caspi & Elder, 1988). When these children become adults, their behavior patterns may include selecting environments and relationships that reinforce within them behaviors similar to their parents, resulting in similar situations. Factors that seem to place children at high risk for divorce include marriages at younger ages, brief periods of going steady before marriages, pregnancy before marriage or shortly thereafter, four or more children, and no religious ceremony at the marriage (Richards, 1988).

The most desirable arrangement for children of divorce is joint custody, when both parents are involved and are able to maintain a close relationship with the children. Joint custody, however, requires the parents to have trust and respect in their relationship, effective communications, and skill in involving the child in decision making. If the divorced parents' relationship is one of turmoil and conflict, joint custody can be a disaster and should not be considered (Derdeyn & Scott, 1984). The best interest of the child should be uppermost, although this often is not the case within the legal system.

The Grieving Process

Children need support and guidance throughout crises of death, loss, and divorce. Gaffney (1988b) identified five seasons of grief for children: "the first days after the death occurs; the time surrounding funeral or memorial services; the period of re-entry following the crisis; the first year; and the significant life events of years ahead" (p. 4). The stages identified by Kubler-Ross (1974) occur throughout the above seasons.

Grief is not programmed for children to move neatly through stages or particular feelings. Intensity of feelings vary and fluctuate in children (Gaffney, 1988b). The grieving process is affected by the particular loss, age, life experiences, individual perceptions, and understanding of what is happening. "If a child is confronted by an actual death at close range such as a significant family member, loved pet, or their own terminal illness, their understanding is enhanced considerably and they are forced into a premature grappling with the subject" (Judd, 1989, p. 19). By understanding the grief process nurses can help children, adolescents, and families cope more effectively with losses.

Often children believe that they should not grieve. They feel guilty and overwhelmed by their feelings and need assistance, support, and approval from significant adults to experience their grief. In bereavement groups of inner city youth, Opie, Goodwin, Finke, Beatty, Lee, and Van Epps (1992) found that although most of the subjects experienced affective distress and somatic complaints, parents and guardians rarely connected these symptoms to grief responses. Children are more prone than adults to pathologic grief reactions (Raphael, 1983). The nature of events, developmental stage, age, severity of the loss as determined by the intensity or closeness of the relationship, and effect on the child's overall environment have been shown to influence the course of emotional disorders later in life, especially as young adults (Miller, Ingham, Kreitman, Surtess, & Sashidaran, 1987). Other important factors include the stability of life circumstances, previous relationships with the deceased, and the presence of supportive, understanding adults who assist the child and give him or her approval to grieve.

Black and Urbanowitz (1982) found that children older than 5 years of age who cry and talk about their loss in the immediate month following the loss demonstrate less emotional and behavioral difficulties. Crying is very "therapeutic in times of stress" (Amadeo, 1988, p. 969). Avoidance of talking about the loss increases children's risk for unforeseeable outcomes. "The therapeutic potential for the child of an emotional display, together with discussing the loss can be inhibited by disturbed parents," suggesting that parents' well-being is of considerable significance to a child's well-being in bereavement (Goodyer, 1990, p. 182). Recent research on the long-term effects of bereavement during childhood suggests that the long-term effects of bereavement may be due to the care the child received, rather than the impact of the loss (Brown, Harris, & Bifulco, 1986).

STAGES OF LOSS

Denial is a way of blocking out reality when a child is unable to accept or cope with a loss. It is a common coping mechanism among children of divorce. Temporary denial is considered to be a normal response; ongoing denial is not and may lead to further problems. When children express, "My parents aren't getting a divorce"; "My sister isn't dead. She'll be back to play with me"; and "This can't be happening to me," they are using denial.

Anger is an intense emotional response and a characteristic, normal part of the grief process. Although children call out for help through anger, their behavior is often inappropriate and pushes people away. They often strike out at those closely involved with the loss. They may express feelings such as "I hate you"; "I don't ever want to see him again"; or "Get away from me—leave me alone!"

Bargaining is a manipulative coping mechanism children use when denial and anger are not productive in getting what they want. Children may bargain, "If I make A's in school, this loss won't really be true"; "If I wash behind my ears everyday, Daddy will come back"; "I know what I can do to get my way"; or "I'll get sick, and things will change."

Depression is a normal part of healthy grief. Children, however, may show increased anxiety and worry about their health. Prolonged depression, or dysfunctional grieving, should be cause for concern. When children realize that they have no control over the loss situation, mourning sets in. Children may internalize their sadness, blame themselves, and become miserable. Or they may externalize their depressive symptoms through lying, cheating, stealing, and striking out at others. "In their attempt to understand events around them, children often assign responsibility to themselves for events over which they have no control," intensifying their feelings of guilt (Rosen, 1986, p. 15). Children may say, "Nobody loves me," "I'm so stupid," "Nothing good happens to me," and "It's all my fault."

Acceptance takes place when children admit that the loss actually happened, and even if they don't like it, the reality does exist. They are no longer angry, depressed, or preoccupied with it but neither do they forget the lost person. Thoughts are more balanced, and they begin to renew interest in other relationships. They may express, "I guess I just have to make the best of the situation," and "I'll just have to find ways to make it."

Children experiencing grief exhibit certain feelings and behaviors (Table 9-3). Rosen's (1986) framework on functions of coping behaviors suggests that certain behaviors are useful in assisting children by helping them to cope with loss. These behaviors help them to "maintain a sense of continuity and safety" (p. 37) (Table 9-4).

How children cope with early losses has a significant impact later in their lives. Entering new schools, graduations, weddings, family reunions, moving, and having a child are changes that influence behavior and are affected by losses. Often early losses need to be regrieved "in light of the experiences in their lives" (Gaffney, 1988b, p. 125).

When death or divorce is related to violence in the family, fear often overshadows grief. Anger and resentment may overwhelm the child. Immediate intervention and long-term support are important to help children through these complicated and difficult situations (Gaffney, 1988b).

The Nursing Process

Nurses come into contact with children experiencing losses in a variety of settings and must be familiar with implementing the nursing process to maximize their care. Through the nursing process, the nurse assesses and diagnoses the health status of children and adolescents after the loss of a significant person from death or divorce. Following assessment and formulation of nursing diagnoses,

TABLE 9–3 Grief in Children: Emotional and Behavioral Responses

Denial	Anger	Bargaining	Depression	Acceptance
Will not discuss the loss	Blames others for their difficulties	Sickness	Isolation	Sense of relief
Hyperactivity	Sullen	Hypermaturity	Sadness	Self-responsibility
Overachiever	Withdrawn	Guilt	Feeling of worthlessness	Trusts others
Does not express sadness	Resentment toward lost one	Doing "A" work	Regression	Improved self-concept
Withdraws	Projects emotions onto teacher	Troublemaker	Crying episodes	Realization that self is not to blame
Easily embarrassed (by loss)	Irritability	Crying	Passive behavior	
Poor school grades	Sleep disturbances	Temper tantrums	Withdrawn	
Decreased eye contact	Enuresis	Attention seeking behavior	Guilt	
Argumentive	Impatience	Refusing to eat	Fears of abandonment	
Fear	Fear	Overeating		
Relief (they'll work it out)	Self-blame	Overtalkative		
	Lowered self-concept	Quiet and withdrawn		

TABLE 9–4 Functions of Coping Behaviors

	Function			
Behavior	***Acceptance of Loss***	***Extinction of Nonadaptive Behaviors***	***Dissipation of Emotions Anger, Grief, Anxiety***	***Maintenance of Continuity and Safety***
1. Focusing on school activities			•	•
2. Keeping object of deceased				•
3. Sibling's religious faith			•	
4. Attending services	•			
5. Crying			•	
6. Observing grief of others	•			
7. Engaging in fate-provoking behavior			•	
8. Talking with therapist	•		•	•
9. Writing "dead" on coloring book	•	•	•	
10. Observing parents' faith	•			
11. Looking at picture of deceased			•	•
12. Maintaining normal routine		•		•

(Rosen, H. [1986]. *Unspoken grief: Coping with childhood sibling loss.* Lexington, MA: D.C. Heath. [Used with permission]) interventions are determined and outcome criteria evaluated. Promotion of health and prevention of developmental and psychologic problems are the main foci of nursing these children and adolescents.

ASSESSMENT

Assessment of children and adolescents requires the nurse to assess the physical, mental, spiritual, and emotional well-being of each individual and the family. The nurse must recognize feelings associated with grief to determine whether health-promoting needs or problems requiring intervention are required. Questions related to problematic issues should be addressed (Box 9-1).

NURSING DIAGNOSIS

Nursing diagnoses are formulated after the assessment data are collected and analyzed for potential and existing problems related to the loss (Box 9-2).

OUTCOME CRITERIA

After establishing a nursing diagnosis, objective and measurable outcome criteria are developed. These criteria are used to evaluate the effectiveness of nursing interventions in resolving problems related to loss.

NURSING INTERVENTIONS

There is little research to guide practice in this area of child and adolescent mental health nursing. Nursing interventions for the care of children who have experienced losses are aimed at prevention and remedy of problems. The main goals of nursing interventions for uncomplicated grief reactions are to support each child and to help him or her mourn. (A list of books recommended for grieving families appears in Box 9-3.) Specific problems are identified through assessment of unresolved grief reactions, and nursing interventions are directed toward resolution of these problems. Examples of application of the nursing process are presented in Table 9-5.

BOX 9–1 • SAMPLE OF INTAKE ASSESSMENT QUESTIONS OF BEREAVED CHILDREN

1. How old is the child? Is it a boy or girl?
2. How old was the child when the loss occurred?
3. Who told the child? What was the child told? When was the child told?
4. What changes have occurred within the family?
5. Does the family or child talk about the loss?
6. Are there any new people involved in the child's life since the loss?
7. Does the child blame himself or herself?
8. How has the child's behavior changed? How long have you noticed behavior changes?
9. What changes have been noticed in eating, sleeping, and self-care patterns?
10. Has performance at school changed? Have grades decreased or improved?
11. Has the child developed any new fears, such as fear of the dark?

BOX 9–2 • POTENTIAL PROBLEMS OF UNRESOLVED GRIEF

1. Dramatic decline in school work
2. School phobia
3. Increased performance in school with perfectionism and "going overboard" in doing good
4. Child not told the truth about the loss
5. Child pretends nothing has happened
6. Suicidal tendencies
7. Anxiety attacks
8. Extreme fears or phobias
9. Physically assaults others
10. Cruelty to animals
11. Drug and alcohol involvement
12. Socially delinquent acts (such as lying, stealing, or cult involvement)
13. Problem socializing with peers
14. Breakdown of communication within the family
15. Running away

Diagnostic and Statistical Manual of Mental Disorders Diagnoses

Problems that develop as a consequence of unresolved grief may be correlated with a number of categories in the *Diagnostic and Statistical Manual of Mental Disorders* (DSM-IV). Phase-of-life problems and other life circumstance problems not attributed to mental disorders and classified as V codes also may be used.

BOX 9–3 • A BIBLIOGRAPHY FOR BEREAVED FAMILIES

FOR BEREAVED PARENTS:

- *The Bereaved Parent,* by Harriet H. Schiff (New York: Crown, 1987). A sensitive and helpful resource, this book explores the feelings parents may have at the death of a child.
- *Living With Death and Dying,* by Elizabeth Kubler-Ross (New York: Collier, 1981). A sensitive book offering comfort and courage to families of terminally ill children who are still afraid to talk about death.
- *Song for Sarah: A Young Mother's Journey Through Grief, and Beyond,* by Paula D'Arcy (Wheaton, IL: Harold Shaw Publishers, 1979). This poignant story is a mother's diary of the lives and accidental deaths of her young child and husband.
- *When Bad Things Happen to Good People,* by Harold S. Kushner (New York: Avon, 1983). A rabbi whose son died of a rare disease explores many of the questions and feelings surrounding the death of a child.
- *The Seasons of Grief: Helping Children Grow Through Loss,* by Donna A. Gaffney (New York: Penguin Books, 1988). A helpful guide for parents with specific actions to help children express their emotions throughout the entire mourning period.

FOR PARENTS AND CHILDREN:

- *A Summer to Die,* by Lois Lowry (New York: Bantam, 1979). A good resource for adolescent girls, this story is about the illness and death of a young girl's sister.
- *Death in the Family,* by James Agee (New York: AMSCO School Publications, 1970). This book for parents and older children tells how a young boy responds to his father's death.
- *A Taste of Blackberries,* by Doris Buchanan Smith (New York: Scholastic, 1973). The response of a young boy to the sudden death of his closest friend is related objectively. The boy comes to grips with the tragedy and learns to manage his grief.
- *Fall of Freddie the Leaf,* by Leo Buscaglia (New York: Slack, Inc., 1982). This warm and simple story tells how Freddie and his friends change with the seasons. It focuses on the delicate balance between life and death and may be helpful in explaining death to children.
- *How it Feels When a Parent Dies,* by Jill Krementz (New York: Knopf, 1986). Eighteen children—boys and girls, black and white, from 7 to 16 years old—speak openly, honestly, and unreservedly of their experiences when either a mother or father has died.
- *I Had a Friend Named Peter,* by Janice Cohn (New York: William Mow, 1987). Betsy's story about the sudden death of her friend Peter can be shared by children and parents to help them cope with a difficult time and to show children that, as Betsy learned, people may die, but memories are forever.
- *It Must Hurt a Lot,* by Doris Sanford (Portland: Multnomah, 1986). A book about death, learning, and growing with emphasis on feelings a child feels after the death of a pet dog.
- *Lifetimes,* by Bryan Mellonie and Robert Ingpen (Toronto: Bantam, 1983). This book explains death to children of all ages with colorful nature pictures explaining that there is a beginning and an ending for everything that is alive.
- *Remember the Secret,* by Elizabeth Kubler-Ross (Berkeley: Celestial Arts, 1982). This book for young children is a story about love, caring, and loss when a young child's close friend dies.
- *The Tenth Good Thing About Barney,* by Judith Viorst (New York: Macmillan, 1988). A good introduction to death for children age 5 through 10, this story tells how a young boy overcomes the sadness he feels when his cat dies by thinking of the 10 best things about him.
- *Tiger Eyes,* by Judy Blume (New York: Bradbury Press, 1981). For girls age 8 to 17, this book recounts the feelings of a daughter whose father has been murdered.
- *When a Pet Dies,* by Fred Rogers (New York: G. P. Putnam's Sons, 1988). This book is written with gentleness and honesty about some of the questions and emotions children may have when their pet dies.

FOR WIDOWS AND WIDOWERS:

- *But I Never Thought He'd Die: Practical Help for Widows,* by Miriam B. Nye (Louisville: Westminster John Knox, 1978). This guide may help widows, their children, friends, and pastors cope with death.
- *Widow,* by Lynn Caine (New York: Bantam, 1987). A young widow with two small children gives a personal and honest portrayal of widowhood.

GENERAL:

- *The Courage to Grieve: Creative Living, Recovery, and Growth Through Grief,* by Judy Tatelbaum (New York: Harper & Row, 1984). This book explores common feelings and reactions to the loss of a loved one. It's a self-help book with creative suggestions for recovery and growth.
- *Grief, Climb Toward Understanding,* by Phyllis Davies (New York: Carol Communications, 1988). This is a self-help book when you are struggling, including checklists of what you can do.
- *When Going to Pieces Holds You Together,* by William A. Miller (Minneapolis: Augsburg Publishing 1976). The author examines how helpful grief behaviors can be to the healing process.

(*continued*)

BOX 9–3 • A BIBLIOGRAPHY FOR BEREAVED FAMILIES (*Continued*)

FOR CHILDREN OF DIVORCE:

- *Dinosaurs Divorce,* by Laurence Krasny Brown and Marc Brown (Boston: Little Brown, 1986). This is a guide for children of changing families, explaining new terms and relationships. It can be a real security blanket for young children in need.
- *Sometimes A Family Has to Split Up,* by Jane Werner Watson, Robert E. Switzer, and J. Cotter Hirschberg (New York: Crown, 1988). A read-together book for parents and children—in the form of a very simple, nonjudgmental story—attempts to provide a framework for calm discussions, bringing feelings and fantasies into the open.

FOR CAREGIVERS AND FRIENDS:

- *How Can I Help? Stories & Reflections on Service,* by Ram Dass (New York: Alfred A. Knopf, Inc., 1985). This book—a guide for personal growth, inspiration, and wisdom—offers both practical and philosophical suggestions to those who wish to help.

(Reprinted by courtesy of The Family Tree Counseling Center, Inc., Arlington, TX.)

TABLE 9–5 Application of the Nursing Process for Children Experiencing Losses

Assessment	Nursing Diagnosis	Outcome Criteria	Nursing Interventions
Age and sex: 5-year-old boy Loss experienced: death of 7-year-old sister Parents preoccupied with their own grief Child not permitted to express feelings Social withdrawal Feels he should have died Pretends sister is still alive Expresses guilt	Family unresolved grief related to feelings of guilt and shame about sibling's death	Work through the grieving process as evidenced by: 1. Realistic understanding of death 2. Abandonment of social withdrawal behavior 3. Parent's helping child express feelings 4. Family members talking about child and sharing memories	1. Provide child with honest and truthful information about the death. 2. Answer questions honestly. 3. Help the child to talk about the loss, and use art and play for ventilation of feelings. 4. Provide parents with support, and sensitize them to child's needs. 5. Encourage family to share memories and select special keepsake memento for child.
Age and sex: 9-year-old girl Loss experienced: Parents divorced; father moved out Expresses fear of leaving home Cries excessively Nightmares Enuresis Unrealistic fears of common daily activities Regression	Anxiety reaction related to feelings of loss and abandonment since parents' divorce	Adaptation to father's absence as evidenced by: 1. Talking about the loss and using art and play for ventilation of feelings 2. Gradually confronting fears 3. Parental support 4. Pursuing age-appropriate behaviors	1. Provide parent education on empathetic listening and nurturing. 2. Sensitize parents to child's needs. 3. Give reassurance. 4. Show parents how to use relaxation techniques with child to reduce anxiety.

(continued)

TABLE 9–5 Application of the Nursing Process for Children Experiencing Losses *(Continued)*

Assessment	Nursing Diagnosis	Outcome Criteria	Nursing Interventions
Age and sex: 12-year-old boy Loss experienced: Taken from family and placed in foster home Poor performance in school Stealing Lying Aggressive and belligerent behavior	Child's dysfunction related to perceived loss of biologic family	Child adapts to placement as evidenced by: 1. Decrease of antisocial behavior, then gradually eliminates such behavior 2. Improved school performance 3. Expression of feeling accepted	1. Sensitize foster parents, and counsel them in parenting child with negative behaviors. 2. Encourage and help to express feelings verbally rather than acting out.

Summary

Losses through death and divorce cause an understandable degree of stress in children's lives. The intensity of bereavement and whether children progress through a normal grieving process or develop problems related to unresolved grief depend on several factors, including age, what the child is told, quality of relationship prior to the loss, support systems, family dynamics, culture, and subsequent relationships. As children grow, develop, and face milestones throughout life, old losses will resurface and will be grieved again. "Adults have been through many milestones; children have not" (Gaffney, 1988b, p. 127). Professional nurses can help children in their care learn how to express their feelings and help them face milestones and changes throughout their lives in a healthy manner.

REFERENCES

Amadeo, D. M. (1988). A time for tears. *American Journal of Nursing, 7,* 967–969.

Black, D., & Kaplan, T. (1988). Father kills mother: Issues and problems encountered by a child psychiatric team. *British Journal of Psychiatry, 153,* 624–630.

Black, D., & Urbanowitz, M. (1987). Family interventions with bereaved families. *Journal of Child Psychology and Psychiatry, 28,* 467–476.

Block, J., Block, J., & Gyerde, P. F. (1988). Parental functioning and home environment in families of divorce: Prospective and concurrent analysis. *Journal of the American Academy of Child and Adolescent Psychiatry, 27,* 207–213.

Brown, G. W., Harris, T., & Bifulco, A. (1986). Long-term effects of early loss of parents. In M. Rutter, C. Izard, & P. Read (Eds.), *Depression in young people—developmental and clinical perspectives.* London: Guilford Press.

Caspi, A., & Elder, G. H. (1988). Emergent family patterns: The intergenerational construction of problem behavior and relationships. In R. Hinde & J. Stevenson-Hinde (Eds.), *Relationship within families.* Oxford: Oxford University Press.

Derdeyn, A. P., & Scott, E. (1984). Joint custody: A critical analysis and appraisal. *American Journal of Orthopsychiatry, 54*(2), 199–209.

Furman, R. (1964). Death and the young child. *Psychoanalytic Study of the Child, 19,* 321–333.

Gaffney, D. A. (1988a). Death in the classroom: A lesson in life. *Holistic Nursing Practice, 2*(2), 20–27.

Gaffney, D. A. (1988b). *The seasons of grief: Helping children grow through loss.* New York: Penguin Books.

Goodyer, I. M. (1990). Family relationships, life events, and child psychopathology. *Journal of Child Psychology and Psychiatry, 31*(1), 161–192.

Hetherington, E. M. (1988). Parents, children, and siblings: Six years after divorce. In R. A. Hinde & J. Stevenson-Hinde (Eds.), *Relationships within families.* Oxford: Oxford University Press.

Hetherington, E. M. (1989). Coping with family transitions: Winners, losers, and survivors. *Child Development, 60,* 1–14.

Hodges, W. F., & Bloom, B. D. (1984). Parents' report of children's adjustment to marital separation: A longitudinal study. *Journal of Divorce, 8,* 33–50.

Jackson, E. (1982). The pastoral counselor and the child encountering death. In H. Wass & C. Carr (Eds.), *Helping children cope with death* (pp. 33–48). Washington, DC: Hemisphere Publishing.

Jozefowski, J. (1983). Children's concepts of death. In D. M. Moriarty (Ed.), *The loss of loved ones: The effects of a death in the family on personality development.* St. Louis: Warren H. Green.

Judd, D. (1989). *Give sorrow words: Working with a dying child.* London: Free Association Books.

Lester, A. D. (1987). *When children suffer.* Philadelphia: Westminister Press.

Koocher, G. (1974). Talking with children about death. *American Journal of Orthopsychiatry, 44,* 45–52.

Kubler-Ross, E. (1974). *Questions and answers on death and dying.* New York: MacMillan.

Kuntz, B. (1991). Exploring the grief of adolescents after the death of a parent. *Journal of Child and Adolescent Psychiatric and Mental Health Nursing, 4*(3), 105–109.

Miller, P. M., Ingham, J. G., Kreitman, N. B., Surtees, P. G., & Sashidharan, S. P. (1987). Life events and other factors implicated in the onset and remission of psychiatric illness in women. *Journal of Affective Disorders, 12*, 73–88.

Nagy, M. (1948). The child's theories concerning death. *Journal of Genetic Psychology, 73*, 3–27.

Opie, N. D., Goodwin, T., Finke, L. M., Beatty, J. M., Lee, B., & Van Epps, J. (1992). The effect of a bereavement group experience on bereaved children's and adolescent's affective and somatic distress. *Journal of Child and Adolescent Psychiatric and Mental Health Nursing, 5*(1), 20–26.

Piaget, J. (1970). *The science of education of the psychology of the child.* New York: Grossman.

Raphael, B. (1983). *The anatomy of bereavement.* New York: Basic Books.

Richards, M. P. M. (1988). Parental divorce and children. In G. Burrows (Ed.), *Handbook of studies in child psychiatry.* Amsterdam: Elsevier.

Rosen, H. (1986). *Unspoken grief: Coping with childhood sibling loss.* Lexington, MA: D.C. Heath.

Royes, A. (1990) *Preschool children's beliefs about health and illness* [unpublished thesis]. Arlington, TX: University of Texas at Arlington.

Rutter, M. (1985). Family and school influences on behavioral development. *Journal of Child Psychology and Psychiatry, 26*, 349–368.

Rutter, M. (1989). Pathways from childhood to adult life. *Journal of Child Psychology and Psychiatry, 30*, 23–52.

Salladay, M., & Royal, M. (1981). Children and death: Guidelines for grief work. *Child Psychiatry and Human Development, 11*(4), 203–212.

Spinetta, J., & Deasy-Spinetta, P. (1981). Talking with children who have a life threatening illness. In J. Spinetta & P. Deasy-Spinetta (Eds.), *Living with childhood cancer.* St. Louis: C.V. Mosby.

Wahlstrom, C. (1983). Children of divorce. In D. M. Moriarty (Ed.), *The loss of loved ones: The effects of a death in the family on personality development.* St. Louis: Warren H. Green.

Wass, H., & Scott, M. (1978). Middle School students: Death concepts and concerns. *Middle School Journal*, 10–12.

Wallerstein, J. S., & Kelly, J. (1980). *Surviving the breakup: How children and parents cope with divorce.* New York: Basic Books.

Zambelli, G. C., Clark, E. J., Barile, L., & de Jong, A. F. (1988). An interdisciplinary approach to clinical intervention for childhood bereavement. *Death Studies, 12,* 41–50.

CHAPTER

10

Victimization of Children and Adolescents

Joyce Swegle and Rebecca Personett

Victimization is an issue that transcends individual and family boundaries and must be viewed as a community, social, and legal problem. In nurses' various roles, they are accountable to prevent victimization and identify and care for child and adolescent victims. Nurses are frequently in contact with families during periods of stress and are the first people to detect and interact with an abused child at home, school, or in a health care setting. They provide nursing care for the victims, families, and communities.

Pender (1987) described prevention as having three distinct levels. Each level is unique to a single point in an occurrence and requires specific nursing interventions. Spradley (1990) stated that the prevention of problems is a major part of a community practice. Victimization of children and adolescents is a community issue and should be addressed through a framework that will allow a broad focus (i.e., the three levels of prevention). The nursing assessment, diagnosis, planning, intervention, and evaluation of child and adolescent victimization are described in this chapter through the levels of primary prevention (identification of individuals at risk), secondary prevention (acute treatment of victims), and tertiary prevention (rehabilitation of victims) (Table 10-1).

Scope of Victimization

TYPES OF ABUSE

Child abuse is defined in the Child Abuse Prevention and Treatment Act (PL 93–247) of 1974. It includes physical or mental injury, sexual abuse, and negligent treatment or maltreatment of a child younger than age 18 by a person who is responsible for the child's welfare under circumstances that indicate that the child's health or welfare is harmed or threatened thereby (Box 10-1).

Kempe, Silverman, Steele, Droegemueller, and Silver (1962) first introduced the term "battered child syndrome" to an unbelieving professional community. Subsequently, child abuse and neglect have been recognized as major social problems.

Physical abuse is nonaccidental trauma inflicted by a caretaker (Schmitt & Kempe, 1979). Physical abuse may be indicated by a variety of forms of injury including fractures; internal injuries; lacerations, bruises, and welts; swelling, dislocations, and sprains; choking, twisting, and shaking; burns and scalding; and poisoning (Mooney, 1989).

TABLE 10–1 Prevention Framework

Nursing Process	Primary Prevention	Secondary Prevention	Tertiary Prevention
Assessment	Risk factors	Index of suspicion Clues to abuse and neglect	Dysfunctional behavioral patterns
Planning	Obviating the cause	Early detection and treatment	Rehabilitation to minimize the impact
Intervention	Potential for abuse Identify special child Crisis intervention	Provision of safety for the victim Mandated reporting	Promotion of developmental progression Education of abusers and victims
Evaluation	Absence of abuse or neglect	Safety assured	Adaptation of dysfunctional patterns Cycle broken

John, age 3, is brought to the emergency room with circumferential, second-degree burns on both hands. The burns are infected. The mother stated that the child spilled hot water on himself 1 week ago, and the burns have failed to heal.

Neglect can be delineated into four different types: physical, emotional, medical, and educational. Unexplained weight loss, malnutrition or failure to thrive, and dehydration under unusual circumstances all signal neglect. Inadequate care, such as severe hunger, diaper rash, inappropriate clothing, and poor hygiene, also indicate neglect. Neglectful care may be evidenced by abandonment for days or weeks or repeated shorter periods of time (Schwab, 1989).

Mary, age 9, frequently comes to school early and stays late. She is watchful of her 5-year-old brother, Jack, during these times. The school nurse discovers that the children's mother works nights, leaving the children unattended while she works and sleeps.

Sexual abuse has been divided into two categories depending on the relationship of the victim and perpetrator. *Intrafamilial sexual abuse* is defined as any kind of exploitative sexual contact that occurs between relatives, no matter how distant the relationship, before the victim turns 18 years old (Russell, 1983).

Melinda, 13 years old, is admitted to a psychiatric unit after attempting suicide by drug ingestion. She discloses in individual therapy that she has been incested by her father since age 10.

Extrafamilial sexual abuse involves one or more unwanted sexual experiences with people unrelated by blood or marriage, ranging from petting (touching of breasts or genitals or attempt at such touching) to rape before the victim turns 14 years and completed or attempted forcible rape experiences from the ages of 14 to 17 (Russell, 1983).

Doug, age 8, is seen in an outpatient clinic for increased discipline problems at home and school. His parents state he has few friends. Recently a neighbor reported that Doug was playing with her 3-year-old son's genitals. Doug discloses that his adolescent sister's boyfriend had sodomized him on repeated occasions.

Emotional abuse is defined as continual rejection or scapegoating of a child by a caretaker with verbal abuse and berating (Schmitt & Kempe, 1979).

Susan, age 10, was seen in a physician's office for evaluation of enuresis. She was withdrawn, had dark circles around her eyes, and sucked her thumb. No physical basis was found for her enuresis, and a referral to a mental health clinic was made. After several sessions, Susan revealed that her parents argued constantly, and both parents were verbally hostile and blamed her for the argument.

INCIDENCE

The number of reported cases of child maltreatment has been influenced by social changes that developed during the 1960s concerning the treatment of children, the mandatory reporting system (1974), and the legitimatization of neglect as a con-

BOX 10–1 • TYPES OF ABUSE

Physical abuse
Neglect
Sexual abuse
  Intrafamilial
  Extrafamilial
Emotional abuse

cern. Dramatic increases in reports of abuse and neglect have occurred, with approximately 6000 in 1967 compared to 2.2 million reports of child abuse in 1986.

The true number of children and adolescents who are victimized each year is unknown. Several factors bear on the determination of the number of children and adolescents who are affected. Abuse and neglectful incidents are concealed as family secrets. Historically, children have been considered family property. As a result, maltreatment of children has been viewed as a family issue and as such not open to outside intervention. Abusive incidents also may be intertwined with many other family issues, such as substance abuse. Unfortunately, many abusive incidents are never identified.

In addition to the failure to identify abuse, a reluctance to report abusive and neglectful incidents continues. Inadequate validation of reported instances also continues to be a problem. Successful identification and validation depends on a willingness to admit that the condition exists.

Knudsen (1988) outlines the three methods used to obtain information about child abuse. These are self-report from participants, either victim or perpetrator; unevaluated reports of maltreatment made by nonparticipant observers; and substantiated reports of maltreatment by agencies or people designated to investigate complaints.

The ability to validate the incidence of abuse is problematic particularly with self-reports and nonparticipant reports. Validity of these reports range from 25% to 40%. Substantiated reports eliminate duplication and frivolous and malicious reports but, at best, are validated only 40% to 60% of the time. Still many cases go undiscovered or unreported until serious injury or death results.

PATTERNS OF CHILD ABUSE AND NEGLECT

A description of the characteristics of victims and perpetrators remains as elusive as a true accounting of cases. Even in case reports of substantiated incidents of child abuse, the data remain ambiguous. This is especially difficult if reports contain more than one victim, different types of injuries, or multiple perpetrators (Rosenthal, 1988).

Fisher and Berdie (1978) found that the majority of reported cases involved children from 10 to 18 years of age. The National Incidence study (1981) confirmed this finding and indicated that the incidence of reporting increased with the victims' age. This study also identified the interaction between age, severity of abuse, and fatalities associated with younger children. For example, preschoolers account for 17% of reported cases and 74% of fatalities.

In general, characteristics of an abusive parent mirror commonalities in the general population (Millor & Josten, 1986). However, some gender-associated patterns have been identified for both victims and perpetrators.

Rosenthal (1988) conducted an exploratory analysis of confirmed cases of child abuse reported to one state registry for an 8-year period. He found that male children sustained a greater number of major injuries and fatalities across all age groups, infant to 12 years. In contrast, adolescent victims were more often female. Even excluding sexual abuse, females from 13 to 17 years of age were the more frequent victim of all types of maltreatment.

When maltreatment resulted in an injury, the perpetrator was predominantly male. Females were more often identified as the perpetrator in situations of neglect. A significant opposite sex relationship between victim and perpetrator was identified, even when sexual abuse cases were excluded. Males were identified as the perpetrator more often in cases of adolescent abuse in samples with and without sexual abuse cases.

Sexual abuse victims are overwhelmingly female. This is most often an intrafamilial victimization by a male perpetrator, usually a biologic father or stepfather. In comparison, sexual abuse of male victims comprises less than 20% of total reports. Males are more likely to be victimized outside the home by either male of female perpetrators (Faller, 1989). Faller (1989) cautioned that these statistics may be biased by the socialization of males not to report weaknesses, doubts, fears, or by the taboo of homosexuality.

Primary Prevention

Spradley (1990) describes primary prevention as obviating the occurrence of a health problem. This is accomplished by anticipatory planning, envisioning potential needs, and intervening before problems occur. Primary prevention of victimization therefore must take place prior to the abusive event.

PRIMARY ASSESSMENT

To gather data for primary prevention, the population at risk must first be identified. Helfer (1973) identified necessary and sufficient components for abuse to occur: potential for abuse, a special child, and a crisis situation.

Several factors contribute to the potential for abuse. First, is the cyclic nature of abuse. Goodwin, McCarthy, and DiVasto (1981) reported 24% of mothers identified as abusive had a history of incest, compared with 3% of mothers in a nonabusive group. Role reversal, parents expecting their needs to be met by the child, also is a factor for potential abuse (Millor & Josten, 1986). Dysfunction in the marital system can lead to dysfunction in the parent–child relationship, which can accompany abuse (Houck & King, 1989). Poor self-concept culminating in low self-esteem may further contribute to maltreatment. Social isolation from other adults or residential mobility as a family pattern, both of which reduce support systems, can predict abusive actions. Unrealistic expectations of the child or adolescent's behavior and lack of knowledge regarding developmental milestones are potential stressors that can result in abuse (Millor & Josten, 1986).

A special child situation that produces stress on the family precipitating abusive behaviors may be real or imaginary. High incidence of child abuse among children born prematurely, with mental or physical anomalies, adopted children, or children with temperaments described as bothersome provide examples of children perceived as special. An adversely perceived child is a continual stress, and interactions with this child may increase vulnerability toward harmful victimizing behaviors (Millor & Josten, 1986).

Caplan (1964) defined crisis as a temporary state of disequilibrium for people who face a situation they find threatening and that they can neither escape nor solve with usual coping mechanisms. A crisis results from inappropriate coping skills, inadequate social supports, or the perception of an event as a crisis. Parents facing a crisis or series of crises are then at high risk for victimization of offspring.

PRIMARY NURSING DIAGNOSES

Nursing diagnoses for primary prevention are numerous. The following is a list of suggested NANDA-approved diagnostic responses:

- Family Coping: Compromised, Ineffective
- Ineffective Individual Coping
- Altered Family Process
- High Risk for Injury
- Parental Role Conflict
- High Risk for Altered Parenting
- Altered Role Performance
- Sexual Dysfunction
- Social Isolation
- High Risk for Violence: Self-Directed or Directed at Others
- Powerlessness

The following is a list of suggested possible etiologies for responses:

- Cyclic nature of abuse behavior
- Dysfunctional marital relationship
- Role reversal
- Poor self-concept
- Social isolation
- Residential mobility
- Unrealistic expectations for child behaviors
- Lack of knowledge regarding developmental milestones
- Ineffective bonding with premature child
- Preadoptive stress
- Adversely perceived characteristic of child
- Temperamental differences
- Inappropriate coping skills
- Ineffective support systems
- Perception of crisis event

Neither the listing for responses nor the etiologies are conclusive but suggestive possible diagnostic combinations.

PRIMARY PLANNING

Planning of primary prevention of child or adolescent victimization must be goal directed with a specific predictable outcome of obviating the occurrence. Successful prevention at the primary level will result in the absence of abuse or neglect. The major step in planning is identification of these families at risk and intervening to alleviate the risk factors before the abuse occurs.

PRIMARY INTERVENTION

Nursing interventions are targeted toward potential for abuse, identification of the special child, and crisis intervention.

Interruption of the abuse cycle can prevent formerly abused individuals from abusing their offspring. Dysfunctional families can be guided toward improving marital and parent–child relationships. Children who are expected to meet the needs of their parents can be relieved from that role reversal. Measures can be provided to improve self-concept and self-esteem of parents. Families who are new to the community following residential mobility can be provided social supports. Education of parents toward realistic expectations and developmental milestones of the children and adolescents can be offered.

Taylor and Beauchamp (1988) reported findings regarding the effectiveness of one hospital-based primary prevention model initiated for primiparous women following delivery. Topics explored with the mothers were stress management, family adjustment, parenting patterns, use of community resources, child development, and child management (Taylor & Beauchamp, 1988).

Mothers involved in this program demonstrated a greater understanding of physical and psychosocial development, and provided a significantly greater amount of verbal stimulation for their infants. In addition, these mothers demonstrated greater versatility in dealing with current and projected parenting concerns. They also recognized greater numbers of resources available for assistance (Taylor & Beauchamp, 1988).

Parental support must be offered to those with identified special characteristics. Such groups would target adoptive parents, parents of premature infants, and those with physical and mental anomalies. Children labeled as temperamentally different can be recognized as potential victims of abuse or neglect.

Crisis intervention can be offered for families presenting with inappropriate coping skills, inadequate support systems, and adversely perceived events. Follow-up for these families would be instituted for a minimum of 4 to 6 weeks following the crisis event to allow for crisis resolution.

PRIMARY EVALUATION

The ultimate evaluation of primary prevention of child or adolescent victimization is the absence of abuse or neglect. More specifically, risk factors will be modified as evidenced by increased coping mechanisms, positive parenting skills, participation in special support groups, and crisis resolution.

Secondary Prevention

Secondary prevention seeks to detect and treat existing health problems at the earliest possible stage (Spradley, 1990). The nurse must be aware of the vastness of child victimization and of the ways in which victimization might be manifested. Table 10-2 lists some physical and behavioral indicators of child abuse and neglect.

SECONDARY ASSESSMENT

There is no single pattern that will signal the occurrence of child and adolescent victimization. There are as many different arrays of findings as there are victims and victimizers. Therefore, the nurse must be cognizant of normal childhood development and be constantly alert to the age, developmental level, and family and social issues relative to each child. This information, in conjunction with an awareness of the different types and extents of victimization, provide a cluster of data from which a conclusion of abuse may be drawn.

INDEX OF SUSPICION

Child abuse must be suspected whenever there is a discrepancy between the medical history and the degree of trauma seen in the child. The nurse must ask, "Is the child old enough, strong enough, or developmentally aware enough to sustain the injury?" (Mooney, 1988). The nurse's answer to the question leads him or her to the decision of whether this could represent an abusive incident. For example, is a 5-year-old sexually aware enough to have contracted gonorrhea?

The nurse also needs to evaluate whether the explanation for the injury seems to fit with the nature of the injury. Could a 3-week-old sustain a spiral fracture of the femur from catching his or her leg between crib spindles? Table 10-3 describes patterns of normal growth and development that provide a point of reference for nursing assessment.

Other assessment factors include how soon the injury is reported, parental patterns in seeking medical attention for the child, and parent–child interactions.

The nurse who sees a child with repeated injuries must consider if the injuries were deliberately inflicted, the result of failure to provide a safe environment, or simply clumsiness on the child's part. Generally, children older than 2 years are allowed some freedom of activity, which would predispose them to greater risk for injury. Natural clumsiness may be seen at certain development stages. A comparison of the nurse's assessment with normal growth and development patterns provides the nurse with data necessary to arrive at the appropriate conclusion.

TABLE 10–2 Physical and Behavioral Indicators of Child Abuse and Neglect

Type of Child Abuse and Neglect	Physical Indicators	Behavioral Indicators
Physical Abuse	Unexplained bruises and welts: On face, lips, mouth On torso, back, buttocks, thighs In various stages of healing Clustered, forming regular patterns Reflecting shape of article used to inflict (electric cord, belt buckle) On several different surface areas Regularly appear after absence, weekend, or vacation	Wary of adult contacts Apprehensive when other children cry Behavioral extremes: Aggressiveness Withdrawal
	Unexplained burns: Cigar, cigarette burns, especially on soles, palms, back, or buttocks Immersion burns (sock-like, glove-like, doughnut-shaped on buttocks or genitalia) Patterned like electric burner, iron, etc. Rope burns on arms, legs, neck, or torso	Frightened of parents Afraid to go home Reports injury by parents
	Unexplained fractures: To skull, nose, facial structure In various stages of healing Multiple or spiral fractures	
	Unexplained lacerations or abrasions: To mouth, lips, gums, eyes To external genitalia	
Physical Neglect	Consistent hunger, poor hygiene, inappropriate dress Consistent lack of supervision, especially in dangerous activities for long periods of time Unattended physical problems or medical needs Abandonment	Begging, stealing food Extended stays at school (early arrival and late departure) Constant fatigue, listlessness, or falling asleep in class Alcohol or drug abuse Delinquency (e.g., thefts) States there is no caretaker
Sexual Abuse	Difficulty in walking or sitting Torn, stained, or bloody underclothing Pain or itching in genital area Bruises or bleeding in external genitalia, vaginal, or anal areas	Unwilling to change for gym or participate in physical education class Withdrawal, fantasy, or infantile behavior Bizarre, sophisticated, or unusual sexual behavior or knowledge

(continued)

TABLE 10–2 Physical and Behavioral Indicators of Child Abuse and Neglect *(Continued)*

Type of Child Abuse and Neglect	Physical Indicators	Behavioral Indicators
Sexual Abuse (continued)	Venereal disease, especially in preteens Pregnancy	Poor peer relationships Delinquent or runaway behavior Reports sexual assault by caretaker
Emotional Maltreatment	Speech disorders Lags in physical development Failure to thrive	Habit disorders (sucking, biting, rocking, etc.) Conduct disorders (antisocial, destructive, etc.) Neurotic traits (sleep disorders, inhibition of play) Psychoneurotic reactions (hysteria, obsession, compulsion, phobias, hypochondria) Behavior extremes: Compliant, passive Aggressive, demanding Overly adaptive behavior: Inappropriately adult Inappropriately infant Developmental lags (mental, emotional) Attempted suicide

(Reproduced from Heindl, C., Krall, C., Salus, M., Broadhurst, D. [1979]. *The nurse's role in the prevention and treatment of child abuse and neglect.* Washington, DC: HEW publication #(OHDS) 79-30202.)

The evaluation of developmental awareness is crucial to the detection of maltreatment. Children who have been victimized have difficulty achieving cognitive, social, and emotional competency. The relationship between the age or developmental level of the child at the time of victimization and the physical and psychosocial developmental factors provide a point of reference for the nurse in assessing children and adolescents.

Early developmental disturbances are likely to contribute to later disturbances in functioning. However, a true linear relationship between developmental level and outcomes cannot be projected because of the variety of mediating factors, such as physical differences and familial and sociologic factors (Houck & King, 1989).

Sink (1986) addressed several problematic areas in the assessment of abuse in a health care setting. First, health care providers need to consider psychosocial information that might point to past abuse or imminent risk of abuse.

Second, victims may be stereotyped by their behavior with parents or in interactions with staff. There also is a tendency to blame prematurely when parents' behavior is not in line with staff expectations. Biases can cloud the protective measures taken and clinical decisions made on behalf of the child.

Finally, the nurse must recognize his or her reluctance to act alone in the face of the family's reaction to allegations of abuse. Unintentional collusion with the parents' denial following alleviation of symptoms may provide road blocks to child protection and advocacy. Other factors that may contribute to the nurse's failure to advocate for the child include parental hostility, rejection of further services, or threats of litigation. Anticipating parental reactions rather than fearing them can help the nurse take a stronger protective stance toward the child (Sink, 1986).

(*text continues on page 138*)

TABLE 10–3 Growth and Development Patterns

Age	Physical Development	Psychosocial Development	Sexual Development
0–1 month	Moves extremities in random, uncoordinated way Turns head side to side		*Infancy* Gender-specific response created through mother's interaction Undifferentiated sensuosity through sensations of warmth, cuddling, caressing, and stroking. Intimacy experience through breastfeeding, bathing, and bodily contact
2 months	May roll over Cannot open hand purposefully but will grasp	Smiles in response to stimuli Coos and squeals Responds to speaking voice	
3 months	Purposefully puts hand in mouth Able to swallow solid foods Crawling movements in prone position Holds head up while in prone position Strikes at toys	Laughs, blows bubbles Seems to enjoy noises Smiles at mother's face	
4 months	Seizes object and puts into mouth Turns from back to side Reaches out and plays with hands	Initiates social play	
5 months	No head lag Rolls back to side Transfers hand to hand	Lifts arms to be picked up Turns head toward voice Splashes bathwater	
6 months	Sits alone briefly	Begins to act coy	
7–9 months	Sits alone Pulls into standing position	Says first words Shy with strangers Waves bye-bye and plays pat-a-cake	
10–12 months	Takes few steps alone Holds cup Tries to use spoon	Enjoys simple games Negative, tantrums Says two or three words	
12–18 months	Walks and runs Climbs stairs Pulls toy Seats himself in small chair	Ten words Rapid shift in attention Begins tantrums Enjoys solitary play Selects favorite toy or object	*Toddler* Gender differences are reinforced Self-concept as girl or boy is completed Asserts control over body functions Discovers genitalia Increased genital stimulation may be observed Nonverbal sex education from parents
19–24 months	Steady gait Runs in controlled manner with fewer falls Begins alternating feet Opens doors Jumps crudely Daytime toilet training accomplished	Enjoys parallel play Does not ask for help Treats other children as objects Cannot share Mimics parents	

(continued)

TABLE 10–3 Growth and Development Patterns *(Continued)*

Age	Physical Development	Psychosocial Development	Sexual Development
25–36 months	Walks on tip toe Stands on one foot Voluntary control of sphincters	Spends time away from mother with another caretaker Begins sense of right and wrong	
3 years	Rides tricycle Walks backward Walks downstairs alone using handrails Tries to dance	Talks in sentences Ritualistic behaviors Jealous of siblings Afraid of dark or animals	Learns sex differences and sexual modesty Develops a body image and a body boundary May ask simple questions about sex
4 years	Climbs and jumps well Goes up and down stairs without holding rails Buttons buttons Lace shoes	Exaggerates, boasts, and tattles Tells family stories without constraint Cooperative in play Knows age Counts to 3 Imaginative—may have imaginary companion	
5 years	Runs and jumps skillfully Balances on one foot Skips Writes first name Ties shoes	Internalizes social norms Talks constantly Asks questions Interested in relatives	
6–12 years	Motor skills become refined Clumsiness and incoordination gradually diminish Works and plays hard Tires easily	Learns to get along with age mates Chooses best friend of same sex Family primary agent of socialization Developing independence Sportsmanship Loyal to friends Uses good manners Will subordinate own goals to group	Learns appropriate masculine or feminine social role Plays games with male–female roles Asks more probing questions May play kissing games Secondary sex characteristics begin for girls
12–18 years	Gangly appearance and awkwardness Reaches physical maturity	Develops relationships with age mates of both sexes Achieves social role Achieves emotional independence Considers possibility of marriage and family Prepares for meaningful work Socially responsible behavior	Menarche and ejaculations May experiment with kissing, petting, and intercourse May involve genital examination, sexual play, and experimentation with same sex Not yet sexually mature but physically capable of reproduction

LEGAL IMPLICATIONS OF ASSESSMENT

Child and adolescent nurses may frequently provide assessment of abuse situations. Knowledge of the legal implications of therapeutic assessment can maximize admissible evidence at a trial and minimize trauma for the child (Yorker, 1988).

Conflicts between Constitutional rights of defendants and protection of children have been identified by Yorker (1988). Generally, children are not prepared for the adversarial role imposed by the trial process. Recognizing this and the threat created for the child by a face-to-face confrontation with the defendant, the courts have granted some latitude in the prosecution of sexual abuse cases. However, many of the novel approaches used have been successfully challenged in a higher court.

First, the Supreme Court found that the use of videotaped child witness testimony violates the defendant's constitutional right to confrontation and due process. In various other cases, the courts have placed a burden on prosecutors to demonstrate the child's incompetence before exempting his or her appearance in court.

In another vein, some states have recognized that victims have no reason to fabricate abusive incidents and have protected the child by the inclusion of hearsay evidence under an excited utterance exception. In this exception to evidentiary rules, an adult having heard the child's statement may report the statement as testimony provided there is not an unacceptable time lapse between the event and the statement. This exception provided the means for physicians to testify about the causation of injury for the purpose of diagnosis and treatment, as well as expert interpretation of play using anatomically correct dolls. However, this exception does not extend to the identification of the perpetrator (Yorker, 1988).

SECONDARY NURSING DIAGNOSIS

The following is a suggested list of NANDA-approved diagnostic responses:

- Family Coping: Compromised, Ineffective
- Family Coping: Disabling, Ineffective
- Ineffective Individual Coping
- Defensive Coping
- Ineffective Denial
- Altered Family Processes
- Fear
- Altered Growth and Development
- High Risk for Injury
- Parental Role Conflict
- Altered Parenting
- Powerlessness
- Altered Role Performance
- Body Image Disturbance, Altered Role Performance, Personal Identity Disturbance
- Self-esteem Disturbance
- Situational Low Self-Esteem
- Sexual Dysfunction
- Altered Sexuality Patterns
- Impaired Social Interaction
- Social Isolation
- Violence

The following is a suggested list of possible etiologies for responses:

- Parental hostility
- Rejection
- Parental feelings of inadequacy
- Undisclosed secrets
- Lack of personal boundaries
- Threats of retribution
- Dysfunctional attachment
- Avoidance
- Lack of ego control
- Poor impulse control
- Inappropriate adjustment patterns
- Poor peer relations
- Inability to establish relationships

Neither the listing for responses nor etiologies are conclusive but suggest possible diagnostic combinations.

SECONDARY PLANNING

Planning for primary prevention focused on the identification of the families at risk. This allowed for interventions to alleviate risks before occurrence of the abuse. In contrast, secondary planning must be directed toward early detection and treatment of incidents of child and adolescent victimization. Planning at the secondary level takes place after the abuse has occurred and the symptoms are present.

Foremost, the goal of secondary prevention is the provision of safety for victims. Nurses have a statutory obligation to report incidents of suspected and actual abuse. After the victim's safety is assured, nurses can intervene to identify and alleviate dysfunctional patterns.

SECONDARY INTERVENTION

NURSING INTERVENTIONS WITH THE VICTIM. Guidelines for nursing interactions with the victimized child were developed by Stanley (1989a). Initially, it is important to provide reassurance to the child. The nurse must communicate to the child that sharing of information is the appropriate choice. Disclosure is risky for the child because the secret of abuse has become a source of fear and a source of safety (Summit, 1983).

Stanley (1989b) provided a guide for helping children compare undisclosed events, such as secrets and surprises. Secrets were described as occurring between the child and one other person. The child has responsibility for keeping the secret. Disclosure of the secret would result in terrible consequences. Therefore, the child is bad if the secret is disclosed. On the other hand, surprises usually involve more than two people who share the responsibility for nondisclosure. Disclosure of a surprise usually results in happiness or possible disappointment if a person is told the surprise beforehand. A similar conceptualization of secrets as both good and bad is presented in written and audiovisual material (Lenett & Barthelme, 1986). These aids serve as a resource to reinforce the child's disclosure and educate for prevention.

It is paramount that the nurse believe the child. By practicing good listening skills, the nurse may collect data about family dynamics, which may require intervention with or without substantiation of abuse. It is essential that the nurse reassure the child that he or she will be kept safe.

The nurse must recognize the guilt that the child or adolescent may experience by disclosing incidents of abuse. The guilt feelings may arise from several different sources. In incidents of sexual and physical abuse, the child may feel that he or she was responsible for the adult's behavior—that he or she behaved in such a way as to deserve the abuse. Also, the child may feel guilty about the role he or she played or will play in splitting the family apart. It is important that the nurse emphasize that the adult or older person, in the case of an adolescent perpetrator, was responsible for the abuse. Feelings of shame or embarrassment can be minimized by maintaining confidentiality and recognizing the child's right to privacy. However, within the context of keeping the child safe, the nurse also must communicate to the child the need to report the incident to the child protective services. The child's feelings of guilt coupled with real or potential threats or fears of retribution often result in a retraction of the disclosure.

To respond and interact therapeutically with the child or adolescent, the nurse must recognize his or her own feelings about abuse. Travelbee (1979) wrote about the uniqueness a practitioner brings to a relationship and that this uniqueness includes not only strengths, but also weaknesses, problems, and deficits. If the practitioner's past is similar, this may contribute to his or her inability to relate to the client's issues and therefore to his or her inability to focus on such issues in-depth.

NURSING INTERVENTIONS WITH THE PARENTS. A nonaccusatory attitude on the part of the nurse is paramount at all interactions with the parent. The nurse must be aware that not every injury is the result of maltreatment. By contrast, there may be no physical evidence of trauma but yet significant sexual or emotional abuse. The nurse's interaction with the parent may be critical in establishing suspicion. On the other hand, the parents may provide information that eliminates reasonable suspicion (Schwab, 1989).

The nurse needs to anticipate the parent's responses. Anger, denial, remorse, ambivalence, and overprotectiveness are all common parental reactions. These various reactions may be intensified or diminished at different times as the issue of abuse unfolds (Stanley, 1989b). Given the cyclic nature of abuse, the nurse also must anticipate the parent's response from the standpoint of having also been a victim.

As with the child, the nurse must honestly communicate to the parent his or her professional responsibility to report suspected or actual abuse. When the parent has a history of threatening or abusive behaviors, it may be prudent to have another team member, a representative from child protective services, or the police present at the time of the interview (Schwab, 1989).

MANDATED REPORTING. A major issue in dealing with child and adolescent victims of abuse is the mandatory reporting required of health professionals. In 1974 Congress passed the Child Abuse Prevention and Treatment Act. Although state child abuse statutes differ, all mandate the reporting of suspected child abuse and neglect by professionals involved in the care of children.

Legal implications of mandated reporting as they relate to school nurses have been identified by Schwab (1989). However, these implications may be generalized to other settings as well. First, the nurses must have knowledge of the law. Lack of knowledge is not an acceptable defense against civil or criminal penalties.

Second, reports must be made in good faith of any suspicion of abuse or neglect. The obligation is for the individual to report, and this obligation cannot be satisfied by reporting to a higher authority. Further, the nurse has a duty to meet professional standards of practice. Nurses are held accountable at a different level than lay people because of their specialized knowledge and skill.

Historic and clinical data should be objective and accurately documented on the formal report form and the child's health or medical record. These may serve as primary evidence in a court action to protect the child.

In contrast to various professional standards, confidentiality is superceded by the duty to report and by such reporting, protect the child from risk of harm. The nurse may share information with an outside agency, which is necessary for the child's protection; this should not be construed to mean that information beyond the scope of the nurse's assessment and management records should be released.

Finally, decisions might be made to act on the parent's behalf to protect the child from imminent danger or further harm. The obligation is to assure treatment and evaluation of medical emergencies. Discussing the incident with the parent is secondary to ensuring the child's safety. However, it must be recognized that notification of parents provides an opportunity to conduct further assessment, which could substantiate or eliminate reasonable suspicion.

SECONDARY EVALUATION

The effectiveness of secondary prevention interventions must be evaluated in relation to the safety of the victim. Early detection and reporting are necessary but not sufficient conditions for victim safety.

Initiation of measures designed to provide for the child's safety indicate successful secondary prevention and could include heightened parental awareness of the child's safety needs, investigation and monitoring of family dynamics, hospitalization, or removal of the child to foster care.

In addition to the evaluation of predicted client outcomes, the nursing process should be evaluated. This evaluation should consider to what extent the planned actions were completed and the extent that the etiology was actually modified (Ziegler, 1989).

Tertiary Prevention

Tertiary prevention is the reduction of the severity of a problem to the lowest level (Spradley, 1990). The goal is one of rehabilitation to lessen the impact or to minimize the effect of an unhealthy condition.

TERTIARY ASSESSMENT

Assessment at the tertiary level must project long-term needs. The tertiary level is entered after the stressor has impacted the victim, and the reaction occurred. The assessment reveals the long-term effects and resulting disequilibrium. As noted in the discussion of secondary assessment, early developmental disturbances that occur at the time of the victimization contribute to later disturbances in functioning. Erikson (1963) described a theory of psychosocial development that can serve as a framework for comparison of normal tasks and the abnormal dysfunctions assessed in the victims of abuse. These disturbances, identified in Table 10-4, can be assessed during tertiary assessment.

The infant's task is to develop trust. When this stage is interrupted, mistrust results in dysfunctions of attachment. The toddler tries to attain the task of autonomy, but if halted, shame or doubt results. Avoidant social reactions then occur. The preschooler strives for initiative but will be halted with guilt, which precedes educational unreadiness. The school-age child works toward industry. When dysfunction occurs at this level, inferiority evolves into inappropriate adjustment patterns. The adolescent is ready for identity to be recognized, but when stopped, role diffusion and antisocial behaviors result.

TERTIARY NURSING DIAGNOSIS

Nursing diagnoses for tertiary prevention also are numerous. The following is a suggested list of NANDA approved diagnostic responses:

Impaired Adjustment
Ineffective Individual Coping
Altered Family Process
Altered Growth and Development
Knowledge Deficit
Altered Parenting
Post-Trauma Response
Powerlessness
Rape Trauma Syndrome
Altered Role Performance
Self Esteem Disturbance
Body Image Disturbance
Sexual Dysfunction
Altered Sexual Patterns
Impaired Social Interaction
Social Isolation
Altered Thought Processes

The following is a suggested list of possible etiologies for responses:

TABLE 10–4 Signs of Developmental Dysfunction

Stage	Task	Dysfunction
Infancy (0–1 year)	Trust versus mistrust	Impaired parent or offspring Dysfunctional attachment Avoidant or ambivalent Proximity seeking avoidance Disorganization
Toddler (1–3 years)	Autonomy versus shame/doubt	Avoidant social interaction Inability to show sadness or empathy Approach/avoidance Lack of impulse control Aggression Self-doubt Delayed language acquisition Poor boundary identification
Preschool (3–6 years)	Initiative versus guilt	Educational unreadiness Poor self-esteem Social failure Lack of ego control Motor awkwardness Poor sphincter control Lack of persistence
School age (6–12 years)	Industry versus inferiority	Inappropriate adjustment pattern Lack of academic achievement Dependent behavior Difficulty establishing relationships Low self-esteem Failure cycle
Puberty/adolescence (12–19 years)	Identity versus role diffusion	Antisocial behavior Lack of coping skills Poor peer relations Alienation Somatic complaints Inappropriate self-image

Inability to trust
Denial of feelings
Difficulty expressing feelings
Feelings of insecurity
Guilt feelings
Impulsive behavior
Feelings of failure
Unsatisfactory relationship building
Inability to set limits
Inability to make choices
Inability to recognize consequences
Difficulty accepting authority
Lack of role understanding
Lack of positive experiences

Neither the listing for responses nor etiologies are conclusive but suggest possible diagnostic combinations.

TERTIARY PLANNING

Tertiary planning affects the entire system, which is involved in the recognition, intervention, and rehabilitation of the victims. Developmental processes that have been delayed must be facilitated. This is now a time to look to the future. Planning must look at what the nurse can do to help the victim move forward in as normal a progression as possible.

Plans must be made for education, not only for the child or adolescent, but also for the abusers. The discrimination between normal and abnormal relationships and the ability to establish personal boundaries are examples of tertiary prevention goals for the child. Reinforcement and rewards for behavioral choices made in relation to the new skills must be provided. Goals for parents might include the demonstration of acceptable parenting skills and appropriate behavioral approaches with their children and adolescents.

TERTIARY INTERVENTION

NURSING INTERVENTION WITH THE VICTIM. No set interventions are appropriate for the victims of child and adolescent abuse. There have been no empirical investigations comparing treatment modalities. As a result, the nurse must intervene on the basis of the age of the child, his or her assessment of the child's developmental dysfunction, quality and quantity of relationships, and behavioral manifestations.

First, the child must be in an emotionally and physically safe environment. The nurse creates an environment conducive to the development of a trusting relationship and protects the child from his or her own poor impulse control. This environment also must be conducive to change. Behavioral change takes time, and the demonstration of new behaviors is uncertain. The child or adolescent must be given the opportunity to try different behaviors and to make some mistakes without fear of retribution.

The nurse assists the child in the identification of feelings. Initially this may be simply to label the feeling. This can progress to the identification of events that precipitate feelings and then to feelings that precipitate behaviors. Furthermore, children may need assistance in articulating feelings or assistance in ventilating feelings in a socially acceptable manner.

In addition to providing a physically safe environment for impulse control, the nurse can provide verbal and physical redirection. Behavioral choices and consequence must be articulated clearly. These choices and consequences need to be age appropriate. Reinforcement for positive behavioral choices, completion of projects or tasks, accepting responsibility for his or her own actions, and appropriate attention-seeking behaviors can range from reward charts to verbal recognition.

Nursing interventions may be directed at establishing and maintaining social relationships. Victims may require assistance in their identification of feelings toward others. Role relationships may need to be explored and reestablished for the child who has assumed the parent role in physically or sexually abusive situations.

Social skills may need further development before peer relationships can be established. Role modeling can be an effective means of demonstrating social skills, such as giving and receiving compliments, confrontational and conflict resolution skills, and appropriate attention-seeking behaviors.

Personal boundary issues are an important component of social skill development. Child and adolescent victims frequently have difficulty discriminating their own boundaries from others because of the assaultative experiences. The nurse must recognize that the only nurturance a child has received may have been within the context of an abusive relationship. The nurse can assist through discussions related to personal space and by demonstrating appropriate physical contact.

The victim may require assistance in learning age-appropriate relaxation techniques and stress management skills. This can be an asset to children who demonstrate hypervigilance, aggression, angry outbursts, difficulty sleeping, or concentration deficits. Alternative outlets for overzealous activity can be identified.

Finally, the nurse can intervene by teaching age-appropriate prevention skills. Avenues for reporting subsequent abusive attempts or incidents should be explored with the victim. A plan can be developed with the child outlining assertive behaviors he or she can use to maintain safety.

The sequelae of ritualized, cult, or severe abuse may be long-term and disabling. Dissociative disorders and in particular dissociative identity disorder may result from childhood experiences of trauma and abuse (Box 10-2).

NURSING INTERVENTION WITH THE PARENT. Caregiver attitudes have a distinct impact on outcomes in nurse–patient interaction. The nurse may reduce parental feelings of inadequacy by discussing the frustration experienced by all adults when dealing with children and by exploring various problem-solving strategies with the parent. This provides an opportunity to role model successful approaches. It also assists in promoting parental self-esteem. Nurses must recognize that a critical attitude toward the parent may precipitate a withdrawal from

BOX 10–2 • DISSOCIATIVE IDENTITY DISORDER

Sheryl Tyson, MN, RN and Nancy Hornstein, MD

Society has witnessed an increased awareness of issues related to abuse. Identifying, exploring, and reaching resolution of childhood trauma have long been the cornerstones of treatment for a variety of disorders of adulthood.

In recent years health care providers have noted that significant numbers of children experience trauma and abuse. Children who had previously been treated for disorders other than abuse (i.e., ADHD, conduct disorder, oppositional defiant disorder, and psychosis) have, on further investigation, frequently been found to have experienced some form of physical or sexual abuse.

Clinicians have learned that dissociative disorders (DDs) are rooted in abusive histories, with abuse occurring at a young age. It is important, therefore, that children who are receiving a psychiatric or developmental disability evaluation also undergo an evaluation for the presence of dissociative disorders. The child's behavioral problems often become severe and require inpatient hospitalization. The inpatient setting provides an opportunity for a thorough psychiatric evaluation.

Evaluation, recognition, and treatment of dissociative disorders in general, and dissociative identity disorder (DID) in particular, are critical for several reasons. First, recognition of these disorders ensures that many of the behavioral problems that lead to hospitalization are dealt with at the etiologic level. Second, recognition enables intervention to assist discontinuation of abuse. Third, in the case of incest, a window of opportunity opens in which intergenerational dysfunction may be terminated and replaced with a plan for family recovery. Finally, children with DID, unlike their adult counterparts, respond rapidly to skilled intervention.

The Diagnostic and Statistical Manual of Mental Disorders (DSM-IV) identifies the essential feature of dissociative disorders as a disruption in the usually integrated functions of consciousnous, memory, identity, or perception. DID occurs when the integrative functions of identity are so impaired that two or more distinct personality states develop.

Children who suffer from DID are frequently misdiagnosed. Misdiagnosis occurs for several reasons: children with DID exhibit behavioral symptoms that meet criteria for other DSM-IV diagnoses; dissociative symptoms (switching behaviors) may be particularly subtle and difficult for the untrained observer to detect; and length of stay in the inpatient setting has become relatively short. Children with DID have, of necessity, become quite adept at hiding their "alters" from others. Typically, DID children require 1 month or longer in the inpatient treatment environment to feel safe enough to allow staff to begin to "meet their alters."

The removal of any child from his or her home is a traumatic event that needs careful evaluation before undertaken. The inpatient setting, however, is recognized as being perhaps the most effective way to ensure the physical safety of the child from himself or others, make the continuous behavioral observations necessary to arrive at a diagnosis, provide the physical proximity to others over time to allow sufficiently for the development of therapeutic alliances, and provide the consistency and intensity of intervention that will be an integral part of treatment. The intensity of the inpatient setting affords a bolus of intervention so that future long-term treatment may occur on an outpatient basis.

Evaluation and treatment of DID in children are multidisciplinary efforts. Nursing staff, by virtue of providing care 24 hours a day, have the most contact with the children and as such, are in an ideal position to make behavioral assessments and follow through with nursing interventions specific to the disorder. Observations of the child should include not only the presence of dissociative symptomatology and switching, but the absence of behaviors as well. Behaviors result from complex psychodynamic processes; behavioral changes that persist indicate changes in the underlying psychodynamics of the child (Hornstein & Tyson, 1991). Behavioral observations that may indicate dissociative symptoms include amnestic periods, switching between alters, affect disturbances, thought process disturbances, somatoform symptoms, and anxiety post-traumatic stress disorder.

Nurses cluster and categorize behaviors with similar theoretical orientation. Then they review the categories to determine relative function and dysfunction. In addition, they examine each category for its relationship to other categories and to intervening variables. Intervening variables include the family, the biopsychosocial state and developmental level of the child, and the physical environment in which the child has lived. Theory-based nursing process facilitates systematic behavioral observation necessary to formulate diagnoses. Knowledge of psychiatric nursing theory and its application to clients with DID enable the nurse to arrive at and prioritize several diagnostic statements. A system-based nursing model promotes a holistic intervention approach that makes an impact on all subsystems of the person and environment.

Goals of intervention are to achieve compatibility between and within behavioral categories and to help the child develop a sense of mastery over his or her internal state. Specific interventions useful in treating children with DID include continually reassuring the child of physical safety, encouraging the child's acknowledgement of his or her various alters, assisting

(*continued*)

BOX 10–2 • DISSOCIATIVE IDENTITY DISORDER (*Continued*)

the child to enlist the aid of his or her alters when difficult situations arise, and helping the child make the alters equally accountable for problematic situations that they generate.

Cooperation among the alters should be encouraged. No one alter, including the one that presents the most often, should be given a greater stature than any other. All alters should be validated as significant and assured of safety. Cooperation among alters leads to integration of ego functioning. As the acute crisis resolves and the child becomes more comfortable with himself or herself, treatment can focus on long-term outpatient intervention.

REFERENCES

Aauger, J. R. (1976). *Behavioral Systems and Nursing.* Englewood Cliffs, NJ: Prentice-Hall.

American Psychiatric Association (1994). *Diagnostic and Statistical Manual of Mental Disorders, (4th Ed.).* Washington, DC: Author.

Grubb, J. (1980). An interpretation of the Johnson behavioral systems model for nursing practice. In R. Riehl (Ed.), *Conceptual models for nursing practice.* New York: Appleton-Century-Crofts.

Hornstein, N. L., & Tyson, S. (1991). Inpatient treatment of children with multiple personality/dissociative disorders and their families. *Psychiatric Clinics of North America, 14*(3), 631–648.

Kluft, R. P. (1985). Childhood multiple personality disorder: Predictors, clinical findings and treatment results. In R. P. Kluft (Ed.), *Childhood antecedents of multiple personality,* (pp. 121–134). Washington, DC: American Psychiatric Press.

Kluft, R. P. (1984). Multiple personality in childhood. *Psychiatric Clinics of North America, 7,* 167–196.

Kluft, R. P. (1986). Treating children who have multiple personality disorder. In B. G. Braun (Ed.), *Treatment of multiple personality disorder* (pp. 81–105). Washington, DC: American Psychiatric Press.

Putnam, F. W., Guroff, J. J., & Silberman, E. K., et al. (1986). The clinical phenomenology of multiple personality disorders: A review of 100 cases. *Journal of Clinical Psychiatry, 47,* 285–293.

contact with the caregiver and the child. This can be prevented by acknowledging areas of parental expertise. Parents can provide information regarding the child's likes and dislikes and can be approached as an equal in the planning process (Millor & Josten, 1986).

NURSING INTERVENTION WITH THE FAMILY. Amundson (1989) described a home-based intervention model program for child abuse. This program offers intensive intervention to families experiencing abuse or neglect.

Family crisis care provides services in three phases: intensive crisis intervention, stabilization, and follow-up. During the first phase, a comprehensive family history is developed with the family and outside service providers. A behavior-specific goal attainment scale is developed for the family's self-monitoring and the therapists' evaluation. Networking with other service providers is accomplished, and regular in-home contact provided during this phase, which lasts approximately 6 weeks.

The second stage lasts 2 to 6 weeks, and regular therapist contact continues. The treatment goals during this phase are maintenance of a new level of functioning, support, concrete services, and facilitation of linkages with out-of-home services.

During the 4- to 12-week follow-up phase, a therapist remains on 24-hour call and continues to visit and provide concrete services. The family is monitored for follow-through with other service providers.

Evaluations are conducted at termination of service and at 3- and 6-month intervals. Indicators for evaluation include stabilization of the child in the home, improved family interaction and problem-solving skills, change in problem behaviors, and ability to use community resources.

Programs of this type provide an alternative to the limited options of outpatient therapy or institutional or foster care. Home-based intervention provides more intensive service than outpatient therapy and is less restrictive than institutional care. This type of program also addresses the need to treat the entire family in its own environment. Additionally, this alternative has been reported to have a higher success rate at significantly lower costs than foster and institutional care.

TERTIARY EVALUATION

One goal of tertiary prevention is to halt dysfunctional patterns and to promote developmental adaptation. Evaluation should compare the predicted outcomes with what was actually achieved. Successful adaptation can be measured by the development of age-appropriate behaviors, adequate social and peer relationships, and prevention skills. The ultimate goal of tertiary prevention is to break the cycle of abuse. This, however, requires longitudinal analysis and eludes measurement at a single point in time.

REFERENCES

Amundson, M. (1989). Family crisis care: A home-based intervention program for child abuse. *Issues in Mental Health Nursing, 10*, 285–296.

Bernette, C. (1993). Sexually abused boys: Awareness, assessments, and invention. *Journal of Child and Adolescent Psychiatric and Mental Health Nursing, 6*(2), 29–35.

Caplan, G. (1964). *Principles of prevention psychiatry.* New York: Basic Books.

Erikson, E. H. (1963). *Childhood and society.* New York: Norton.

Faller, K. (1989). Characteristics of a clinical sample fo sexually abused children: How boy and girl victims differ. *Child Abuse and Neglect, 13*, 281–291.

Fisher, B., & Berdie, J. (1978). Adolescent abuse and neglect: Issues of incidence, intervention, and service delivery. *Child Abuse and Neglect, 2*, 173–192.

Goodwin, J., McCarthy, T., & DiVasto, P. (1981). Prior incest in mothers of sexually abused children. *Child Abuse and Neglect, 5*, 87–96.

Helfer, R. (1973). The etiology of child abuse. *Pediatrics, 51*, 777–779.

Houck, G., & King, M. (1989). Child maltreatment: Family charateristics and development consequences. *Issues in Mental Health Nursing, 10*, 193–208.

Johnson, T. (1989). Female child perpetrators: Children who molest other children. *Child Abuse and Neglect, 13*, 571–585.

Kempe, C., Silverman, F., Steele, B., Droegemueller, W., & Silver, H. (1962). The battered child syndrome. *Journal of the American Medical Association, 181*, 17–24.

Knudsen, D. (188). Child maltreatment over two decades: Change or continuity. *Violence and Victims, 3*, 129–144.

Lenett, R., & Berthelme, D. (1986). *Sometimes it's O.K. to tell secrets!* (film). Hollywood, FL: Kid Stuff Records and Tapes.

Millor, G., & Josten, L. (1986). Child abuse. In D. Kjervik & I. Martinson (Eds.), *Women in health and illness: Life experiences and crisis* (pp. 150–166). Philadelphia: W.B. Saunders.

Mooney, A. (1989). Physical child abuse. *Orthopaedic Nursing, 8*, 29–32.

National Study of Incidence of Child Abuse and Neglect (1988). (Executive Summary) DHHS Pub N(OHDS) 81-30329. Washington, DC.

Pender, N. (1987). *Health promotion in nursing practice* (2nd ed.). Norwalk, CT: Appleton and Lange.

Rosenthal, J. (1988). Patterns of reported child abuse and neglect. *Child Abuse and Neglect, 12*, 263–271.

Russell, D. (1983). The incidence and prevalence of intrafamilial and extrafamilial sexual abuse of female children. *Child Abuse and Neglect, 7*, 133–146.

Schmitt, B., & Kempe, C. (1979). Abuse and neglect of children. In V. Vaughn, R. McKay, & R. Behrman (Eds.), *Nelson textbook of pediatrics* (11th ed.). (pp. 120–126). Philadelphia: W.B. Saunders.

Schwab, N. (1989). Child abuse and neglect: Legal and clinical implications for school nursing practice. *School Nurse, 5*, 17–28.

Sink, F. (1986). Child sexual abuse: Comprehensive assessment in the pediatric health care setting. *Child Health Care, 15*, 108–113.

Spradley, B. (1990). *Community health nursing concepts and practice* (3rd ed). Glenview, IL: Scott, Foresman.

Stanley, S. (1989a). Child sexual abuse: Recognition and nursing intervention. *Orthopaedic Nursing, 8*, 33–40.

Stanley, S. (1989b). Disclosure of sexual abuse: The secret is out—what now? *Journal of Child and Adolescent Psychiatric and Mental Health Nursing, 2*, 154–160.

Summit, R. (1983). The child abuse accommodation syndrome. *Child Abuse and Neglect, 7*, 177–193.

Taylor, D., & Beauchamp, C. (1988). Hospital-based primary prevention strategy in child abuse: A multi-level needs assessment. *Child Abuse and Neglect, 12*, 341–354.

Travelbee, J. (1979). *Intervention in psychiatric nursing* (2nd ed.). Philadelphia: F.A. Davis.

Valente, S. M. (1992). The challenge of ritualistic child abuse. *Journal of Child and Adolescent Psychiatric and Mental Health Nursing, 5*(2), 37–46.

Yorker, B. (188). The prosecution of child sexual abuse cases. *Journal of Child and Adolescent Psychiatric and Mental Health Nursing, 1*, 50–57.

Ziegler, S. (1989). Strategy for practice-oriented theory in nursing. In S. Ziegler (Ed.) *Practice-oriented theory in nursing.* (Fall 1989) Denton, Texas: Texas Woman's University, College of Nursing.

CHAPTER

11

Disability and Chronic Illness

Sally Francis

Approximately 7.5 million families, or 10% to 15% of children, in the United States face the daily challenge of living with a child's chronic condition (Gortmaker & Sappenfield, 1984). For some families, the challenge leads to coping, adaptation, and resilience (Cadman, Rosenbaum, & Boyle, 1991; Drotar, Doershuk, Stern, Boat, Boyer, & Matthews, 1981; Tavormina, Boll, Luscomb, & Taylor, 1981); for others, the challenge interacts with additional life disadvantages and results in continuing despair (Garmezy, 1991; Pless & Wadsworth, 1989; Stein & Jessop, 1982). There are numerous opportunities for health care providers to influence the day-to-day lives of children and families with chronic conditions—opportunities to assist in the development of resilience, instead of psychosocial disruption and despair (Bolig & Weedle, 1988; Patterson & Geber, 1991; Ritchie, 1985; Rutter, 1987).

Chronic illness and disability as a phenomenon in modern life has a past, present, and future. Nursing and other health care professions must address the present challenges by building on the research and clinical work of the past in preparation for the newfound future of children with chronic illnesses and disabilities. This new future results from the increased survival of children with chronic conditions into adulthood (Gortmaker & Sappenfield, 1984). The conditions include 5% of children with conditions that cause a marked degree of functional impairment; 6% of children identified as having impairments such as mental retardation, sensory disabilities, and speech problems; and 3.7% who are limited in the amount or kind of usual activities of childhood in which they can participate (Brewer, McPherson, Magrab, & Hutchins, 1989). The challenge to health care is to assist children to be prepared to participate to the maximum extent possible in the activities of our society (Stein, 1989).

This chapter will discuss chronic illness and disability from a mental health perspective for assisting children and families. The process of assessment, nursing diagnosis and planning, carrying out interventions, and evaluating will be grounded in a developmental approach and will build on a stress–coping–resilience theoretical perspective.

Definition

What is a chronic illness or disability? Stein (1989) describes chronic illness as a framework for thinking about a range of conditions that threatens the health and developmental potential of infants, children, and adolescents and that requires special treatments and health care services. This framework evolved from research and clinical descriptions that were initially focused on specific conditions (Drotar, 1981; Pless & Rohgmann, 1971). With time, similarities in psychosocial challenges were

Barbara Schoen Johnson: CHILD, ADOLESCENT AND FAMILY PSYCHIATRIC NURSING, © 1994 J.B. Lippincott Company

identified across disease categories (Stein & Jessop, 1982; Perrin & MacLean, 1988). In the 1970s, chronic illness was defined as an illness or condition that lasted 3 or more months or that required at least 1 month of hospitalization (Pless & Douglas, 1972; Pless & Pinkerton, 1975). An expanded definition describes chronic illness as serious, ongoing, physical health conditions that cause stress on the family unit and require investment of time, energy, and personal resources to cope. The conditions continually or repeatedly threaten to disrupt normal development in the physical, intellectual, emotional, or social sphere (Ireys, 1981; Silverman & Koretz, 1989). The chronic illness framework has moved from a strict medical model (i.e., a deficit model of individual conditions) to a broad look at conditions that extend over time and produce stress in the individual and family that influences both the physical status and the psychosocial functioning of the individual and family (Eiser, 1990; Nolan & Pless, 1986). Concern now focuses on the consequence of the disease or disorder to the person, family, *and* health care provider (World Health Organization, 1980).

Three additional definitions are needed to consider chronic conditions: impairment, disability, and handicap. *Impairment* refers to the loss of function or to an abnormality of psychologic, physiologic, or anatomic structure or function. *Disability* is a restriction or lack of ability resulting from an impairment to perform an activity within the normal range. *Handicap* results when the impairment or disability prevents or limits the fulfillment of a role that is usual for the individual and thereby places the individual at disadvantage for performance of life expectations (WHO, 1980). The sequence from disease or disorder can progress or be modified at any step, from impairment, to disability, to handicap. For example, technologic engineering advances enable physically impaired individuals to be mobile in wheelchairs, automobiles, and the workplace. This intervention has limited disorder to impairment, rather than handicap.

Epidemiology in childhood chronic illness and disability is complex to study, particularly considering the sequence, or possible sequence, from disorder to handicap. Some chronic conditions require special care but do not render the child too ill to function unless the care is inadequate (Stein, 1989), for example, renal disease. Some conditions may require special care but allow the child to continue normal activities for varying lengths of time until the condition progresses to greater physiologic involvement, for example, cystic fibrosis. Some conditions, such as muscular dystrophy and arthritis, require functional assistance over time. Other chronic conditions extend for long periods but may resolve, such as asthma. Some conditions, such as childhood leukemia, may achieve a cure designation but the long-term effects of uncertainty may handicap the individual in psychologic, economic, and work areas.

Eleven conditions have been designated "marker" conditions for research and public policy efforts and represent the larger class of childhood chronic illnesses. These include juvenile-onset diabetes, muscular dystrophy, cystic fibrosis, spina bifida, sickle cell anemia, congenital heart disease, chronic kidney diseases, thalessemia and hemophilia, leukemia, craniofacial birth defects, and asthma. Additional chronic conditions include rare congential defects, cerebral palsy, bronchopulmonary dysplasia, and other conditions that require long-term technologic assistance for survival and functioning. A final group includes children with mental retardation, sensory disabilities, and speech problems. The total group is referred to as "children with special health care needs" (Koop, 1987). For brevity, the term chronic condition is used throughout this chapter unless the reference is specifically to an illness, such as one of the marker diseases.

There is general agreement that 10% to 15% of children have or will experience special health care needs. Of the total child population, 1% to 2% have severe conditions that limit the child's daily functioning. This translates to approximately 7.5 million children in the United States (Gortmaker & Sappenfield, 1984). In addition, there is the emergence of pediatric acquired immunodeficiency syndrome (AIDS) and the growing number of medically fragile, technology-assisted children (Stein, 1989).

Existence of psychosocial problems in children with chronic conditions has been recognized and documented (Cadman et al., 1991; Walker, Gortmaker, & Weitzman, 1981); however, prevalence has been difficult to determine. Consider the following: *John,* diagnosed with acute myelogenous leukemia at 12 years of age, completed required protocols in 2 years with a continuous remission for an additional year and a half. At relapse, the reinduction of treatment was complicated by John's drug and alcohol abuse. *Alex,* recipient of a liver transplant at age 14, was admitted for psychiatric care following a school counselor's concern for Alex's suicidal thoughts in his senior year of high school. *Mirah,* raised by her grandmother in a public housing project, joined the long-term, follow-up oncology clinic as she began a 4-year music scholarship at a state university. *Stephen,* at age 16, proudly shares his academic achievements that propel him toward his goal of becoming a physician. Treatment for lye ingestion begun at age 2 has included numerous, lengthy hospital and intensive care unit stays and now involves esophageal dilatation every 6 weeks in outpatient surgery. *Karen,* a college graduate, has begun a master's degree program in deaf education. Diagnosed with recurring neuromyopathy at age 8, she continued intermittent plasmapheresis throughout elementary and high school. She is interested in working with hearing-impaired infants and has received a scholarship from the children's hospital where she received medical care.

What helps health care and society understand the diversity seen in these young people and their response to chronic conditions? Studies of prevalence of psychosocial dysfunction in children with chronic illness and disability have found psychopathology, as evidenced in John and Alex, to be rare (Cadman, Boyle, Szatmari, & Offord, 1987). However, in these examples and in research, children with chronic conditions represent a vulnerable population. This is seen in study findings of chronic illnesses (Walker et al., 1981), developmental disabilities (Wikler, Wasow, & Hartfield 1981), birth defects (Nolan & Pless, 1986), and physical disabilities (Breslau & Prabucki, 1981; Steinhausen & Wefers, 1976).

Scientific and clinical efforts have addressed the search for prevalence and causation of psychosocial dysfunction leading to handicap and for prevention and intervention strategies for children and their families. How can health care respond to foster the outcomes of Mirah, Stephen, and Karen for all children? As seen in these examples, children can develop from birth, childhood, or adolescence with serious, ongoing health conditions. They may experience multiple hospitalizations, physical limitations in energy and activity, and disruptions in school and peer relations and have challenges to family time, energy, and resources. As Stein (1989) states: "The challenge for all of us is to continue to make our own individual and collective contributions to caring for children with chronic illness and to assume a leadership role in setting a high standard for the provision of comprehensive and humane services to these children and their families" (p. 193). In light of this statement, the clinical application focus of this chapter must be balanced by the realization that the nurse can make contributions to health care delivery systems, public policy, and societal institutions that affect children and families with chronic conditions.

Historic Overview

Since 1967, the number of children identified as having a chronic condition has significantly increased (Gortmaker & Sappenfield, 1984; Newacheck et al., 1986). This increase has been rapid and dramatic. Advances in medical care and available technology have led to survival and longer life into adulthood. Growing attention resulting from this increase has pointed out the threat to the mental health of the ill child, siblings, parents, and the family unit (Breslau & Prabuchi, 1981; Cadman et al., 1987; Gortmaker, Walker, Weitzman, & Sobol, 1990; Mattson, 1972; and Sabbeth & Leventhal, 1984). This threat has been seen in varying degrees of emotional and social maladjustment with secondary social and psychologic maladjustment attributed to physical disorders (Pless & Roghmann, 1971), underachievement in school (Satterwhite, 1978), and later psychologic adjustment difficulties (Mulhern, Wasserman, Friedman, & Fairclough, 1989).

Early research focused on specific disease entities. Frequent hospitalization and progressive deterioration of the child was found to influence maladjustment in children with cystic fibrosis (Gayton, Koocher, Foster, & O'Malley, 1977). Dorner (1976) found children with spina bifida to have anxieties related to their social lives. Other studies of chronic conditions indicating difficulty in psychosocial functioning included hemophilia (Bruhn, Hampton, & Chandler, 1971) and cancer (Lansky, Lowman, Tribhawan, & Gyulay, 1979).

In spite of the disease focus of these early studies, Pless and Pinkerton (1975) questioned the relevance of a disease-specific approach in assisting adjustment of children with chronic conditions. Stein and Jessop (1982) reported a study of 209 families whose child had one of 98 chronic illnesses. The researchers identified the impact of chronic uncertainty and the visibility of the child's condition as affecting the psychosocial functioning of the child and family. This impact was seen across the sample of families and across the disease entities. This cross-incidence of shared issues was labeled the noncategoric approach and has continued to gain support from clinical and research areas. Acceptance of the noncategoric approach can be seen in its effect on public policy initiatives (Brewer et al., 1989; Hobbs & Perrin, 1985) and in clinical application (Blum, 1991).

Negative effects of a child's disability or illness on parents has been documented (Tavormina et al., 1981; Venters, 1981). Some effects include maternal stress and depression (Kazak & Marvin, 1984; Goldberg, Morris, & Simmons, 1990), marital stress (Martin, 1975; Sabbeth & Leventhal, 1984), and responses of fathers (McKeever, 1981). In addition, common themes in parental response across conditions have been identified. These include chronic sorrow (Clubb, 1991; Lemons & Weaver, 1986; Olshansky, 1962; Romney, 1984; Worthington, 1989), stress extending over time with uncertainty (Cohen & Martinson, 1988; Stein & Jessop, 1982), financial demands (Weeks, 1985), and difficulties with professional and support services (Diehl, Moffitt, & Wade, 1991). Research also has identified family and parental strengths, coping, and adaptation (Cadman et al., 1991; Drotar et al., 1981; Kovacs, Iyengar, & Goldston, 1990).

Increased survival rates combined with rapidly increasing health care costs brought government attention to family needs in the 1980s (Hobbs & Perrin, 1985). Earlier discharge from the hospital meant many families were faced with complex caregiving, often without ongoing education and support. The phrase "family-centered care" was introduced through initiatives of the U.S. Surgeon General's Office, the Bureau of Maternal and Child Health and Resources Development, Department of Health and Human Services, and the Association for the Care of Children's Health. This phrase signals a shift in traditional caregiving from provider to patient–recipient to a collaborative partnership between the providers and the recipient defined as the family unit. Parents and professionals are seen "as equals in a partnership committed to the development of optimal quality in the delivery of all levels of health care" (Brewer et al., 1989, p. 1055).

This family-centered approach is outlined as a family systems model of enablement and enpowerment by Dunst, Trivette, and Deal (1988). The model developed in early intervention programs for developmental disabilities can be applied to work in any area of chronic conditions. It emphasizes strengths and growth-producing behaviors rather than focusing on problems. It is accomplished by identifying family functioning style and sources of support and resources appropriate to the functioning style. It requires participation of providers and family in equal roles.

The family-centered focus includes siblings in the family. Once considered the forgotten members of the family, early studies of siblings began to identify the effects of a chronic condition on these members of the family. Tew and Lawrence (1973) found siblings of children with spina bifida four times more likely to be anxious than siblings of control siblings. Gayton et al. (1977) looked specifically at siblings of children with cystic fibrosis and found behavioral distress. Cairns, Clark, Smith, and Lansky (1979) found siblings of children with cancer to have significant anxiety and feelings of social isolation and neglect by parents.

Recent studies of children with chronic conditions and of siblings have seen the negative psychosocial impact of chronic conditions give way to a realization that children, both patients and siblings, may *not* be negatively affected. This change is attributed to larger study populations and refined research techniques. The recent studies of children with chronic conditions identify an increased risk for mental health problems and also identify children who show little or no disturbance (Cadman, et al., 1987; Drotar & Crawford, 1986; Eiser, 1990). The most comprehensive study of siblings to date led its researchers to conclude that clinicians should not expect that siblings of chronically ill children will have mental health or adjustment problems (Cadman, Boyle, & Offord, 1988).

The finding that all children are not negatively affected in psychosocial functioning, coupled with growing evidence of shared issues across chronic conditions (i.e., the noncategoric approach), joined in the 1980s with psychologic research from a variety of areas into a stress-resistant or stress-coping theoretical perspective (Luthar & Zigler, 1991; Pellegrini, 1990; Perrin & MacLean, 1988; Rutter, 1987). There is increasing interest in how most children and families manage to cope with chronic conditions. The focus has moved from a deficit, problem-oriented model to one that looks for coping, competence, and sources of support (Sinnema, 1991).

Stress–Coping–Resilience Framework

Stress is defined as "a particular relationship between the person and the environment that is appraised by the person as taxing his or her resources and endangering his or her well-being" (Lazarus & Folkman, 1984, p. 19). Two processes mediate the person–environment relationship: cognitive appraisal and coping. Cognitive appraisal refers to the process in which the individual evaluates the significance of what is happening for his or her well-being; the harm or loss, threat, and challenge involved; and the judgment concerning what might and can be done. Coping is the process through which the individual manages stress and the emotions generated (i.e., the cognitive and behavioral efforts to manage specific external or internal demands that are appraised as taxing or exceeding the resources of the person). Coping can be directed toward dealing with the environment or with one's thoughts and feelings about the stress. Developing and practicing coping strategies and participating in educational programs are examples of the former. Efforts to deal with thoughts and feelings may include physical exercise to release tension, reappraisal of stress as not harmful, and the use of defense mechanisms.

Coping strategies for children in health care have been described as stress-immunization techniques (Poster & Betz, 1983). Such strategies include relaxation techniques, systematic desensitization, cognitive rehearsal, hospital play, and discussion. Melamed (1988) adds distraction, modeling, imagery, calming self-talk, and reinforcement. Predominant coping styles in children's response to illness and treatments are active, information-seeking, and avoidant, information-denying (Tesler & Savedra, 1981; Peterson, 1989). Peterson and Toler (1986) found parents to be sources of information in assessing their child's information-seeking or avoidance coping style. Information from parents included the child's historic success in coping with medical procedures, the child's typical preferences for acquiring information, and the child's typical coping behaviors. Worchel, Copeland, and Barker (1987) found that behavioral control-related coping strategies were predictive of better emotional adjustment in children and adolescents with cancer. Decisional control, the child's perceived control over treatments, activities, and meals by providing the opportunity to make decisions and have choices, can increase one's sense of efficacy or the belief that one can have an effect on one's environment.

Chronic conditions as stressful life events can be seen as precipitating events, which can have negative outcomes *or* can lead to coping and adaptation. A shift from looking at predisposing to precipitating events provides avenues for interventions within a stress-coping framework (Silverman & Koretz, 1989). For example, if poverty is seen as a predisposing factor, then Mirah should not have left the projects as a young adult cancer survivor to attend college. In spite of poverty, Mirah and her grandmother viewed her condition as another challenge that could be faced and mastered. A family value system that identified education as a way to get ahead in life and social supports gained through school and church allowed Mirah to continue to develop her intellectual and musical skills and receive years of chemotherapy. For Mirah, poverty and cancer were stressors to which she responded with coping and resilience. Although poverty does not condemn a child to mental health problems, it does present an intense, additional stress. Cumulative stressors and fewer protective factors have been found to increase greatly the risk for negative outcomes (Garmezy, 1991).

Understanding a precipitating factor, such as stressful life events, as the "triggering mechanism" for the expression of maladaptive coping behavior sheds light on John's experience. The recurrence of disease can be seen as a stressor to which he responded with inadequate, counterproductive efforts. The stressful life events of chronic conditions place challenges on the child's coping and make the child a source of stress for others in his or her social network—parents, siblings, peers, and school. How the child and support network perceive the stressors will determine how they adapt to the chronic condition (Silverman & Koretz, 1989). While we search for prevention of chronic conditions, we also must look for ways to decrease the negative effects of chronic conditions by increasing coping efforts and resilience.

Resilience refers to the individual's ability to bounce back from stressful events. It is an individual variation in response to risk that is not a fixed attribute but changes as circumstances in an individual's life change and has protective benefits. Garmezy (1983) describes three sets of variables that function as protective factors: 1) dispositional attributes of positive temperament, sociability, hardiness, autonomy, and particularly self-esteem; 2) family cohesion, seen in warmth, harmony, and absence of neglect; and 3) the availability of external support systems that encourage and reinforce a child's coping efforts.

John's family, as an example, was continually changing and had been long before his diagnosis. Mother and father would separate, take new partners, reunite, and then change partners. John was moved back and forth between the parents. Not only were parent–child relationships unstable, but social supports were broken each time John changed communities and schools. The stress of John's recurrence, coupled with an absence of protective factors, resulted in despair, self-devaluation, and self-abusive behavior.

Rutter (1987) describes the protective factors as reduction of the risk impact (for John, the impact of his recurrence could not be reduced); reduction of negative chain responses (family therapy interventions were not successful with John's family); establishment and maintenance of self-esteem and self-efficacy; and the opening up of opportunities through social support networks. In both these areas, John's nomadic life prevented formation of relationships beyond the health care setting that could support his self-esteem and provide opportunities.

Rutter (1987) finds two types of experiences most influential in supporting and strengthening self-esteem: personal relationships and task accomplishment. Task accomplishment is defined as the positive accomplishment of such things as school, success in nonacademic activities, social relations, and management of stressful events. Task accomplishment that aids self-esteem as a protective mechanism includes learning effective coping skills, social problem-solving skills, knowledge of having coped successfully in the past with challenges, and the positive appraisal of one's self and actions by others. For example, the musical talents and academic skills Mirah continued to develop throughout her treatments provided self-esteem, self-efficacy (mastery), and task accomplishment and led to greater opportunities through a music scholarship. Social supports came from school, church, and the health care setting as she participated in an ongoing adolescent support group and summer camp.

Opportunities for self-directed and self-initiated behavior aid self-efficacy and a sense of decisional control. Unstructured play opportunities for children have been described by Bolig and Weedle (1988) as a hospital-based intervention that supports resilience. The opportunity to initiate and self-direct play allows the child to regain a sense of mastery in the environment and to make choices and act on those choices when so many decisions are out of the child's control. This self-initiation and self-direction in unstructured play counteracts feelings of powerlessness, helplessness, and overdependence on others (Bolig & Fernie, 1986).

SELF-CONCEPT, BODY IMAGE, AND SOCIAL STIGMA

While self-esteem is the picture of one's individual worth, self-concept and body image are related concepts that influence self-esteem (Neff & Beardslee, 1990; Harvey & Greenway, 1984). Self-concept, the operational definition of self-esteem, is the individual's mental picture of himself or herself that includes ideas, beliefs, and attitudes about the self, as well as thoughts and feelings about physical appearance (body image) and self-worth or self-esteem (Sieving & Zirbel-Donish, 1990). Body image develops as a result of the reactions of others to one's physical appearance and is a part of self-concept. Negative feelings experienced when rejection of the self is based on physical appearance contribute to a negative self-concept. To establish one's identity, there must be an intact image of one's own body. This process is more difficult for children with chronic conditions, such as disability, because they encounter social stigmatization (Richardson, 1970). Children with no handicaps were viewed as most liked as children grew older; children with cosmetic handicaps (limb missing, facial deformity) were liked less than children with functional handicaps (requiring braces, crutches, or wheelchair). Changes in body image are seen as losses to which the individual responds with changes in self-concept (Varni & Setoguchi, 1991). The long-term effect of social isolation, or social stigmatization, resulting from cosmetic or functional difference, and loss experienced with changes in the body's physical appearance may result in a handicapping self-image. Strax (1991) states the following:

> The social ostracizing of youths with disabilities further reinforces the individual's sense of difference. By the time a child with a physical disability becomes an adolescent, he or she is aware of society's ideal physical image. Like his or her ablebodied peers, the child will reject a physically disabled adolescent and will also reject him- or herself. As more and more children with chronic illnesses and disabilities survive into adulthood, the hope is that they can develop the skills to be resilient (pp. 510–511).

The handicap resulting from the disability that involves physical difference arises from the rejection of one's self, from social isolation or stigma, and from restricted opportunities for task accomplishment and independence. All of these may combine to influence negatively the evaluation of self-worth and result in decreased self-esteem.

A final area related to self-esteem is that of personal relationships. Relationships that develop and strengthen self-esteem are harmonious and secure parent–child relationships and in older children and throughout adulthood, intimate relationships (Rutter, 1987).

Coping efforts and resiliency influence the outcome of the response to the stressful life events of chronic illness and conditions. How can we influence coping and resilience? What individual and institutional efforts can support self-esteem and self-efficacy, the development of social supports, family functioning, and the unfolding of opportunities?

First, a search for interventions to foster resilience must be seen within a dynamic, transactional, developmental, and ecologic perspective: *Dynamic* means that change occurs, and the chronic condition is not a fixed attribute but changes due to the medical course or as it influences the child's developmental progress and developmental task accomplishment. *Transactional* means that interactions between the child and others (parents, health care providers, peers) influence the development of resiliency. *Developmental* means that at each stage of cognitive, social, physical, and emotional development, challenges are presented that influence future development. *Ecologic* means that the child and family do not live in a vacuum, but rather are a system that interacts with, influences, and is influenced by other systems such as health care, school, and social systems.

Second, the search can take many directions. It can be specific or global. It can include analyses of behavioral programs to increase chronically impaired children's social skills (Clark, 1989), techniques to enhance marital adjustment and family functioning (Griffith & Griffith, 1987), or public policy efforts to provide financial assistance and medical insurance to families (Weeks, 1985).

Several conceptual models and theories have been applied to pediatrics. Among them are Hymovitch's Family Developmental Task Model (1979) and the Double ABCX Model of Family Adaptation (McCubbin & Patterson, 1983). The stress–coping framework has been used in research by Tesler and Savedra (1981) and in clinical application by Poster and Betz (1983). The stress–coping–resilience framework used in a mental health perspective has been discussed by Drotar and Bush (1985), Silverman and Koretz (1985), and Patterson and Geber (1991).

DEVELOPMENTAL CONSIDERATIONS

Certainly, the child's progression through cognitive, social, emotional, and physical development influences coping and resilience. Coping strategies used by toddlers will be different from those of an adolescent. The younger the child, the fewer the available strategies. For example, a preschool child can learn a coping technique through modeling and imitation; a 10-year-old can add reading a book, writing a story, and teaching another child to his or her repertoire of learning techniques. Developmental progression may be uneven across the realms, particularly when considering a chronic condition. A preschool child confined to a wheelchair may have more developed social skills and language, far beyond the development of gross motor skill. Table 11-1 presents major concepts to summarize the vast array of developmental information that relates to chronic conditions. Some concepts appear in more than one stage of development; others evolve and transform. Understanding cognitive development is crucial (Bibace & Walsh, 1981; Brewster, 1982; Hauck, 1991; Perrin, Sayer, & Willett, 1991). Each developmental stage presents challenges to the child. Vulnerability evident in the infant's dependence on the world for physical and emotional sustenance resurfaces but is transformed in adolescents with chronic conditions (Ell & Reardon, 1990). Increased noncompliance (which can be as high as 50%), coupled with increased behavioral distress, renders adolescents vulnerable to physical and emotional security.

Self-Assessment

Before accepting responsibility to work with children with chronic conditions, each health care professional should contemplate his or her technical and emotional preparedness. Professional training is one aspect that influences outcomes in children with chronic conditions (Hobbs & Perrin, 1985). Professional training across disciplines should result in abilities to provide technically competent services, communicate with families, participate as an effective team member, be sensitive to ethical issues (respect for multicultural issues and confidentiality, for example), and the ability to conceptualize problems in ecologic terms—to view the child and family in the complexity of their overlapping worlds of home, school, health care, work, and social relationships.

Perhaps the most important ability all professionals must have and share is the ability to see the child as a child. "All too often a child with, for example, cystic fibrosis is referred to as a 'cystic.' This generalization of the disease to characterize the whole child limits, in a profound but subtle fashion, the future one might envision for that child" (Hobbs, Perrin, & Ireys, 1985, p. 55).

Self-assessment includes questioning one's thoughts, feelings, attitudes, and values. Do they lead to an "opening up of opportunities," as Rutter describes resilience (Rutter, 1987), or do they lead to a limited vision of the child's future? There are additional challenges for the nurse who provides direct care that require self-assessment and continuing reflection. These challenges can be described as boundary issues and dependency (or codependency) concerns. The impact of each is heightened in the hospital setting, particularly in tertiary care centers where the majority of children with chronic conditions are diagnosed and often receive ongoing medical management. For example, a child with a chronic condition may have several hospital admissions. The number of disciplines involved in the child's care and the even greater number of people in those disciplines, coupled with their varying levels of knowledge and experience, make agreement on goals for a child and family difficult. Consistency in carrying out goals is even more difficult to achieve.

Psychosocial understanding is a complex process built on theories, research, and clinical study and experience. Too often a significant number of

TABLE 11–1 Developmental Concepts

Infant	Toddler	Preschool	Schoolage	Adolescent
Trust	Autonomy (shame, doubt)	Initiative (guilt)	Industry (inferiority)	Identity (autonomy and independence)
Begin cause, effect	Preoperational thought Egocentric → Fantasy →	Intuitive transductive reasoning	Concrete operations	Formal operations
Perception of condition → pain/distress seen as responses	Pain, discomfort, distress	Magical thought Illness as punishment, self-causation	Can infer intent of treatment Can state one physical cause	Can infer intent and empathy Understands multiple causes
Play begins →	Parallel play—interactive	Cooperative play —	Rule-bound, games —	Recreation
Loss →	Self-concept emerging	Body image Fears of mutilation, penetration	Body image Concern, threat/loss of control	Can be extreme, noncompliant
Parental grief	Chronic sorrow continues →	→	→	
Temperament →	→	Temperament with developing optimism/pessimism →	→	
Attachment parents →	→	→	Peers	Peers/intimacy/adult mentors
Regression may be seen in loss of interest in physical surroundings	Regression may be seen in loss of newly acquired body functions, toileting	Regression may be seen in insecure behaviors, clinging, easily upset, whining, crying	Regression may be seen in hypercontrolling behaviors	Regression may be seen in cognitive regression, withdrawal, control issues

direct care providers in tertiary settings are young and less experienced. With inexperience, many are inclined to use their own personal life experience as a frame of reference for understanding and relating to others. In a survey of 243 pediatric nurses, marital and parental status, experience, and further education were significantly correlated with more accepting attitudes of, and participation with, parents in pediatric units (Gill, 1987). Regardless of age or experience, many disciplines bring skills based on a deficit model, rather than based in a mental health, developmental perspective. Issues of boundaries and dependency must be explored before initiating the nursing process.

BOUNDARIES

Although a child is in our care, the child is not ours. The child is a member of a family, and this membership continues in spite of a chronic condition and resulting hospitalization. Respect for the child and family is fully integrated when a nurse says "your child" rather than "my patient." Family boundaries are necessary for individuals in the family and the family as a system to effectively fulfill the tasks required of a family—physical and emotional security that allows each member to function in society. Studies of medically fragile children found family boundaries and integrity most effective in families who maintained a professional, versus friendship, relationship with providers (Patterson, 1991). In describing work with children who have cancer, Fochtman (1991) discussed the need to recognize when clinical judgments may be compromised if professional–family boundaries become blurred.

Within the framework of caring for children and families with chronic conditions, consistency and continuity are powerful supports to families. To be consistent, physically present, and emotionally available with time, caregivers must continually assess their own boundaries with families and be wary of enmeshment that can cloud judgment and deplete energy. Instead nurses can rejoice in the strides children and families make with our support *and* with their own efforts and strengths.

DEPENDENT AND CODEPENDENT BEHAVIORS

We choose to work with children with chronic conditions because we want to make a positive difference in life. However, our needs may interfere with the needs of the child and family. This is easily seen when a caregiver rushes to "rescue" a frustrated child: "Don't get upset; I'll button your shirt for you/move your wheelchair/tell those kids not to bother you." The hidden message is a debilitating one: The child is not expected to be able to do these things. The child is seen as dependent, and only others can do and control life and events. Efforts to be helpful may be less helpful if they deprive the child of opportunities to be active in his or her own behalf.

Other behaviors that reward dependency may be seen in the hospital setting when caregivers reward child–adult interactions to the exclusion of developmentally beneficial, child–child interactions. "Stay with me while I finish my charting and then I'll take you to get a snack." The caregiver feels good being with the child (and perhaps it is an easier way to add medication to the child's IV at the appropriate time). However, the child may miss opportunities for developmental activities and interactions with peers. Continually, we must ask ourselves: Whose needs am I meeting? Am I reinforcing passivity and dependency to meet my needs, and what is the possible effect on the child? In singling out this child, what message am I conveying to other patients and families? There may be times when the answer, truthfully told, is "I am meeting my needs. I just came from a patient's room where the child has been placed on 'do not resuscitate' status. I need the closeness and hug of a more healthy child to renew my spirit." This answer reflects the commitment necessary to care for children with chronic conditions and self-awareness that signals emotional health. However, an answer that supports a habitual need for self-enhancement and validation or convenience is not in the best interests of a developing child. The child needs encouragement to move into the world rather than retreat from the challenges of a chronic condition. Comparison of locus of control in 71 healthy children with 207 children divided into four chronic condition groups found internal locus of control less present in chronically ill children and in their mothers (Perrin & Shapiro, 1985). The researchers concluded that health care providers should assist young children in recognizing, even in small ways, the efforts they can take to increase control over their health. Reliance on providers may be detrimental for the child and mother to learning effective skills for independent health-related decision making.

Several reports of parents' experiences of stress indicate the conflicts that arise between dependent and independent needs. Hayes and Knox (1984) found that role conflict with staff was a major source of stress for parents during their disabled child's hospitalization. Parents felt their expertise in caring for their child at home was ignored in the hospital. While the parents felt responsible for their child, they did not feel they had control. Robinson (1984) reports similar findings, which are described as the "double-bind" of parenting in health care settings. Identifying stressful and rewarding events that have been experienced in professional and personal areas and one's responses to them are suggested as catalysts for a personal inventory to distinguish between codependent, accommodating, and independent professional practices (Sherman, Cardea, Gaskill, & Tynan, 1989).

Reflection is the process used to increase self-awareness and evaluation. "What am I doing? Why? What else do I need to consider?" This reflection-in-action leads to greater competence and increased benefits for self and clients (Schon, 1987). Reflection combined with evaluation of scientific components of care maximizes effectiveness of practice (Aita, 1990; Saylor, 1990).

Loss and Grief

Loss occurs throughout life and is an accepted reality. The birth or diagnosis of a child with a chronic condition, however, is neither usual nor expected and is difficult to accept. Throughout the life of a child with a chronic condition, loss occurs but with added meaning. Grief can be expressed by the child, the parents, and other family members and by health care personnel.

Parents mourn the loss of their fantasized "perfect" baby. They mourn the loss of what their child could have been, or was, and the loss of their fantasies for the child's future and the family's future (Edwards, 1987; Lemons & Weaver, 1986).

For children, the chronic condition presents changes in self-concept, which occur in response to body changes, such as hair loss, extreme weight gain or loss, limb amputation, and loss of physical functioning. The change in self-concept results from the loss of the healthy self, to which grief is a normal reaction (Seagull, 1990). Other losses abound throughout treatment—loss in normal routines and family life, loss of relationships due to hospitalization and separation from home and school, and loss of support as family members experience their own grief and may be less emotionally available. Olshansky (1962) used the phrase "chronic sorrow" to describe loss experienced over time, a natural response to a tragic event. "Chronic sorrow" implies functional adaptation to, but not closure or final acceptance of, the child's condition (Clubb, 1991). Copley and Bodensteiner (1987) proposed that parents have two phrases of adjustment. The first is a cycle of high and low emotions; the second focuses outward, with functioning coping strategies and acceptance of the child as he or she is. Wikler et al. (1981) found chronic sorrow to be a coping mechanism that allows for periodic grieving at points related to developmental milestones and points that have special meaning to the family. This formulation, coupled with the two phases of adjustment discussed previously, give direction to nurses as they interact with families, particularly as they strive to understand parents. For example, a mother who usually arrives at the hospital in a cheerful, coping stance presents as angry and withdrawn; she may have just had a fight with her husband, or she may be mourning the loss of a developmental milestone (e.g., her son's inability to dance at the prom because of his muscular dystrophy).

Parents have different responses to loss (Fraley, 1986). Differences between mothers and fathers have been identified (Damrosch & Perry, 1989), as have differences between children. Adolescents' experiences may be intensified by their cognitive skills of formal operations and resulting abilities to project into the future about what they may be and what might have been.

"Disenfranchised grief" has been used to describe losses experienced, which are not openly acknowledged, publicly mourned, or socially supported (Doka, 1989). The term connotes the societal norms that regulate grieving. These norms, however, may not reflect the nature of attachments, sense of loss, and feelings of everyone in society. For example, a wife grieves for her husband's death and receives support from many sources. The husband's golf partner for the past 10 years also mourns but does not receive the same level of support and is expected to support the widow. Mourning a pet companion is another example of disenfranchised grief. There are few public rituals or acknowledgments of the loss; the loss is disenfranchised because it is not recognized as important or significant.

Nurses may encounter parents and children with chronic conditions who are disenfranchised grievers. The nurse is in a unique position to validate the feelings of the child and family as they respond to losses in chronic conditions. Who, then, supports the disenfranchised grief of the nurse and other health care personnel? Nurses also experience sadness when a child is born "less than perfect," is diagnosed or relapses with cancer, and is confined to a wheelchair with juvenile arthritis. In discussing disenfranchised grief in nurses who work with dying patients, Lev (1989) states, "Support a caregiver receives from others may be the additional ingredient necessary to enable him or her to enter into therapeutic relationships without risk to one's self" (p. 292). Such support from others may be a critical ingredient in preventing job dissatisfaction and burnout. Coping with caregivers' grief related to death has recently received increased attention (Lev, 1989). Feelings of loss and grief related to care of children with chronic conditions have not been explored.

Nurses who conceal job-related stress exhibit reactions such as physical and emotional distancing from patients and other staff and experience feelings of inadequacy, anger, frustration, and impatience (Larson, 1987). Suggestions for supports to nurses include expression of feelings through collegial support groups; clinical supervision; continuing education about grief, loss, and bereavement; and following good personal health care practices. As suggested for children, the nurse also can use coping strategies of cognitive appraisal and attribution, that is, finding meaning in his or her efforts as supports for personal coping and resilience.

Supportive Communication

Unique skills of communication can assist the nurse's work with children who have chronic conditions. These skills, labeled here as supportive communications, include nonthreatening language, descriptive praise, mediated learning experience, and positive self-talk.

NONTHREATENING LANGUAGE

Gaynard, Wolfer, Goldberger, Thompson, Redburn, and Laidley (1990) present an extensive discussion and examples of nonthreatening language, involving the selection of words and expression of concepts that are concrete and have little ambiguity and the use of "soft" rather than "hard" words.

Supportive, nonthreatening communication also allows the child to bring his or her own experience into the exchange. For example, in describing an injection, the word injection is softer than "shot"; however, it is not as concrete and can be better described as a "sting." More helpful for the child is to ask how he or she thinks it will feel and then provide a range of possibilities, such as "Some children have told me the injection feels like a mosquito sting; some say they don't really feel anything; some say it's a little sting but doesn't last long. After we do this, you can tell me what it was like for you." This range does not predispose the child to the experience and supports the uniqueness of the child and the child's experience.

DESCRIPTIVE PRAISE

Too often global value judgments are used as praise and reinforcement of a child's actions. This can be confusing to the child and nonreinforcing. For example, health care settings are replete with "What a good girl!" when a child has completed a painful procedure. The child may wonder, "If they think I'm good now, what happens when they think I'm bad? Am I bad? Is it because I have bad blood? What if I'm not so good the next time? Will they still be my nurses if I'm not good?" It is more helpful to be specific and descriptive when praising a child and acknowledge degrees of effort (Faber & Mazlish, 1980; Bolig & Weedle, 1988). "You were really working hard to hold your arm still when I started your IV. I could tell! You helped me when your arm didn't move. That really helped me get the needle in quick. Thank you for helping!"

MEDIATED LEARNING EXPERIENCES

Mediated learning experiences refer to adult actions that assist the child in organizing and learning from an experience (Feuerstein, 1979; Mearig, 1985). To have meaning, experience must be organized into cognitive schemata. This is seen in infants from a Piagetian perspective as early cause and effect; the infant organizes novel actions through repetition into beginning cause and effect. A fling of an arm caused a toy to rattle. With repetition, the fling becomes purposeful: "I want the toy to rattle, so I will move my arm." Many experiences in health care have no relation to the child's existing cognitive schemes; they have not been encountered before, or the sequences and people involved are novel, and generalization from past experience to the present is difficult. Children with chronic conditions may learn to expect treatments to be one sequence of events, which is not replicated when the child is hospitalized because new people, with new routines and possibly different equipment, are involved in the experience. Without support, the child will have difficulty making sense of the experience. The nurse can provide mediation, adding information that links the present experience to past experiences and to the future.

"This time when you go to x-ray to have a picture taken, the camera will be different. It won't be like the last time you went. Remember when you got on the table and had to hold very still? This time the table will move. You will have to hold real still again, but the the table will move so the camera can take a new picture. This new picture will show the doctor how she can help your stomach when it hurts." The nurse, through communication, has mediated the learning, connecting the experience to the past and extended it into the future.

POSITIVE SELF-TALK

Children learn from experience and through imitation. Rather than silently carrying out nursing tasks, the nurse can model positive self-talk:

"Let's see, I'm going to check this IV. I made sure I know the time to put the medicine in and I have everything I need, so I am really organized!"

"I did a pretty good job getting that breakfast tray here, and I didn't spill a drop. Good for me!"

"Oops, I dropped my papers. Oh well, I do that sometimes. I can pick them up; it's not the end of the world."

Most importantly, an optimistic outlook, as Gudas, Koocher, and Wypij (1991) found related to compliance with medical treatments, can be modeled:

"You and I have a busy day today—lots of tests and things to do. I wonder if I can get all my work done? I'll bet I can."

"Let's see now, you are really good at playing checkers. I wonder if I can play OK. I'll bet I can play as good as I possibly can. I'm going to give it a try. I'll have fun playing with you."

This optimistic outlook can be fostered by combining verbal communication and action. For example, "You are having your operation in the morning. You will come back from your operation, and you will need to stay in bed. What would you like to do when you are back in your bed? Let's plan something very special that you would like to do!"

The optimistic view is that the child is expected to return from surgery and then will be able to act on his or her choices and plans.

Nursing Process

During a child's hospitalization, families have intense contact with health care, which offers opportunities to influence coping and resilience; Hymovitch (1985) has identified additional placements, such as community-based clinics, schools, community agencies, and homes, in which nurses care for children with chronic conditions. Regardless of the setting, however, the stress–coping–resilience framework can be applied. Nurses, child-life specialists, social workers, physical therapists, and others in the setting should collaborate to develop a mental health program of support for children.

Drotar and Bush (1985) state the following goals for a systems approach to the promotion of coping and resiliency: mastery of potentially disruptive anxiety related to the condition and its physical management; understanding of and adherence to necessary medical regimens; integration of the illness or condition into family life, particularly reconciliation of family needs with those of the ill child; and adaptation to hospital, home, school, and peers. A "reasonable level of adaptation" by the child and family arises from trust developed through the following:

- Continuity of relationships
- Active participation by professional caregivers
- Mutual participation of child and family
- Advocacy
- A focus on coping and competence
- A developmental perspective
- Family-centered care

This approach focuses on the stressful, yet potentially manageable, prospect of living with a chronic condition and views the condition as an opportunity for mastery rather than an inevitable disruption (Drotar & Bush, 1985).

ASSESSMENT

A positive expectation bias for a child's and family's coping is required as a first step in assessment. This positive expectation bias also includes the knowledge that there is an increased risk for mental health problems in children with chronic conditions. Assessment should identify strengths, needs, and the presence or absence of protective factors of resilience, including self-esteem and self-efficacy, social supports, family functioning, and opportunities. This assessment should be carried out with an overriding goal of care: "to confine the consequences of the biologic disorder to its minimum manifestation, to encourage normal growth and development, to assist the child in maximizing potential in all possible areas, and to prevent or diminish the behavioral and social consequences" (Stein & Jessop, 1982, p. 193).

The assessment is complicated by the complex interaction of changes that occurs in the life of a child and family. These simultaneous changes occur in the child's developmental progress, the medical condition, the evolving family, and adaptation by the child and family to the child's chronic condition. Assessment begins with information gathered about the child's developmental status; the medical diagnosis and required or expected treatments and medications; the family; the appraisal by child and family of the stress; and existing, available coping strategies, self-esteem, and social supports. Age at onset, impact on mobility, and impact on cognitive abilities are developmental considerations that influence assessment (Perrin & MacLean, 1988). Predictability versus uncertainty (Stein & Jessop, 1984) also influence cognitive appraisal and stress.

Leventhal (1984) suggests six questions that should be addressed in assessment: 1) What is the extent of the disease, condition, and its complications for the child? 2) What are the physical effects on the child? 3) How has the illness or condition affected the child's performance at home, with peers, in school, or other settings? 4) How has the child adjusted to the condition? 5) What impact does the illness have on the family and its members? 6) How has the family adjusted to the special impact or burden of the illness?

The detailed assessment outline in Box 11-1 includes information to be gathered about the condition, the child, and the family, first identifying general information as a baseline against which to compare specific information with normative information. Identification of needs specific to the child and family can be made, and from these data are formulated nursing diagnoses that guide the planning of interventions. (See Box 11-2 for a thorough assessment of a 14-month-old with cystic fibrosis.)

Planning and Intervention

Assessment and identification of needs and nursing diagnoses lead to planning of interventions. Within the stress–coping–resilience framework, in-

BOX 11–1 • ASSESSMENT OUTLINE

I. Assessment—general
 A. Pertinent medical information
  1. Diagnosis/presenting problems
   a. Information obtained from patient's physical assessment
   b. Information obtained from patient's and parent's interviews
  2. Procedure(s) child can be expected to experience (based on diagnosis)
  3. Medications that could behaviorally affect child
 B. Developmental (normative)
  1. General physical development
  2. Psychosocial stages (Erikson)
  3. Cognitive development (Piaget stages, health beliefs)
 C. Issues or challenges to coping—anticipated
II. Assessment—specific
 A. Medical information
  1. Child's or family's reason for hospitalization and why (in their words)
  2. Child's or family's understanding of what will happen and why
  3. Child's or family's assessment of threat or discomfort
  4. Previous hospitalizations
   a. If yes, where and when?
   b. Child's or family's memories of previous hospitalization
   c. Child's or family's assessment of coping with previous hospitalization
  5. Child's experiences with procedures to date
  6. Planned medical experiences or procedures during this hospitalization
 B. Developmental information
  1. General physical development of *this* child; any known limitations—motor, sensory, developmental
  2. This child's stage of psychosocial development (with examples)
  3. This child's stage of cognitive development (with examples)
 C. Environmental—family information
  1. Structure and functions: members, problems, available supports
  2. Sociocultural
  3. Physical availability during hospital stay
  4. Recent family stressors
  5. Coping strategies
 D. Idiosyncratic (personal to this child)
  1. Temperament or personality
  2. Preferred coping stance (avoidant—actively seeks information)
  3. Coping strategies
  4. Comfort preferences
  5. Previous separation experiences and responses
  6. Prehospital routines of daily living
III. Issues for this child and family
 A. Identified needs
 B. Goals
 C. Plans

terventions are grouped into three major categories:

- Those that decrease stress and increase coping
- Those that support self-esteem, mastery, and social support
- Those that foster family functioning

STRESS AND COPING

Assisting the child and family in viewing the immediate stress and the long-term process as manageable is an intervention related to cognitive appraisal. Obtaining information about the condition and treatments reduces uncertainty and ambiguity with decreases in stress and anxiety (Vulcan & Nikulich-Barrett, 1988). Educational efforts are widespread and useful interventions (Conatser, 1986); however, a caution exists. Having educational material available does not guarantee knowledge and understanding. Careful review and analysis of written materials must be combined with knowledge of the child and family (Glazer-Waldman, Francis, & Smith, 1987). Does the parent read? At what grade level? In what language? These answers should direct selection of materials (Lynn, 1989) and can apply to audio and videotape materials and computer-assisted learning (Rubin, 1989).

The most common vehicle for information to children is referred to as preparation, the development of emotional and cognitive understanding of events and treatments during hospitalization. Preparation using stress point information, filmed modeling, and coping skills training is beneficial to decrease stress and increase coping. Preparation should always be engaged with a child by using a developmental, interactional style based on knowl-

BOX 11–2 • ASSESSMENT OUTLINE

I. Assessment—general
  A. Medical information
    1. Diagnosis: Wesley, a 14-month-old white boy, admitted for newly diagnosed cystic fibrosis; may have recurrent respiratory infections, failure to thrive, electrolyte imbalances, malabsorption
    2. Procedures—expected: IV antibiotics and respiratory therapy (CPT), nutrition and dietary needs evaluation
  B. Developmental (normative)
    1. Physical: weight since birth tripled; length increased 50%; can breathe through mouth when nose is occluded
      a. Pincer grasp mastered
      b. Can play pat-a-cake with hands brought to midline
      c. Drinks from a cup
      d. Beginning skill with a spoon
      e. Walks well; able to stoop and recover toys
      f. Builds two- to three-cube tower; enjoys environment that allows active exploration and manipulation
      g. Two- to three-word vocabulary other than "mama" and "dada"; enjoys imitating, speech games
    2. Psychosocial: stage of basic trust versus mistrust
    3. Cognitive: sensorimotor stage—tertiary circular reactions and internalization of schemes; recognizes objects by name—beginning symbols; understands simple commands
  C. Issues or challenges to coping—anticipated
    1. Separation anxiety; fear of strangers
    2. Need for consistency in caregivers and routine
    3. Need for physical exploration and interaction with objects and environment
    4. Need for caregivers to recognize and provide child's comfort measures
    5. Need for parents to be taught about chronic care of cystic fibrosis

II. Assessment—specific
  A. Medical information
    1. Child/family's reason for hospitalization
    2. Understanding of events and rationale
    3. Assessment of threat
      a. Mother—states feelings of being overwhelmed and inadequate
      b. Wesley—too young for verbal cognitive assessment; however, displays fear of strangers, medical personnel, and treatment
    4. Previous hospitalizations: none other than related to this admission—emergency room at another hospital, then transfer to children's hospital
    5. Child's experience of procedures to date: responds with physical responses (crying, withdrawal) to procedures of respiratory therapy and IV antibiotics
    6. Planned procedures: continue CPT and IV antibiotics
  B. Developmental information
    1. Physical development
      a. Good use of hands—manipulates toys
      b. Holds and drinks from cup
      c. Jabbers; says "hi," "no," "ma," and imitates sounds
      d. Observations in playroom raised questions about visual ability
      e. Within normal range of growth but at 10th percentile
    2. Psychosocial development
      a. Erikson's stage of basic trust versus mistrust evidenced in Wesley's attachment to significant caregivers and separation anxiety
      b. Displays curiosity and exploration; socially responsive when with mother or other well-known person
    3. Cognitive development: Piaget's sensorimotor stage as seen in use of objects, play, and language development to date; development of object permanence seen when Wesley dropped a toy and searched for it with his hands
  C. Environmental
    1. Family: mother and patient make up household; mother 17 years old, unemployed, not in school; maternal grandmother and aunt visit; father not involved with family
    2. Sociocultural: economically impoverished; somewhat isolated—no church, work, or school affiliations to offer support
    3. Physical availability: limited due to transportation (no car, and relatives work during the day)
    4. Recent family stressors: nothing specifically known other than chronic stressors of poverty and isolation
    5. Coping strategies of family: undetermined to date; question of impulse control of mother
  D. Idiosyncratic
    1. Temperament or personality: described by grandmother as easy going, quick to warm up, happy
    2. Preferred coping stance: actively explores environment and objects

(continued)

BOX 11–2 • ASSESSMENT OUTLINE *(Continued)*

3. Comfort preferences: mother reported that Wesley likes to be rocked and have a bottle when upset
4. Previous separation experiences and responses: unknown at this time; is not involved in day care program or other early childhood program
5. Prehospital routines of daily living: appears to have had few routines and little consistency in wake, sleep, and feeding patterns

III. Issues for this child and family
 A. Identified needs
  1. Questions of visual ability raised by observations in playroom; further assessment of vision needed
  2. Consistency and attachment needs for secure, predictable responses
  3. Ability of patient to cope with hospital (need to reduce, redirect negative behaviors, such as biting)
  4. Ability to cope with procedures
  5. Parent and family teaching about diagnosis, treatments, and chronic care
  6. Financial support
  7. Parent-to-parent support
  8. Ongoing developmental support and parenting education
  9. Potential referral to early intervention program as chronic condition places Wesley in "at-risk" category for developmental progress

edge of the child's previous coping efforts, preferences, and style. This approach can then be combined with filmed modeling (the most successfully researched intervention to date for surgery) or other modalities (Visintainer & Wolfer, 1975; Melamed & Siegel, 1975). The developmental, interactional stance with the child allows monitoring and response to the child as the child deals with potentially stressful stimuli. Involvement of parents has been found to be successful (Peterson & Toler, 1986); parents can continue to practice coping skills with the child beyond the specific preparation.

SELF-ESTEEM, MASTERY, AND SOCIAL SUPPORTS

The three concepts of self-esteem, mastery, and social supports are presented together, although interventions are not limited to one area but foster the development of each. For example, planning group playtime for a 5-year-old hospitalized for chronic renal failure provides opportunities for the child. The child may choose what toys and paints to use (making choices that give a sense of control, self-efficacy, and mastery), carry out a craft project (task accomplishment, which aids self-esteem), and interact with peers and supportive adults (social supports). School also gives the child opportunities to accomplish tasks and support self-esteem and provide social supports through peers and teachers.

PLAY AND RELATED ACTIVITY

Play generally refers to activities of infants and children; related activity refers to the play and recreational activity of adolescents. These activities fuel a child's development and provide countless hours and opportunities for self-direction and control over the environment (mastery and self-efficacy); release of tension (decreased stress); practice of new behaviors (increased coping); accomplishment of tasks through art, crafts, and games (self-esteem); and interaction with others for social support (Bolig & Weedle, 1988). As an intervention, the hospital nurse should organize physical care routines so that ample time is available for play and activity; use available resources, such as a child-life department and activity rooms; and monitor the provision of issue-specific play and unstructured, self-directed play. Guidance and information can be discussed with parents about the value of play and activity for the child and how it can be carried out at home and in the family's community. Encouragement for and referrals to community agencies, such as YMCA, YWCA, scouting, and other recreation programs may assist the play and leisure needs of the child. Some communities have specific therapeutic recreation programs and facilities to accommodate children with special health care needs.

Environmental Considerations

Environments give powerful messages and structure behavior. Dependence or independence can be facilitated through environmental organization and design. The environment can foster coping and social relationships or encourage isolation, rigidity, and depersonalization (Olds, 1978; Piserchia, Bragg, & Alvarez, 1982).

Six dimensions of supportive physical environments are important to consider in fostering coping and resilience: safety; comfort; personalization; normalization; the continuum from active to passive, directed to self-initiated activity; and family-centered care (Box 11-3).

SAFETY

Is the physical environment designed to meet developmental needs of children and adults? Is there ample space for movement and movement with assistive devices and medical equipment? Is space adequate for safe movement in patient rooms and activity rooms? Are materials in patient and activity room safe for the ages served? Are infection control concerns determined and carried out? A survey of three pediatric settings found hazards in every safety category examined. The majority of hazards were due to carelessness in day-to-day routines or lack of knowledge of potential hazards to hospitalized children (Banco & Powers, 1988).

COMFORT

The environment should be designed for comfort, including beds, chairs, and space in which to comfortably move. The space should be adaptable to meet changing needs as children progress through treatments and have changing functional assistance needs.

PERSONALIZATION

The environment should have ways in which a specific child or group of children can demonstrate their unique presence in the environment. For example, one setting uses the child's picture, taken during the admission process, to signify the child's room. A small bulletin board by the patient's door displays the picture along with necessary medical information, such as isolation precautions. Another setting has Plexiglas art frames in corridors and playrooms, which easily provide a rotating art exhibit produced by current patients. Permission and places to display greeting cards, artwork, and other memorabilia in the patient's room imparts a sense of belonging and uniqueness that aids self-esteem.

BOX 11–3 • CHECKLIST FOR THE ENVIRONMENT

Does the environment for children and adolescents provide for the following:

- Safety
- Comfort
- Personalization
- Normalization
- Active and passive, directed and self-initiated play and activity
- Family-centered care

NORMALIZATION

The environment of the unit, patient's room, and activity room should have consonance with the child's previous experiences and a connection with the child's prehospital life. Playrooms can easily contain familiar materials and objects and favorite toys and games. Play telephones allow children to pretend to talk to absent family and friends and extend the present experience into a connection with usual experiences of home. Colorful posters on infants' cribs can have routines approximating home routines as closely as possible. Clocks, calendars, and daily schedules of events assist in structuring time for older children, increasing predictability and decreasing feelings of loss of control and boredom (Voltz, 1981).

ACTIVE–PASSIVE, DIRECTED–SELF-INITIATED CONTINUUM

The environment should have spaces for very active robust play and places to retreat for quiet reflection for the child and parent. Activity rooms should have places for children to watch passively and vicariously benefit from the play of other children. This is helpful for children with limited physical energy or who are new to the environment or peer group and beginning the development of trust. The activity room should be arranged so that reliance on adults is not a prerequisite to play. Safe materials should be easy to access, even with wheelchair confinement or medical equipment limiting the child's movement. Most importantly, the room, through the arrangement, materials, and furniture, should address and promote the developmental needs of the children or adolescents using the room (Francis, Myers-Gordon, & Pyper, 1988). There should be a balance between activities on the unit and playroom that are directed by an adult and those that are unstructured and allow the child to be the initiator in self-directed play and activity.

When a hospital playroom was specifically designed to meet developmental play needs of physically handicapped children, the design–researchers found a significant increase in total play behavior and a significant decrease in unoccupied "wandering" in the room (Eisert, Kulka, & Moore, 1988).

FAMILY-CENTERED

The environment should provide for the needs of all family members: places for parents to comfortably sleep and shower, places for siblings to visit with patient and parents, places for parents to continue parenting roles. For example, playrooms should have furniture for adults and children. A sofa that allows a child and parent to curl up together and read stories provides comfort, normalcy, and clearly gives the message that the setting is family centered.

SCHOOL: OPPORTUNITIES FOR SELF-ESTEEM, MASTERY, AND SOCIAL SUPPORT

As children with chronic conditions mature or older children are diagnosed with a chronic condition, school becomes a focal point for social support, self-esteem, and the acquisition of skills and knowledge necessary for future roles in society (Weitzman, 1984). The opportunity to benefit from school is challenged by the presence of a chronic condition. Children with chronic conditions have increased school absences which can lead to social, behavioral, and learning problems. Reasons for absence are varied and not limited to the health condition. Children who have chronic conditions and psychosocial problems have been found to miss more school than children with a chronic condition alone (Weitzman, Walker, & Gortmaker, 1986). School-related problems of children who have been off therapy for cancer for 2 or more years have been found to be increased fourfold when compared with peers in the general population. Related to cancer, the presence of functional impairment (but not cosmetic impairment) increased the risk for academic problems (Mulhern et al., 1989). In other conditions, cosmetic impairment has been found to increase problems in psychosocial adjustment (Richardson, 1970; Harper, Wacker, & Cobb, 1986; Stein & Jessop, 1982).

Decreased academic performance related to school absence places the child at risk for successful task accomplishment. Failure experienced by the child and acknowledged by peers and others decreases self-esteem. Decreased esteem, in turn, can lead to fewer efforts by the child, which further limits opportunities for mastery. This downward spiral is influenced by peers reacting to other differences the child may have resulting from the chronic condition and treatments. School personnel and peers may react negatively to the child's decreased energy or limited activity. Their attributions may be erroneous; limitations may be seen as lack of motivation rather than as functional (Walker, 1984). Peer relations are further strained as children react to changes in the child's body image or to misinformation about the condition. Teasing, bullying, and social isolation may be experienced (Katz, Rubinstein, & Hubert, 1988; Varni & Setoguchi, 1991).

Interventions to increase positive experiences with school can come from a systems approach and from direct child–parent interventions. A systems approach includes increasing the quality of communication between the school, family, and health care team. Coordination between the school nurse and hospital clinic or community health nurse and between the hospital or homebound teacher and school teacher are examples. Education efforts to increase understanding about health needs and school needs also have been successful (Benner & Marlow, 1991; Pollard, Ellingwood, Markwood, Norville, & Pryor, 1985).

Direct interventions during a child's hospitalization can include continuation of academic experiences through the hospital teacher and tutors. Recognition of the child's academic efforts by the nurse also supports positive associations with school. Nurses must realize that schoolwork needs time and space and should therefore organize care to provide uninterrupted time for the child to attend school and complete assignments. Discussion about school, peers, and activities with the child may bring expression of negative feelings and insecurities, thus indicating areas for behavioral interventions, such as behavioral coping strategies and social skills training (Ross & Ross, 1986; Katz, Rubinstein, & Hubert, 1988).

When children have extended absences from school, re-entry can be an additional source of stress. The transition from hospital or home back into school can be eased by a school re-entry program (Treiber, Schramm, & Mabe, 1986). The program should be tailored to the needs and preferences of the child and family and the perceived needs of the school. It can include desensitization and information sharing and elicit social support of the classmates for the child by exploring their ideas about the condition.

During hospitalization the process of preparing for school re-entry can be facilitated by encouraging ongoing contact with school and classmates. School visitors should be warmly greeted, put at ease, and recognized for their efforts to support the child. The nurse can suggest making and sending cards to classmates and using the hospital experience for a science or social studies project as additional ways to foster contact with school. Most of all, the nurse supports school by modeling an interest in school, cognitive activities, and accomplishments.

Parents can be supported to assist in their efforts to collaborate with the school through discussion and exploration of feelings. Parents may need additional support as they acquire advocacy skills and access services available through special education and school health services provided through Public Law 94–142.

DEVELOPMENTAL PROGRAMS FOR INFANTS

Public Law 94–142, the Education for All Handicapped Children Act of 1975, was amended in 1986 to include children from birth to 3 years of age in Public Law 99–457 (Walker, 1989). Chronically ill infants at risk for developmental delays and infants with handicapping conditions became eligible for early childhood intervention programs. These programs provide a variety of developmental services for infants and parents. Financial allocation and availability vary from state to state, as do the models for program delivery (Brown, Pearl, & Carrasco, 1991). Several hospitals have developed programs following federal guidelines, specifically the inclusion of parents as members of the developmental team and the establishment of individualized treatment goals (Korteland & Cornwell, 1991) (Box 11-4). Nursing roles with early intervention can be hospital or community based. The nurse should be aware of referral opportunities, supportive of program efforts in the hospital and community, and supportive of parents as they transition from hospital to community services (Forness & Hecht, 1988; Kilgo, Richard, & Noonan, 1989).

FAMILY FUNCTIONING

As Rutter (1987) states, harmonious family relationships serve as a protective factor for children. A child's chronic condition places stress on the family unit and individuals in the family (Shapiro, 1983). The responses to the stress may increase vulnerability to psychosocial problems or increase the child's resilience (Dyson, 1991). As seen in studies of outcomes with children and their siblings, the findings have been diverse related to families. Increased stress has been documented in mothers (Breslau & Prabucki, 1981), while atten-

BOX 11–4 • A HOSPITAL MODEL FOR EARLY INTERVENTION: THE INFANT EDUCATION PROGRAM

To demonstrate that family-centered, coordinated, developmental support for children up to 3 years of age can follow the federal guidelines of P.L. 99-457 without dependence on outside funding, Children's Medical Center of Dallas initiated a multidisciplinary exploration that resulted in The Infant Education Program. The key to using existing resources was educating ourselves about the guidelines of P.L. 99-457. This included literature review, discussion seminars with the community, early intervention programs, gaining support from administrative and clinical areas affected, and piloting a process.

The Infant Education Program includes enrollment; assessment, which includes parents in establishing individualized treatment goals; service delivery; and evaluation. Begun in 1988, we have enrolled 76 infants to date. Carrying out a planned process for developmental intervention in a tertiary, crisis-oriented setting is challenging. However, our experience validates our belief in success of the concept for infants and families, for a hospital developing family-centered care, and for transitions, coordination, and collaboration between hospital, family, and community.

tion to fathers has been limited (McKeever, 1983). Increased risk of marital stress has been found (Martin, 1975). Further analysis of 34 studies found no support for the hypothesis that a child's chronic condition necessarily leads to dysfunction or divorce (Sabbeth, 1984).

Family structure has been found to be a risk factor for children. Mulhern et al. (1989) found a twofold risk for children with chronic conditions to have school problems when living in a single-parent household and a greater risk for showing fearful, inhibited, or overcontrolling behavior. Socioeconomic status was not related to the increased risk. Varni, Rosenfeld, Talbot, and Setoguchi (1989) found higher psychologic and social adaptation in children with congenital or acquired limb loss when there was more family cohesion and moral–religious emphasis in combination with less family conflict. The finding of positive, direct effects of family cohesion on child psychologic and social adjustment is consistent with studies of children with juvenile arthritis and diabetes (Varni, et al., 1989). These studies point out the need to support existing two-parent families so they will continue in harmony and to support efforts that impact family cohesion. The public policy emphasis on family-centered care is a reflection of this need.

Patterson (1991) and McCubbin and Patterson (1983) identify aspects of resilient family processes. These include attribution of meaning that is positive (cognitive appraisal that falls in the moral–religious emphasis found in the Varni, et al. 1989 study), maintaining clear boundaries, balancing the illness with other needs of the family, open expression, and family cohesion. Analysis of 500 families with children affected by cytic fibrosis, cerebral palsy, or myelomeningocele identified three coping patterns, each of which is made up of several coping behaviors (McCubbin, McCubbin, Nevin, & Cauble, 1979). These coping patterns are maintaining integration, cooperation, and an optimistic definition of the situation; maintaining social support, self-esteem, and psychologic stability; and understanding the medical condition through communication with other parents and medical staff. The impact of cognitive appraisal is further identified by Venters (1981). In studying families affected by cytic fibrosis, families with a belief system (a philosophy that explains and makes sense out of the circumstance of the chronic condition) who were able to endow meaning to the illness, were better able to cope.

INTERVENTIONS FOR THE FAMILY

Organizing delivery of care around a family-centered care philosophy means that families will be involved in all aspects of care involving their child (Shelton, Jeppson, & Johnson, 1987). It includes consideration for the family's cultural and ethnic orientation and the effect on family functioning (Randall-David, 1989). It also must decrease gatekeeping behaviors and role conflicts between medical staff and parents (Diehl et al., 1991). Family-centered care must be sensitive to the impact of grief, whether it occurs at initial diagnosis (Fraley, 1986; Goldberg et al., 1990) or continuing grief (Cohen & Martinson, 1988). Loneliness and social isolation are prevalent in mothers of chronically affected children (Florien & Kralik, 1991). For this reason and for education and coping strategy development, support groups have been extremely helpful to families (Iscoe & Bordelon, 1985). Stein and Jessop (1989) have identified the assistance of a family-support person who is available to negotiate the course of the condition and delivery systems with the family.

SIBLINGS AND INTERVENTION

Siblings are a part of the family and must be included in the process of caring for a child with a chronic condition (Drotar & Crawford, 1986; Breslau & Prabucki, 1981; Gogan, Koocher, & Foster, 1977). Siblings, too, must be viewed within a developmental, mental health framework of coping and resilience. Efforts for siblings can include education, support groups, and involvement in activities at the health care setting. Anticipatory guidance can assist parents in recognizing potential needs of siblings and in planning to support siblings.

Support groups for siblings use a variety of formats, for example, session-limited with an education focus (Kramer & Moore, 1983; Kinrade, 1985); session-limited with a support as opposed to education format (Cunningham, Betsa, & Gross, 1981; Heiney, Goon-Johnson, Ettinger, & Ettinger, 1990); and single-session, psychoeducational format (Adams-Greely, Shiminski-Maher, & McGowan, 1986). While research findings related to sibling support groups are limited, clinical assessments consistently find the groups to be beneficial. One study in progress is investigating the effects of a time-limited, psychoeducational format for siblings of children with cancer on the participants' self-report of anxiety and coping and the parents' perceptions of the siblings' anxiety and coping (Sally Francis, personal communication). In Heiney, et al. (1990), anger was found as a focus of three of seven sessions, and denial, avoidance, and interaction with peers were the most commonly used coping mechanisms of the siblings. This points to the need for siblings to have a place and structure for support. Siblings have a myriad of experiences and feelings related to coping (Hannah & Midlansky, 1985), which the nurse can support through advocacy and program development (see the Clinical Example).

Evaluation

At each step of the nursing process, assessment of progress in accomplishing observable outcomes must be made. For example, interventions to decrease stress will be observed in more relaxed body stance and greater variety in facial affect. Interventions to increase coping will be seen in application of coping technique learned. Outcomes in self-esteem, mastery, and social support will be seen in increased efforts, greater verbalizations, and increased play contacts with other children. Family functioning can be observed in successful problem-solving efforts of parents and increased participation in a family support group.

Self-assessment and monitoring of the nurse's individual stress and coping also should be continuous. Reflection-in-action and using peers as sources of feedback assist evaluation. Evaluation also can be carried out in organized activities of the health care team through staff conferences, chart reviews, and research activities.

The Future: Our Challenge in Health Care

A FUTURE CONCERN IN THE PRESENT: PEDIATRIC AIDS

The emergence of AIDS or human immunodeficiency virus (HIV)-related diseases in children has introduced a new chronic, potentially fatal disease. Psychosocial issues are similar to those found within a noncategoric approach; however, the risk for severe problems may be great. Many children with perinatally transmitted AIDS may be from families who have more dysfunction, as seen in extreme poverty, drug abuse, social isolation, or homelessness. For other families for whom transmission is from medical treatment-related causes, the expected challenges of living with a chronic condition are amplified. This is a result of the parent's ill health or social stigmatization. Close monitoring of the family and child coping and the use of community resources are needed. Some communities have developed respite programs for families with AIDS, which offer a variety of services for child, siblings, and parents. The nurse in pediatrics needs to be familiar with existing resources and support the development of services, because the incidence is expected to increase as more individuals who are HIV positive develop AIDS. The needs are magnified when one realizes that cure and prevention are not in the foreseeable future (Cohen, 1991).

The Future

What does the future hold for children with a chronic illness or disability and their families? We hope that the future will bring as much progress as the last 25 years have had in medical advancements, societal awareness, public policy change, and educational reform. There is still much to learn about the forces, processes, and events that lead to successful outcomes seen in adult satisfaction with love, work, life, and generativity. We can hope that new conditions will not arise as pediatric AIDS has in this decade. We can hope for and encourage the development of children and families with chronic conditions through day-to-day efforts, health care delivery, and advocacy. We can promote research, participate in the application of findings, and use new technology, particularly computer applications to chronic conditions. Most importantly, we can collaborate with families and community systems to integrate fully the concepts of comprehensive, coordinated, family-centered care.

Summary

While most children with chronic conditions do not develop psychopathology, the risk for mental health problems exists. Support and prevention can come from viewing the chronic condition as a life stressor. The stressor precipitates coping efforts by the child and family. Interventions can be organized to support coping and resilience. Through

(*text continues on page 169*)

CLINICAL EXAMPLE: MICHAEL

Michael is a 7-year-old diagnosed with acute lymphocytic leukemia (ALL). Many caregivers are involved with Michael and his family and have been since his diagnosis 2 months prior to this hospital admission. The current admission is one step in Michael's overall care; however, Michael's primary nurse must organize his daily physical care, assess for coping and adaptation, and plan for fostering resilience. Assessment and planning during the hospital admission should coordinate with long-term goals for physical and psychosocial development. Communication with other staff (physicians, clinical nurse specialists and clinic nurses, child-life specialist, social worker) and with Michael and his family can aid coping and resilience.

The nursing process begins with an assessment of Michael and his family. Remembering the interaction of change, the dynamic elements of the framework, the nurse will not make assumptions based on information from prior admissions, but will carry out the assessment knowing that, for example, Michael's assessment of threat or understanding of this admission may be very different from his last admission. For example, he may have had complete hair loss and experienced teasing and be concerned with body image changes. New information will lead to new plans and interventions.

I. Assessment: general
   A. Medical information
      1. Michael is a 7-year-old white boy admitted for his fifth course of chemotherapy treatment for ALL.
      2. Expected procedures: IV will be started within 2 hours of admission for administration of chemotherapy.
      3. Chemotherapy will be given, which frequently has side effects of nausea and vomiting.
   B. Developmental—normative
      1. Physical: Gross motor coordination is well-developed; fine motor coordination is integrated with gross motor.
      2. Psychosocial: A 7-year-old is in Erikson's stage of industry versus inferiority.
      3. Cognitive: Seven-year-olds typically are in concrete operations stage of cognitive development or in transition from preoperational thought to concrete operations.
      4. Expected issues:
         a. Coping with chronic illness
         b. Fears of body mutilation and loss of control
         c. Disruption in peer relations and usual peer activity
         d. Disruption in school attendance and performance
         e. Threat to feeling of mastery, accomplishment, ability to be productive and industrious
         f. Stress or disruption in family functioning resulting from chronic illness

II. Assessment: specific
   A. Medical information:
      1. Reason for hospitalization: Michael and his mother have accurate understanding of leukemia and reason for hospitalization (chemotherapy).
      2. Understanding: Because this is fifth course, parent and child feel they have understanding of what will happen and why.
      3. Cognitive appraisal: Michael assesses threat as manageable: "I've got to get my chemo. If I don't get too sick I'll play bingo tomorrow. Can we make nachos? I didn't get to last time."
      4. Previous hospitalization: Michael was last admitted here 3 weeks ago. Admission went according to medical plan. Mother states no problems.
      5. Child's experiences to date: Michael has had numerous intrusive procedures to date (IVs and bone marrows). He has developed a coping strategy (blowing) for procedures.
      6. Planned experiences/procedures: Once IV is started in this admission, Michael will probably sleep for the rest of the afternoon and night. If nausea and vomiting are experienced, he will stay in bed most of second day. If not, he will be in the playroom. The third day of admission, IV will be removed, and he will be discharged.
   B. Developmental
      1. Physical: Michael is small for his age but within normal growth curve. Gross and fine motor skills are intact; coordination is good. He enjoys playing soccer. No identified problems or limitations in physical development, to date.
      2. Psychosocial: Play choices indicate a strong drive to be productive (industry).
      3. Cognitive: He demonstrates conservation, seriation, and tells time.

(continued)

CLINICAL EXAMPLE: MICHAEL (*Continued*)

C. Environmental
   1. Family: Mother and father have an intact marriage. Michael is the only child. Family lives 45 minutes from hospital. The father is employed; the mother is a homemaker. Maternal and paternal relatives live within 1 hour's drive of family and assist with hospital and clinic visits. No marital discord per social work report.
   2. Sociocultural: Stable economic conditions; church affiliation is source of support by mother's report. No problems noted in this area.
   3. Availability: Mother will be present throughout hospital stay. Father visits in evening after work. Aunts and uncles may visit. No siblings to consider.
   4. Stressors: No recent stressors on family and no stressors on family within 6 months prior to initial diagnosis.
   5. Coping strategies: Mother usually attends "morning support group—coffee meeting" for parents of children on hematology–oncology service. Mother states she enjoys the opportunity to talk with others about how things are going.

D. Idiosyncratic
   1. Personality or temperament: Michael appears shy and is slow to warm up to strangers. He talks most when there are only a few people around and if he knows them well.
   2. Coping: Michael uses activity as a coping strategy and seeks information when anything unexpected occurs. He has developed several rituals, preferences, for managing hospital stay.
   3. Comfort and separation: This is one of several admissions, and Michael handles separation well; separates from mom to come to playroom. Allows mom to hug and hold him when he is upset. Does not seek other adults' body contact as comfort measure.

III. Issues for this child and family
   A. Identified needs:
      1. Maintenance of predictability, if at all possible, for example, bingo and making nachos. Michael uses these preferred activities as rituals, signaling that all is going well and according to plan.
      2. During last admission, Michael enjoyed "Hospital Bingo" variation. Use again to reinforce cognitive understanding of hospital events.
      3. No children are admitted now who are known to Michael. Facilitate entry into playroom and interaction with other children.
      4. Discuss body image changes; opportunity to explore coping with feelings and with peers.

IDENTIFIED NEEDS

Within a stress–coping–resilience framework, what needs have been identified with Michael and his family from the assessment for decreasing stress and increasing coping, for self-esteem, for mastery and social support, for family functioning? What nursing diagnoses (based on the North American Nursing Diagnosis Association taxonomy) encompass the needs and lead to interventions, and the protective factors of resilience?

DECREASE STRESS

Nursing Diagnosis: Powerlessness related to knowledge deficit

Interventions

1. While Michael and his family have cognitively appraised this admission as manageable and thereby decreased stress, this appraisal should continue to be monitored. Cognitive activities are planned to support appraisal.
2. Ask parents if they have their copy of the "Family Information Handbook" and what questions, if any, they now have.
3. During the last admission, Michael enjoyed "Hospital Bingo" in the child life program. Involve him again to reinforce cognitive understanding of hospital and treatment events.
4. Maintenance of predictability: While the uncertainty involved with the diagnosis cannot be negated, any other ways that Michael and his family can control and predict events during the admission will decrease feelings of powerlessness. Decisional control exists through menu selection, scheduling of daily activities, and choices about activities.
5. Michael looks forward to bingo and cooking during each admission. He uses these preferred activities as rituals, signalling that all is going well and according to plan (Geist, 1979).

Schedule times with child-life specialist.

INCREASE COPING

Nursing Diagnoses: High Risk for Activity Intolerance, Pain, Ineffective Individual Coping, Impaired Physical Mobility

(*continued*)

CLINICAL EXAMPLE: MICHAEL (*Continued*)

Interventions

1. With Michael, plan activities to do after chemotherapy has begun, and he is in bed; he usually spends his second day with decreased energy. Videogames can be easily used or fantasy stories can be read (Johnson, Whitt, & Martin, 1987).
2. Discomfort, possible nausea and vomiting with chemotherapy may be alleviated with distraction. Again, plan pleasurable activities for Michael to do in his room.
3. Involve Michael in as many self-care activities as possible. Recognize his acts, and give specific feedback and specific praise.
4. Mobility may be limited by IV pump; organize care so Michael can move easily with his pump and not worry about safety or functioning of the pump.

SUPPORT SELF-ESTEEM AND MASTERY

Nursing Diagnoses: Disturbance in Self-Concept: Body Image Disturbance, Identity Disturbance, Situational Low Self-Esteem

Interventions

1. Use communication skills to determine how Michael is coping with hair loss.
2. Discuss progress of homebound school with Michael and parents.
3. Provide activities with end-products (crafts, cooking) that give Michael a sense of accomplishment and of being productive to enhance developmental task of acquiring a sense of industry.
4. Discuss possible scheduling of school reentry program with clinic nurse, social worker, and child-life specialist (Chekryn, Deegan, & Reid, 1986).
5. Acknowledge Michael's "products" (art, crafts, cooking). Encourage him to display products in his room. Use communication techniques to praise his efforts (Faber & Mazlish, 1980).

PROMOTE SOCIAL SUPPORT

Nursing Diagnoses: Impaired Social Interaction, Social Isolation

Interventions

1. Encourage telephone contact with school friends. Ask family if cousins or friends would like to visit and encourage them.
2. Facilitate peer interactions at bedside with videogames.
3. Introduce Michael to bibliotherapy (Fosson & Husband, 1984). Take Michael and mother to family library and suggest books in which Michael might be interested that have coping themes. When Michael is in his room and in bed, plan time to let him tell you some of the stories he has read, thereby reinforcing the benefits of the coping models.
4. Explore with Michael and his mother what time at home is like: Is he isolated, or have they arranged for visits from his favorite neighbors? Provide anticipatory guidance about the need to stay involved with others.
5. Suggest that classmates make audio or videotapes for Michael, and suggest Michael do the same to provide a continuing connection with his prediagnosis social contacts.

PROMOTE FAMILY FUNCTIONING

Nursing Diagnoses: Family Coping; Potential for Growth; Anticipatory Grieving; Spiritual Distress; High Risk for Altered Parenting; Parental Role Conflict

Interventions

1. Reinforce mother's attendance at morning parent group meeting; if she has any concerns about leaving Michael during this time, elicit problem-solving, and give mother opportunity to solve the problem herself. If necessary, enter into mutual problem-solving.
2. Arrange a time to meet with both mother and father (father usually visits in the evening).
3. Encourage Michael to make some particular craft projects for his mom and dad, thus promoting a more normal, yet meaningful, exchange among the family.
4. Organize care so that you and mother have opportunities to talk while Michael is in the playroom to allow the mother expression of feelings of grief and loss.
5. Make a referral to the hospital chaplain if agreeable to the mother, and let her know how to access the chaplain.
6. Explore with the mother the need to have rest and relaxation; provide anticipatory guidance about the need for parents to have some private time together.

supportive communication, the nurse builds on attributes of commitment, optimism, and realism to support adaptation. Nursing care is provided that is sensitive to the issues of loss and grief; is family-centered; fosters resilience through the developing child's self-esteem, mastery, and social support; decreases stress and increases coping; and supports family functioning.

REFERENCES

Adams-Greenly, M., Shinimsky-Maher, T., & McGowan, N. (1986). A group program for helping siblings of children with cancer. *Journal of Psychosocial Oncology, 4,* 55–67.

Aita, A. (1990). The art of nursing. *Nursing Educator, 15* (16), 24–28.

Banco, L., & Powers, A. (1988). Hospitals: Unsafe environments for children. *Pediatrics, 82* (5), 794–797.

Barnsteiner, J. H., & Gillis-Donovan, J. (1990). Being related and separate: A standard for therapeutic relationships. *Maternal Child Nursing, 15,* 223–228.

Benner, A. E., & Marlow, L. S. (1991). The effect of a workshop on childhood cancer on student's knowledge, concerns, and desire to interact with a classmate with cancer. *Children's Health Care, 20*(2), 101–107.

Bibace, R., & Walsh, N. E. (Eds.). (1981). *New directions for child development.* San Francisco: Jossey-Bass.

Blum, R. W. (Ed.). (1991). *Pediatic Annals* (complete issue). *20*(9), .

Bolig, R., Fernie, D., & Klein, E. (1986). Unstructured play in hospital settings: An internal locus of control rationale. *Children's Health Care, 12*(3), 122–129.

Bolig, R., & Weedle, K. D. (1988). Resiliency and hospitalization of children. *Children's Health Care, 16*(4), 225–260.

Breslau, N., & Prabucki, K. (1981). Psychological functioning of siblings of disabled children. *Pediatrics, 67,* 334–353.

Brewer, E. J., McPherson, M., Magrab, P. R., & Hutchins, V. L. (1989). Family-centered, community-based, coordinated care for children with special health care needs. *Pediatrics, 83*(6), 1055–1060.

Brewster, A. B. (1982). Chronically ill hospitalized children's concepts of their illness. *Pediatrics, 69*(3), 355–362.

Brown, W., Pearl, L. F., & Carrasco, N. (1991). Evolving models of family-centered services in neonatal intensive care. *Children's Health Care, 20*(1), 50–55.

Bruhn, J. G., Hampton, J. W., & Chandler, G. C. (1971). Clinical marginality and psychological adjustment in hemophilia. *Journal of Psychosomatic Research, 15,* 207–213.

Cadman, D., Boyle, M., & Offord, D. R. (1988). The Ontario child health study: Social adjustment and mental health of siblings of children with chronic health problems. *Developmental and Behavioral Pediatrics, 9,* 117–121.

Cadman, D., Boyle, M., Szatmari, P., & Offord, D. R. (1987). Chronic illness, disability and mental and social well-being: Findings of the Ontario Child Health Study. *Pediatrics, 79* 805–813.

Cadman, D., Rosenbaum, P., & Boyle, M. (1991). Children with chronic illness: Family and parent demographic characteristics and psychosocial adjustment. *Pediatrics, 87,* 884–889.

Cairns, N., Clark, G. M., Smith, S. D., & Lansky, S. (1979). Adaptation of siblings to childhood malignancy. *Journal of Pediatrics, 95,* 484–487.

Clark, H. B. (1989). A social skills development model: Coping strategies for children with chronic illness. *Children's Health Care, 18,* 19–29.

Clubb, R. L. (1991). Chronic sorrow: Adaptation patterns of parents with chronically ill children. *Pediatric Nursing, 17*(5), 461–465.

Cohen, M. H., & Martinson, I. M. (1988). Chronic uncertainty: Its effect on parental appraisal of a child's health. *Journal of Pediatric Nursing, 3*(2), 89–96.

Cohen, D. G. (1990). Similarities between the nursing care needs of children with cancer and children with human immunodeficiency virus infection. *Journal of Pediatric Oncology Nursing, 7*(4), 149–153.

Conatser, C. (1986). Preparing the family for their responsibilities during treatment. *Cancer, 58(2),* 508–511.

Copley, M. F., & Bodensteiner, J. B. (1987). Chronic sorrow in families of disabled children. *Journal of Child Neurology, 2,* 67–70.

Cunningham, C., Betsa, N., & Gross, S. (1981). Sibling groups: Interactions with siblings of oncology patients. *American Journal of Pediatric Hematology & Oncology, 3,* 135–138.

Damrosch, S. P., & Perry, L. A. (1989). Self-reported adjustment, chronic sorrow and coping of parents of children with Down's syndrome. *Nursing Research, 38,* 25–30.

Diehl, S. F., Moffitt, K. A., & Wade, S. M. (1991). Focus group interviews with parents of children with medically complex needs: An intimate look at their perceptions and feelings. *Children's Health Care, 20*(3), 162–169.

Doka, J. (Ed.). (1989). *Disenfranchised grief: Recognizing hidden sorrow.* Lexington, MA: Lexington Books, D.C. Heath.

Dolgin, M., Katz, E., Doctors, S., & Siegel, S. (1986). Caregivers' perceptions of medical compliance in adolescents with cancer. *Journal of Adolescent Health Care, 7,* 22–27.

Dorner, S. (1976). Adolescents with spina bifida: How they see their situation. *Archives of Diseases of Childhood, 51,* 439–444.

Drotar, D. (1981). Psychological perspectives in chronic childhood illness. *Journal of Pediatric Psychology, 6,* 211–228.

Drotar, D., & Bush, M. (1985). Mental health issues and services. In N. Hobbs & J. M. Perrin (Eds.), *Issues in the care of children with chronic illness* (pp. 514–550). San Fransico: Jossey-Bass.

Drotar, D., & Crawford, P. (1986). Psychological adaptations of siblings of chronically ill children: Research and practice implications. *Developmental and Behavioral Pediatrics, 6*(6), 355–362.

Drotar, D., Duerchuk, C. F., Stern, R. C., Boat, T. F., Boyer, W., & Matthews, L. (1981). Psychosocial functioning of children with cystic fibrosis. *Pediatrics, 67,* 338–343.

Dunst, C., Trivette, C., & Deal, A. (1988). *Enabling and empowering families: Principles and guidelines for practice.* Cambridge, MA: Brookline Books.

Dyson, L. L. (1991). Families of young children with handicaps: Parental stress and family functioning. *American Journal of Mental Retardation, 95*(6), 623–629.

Edwards, D. R. (1987). Initial psychosocial impact of insulin-dependent diabetes mellitus on the pediatric client and family. *Issues in Comprehensive Pediatric Nursing, 10*(4), 199–207.

Eiser, C. (1990). Psychological effects of chronic disease. *Journal of Child Psychology and Psychiatry, 31,* 85–98.

Eisert, D., Kulka, L., & Moore, K. (1988). Facilitating play in hospitalized handicapped children. The design of a therapeutic play environment. *Children's Health Care, 16*(3), 201–208.

Ell, K. O., & Reardon, K. K. (1990). Psychosocial care for the chronically ill adolescent: Challenges and opportunities. *Health Social Work, 15*(4), 272–282.

Faber, A., & Mazlish, E. (1980). *How to talk so kids will listen and listen so kids will talk.* New York: Avon.

Ferguson, B. (1979). Preparing young children for hospitalization: A comparison of two methods. *Pediatrics, 64*, 656–664.

Feuerstein, R. (1979). *Instrumental enrichment: An intervention program for cognitive modifiability.* Baltimore: University Park Press.

Fochtman, D. (1991). Therapeutic relationships. *Journal of Pediatric Oncology Nursing, 8*(1), 1–2.

Forness, S., & Hecht, S. (1988). Special education for handicapped and disabled children: Classification, programs, and trends. *Journal of Pediatric Nursing, 3*(2), 75–87.

Fraley, A. M. (1986). Chronic sorrow in parents of premature children. *Children's Health Care, 15*, 114–118.

Francis, S., Myers-Gordon, K., & Pyper, C. (1988). Design of an adolescent activity room. *Children's Health Care, 16*(4), 268–273.

Garmezy, N. (1991). Resilience in children's adaptation to negative life events and stressful environments. *Pediatric Annals, 20*(9), 459–466.

Garmezy, N. (1983). Stressors of childhood. In N. Garmezy & M. Rutter (Eds.), *Stress, coping and development in children* (pp. 43–84). New York: McGraw-Hill.

Gaynard, L., Wolfer, J., Goldberger, J., Thompson, R., Redburn, L., & Laidley, L. (1990). *Psychosocial care of children in hospitals: A clinical practice manual.* Washington, DC: Association for the Care of Children's Health.

Gayton, J. L., Koocher, G. P., Foster, D. J., & O'Malley, J. E. (1977). Children with cystic fibrosis: Psychological test findings of patients, siblings, and parents. *Pediatrics, 59*, 888–894.

Gill, K. M. (1987). Nurses' attitudes toward parent participation: Personal and professional characteristics. *Children's Health Care, 15*(3), 149–151.

Glazer-Waldman, H. R., Francis, S., & Smith, C. (1987). Families' knowledge acquisition and written health materials. *Children's Health Care, 15*(3), 152–155.

Gogan, J. E., Koocher, G. P., & Foster, D. J. (1977). Impact of childhood cancer on siblings. *Health Social Work, 21*, 41–57.

Goldberg, S., Morris, P., & Simmons, R. J. (1990). Chronic illness in infancy and parenting stress: A comparison of three groups of parents. *Journal of Pediatric Psychology, 15*, 347.

Gortmaker, S. L., & Sappenfield, W. (1984). Chronic childhood disorders: Prevalence and impact. *Pediatric Clinics of North America, 31*, 3–18.

Gortmaker, S. L., Walker, D. K., Weitzman, M., & Sobol, A. M. (1990). Chronic conditions, socioeconomic risks, and behavioral problems in children and adolescents. *Pediatrics, 85*, 267–276.

Griffith, J. L., & Griffith, M. E. (1987). Structural family therapy in chronic illness. *Psychosomatics, 28*, 202–205.

Gudas, L. J., Koocher, G. P., & Wypij, D. (1991). Perceptions of medical compliance in children and adolescents with cystic fibrosis. *Developmental and Behavioral Pediatrics, 12*(4), 236–242.

Hannah, M. E., & Midlarsky, E. (1985). Siblings of the handicapped: A literature review for school psychologists. *School Psychology Review, 14*, 510–520.

Harper, D. C., Wacker, D. P., & Cobb, L. S. (1986). Children's social preferences toward peers with visible physical differences. *Journal of Pediatric Psychology, 11*, 323–342.

Hayes, V., & Knox, J. (1984). The experience of stress in parents of children hospitalized with long term disabilities. *Journal of Advanced Nursing, 9*, 333–341.

Harvey, D. H. P., & Greenway, A. P. (1984). The self-concept of physically handicapped children and their non-handicapped siblings: An empirical investigation. *Journal of Child Psychology and Psychiatry, 25*, 273–284.

Hauck, M. R. (1991). Cognitive abilites of preschool children: Implications for nurses working with young children. *Journal of Pediatric Nursing, 6*(4), 230–235.

Heiney, S. P., Goon-Johnson, K., Ettinger, R. S., & Ettinger, S. (1990). The effects of group therapy on siblings of pediatric oncology patients. *Journal of Pediatric Oncology Nursing, 7*(3), 95–100.

Hobbs, N., & Perrin, J. (1985). *Issues in the care of children with chronic illness.* San Francisco: Jossey-Bass.

Hobbs, N., Perrin, J. M., & Ireys, H. (1985). *Chronically ill children and their families: Problems, Prospects, and Proposals from the Vanderbilt Study.* San Francisco: Jossey-Bass.

Honig, R. G. (1982). Group meetings on an adolescent medical ward. *Adolescence, 17*, 99–106.

Hughes, M. C. (1982). Chronically ill children in groups: Recurrent issues and adpaptations. *American Journal of Orthopsychiatry, 52*(4), 704–711.

Hymovitch, D. P. (1983). The chronicity impact and coping instrument: Parent Questionaire (CICI:PQ). *Nursing Research, 32*, 275–281.

Hymovitch, D. (1985). Nursing services. In N. Hobbs & J. M. Perrin (Eds.), *Issues in the care of children with chronic illness* (pp. 478–497). San Francisco: Jossey-Bass.

Ireys, H. T. (1981). Health care for chronically disabled children and their families. In: *The report of the select panel on the promotion of child health for our children: A national strategy, I* (pp. 321–353). Washington, DC: U.S. Government Printing Office.

Iscoe, L. K., & Bordelon, K. J. (1985). Pilot parents: Peer support for parents of handicapped children. *Children's Health Care, 14*(2), 103–109.

Jay, S. M., Elliott, C. H., Ozolins, M., Olson, R., & Pruitt, S. D. (1985). Behavioral management of children's distress during painful medical procedures. *Behavior Research and Therapy, 23*, 513–520.

Kozak, A. E., & Marvin, R. S. (1984). Differences, difficulties and adaptation: Stress and social networks in families with a handicapped child. *Family Relations, 33*, 67–77.

Katz, E. R., Rubenstein, C. L., & Hubert, N. C. (1988). School and social reintegration of children with cancer. *Journal of Psychosocial Oncology, 6*, 123–140.

Kilgo, J. L., Richard, N., & Noonan, M. J. (1989) Teaming for the future: Integrating transition planning with early intervention services for young children with special needs and their families. *Infants and Young Children, 2*(2), 37–48.

Kinrade, L. C. (1985). Preventive group intervention with siblings of oncology patients. *Children's Health Care, 14*, 110–113.

Koop, C. E. (1987). *Surgeon General's report: Children with special health care needs—campaign 87—commitment to family-centered, coordinated-care for children with special health care needs.* Washington, DC: U.S. Department of Health and Human Resources, U.S. Government Printing Office.

Korteland, C., & Cornwell, J. R. (1991). Evaluating family-centered, programs in neonatal intensive care. *Children's Health Care, 20*(1), 56–61.

Kovacs, M., Iyengar, S., & Goldston, D. (1990). Psychological functioning among mothers of children with insulin-dependent diabetes mellitus: A longituudinal study. *Journal of Consulting Clinical Psychology, 58*, 189–193.

Kramer, R. F. (1984). Living with childhood cancer: Impact on healthy siblings. *Oncology Nursing Forum, 11*, 44–51.

Kramer, R. F., & Moore, I. M. (1983). Childhood cancer: Meeting the special needs of healthy siblings. *Cancer Nursing, 6*, 213–217.

Lansky, S. B., Lowman, J. T., Tribhawan, & Gyulay, J. E. (1979). School phobia in children with malignant neoplasms. *American Journal of Diseases of Children, 129*, 42–46.

Larson, D. G. (1987). Helper Secrets. *Journal of Psychosocial Nursing, 25*(4), 20–27.

Lavigne, J. V., & Ryan, M. (1979). Psychologic adjustment of siblings of children with chronic illness. *Pediatrics, 63*, 616–627.

Lazarus, R., & Folkman, S. (1984). *Stress, appraisal, and coping.* New York: Springer Publishing.

Lemons, P. A., & Weaver, D. D. (1986). Beyond the birth of a defective child. *Neonatal Network, 5*, 13–20.

Lev, E. (1989). A nurse's perspective on disenfranchised grief. In J. Doka (Ed.), *Disenfranchised grief: Recognizing hidden sorrow.* Lexington, MA: Lexington Books; D.C. Heath.

Leventhal, J. M. (1984). Psychosocial assessment of children with chronic physical disease. *Pediatric Clinics of North America, 31*(1), 71–86.

Luthar, S. S., & Zigler, E. (1991). Vulnerability and competence: A review of research on resilience in childhood. *American Journal of Orthopsychiatry, 61*(1), 6–22.

Lynn, M. R. (1989). Readability: A critical instrumentation consideration. *Journal of Pediatric Nursing, 4*(4), 295–297.

Martin, P. (1975). Marital breakdown in families of patients with spina bifida cystica. *Developmental Medicine and Child Neurology, 17*, 757–764.

Mattson, A. (1972). Long-term physical illness in childhood: A challenge to psychosocial adaptation. *Pediatrics, 50*, 801–811.

McCubbin, H. I., McCubbin, M., Nevin, R., & Cauble, E. (1979). *CHIP: Coping health inventory for parents.* St. Paul: Family Social Science.

McCubbin, H., Needle, R., & Wilson, M. (1985). Adolescent health risk behaviors: Family stress and adolescent coping as critical factors. *Family Relations, 34*, 51–62.

McCubbin, H. I., & Patterson, J. M. (1983). The family stress process: The double ABCX model of family adjustment and adaptation. In H. McCubbin, M. Sussman, & J. Patterson (Eds.), *Advances and development in family stress theory and research.* New York: Haworth.

McKeever, P. (1981). Fathering the chronically ill child. *Maternal Child Nursing, 6*, 124–128.

McKeever, P. (1983). Siblings of chronically ill children: A literature review. *American Journal of Orthopsychiatry, 53*(2), 209–218.

Mearig, J. S. (1985). Cognitive development of chronically ill children. In N. Hobbs & J. M. Perrin (Eds.), *Issues in the care of children with chronic illness: A sourcebook on problems, services, and policies* (pp. 672–697). San Fransico: Jossey-Bass.

Melamed, B. (1988). Helping children and families cope with hospitalization and outpatient medical treatments. *Feelings, 30*(4), 15–20.

Melamed, B. G., & Siegel, L. J. (1975). Reduction of anxiety in children facing hospitalization and surgery by use of filmed modeling. *Journal of Consulting and Clinical Psychology, 43*, 511–521.

Mulhern, R. K., Wasserman, A. L., Friedman, A. G., & Fairclough, D. (1989). Social competence and behavioral adjustment of children who are long-term survivors of cancer. *Pediatrics, 83*(1), 18–25.

Neff, E. J., & Beardslee, C. I. (1990). Body knowledge and concerns of children with cancer as compared with the knowledge and concerns of other children. *Journal of Pediatric Nursing, 5*(3), 179–189.

Newacheck, P. W., Budetti, P. P., & Halfon, N. (1986). Trends in activity-limiting chronic conditions among children. *American Journal of Public Health, 76*(2), 178–184.

Nolan, T., & Pless, I. B. (1986). Emotional correlates and consequences of birth defects. *Journal of Pediatrics, 109*, 201–207.

Olds, A. R. (1978). Psychological considerations in humanizing the physical environment of pediatric outpatient and hospital settings. In E. Gellert (Ed.), *Psychological aspects of pediatric care* (pp. 111–131). New York: Grune & Stratton.

Olshansky, S. (1962). Chronic sorrow: A response to having a mentally defective child. *Social Casework, 43*, 190–193.

Patterson, J. M. (1991). Family resilience to the challenge of a child's disability. *Pediatric Annals, 20*(9), 491–499.

Patterson, J.M. & Geber, G. (1991). Preventing mental health problems in children with chronic illness or disability. *Children's Health Care, 20*(3), 150–161.

Pazola, K.J. & Gerberg, A.K. (1985). Teen group: A forum for the hospitalized adolescent. *Maternal Child Nursing, 10*, 265–269.

Pearson, J., Cataldo, M., Tureman, A., Bessman, C., & Rogers, M. (1980). Pediatric intensive care unit patients: Effects of play intervention on behavior. *Critical Care Medicine, 8*, 64–67.

Pellegrini, D. S. (1990). Psychosocial risk and protective factors in childhood. *Developmental and Behavioral Pediatrics, 11*(4), 201–209.

Perrin, E. C., Sayer, A. G., & Willett, J. B. (1991). Sticks and stones may break my bones . . . reasoning about illness causality and body functioning in children who have a chronic illness. *Pediatrics, 88*(3), 608–619.

Perrin, E. C., & Shapiro, E. (1985). Health locus of control beliefs of healthy children, children with a chronic psysical illness, and their mothers. *Journal of Pediatrics, 185*(107), 627–633.

Perrin, J. M., & MacLean, W. E. (1988). Children with chronic illness: The prevention of dysfunction. *Pediatric Clinics of North America, 35*(6), 1325–1337.

Peterson, L. (1989). Coping by children undergoing stressful medical procedures: Some conceptual, methodological, and therapeutic issues. *Journal of Consulting and Clinical Psychology, 57*, 380–388.

Peterson, L., Schulthesis, K., Ridley-Johnson, R., Miller, D. J., & Tracy, K. (1984). Comparison of three modeling procedures on the presurgical reactions of children. *Behavior Therapy, 15*, 197–203.

Peterson, L., & Shigetomi, C. (1981). The use of coping techniques to minimize anxiety in hospitalized children. *Behavior Therapy, 12*, 1–14.

Peterson, L., & Toler, S. (1986). An information-seeking disposition in child surgery patients. *Health Psychology, 5*, 343–358.

Piserchia, E. A., Bragg, C. F., & Alvarez, M. M. (1982). Play and play areas for hospitalized children. *Children's Health Care, 10*(4), 135–138.

Pless, I. B., & Douglas, J. W. B. (1971). Chronic illness in childhood: Part 1: Epidemiological and clinical characteristics. *Pediatrics, 47*(2), 405–464.

Pless, I. B., & Pinkerton, P. (1975). *Chronic childhood disorders: Promoting patterns of adjustment.* London: Henry Kimpton.

Pless, I. B., & Roghmann, K. J. (1971). Chronic illness and its consequences: Some observations based on three epidemiological surveys. *Journal of Pediatrics, 79,* 351–359.

Pless, I. B., & Wadsworth, M. E. J. (1989). Long-term effects of chronic illness on young adults. In R. E. K. Stein (Ed.), *Caring for children with chronic illness: Issues and strategies* (pp. 147–158). New York: Springer.

Pollard, A., Ellingwood, G., Markwood, K., Norville, R., & Pryor, A. (1985). School and the child with cancer: A program to assist school personnel. *Journal of the Association of Pediatric Oncology Nurses, 2*(3), 7–10.

Poster, E. C., & Betz, C. L. (1983). Allaying the anxiety of hospitalized children using stress immunization techniques. *Issues in Comprehensive Pediatric Nursing, 6,* 227–233.

Randall-David, E. (1989). *Strategies for working with culturally diverse minorities and clients.* Washington, DC: Association for the Care of Children's Health.

Richardson, S. A. (1970). Age and sex differences in values toward physical handicaps. *Journal of Health and Social Behavior, 11,* 207–214.

Ritchie, J. A. (1985). Gaps in the care of young hospitalized chronically ill children: Can they be closed? In C. Fore & E. Poster (Eds.), *Meeting psychosocial needs of children and families in health care* (pp. 5–11). Washington, DC: Association for the Care of Children's Health.

Robinson, C. A. (1984). When hospitalization becomes an "everyday thing." *Issues in Comprehensive Pediatric Nursing, 7,* 363–370.

Romney, M. C. (1984). Congenital defects: Implications on family development and parenting. *Issues in Comprehensive Pediatric Nursing, 7,* 1–15.

Ross, D. M., & Ross, S. A. (1986). Teaching the child with leukemia to cope with teasing. *Issues in Comprehensive Pediatric Nursing, 7,* 59–66.

Rubin, D. H. (1989). Computer-assisted care. In R. E. K. Stein (Ed.), *Caring for children with chronic illness: Issues and strategies* (pp. 256–267). New York: Springer.

Rutter, M. (1987). Psychosocial resilience and protective mechanisms. *American Journal of Orthopsychiatry, 57*(3), 316–360.

Sabbeth, B., & Leventhal, J. (1984). Marital adjustment to chronic childhood Illness: A critique of the literature. *Pediatrics, 73*(6), 762–768.

Satterwhite, B. B. (1978). Impact of chronic illness: An overview based on five surveys with implications for management. *International Journal of Rehabilitation Research, 1*(1), 7–17.

Saylor, C. R. (1990). Reflection and professional education: Art, sciences, and competency. *Nurse Educator, 15*(2), 8–11.

Schon, D. (1987). *Educating the reflective practioner.* San Francisco: Jossey-Bass.

Seagull, E. A. (1990). Childhood depression. *Current Problems in Pediatrics, 20*(2), 734–739.

Shapiro, J. (1983). Family reactions and coping strategies in response to the physically ill or handicapped child: A review. *Social Science and Medicine, 17,* 913–931.

Shelton, T. L., Jeppson, E. S., & Johnson, B. H. (1987). *Family-centered care for children with special health care needs.* Washington, DC: Association for the Care of Children's Health.

Sherman, J. B., Cardea, J. M., Gaskill, S. D., & Tynan, C. M. (1989). Caring: Commitment to excellence or condemnation to conformity? *Journal of Psychosocial Nursing, 27*(8), 25–29.

Sieving, R. E., & Zirbel-Donish, S. T. (1990). Development and enhancement of self-esteem in children. *Journal of Pediatric Health Care, 4*(6), 290–296.

Silverman, M. M., & Koretz, D. S. (1989). Preventing mental health problems. In R. E. K. Stein (Ed.), *Caring for children with chronic illness: Issues and strategies* (pp.213–229). New York: Springer.

Sinnema, G. (1991). Resilience among children with special health-care needs and among their families. *Pediatric Annals, 20*(9), 483–486.

Stein, R. E. K. (1989). *Caring for children with chronic illness: Issues and strategies.* New York: Springer.

Stein, R. E. K., & Jessop, D. (1982). A noncategorical approach to chronic childhood illness. *Public Health Reports, 97*(4), 354–359.

Stein, R. E. K., & Jessop, D. (1989). What diagnosis does not tell: The case for a noncategorical approach to chronic illness in childhood. *Social Science Medicine, 29,* 769–778.

Steinhausen, H. C., & Wefers, D. (1976). Intelligence structure and personality in various types of physical handicaps in childhood and adolescence. *Neuropaediatrics, 7,* 313–320.

Strax, T. E. (1991). Psychological issues faced by adolescents and young adults with disabilities. *Pediatric Annals, 20,* 507–511.

Tavormina, J. B., Boll, T. J., Luscomb, R. L., & Taylor, J. R. (1981). Psychosocial effects on parents of raising a handicapped child. *Journal of Abnormal Child Psychology, 9,* 121–131.

Tesler, M., & Savedra, M. (1981). Coping with hospitalization: A study of school-age children. *Pediatric Nursing, 7,* 35–38.

Tew, B. J., & Lawrence, K. M. (1973). Mothers, brothers, and sisters of patients with spina bifida. *Developmental Medicine and Child Neurology, 15*(29), 69–76.

Thomas, R. (1988). The struggle for control between families and health care providers when a child has complex health care needs. *Zero-to-Three,* 15–18.

Treiber, F., Schramm, L., & Mabe, P. (1986). Children's knowledge and concerns toward a peer with cancer: A workshop intervention approach. *Child Psychiatry and Human Development, 16*(4), 249–260.

Varni, J. W., Rubenfeld, L. A., Talbot, D., & Setoguchi, Y. (1989). Family functioning, temperament, and psychologic adaptation in children with congenital or acquired limb deficiencies. *Pediatrics, 84,* 323–330.

Varni, J. W., & Setoguchi, Y. (1991). Correlates of perceived physical appearance in children with congenital/acquired limb deficiencies. *Developmental and Behavioral Pediatrics, 12*(3), 171–176.

Venters, M. (1981). Familial coping with chronic and severe childhood illness: The case of cystic fibrosis. *Social Science and Medicine, 15,* 289–297.

Visintainer, M. A., & Wolfer, J. A. (1975). Psychological preparation for surgical pediatric patients: The effect on children's and parents' stress responses and adjustment. *Pediatrics, 56* 187–202.

Voltz, D. D. (1981). Time structuring for hospitalized school-aged children. *Issues in Comprehensive Pediatric Nursing, 5*(4), 205–210.

Vulcan, B. M., & Nikulich-Barrett, M. (1988). The effect of selected information on mothers' anxiety levels during their children's hospitalization. *Journal of Pediatric Nursing, 3*(2), 97–102.

Walker, D. K. (1984). Care of chronically ill children in schools. *Pediatric Clinics of North America, 31*(1), 221–233.

Walker, D. K. (1989). Public education: New commitments and consequences. In R. E. K. Stein (Ed.), *Caring for children with chronic illness: Issues and strategies* (pp. 41–60). New York: Springer.

Walker, D. K., Gortmaker, S. L., & Weitzman, M. (1981). *Chronic illness and psychological problems among children in Genesee County.* Boston: Harvard School of Public Health, Community Child Health Studies.

Weeks, K. H. (1985). Private health insurance and chronically ill children. In N. Hobbs & J. M. Perrin (Eds.), *Issues in the care of children with chronic illness* (pp. 880–911). San Francisco: Jossey-Bass.

Weitzman, M. (1984). School and peer relations. *Pediatric Clinics of North America, 31*(1), 59–69.

Weitzman, M., Walker, D. K., & Gortmaker, S. (1986). Chronic illness, psychological problems, and school absences. *Clinical Pediatrics, 25*(3), 137–141.

World Health Organization (1980). *International classification of impairments, disbilities, and handicaps* (p. 24). Geneva: WHO.

Wikler, L., Wasow, M., & Hartfield, E. (1981). Chronic sorrow revisited: Parent versus profession depiction of the adjustment of parents of mentally retarded children. *American Journal of Orthopsychiatry, 30.*

Worchel, F. F., Copeland, D., & Barker, D. (1987). Control-related coping strategies in pediatric oncology patients. *Journal of Pediatric Psychology, 12*(1), 25–38.

Worthington, R. C. (1989). The chronically ill child and recurring family grief. *Journal of Family Practice, 29,* 397–400.

CHAPTER

12

Mental Retardation

Linda M. Finke

Definitions and procedures for identifying children with mental retardation differ among states and are changing (Frankenberger & Harper, 1988); therefore, accurate counts are difficult to assess. Nevertheless, professionals in mental health are treating increasing numbers of mentally retarded children and their families as the need is recognized. Deinstitutionalization, begun by Federal mandate in the early 1970s, took these children out of segregated facilities, where they were often hidden from society, and placed them into mainstream life. Repeated studies have shown that mentally retarded people have the same range of mental health problems and needs as does the general population (Parsons, May, & Menolascino, 1984). Psychiatric nurses need to develop an understanding of the complex condition of mental retardation and special needs of these children and their families.

The psychiatric nurse working with a mentally retarded child and the child's family will have several roles, including diagnostician, therapist, educator, and advocate. The following chapter delineates the knowledge and skills needed to assist these children and their families with special needs.

Meaning of the Mental Retardation Label

An understanding of mental retardation begins with an understanding of the various labels and definitions of the condition. New labels and definitions are evolving. A term that has gained prominence when referring to individuals previously labeled mentally retarded is "developmentally delayed." The change in label is part of a movement toward social acceptance of these individuals. The new focus is on development with an associated potential for growth.

The American Association on Mental Retardation defines mental retardation as "significantly subaverage general intellectual functioning existing concurrently with deficits in adaptive behavior and manifested during the developmental period, which adversely affects a child's educational performance" (Grossman, 1973, p. 5). This definition is used in all federal legislation and policy development (Federal Register, 1977).

The emphasis of this definition, therefore, is not on I.Q. alone, but more importantly on adaptive behavior. Adaptive behavior includes self-help skills, skills of daily living, and social skills. I.Q. assessment is difficult under the best circumstances. Assessing the I.Q. of a child with poor cognitive skills who also may have perception, vision, and hearing deficits among other problems often is even more difficult. If a child also is experiencing an emotional or psychiatric disorder, the I.Q. assessment could be further altered.

The emphasis on adaptive skills to assess mental retardation is also evident in the Diagnostic and Statistical Manual of Mental Disorders, 4th ed., (DSM-IV) classification (1994). The two components of the diagnosis of mental retardation are an I.Q. below 70 and a deficit or impairment in adaptive functioning with an onset before the age of 18 years. The impairment in social adaptive functioning may be indirect, such as the inability to think abstractly, or it may be represented by a delay in developmental milestones, such as not dressing independently (Menolascino, Gilson, & Levitos, 1986).

Unfortunately, states are increasingly setting I.Q. cutoffs in their educational regulations as they attempt to categorize children for educational programs (Frankenberger & Fronzagillo, 1990). It should be noted, however, that PL 94-142, The Education of Handicapped Children Act, specifically states that I.Q. alone cannot be used in the determination of appropriate education for a child (U.S. Department of Education, 1984).

Assessment

Great care should be taken in the assessment of a child who is mentally retarded. The psychiatric nurse should assess the child's developmental level and adaptive skills instead of focusing on I.Q. level and making distinctions between labels, such as severely mentally retarded, moderately retarded or trainable, and mildly retarded or educable. Mental retardation is, of course, a complex condition with considerable variance and unknowns. Poor communication skills, illiteracy, inappropriate education, and so forth can lead not only to poor performance on I.Q. tests, but also inappropriate social interactions.

The nursing assessment should include a total assessment, including awareness of physical health assessment, neurologic status, educational plan, and behavioral assessment, which includes adaptive skills. The nurse obtains information from the child, family members, teachers, and caretakers if involved. Observation of the child in his or her usual environment also is helpful. Children who are mentally retarded often are uncomfortable with unfamiliar people and unfamiliar settings. Therefore, an unusual amount of time may be needed to build a trusting relationship. Assessment also may be difficult because the child may have limited verbal skills and a lack of social perceptions. The nurse must remember that parents know the child best and often provide needed insight. The child's teachers also are an important resource.

A family assessment is an integral part of any assessment of a child and is vital when assessing a child who is mentally retarded. The assessment should include the effect of the child's behavior on the family and the family's effect on the child's behavior.

The grief parents suffer when they discover they have a child who is mentally retarded is a topic about which much is written. Families progress through a cycle of grieving, which must be assessed by the nurse (Fig. 12-1). The grief cycle begins with a stage of denial and disbelief, which then leads to anger. Searching for causes and solutions follows. (Only approximately 25% of the families find an etiology for the mental retardation.) Families then move from trying to find cures to a phase exemplified by a preoccupation with the child's weaknesses and disability. As families move through the grief cycle, they progress to finding the child's strengths and abilities. The grieving is not a one-time process but a cycle that repeats in some form when a milestone is reached or the child experiences an illness or change in behavior. Examples of these milestones might include delayed walking, beginning school, or reaching adolescence. Other precipitating events may include an illness, hospitalization, acting-out behavior, or self-injurious behavior.

Assessment of the child and family should be ongoing. Family behavior patterns may trigger unacceptable behavior in the child, and the child's behavior may influence family members' reactions, which form a circular situation (Wright & Leahy, 1984).

The nurse must carefully review the child's medication. Many children who are mentally retarded are receiving anticonvulsants for seizure disorders, stimulants for hyperactivity, and beta-blockers for medical problems or behavior control. Any of these medications can have significant side effects, including drowsiness, irritability, dizziness, hyperactivity, and sleep disturbances. These or other side effects could induce symptoms of mental illness or mask symptoms of a mental health problem.

Diagnosis

The complex nature of mental retardation and mental illness; the overlap between neurologic, biochemical, and social influences; and the institutionalization of many of these children make specific diagnostic conclusions difficult. "The symptomatology of mentally retarded individuals often differs from that observed in non-retarded people, and the behavioral manifestations of mental disorders depend on the level of cognitive and neuro

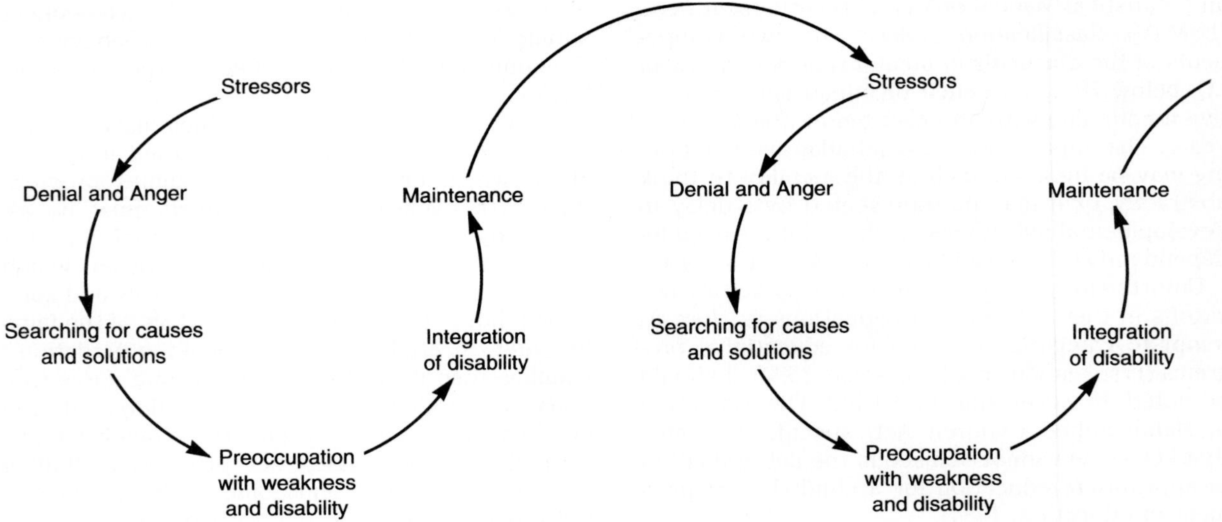

FIGURE 12–1 • Family coping cycle

physical development. Thus, it is difficult to delineate which behavior disturbances are the result of emotional problems and which are the result of mental retardation" (Nihira, Price-Williams, & White, 1988, p. 186).

Regarding diagnosis, the nurse should note that children who have been institutionalized may exhibit symptoms of isolation or separation anxiety rather than psychosis or some other major psychiatric disorder. As caretakers change, pieces of a child's health history may be lost as well, which makes distinction between learned behavior and illness difficult. Parsons et al. (1984) estimate that the frequency of functional psychosis in the mentally retarded is 5% to 12%. Again, because of their developmental level, some mentally retarded children display psychotic behavior, such as poor eye contact, wariness of new situations, and disorganization of thought.

Major depressions and bipolar disorders are difficult to detect in children who are mentally retarded. The regimentation and limit setting that are frequently placed on the lives of mentally retarded children can camouflage symptoms of depression. Feelings of despair, helplessness, and fear of being abandoned by family or caretakers can create suicidal ideation or dependent clinging (Menolascino et al., 1986).

Children with mental retardation and psychosis often are inappropriately diagnosed as autistic. Some children are labeled "autistic-like" because of the symptoms they present, such as self-stimulating behavior and poor social interaction. It is difficult to distinguish symptoms from disease or disorder because a high percentage of autistic children have poor adaptive skills.

Menolascino et al. (1986) suggest that borderline personality disorder is a neglected diagnosis in mentally retarded adolescents. It does seem logical that children with poor boundary maintenance who need self-stimulation to function due to their low developmental level could have borderline personality disorder.

Children who are mentally retarded often carry a dual diagnosis. The first diagnosis refers to the mental retardation, and the second diagnosis refers to the mental illness or emotional diagnosis.

The psychiatric nurse should not be discouraged by the blurring of symptoms and the difficulty in determining distinct diagnoses for children who are mentally retarded and their families. Nursing's approach to holistic care and nursing diagnoses based on treatable symptoms give nurses a unique ability to work effectively with mentally retarded children and their families. Care should be based on the recognition that regardless of the disability, these children and families have the same needs for acceptance, love, nurturing, and growth as other children and families.

Most mental retardation care facilities and mental health facilities find the dually diagnosed child difficult to treat. Mental retardation facilities focus on daily living and job skills, while the mental health facilities focus on diagnosis and treatment of identifiable psychiatric problems. Because of the regulations of funding sources, children who are mentally retarded and have a mental health problem do not fit neatly into either system, and the staff is not prepared to work with a child with such complex needs. Nurses must work with families and health care delivery systems to ensure that children are not denied access to treatment because of a complex diagnosis.

Planning

Planning for appropriate interventions for a child who is mentally retarded should include the child, family members, teachers, and other caretakers. A multidisciplinary approach encourages the various services involved with the family to become active participants in the treatment plan. Treatment must be consistent and realistic. Establishing short- and long-term goals allows progress to be monitored.

Treatment should take place in a familiar setting with family support available. As discussed previously, new settings and unfamiliar people often are sources of fear and anxiety for the child. Frequent changes in staffing, often a part of residential settings, are particularly anxiety producing for a child who is mentally retarded. Flexibility and adaptation often are difficult for a mentally retarded child to achieve.

The psychiatric nurse must serve as advocate and therapist. Coordination of care assists the integration of treatment into everyday life and reinforcement by those who work with the child at home and school. Because cognition is slow for mentally retarded children and change is difficult, consistency and repetition are needed to accomplish a successful outcome. The nurse must protect the rights of these children in and out of the treatment setting. Those planning treatment should remember the complex nature of mental health problems of children who are mentally retarded.

A family focus should dominate intervention planning. Research has shown that families with handicapped children often have high stress levels (Friedrich, Witmer, & Cohen, 1985). These children present increased caretaking responsibilities, and families need additional resources and support (Box 12-1). Margolit, Shulman, and Stuchiner (1989) studied 39 families of mentally retarded children. They found a difference in the causes of stress for fathers and mothers of these children. Isolation and anxiety disorders in their children caused increased stress for fathers, while acting-out behavior caused the greatest stress for mothers.

BOX 12–1 • STRATEGIES TO EMPOWER FAMILIES

- Encourage expression of anxiety.
- Assist to dispel guilt.
- Provide support through grieving cycle.
- Encourage open exchange of information.
- Encourage questions.
- Assist to reframe perceptions.
- Emphasize strengths.
- Mutually set future-oriented, realistic goals.
- Teach assertiveness skills.
- Educate about legal rights and responsibilities.
- Connect with community resources.

Community resources available to provide specialized care and education decreased the stress levels of parents.

Any intervention plan also should include siblings, because they often assume caretaking responsibilities for their brother or sister who is mentally retarded. Siblings may feel they do not receive the attention that the mentally retarded child receives and therefore have feelings of anger, guilt, or resentment.

Intervention

Care providers must carefully choose interventions that take into consideration the unique nature of the child needing treatment. The therapist must allow for time to build a trusting relationship. The child may test the boundaries of the relationship. In addition, mentally retarded children often try to please the adults in their lives and therefore may appear submissive. They are particularly sensitive to others' feelings and sensitive to feedback from others. At the same time, they often lack social and expressive skills, so their behavior, such as frequent hugging, may seem inappropriate. They may display their frustration by hitting, head banging, or self-injury. These behaviors must be assessed by health care professionals when planning interventions.

Care providers frequently need to intervene directly because of the cognitive level of the children and their difficulty recognizing and describing feelings. For example, the caregiver may need to describe a problem for the child, instead of the child identifying the problem. Instead of the child proposing possible actions he or she may need to be given options. Intervention needs to be appropriate to the child's developmental level and adaptive ability. Play, art, and music may be more appropriate therapies than discussion for many mentally retarded children. During verbal exchanges, the child may need gentle guidance to remain on task and may need assistance in clarifying ideas and identifying and labeling feelings. In addition, pictures may serve as a helpful tool to stimulate discussion or label feelings. Discussion of irrelevant material should be discouraged.

Directions to the child need to be clear, brief, and specific. Verbal prompts should include frequent praise to keep the child on task. Physical prompts also may be necessary, such as placing the hand on his or her paper or leading the child to time-out space. The therapist should reinforce socially appropriate behavior and bring inappropriate behavior to the child's attention and give him or her other options.

Group therapy provides a useful treatment modality for children who are mentally retarded. In a group, children have the opportunity to practice appropriate behavior and pool insights and solutions. Role playing can assist group members to anticipate reactions to their behavior and try out new behavior. A group setting helps build relationships with others and diminishes feelings of isolation and rejection. Through the group, children are able to share experiences and to realize that others also have problems or frustrations, and they can begin to form social ties.

Groups for parents and siblings also are helpful. Families can share experiences and normalize feelings in group settings, and parents can learn effective parenting skills to deal with their children.

Self-injury is a problem of significant concern for those who work with mentally retarded children. This behavior often includes hand-banging, biting, tongue-chewing, and hair-pulling. Attempts to extinguish such behavior require behavior modification. Applegate and Barol (1989) suggest a developmental approach to dealing with self-injurious behavior. They view self-injurious behavior disorders as secondary to poor bonding and the behaviors as maladaptive attempts at self-stimulation and social relatedness. These behaviors also could be attempts at self-soothing. The authors propose interventions directed toward attachment, mirroring, and a safe nurturing environment. Treatment aims include acceptance, trust, and consistency. Bonding, rather than completion of a particular task, is the goal. When displaying inappropriate behavior, the therapist redirects the child back to the task and praises his or her attention to the task and his or her relating to the therapist. The child is rewarded for interpersonal participation. The approach of Applegate and Barol (1989) replaces control-oriented behavior modification with positive rewards of bonding and collaborative participation.

As with any child, intervention must be individualized for children who are mentally retarded. Progress may be slow, requiring persistence and patience. The goal of treatment is to assist these children to reach their potential. Because potential is unknown, expectations should be high but attainable.

Evaluation

Evaluation of treatment should be ongoing. Frequent assessment of progress and goal setting help identify progress, albeit slow or delayed progress. Careful notes allow for regular evaluation and needed modification of the treatment plan. Because improvement may be difficult to detect, short-term goals are helpful in measuring progress.

Meetings of all involved in the treatment plan, including the family and the child when appropriate, should take place on a regular basis. Discussing the treatment plan and progressing toward goals are important components of effective treatment and evaluation.

Summary

Intervention with a child who is mentally retarded and has a mental health problem is a challenge to the psychiatric nurse. The nurse must use a variety of skills and serve in a variety of roles. Careful assessment and diagnosis are essential. Intervention should be family centered and appropriate to the child's developmental level. A team approach must include the family and teachers. Ongoing evaluation assists in measuring the effectiveness of the treatment plan. Psychiatric nursing care of a child who is mentally retarded requires creativity and a holistic approach to the child's and family's complex needs.

REFERENCES

American Psychiatric Association. (1994). *Diagnostic and statistical manual of mental disorders* (4th ed.). Washington, DC: Author.

Applegate, J., & Barol, B. (1989). Repairing the nest: A psychodynamic developmental approach to clients with severe behavior disorders. *Clinical Social Work Journal, 17*(3), 197–207.

Federal Register. (August 1977). *42*(163).

Frankenberger, W., & Fronzagillo, K. (1990). *States' definitions and procedures for identifying mentally retarded children: A comparison of 1981–82, 1985–86, and 1989–90 guidelines.* Unpublished manuscript, University of Wisconsin—Eau Claire.

Frankenberger, W., & Harper, J. (1988). States' definitions and procedures for identifying children with mental retardation: Comparison of 1981–1982 and 1985–1986 guidelines. *Mental Retardation*, *26*(3), 133–136.

Friedrich, W., Witurner, L. T., & Cohen, D. S. (1985). Coping resources and parenting mentally retarded children. *American Journal of Mental Deficiency, 90,* 130–139.

Grossman, H. (Ed.). (1973). *Manual on terminology and classification in mental retardation.* Washington, DC: American Association on Mental Deficiency.

Margolit, M., Schulman, S., & Stuchiner, N. (1989). Behavior disorders and mental retardation: The family system perspective. *Research in Developmental Disabilities, 10,* 315–326.

Menolascino, F., Gilson, S., & Levitas, A. (1986). Issues in the treatment of mentally retarded patients in the community mental health system. *Community Mental Health Journal, 22*(4), 314–327.

Nihira, K., Price-Williams, D., & White, J. (1988). Social competence and maladaptive behavior of people with dual diagnosis. *Journal of Multihandicapped Persons, 1*(3), 185–199.

Parsons, J., May, J., & Menolascino, F. (1984). The nature and incidence of mental illness in mentally retarded individuals. In F. Menolascino & J. Stark (Eds.), *Handbook of mental illness in the mentally retarded.* New York: Plenum Press.

U.S. Department of Education (1984). *To assure free appropriate public education of all handicapped children: Sixth annual report to Congress on the implementation of Public Law 94–142: The education for all handicapped children act.* Washington, DC: Author.

Wright, L., & Leahy, M. (1984). *Nurses and families: A guide to family assessment and intervention.* Philadelphia: F.A. Davis.

CHAPTER

13

Homeless Families

Cheryl Taylor

Homelessness is a complex, multidimensional problem that requires solutions. It is increasing nationally, with population estimates ranging from 250,000 to 3 million affected (Bassuk, 1990b; Bingham, Green, & White, 1987; Brickner, Sharer, Conanan, Elvy, & Savarese, 1985; Institute of Medicine, 1988; Peroff, 1987). It is being studied by researchers, written about by scholars, and reported in the news media. The first generation of studies on homelessness has provided researchers, health care providers, and public policy planners with valuable information about contributing factors, demographics, health care, and service needs of homeless people in general (Morrissey & Dennis, 1990; Roth & Bean, 1986; Wright, 1987). Risk factors associated with homelessness pose serious challenges to clients and health care providers, because health care is generally unavailable for homeless people (Brickner, Scanlan, & Conanan, 1986), and their previous experiences make them cautious about using institutional care for health services (Hays, 1987).

The concept of the homeless family may seem a contradiction in terms to many for whom the ideas of "home" and "family" are inseparable, but increasing levels of poverty and violence and higher rates of divorce show a different picture of the face and place of the American home and family. Families with children represent an estimated 35% of the homeless population (Bassuk, 1990b), and single women with children comprise approximately 70% to 85% of homeless families (Bassuk, 1990b; Berne, Dato, Mason, & Rafferty, 1990).

These families represent a growing population at risk for health problems, including a subpopulation—largely consisting of women, infants, children, and adolescents—with their own distinctive demography, epidemiology, history, and health care needs (Bachrach, 1981). Most American families face common developmental stressors in their daily lives (e.g., maintaining employment and financial stability and raising physically and mentally healthy children). How individual family members structure and cope with these ongoing challenges from a housed position will vary based on family history and available internal and external resources, but such challenges are undoubtedly increased when a family loses its home. The family's consistency, physical safety, emotional security, and autonomy are threatened.

Nursing knowledge and intervention can be essential factors in improving the health outcomes for this subpopulation, because of the impact that homelessness has on family structure and the physical and psychosocial growth, development, and health of its members. Psychiatric-mental health nurses participate on treatment teams in planning comprehensive care, developing policies and standards of care, and matching homeless client preferences with available resources. Nursing intervention is particularly important for homeless children and adolescents, who are at risk for emotional and mental disorders and who need access to safe housing, stable parenting, and supportive health care services for a healthy transition into adulthood.

This chapter examines the definitions of, and contributing factors to, homelessness. Model programs and interventions, including health care for homeless families are discussed.

Defining Home and Homelessness

A house in itself is not a home, but it is a structural place for starting and maintaining family development. Conceptually defining home and homelessness is challenging but necessary for understanding homeless populations and their care needs; McChesney's (1987) study of homeless families revealed that residential instability (i.e., temporary housing arrangements) combined with family poverty are primary reasons that families are homeless.

A "What is a home?" survey of 200 people revealed that the meaning of home to men differed strikingly from its meaning to women (Taylor-Walton, 1988). Homeless men consistently included the presence of a woman in their identification of essential criteria for a home. The women surveyed were not so gender specific. They referred to love, support, and caring and consistently included a place of acceptance and support in their definitions of home (Taylor-Walton, 1988).

Definitions of "homelessness" apparently depend on one's perspective. A review of the literature revealed definitions ranging from complete absence of shelter to temporary living and sleeping arrangements. However, in a survey, homeless people described "homelessness" as joblessness, loneliness, being vulnerable, wandering, being outcast, being adrift, being hungry and confused, having no family support, and being homesick (Taylor-Walton, 1988). For the homeless men surveyed, homelessness meant joblessness, not "lack of shelter." Homeless men expressed the feeling that if they could find a job that paid well, they could support their families and afford a place to live. Themes of loneliness, depression, and lack of family support persisted among the responses of homeless people in this survey.

Combining the literature's definitions of home with the concept's currently common usage led to the development of a conceptual model of home. The critical attributes of home according to this model include boundaries, memories, centrality, sharing, self-control of resources, codes of conduct, and security (Taylor-Walton, 1988).

The author's ethnographic research findings (Taylor-Walton, 1988) led to beginning development of a conceptual model of homelessness and houselessness that needs further development and testing. Consider the following propositions. Some people are continually homeless, lacking the basic foundational psychosocial supports of a home. Some people are houseless and homeless, a group possibly at greatest risk for developing or exacerbating psychologic problems or severe mental illness.

Examples of people who are houseless might include hurricane or earthquake victims who experience loss or severe damage to their houses by disaster. However, the healthy family remains intact and works together to restore material loss. People who might be considered homeless have no or a limited sense of boundaries, familiarity, memories, internal and external resources, privacy, and centrality—those essential features of "home." For example, a 3-year-old girl who experiences incest nightly by her father could be considered homeless. People who are homeless and houseless might live on the streets, frequently moving from shelter to shelter, lacking a sense of permanent residence, ownership, emotional autonomy and the essential features of a home.

The Five Senses of Homelessness

People experiencing homelessness have their own particular way of being in the world. They have their own rhythm and pace of movement with which they order their lives (Taylor-Walton, 1988). The author's model, "The Five Senses of Homelessness," represents a contextual view of homelessness that can be further used as a conceptual framework for working with homeless clients. The sources for descriptions of the five unique senses of homelessness come from the author's observation and participation as a researcher in the field of homelessness. These senses include the following:

- *Sense of person.* The sense of person involves the inner feelings of being labeled homeless, of being "on display" in public settings, of having to wear used or soiled clothing, and of being judged by others based on one's appearance.
- *Sense of place.* The sense of place evolves from frequent external reminders that the homeless

person owns little or nothing. Signs, security guards, service providers, and others may remind homeless people of their proper place and of the rules of borrowed space. This sense of place context emphasizes predetermined boundaries and an individual's control or lack of control of the immediate environment.

- *Sense of time and timing.* A sense of time and timing evolves from living as a dependent person and being governed by a public time system, primarily clock time. Adjustments to the preset times for sleeping, waking, eating, and being admitted to shelters and public facilities are requirements for daily survival in the context of homelessness. Waiting for help with a sense of uncertainty seemed to be a dominant theme and an expected activity in the world of being homeless, because waiting in line for food, clothing, health services, job applications, or attention from others is common for homeless people.
- *Sense of community.* A sense of community evolves out of owning little or nothing of material value, coupled with a value of sharing scarce resources among each other. Ritualistic, repetitious group acts of waking up, walking, eating in soup kitchens, and sharing public bathrooms may contribute to this sense of community among homeless people.
- *Sense of humor.* A sense of humor appears to be a way of coping with hard times. Amusement, aloofness, teasing, and light-hearted optimism were some general behaviors observed in the field among homeless adults in shelters, particularly homeless men.

Societal Assumptions about Homelessness

It is critical for nurses and other health care professionals to examine societal and personal assumptions about homelessness because these assumptions influence personal and professional attitudes toward homeless people. Such assumptions often are translated into politics, and they affect how homeless people are perceived and treated.

Myths and assumptions about homeless people are listed in Table 13-1. These assumptions focus on mental ability and productivity issues (i.e., no one "in their right mind" would be homeless) or imply that all homeless people are drug addicts and criminals.

The most damaging assumption suggests that homelessness is a premeditated choice that people make—an option among many, possibly better, options (for example, getting a job), as if such options were equally available to everyone. This assumption labels choices made without clarifying the dynamics of those choices. For example, a woman who decides to stop being beaten by her husband and leaves her home with no place to go is not choosing to be homeless as much as she is choosing not to be beaten. A teenager may run away from home for similar reasons. A homeless man on the streets who does not want to go to a shelter during bad weather may not be choosing to be homeless as much as he may be choosing to be in control, free from shelter rules or shelter atmosphere. The consequence of such choices may *lead* to homelessness, but they are not choices to *be* homeless.

Contributing Factors to Families Becoming Homeless

Homelessness among families results from a combination of factors that leads to disequilibrium within the family. Such factors may include poverty, residential instability, personal stressors, family disruption, a history of psychosocial trauma, and tenuous support systems (Bassuk, 1990; McChesney, 1987). Three fourths of all homeless families are single-parent families with two or three children, most of them younger than the age of 5 (Berne et al., 1990; Bassuk, 1990). Homeless family types also may include two-parent families, adolescent parents, siblings with no parents, and pregnant women; infants, preschoolers, or school-age children may or may not be present or may rotate in and out of the homeless family depending on parental support systems. According to Bassuk (1986), the more disorganized and dysfunctional the family, the more likely they are to become homeless. One family's experience of homelessness is illustrated in the Clinical Example for the Jones family.

Health Care for Homeless Families

Much of the research on homelessness indicates that unemployment, scarcity of low-cost housing, and social service cutbacks are contributing factors to homelessness (Greer, 1985; Hopper, 1983; Jones, 1989; Rossi & Wright, 1987; Roth & Bean, 1986; Sebastian, 1985). Aldwin and Revenson (1986) developed a stress vulnerability model and explored relationships between economic stress and psychologic stress. They concluded that increases in economic stress adversely affected mental

TABLE 13–1 Common Assumptions and Myths About Homelessness

Assumption/Myth	Facts	Analysis
Homeless people are not intelligent.	Populations of homeless people include varying educational backgrounds and socioeconomic classes.	
Most of the homeless are "crazy" or mentally ill.	Approximately one third of the homeless are chronically mentally ill (Wasem, 1991; Dennis, 1990).	Homeless people are a highly visible segment of society. Mentally ill people among the homeless are more visible than mentally ill people who live in houses.
Most of the homeless are alcoholics and drug abusers.	There is a high prevalence of alcohol problems among homeless men (Fischer, 1991). Approximately 10% to 20% of the homeless abuse drugs (Fischer, 1991).	Alcohol and drug abuse is prevalent among housed and homeless people. However, homeless people live in the drug dealers' domain.
Homeless people are dangerous.	Homeless people live in the public domain and are more vulnerable to being victims than perpetrators of personal assaults and crimes (Community Council of Greater Dallas, 1990).	High visibility lends itself to frequent observation and reporting of crimes committed by homeless people.
People choose to be homeless.	Homelessness represents more of an outcome consequence than a choice (Taylor-Walton, 1989). Socioeconomic and political factors contribute to people becoming homeless (Hodnicki, 1990).	People may choose to be houseless and appear to be homeless.

Community Council of Greater Dallas (1990). *Homeless services task force: Community report and recommendations.*

Dennis, D. (1990). Exploring myths about "street people." *Access: A Publication of The National Resource Center on Homelessness and Mental Illness, 2*(2), 1–8.

Fischer, P. J. (1991). *Alcohol, drug abuse and mental health problems among homeless persons: A Review of the literature 1980–1990.* Report to Homeless Demonstration and Evaluation Branch, Division of Clinical and Prevention Research National Institute on Alcohol Abuse and Alcoholism Rockville, MD.

Hodnicki, D. B. (1990). Homelessness: Health care implications. *Journal of Community Health Nursing, 7*(2), 59–67.

health. Individuals with poor mental health prior to economic stress included in their study experienced "difficulty paying off bills, mortgage foreclosure, and unemployment" (p. 167). With increased vulnerability to stress, limited resources, and no permanent living arrangements, homeless people represent subpopulations of men, women, and children at risk for health problems or exacerbated illness problems. Thus, the question arises: If one cannot pay for the basic necessities of shelter, food, and clothing, how can one pay for health care?

The current health care delivery system emphasizes economic efficiency and cost containment measures with a payment-by-illness focus (Feldstein, 1983). The growing numbers of homeless people in need of health care services led to the development of homeless health care demonstration projects in 19 major cities in the United States (Wright, 1987). Grant funding for health care programs for homeless people was initiated and provided in May 1985 by the Robert Wood Johnson Foundation and the Pew Memorial Trust in conjunction with the United States Conference of Mayors (Wright, 1987). The demonstration projects known as the National Health Care for the Homeless Program received 25 million dollars (Wright, 1987).

CLINICAL EXAMPLE: THE JONES FAMILY

Nineteen-year old Susan Jones and her three children, ages 2, 3, and 4 years, were taken to the local hospital emergency room following Susan's collapse while crossing the street with her children. Assessment reveals that she had experienced profuse vaginal bleeding the previous night. She was diagnosed and treated for spontaneous abortion, malnutrition, lice, depression, and gonorrhea. Additionally, her children manifested severe malnourishment, lice infestation, developmental lags, and need for immunization.

Further questioning revealed that Susan had worked as a nurse's aide for an agency that called her on demand. She lived with her children in a two-bedroom house, for which her sympathetic landlord did not charge her rent because the house was in poor condition. She used most of her earnings for child care and food.

When her landlord died, her house was turned over to a real estate company, which eventually evicted Susan after 30 days' notice. Subsequently, the family moved into a garage-like space next to Susan's only relative in the area, with whom she did not get along; 2 days later, it was destroyed by fire after the children "played house" with matches.

Susan was fired from her job due to her unstable living arrangements and lack of a telephone. With no money, the family went to a soup kitchen for food and slept in an abandoned car in freezing weather. When the children developed upper respiratory infections, their mother made them sit in the public library during the day to stay warm and dry; they used the library bathroom to perform self-care activities. In addition, Susan had "felt" pregnant but feared the outcome of going to a clinic for a pregnancy test.

Susan has had a few offers from others to take her children but she does not want to be separated from them. She is very suspicious of the intentions of people who offer her help because she has been taken advantage of, materially and sexually, in the past. With no mailing address, no telephone, no clean clothes, no private bathroom, and no money, she and her children are vulnerable to multiple health hazards.

The studies by Brickner et al. (1986) and Sebastian (1987) specified several health hazards of being homeless. These included exposure to extremes of heat and cold; lack of protection from rain; increased incidence of trauma, infections, and peripheral vascular diseases; and exacerbation of chronic diseases (Brickner et al., 1986; Sebastian, 1987). Bassuk, Rubin, and Lauriat (1986) studied and described the characteristics of 80 homeless families. The majority of the respondents were single parents who had experienced major family disruption. The women lacked supportive relationships; 25% named their child as their major support. Seventy-one percent of the mothers were diagnosed as having personality disorders, and more than half of the children studied showed evidence of developmental problems and learning disabilities. Weiss (1985) investigated the health status practices and service use of 76 homeless women in Seattle, Washington. The women, whose mean age was 33 years, were interviewed in emergency shelters; the majority of respondents were white women caring for young children. Half of the women reported an income of less than $200 the previous month, and 42% of them had not completed high school (Weiss, 1985). Poor general and dental health also were evident. Fourteen percent of the respondents were pregnant, while a significantly large number had experienced a spontaneous abortion. The respondents reported that limited finances and lack of insurance were their reasons for not using health care (Weiss, 1985).

The increased numbers of homeless people and need for housing and health care prompted the federal government to enact legislation to provide services for homeless people. On July 22, 1987, the Stewart B. McKinney Homeless Assistance Act, Public Law 110-77, was signed by President Reagan. The McKinney Act made funds available to cities that submit acceptable grant proposals to provide services to the homeless (U.S. Department of Housing and Urban Development, 1987). Eight major areas (Table 13-2) are included in the McKinney Homeless Act.

The McKinney Homeless Assistance Grants are coordinated by the United States Department of Housing and Urban Development and the Department of Health and Human Services. Religious and nonprofit organizations play a significant role by sponsoring services and providing support to homeless people (Cooper, 1987).

Features of Model Programs

Seven features of model programs providing services to homeless families include (1) community-based outreach and (2) interdisciplinary team

TABLE 13–2 Components of the McKinney Homeless Assistance Act of 1987

- Interagency council comprised of federal, state, local, private, and nonprofit representatives
- Emergency food and shelter
- Transitional and longer-term housing
- Primary and mental health care services
- Adult education and homeless children and youth education grants
- Job training
- Alcohol and drug abuse programs
- Income assistance programs

Source: *The McKinney Act: A Program Guide.* Interagency Council on Homelessness, 1989.

work with (3) ongoing staff development and (4) focus on empowering clients; (5) long-term follow-up care; (6) program evaluation components; and (7) family support centers (Bassuk, 1990; Mead-Fox, 1990).

In addition, special programs designed to address family violence and substance abuse in homeless families may be featured in model treatment programs. There are three dozen model programs for homeless families listed in Bassuk's (1990) Program Design Manual. The National Resource Center on Homeless and Mental Illness (1990) provides information, technical assistance, and telephone consultation to agency personnel and programs providing services to homeless mentally ill subpopulations.

Homeless Children and Adolescents

A child's healthy growth and development depend as much on the *place* and *things* that are part of their environment as they do on the *people* in their environment. Homelessness has a negative effect on children's response to their environment (Berne et al., 1990).

Bassuk (1990) classified homeless infants and children into three groups:

1. Homeless infants responding to frequently changing environments and people
2. Homeless preschoolers experiencing developmental delays
3. School-age children experiencing frequent academic failures (Bassuk, 1990).

Psychologic distress manifested by anxiety, depression, sleep problems, and suicidal ideation was identified among homeless children studied by Bassuk and Rubin (1987).

An estimated 1 million homeless adolescents represent a hidden subpopulation of homeless people living on the streets (Robertson, 1988). Exact ages of homeless adolescents are difficult to prove because of their low profiles as they attempt to steer clear of juvenile authorities, but they are at risk for becoming homeless adults (Robertson, 1988; McChesney, 1987). Some homeless adolescents are forced to work as prostitutes. Others may resort to criminal activities, specifically drug dealing and pornography, to support themselves (Robertson, 1990.) Consequently, homeless adolescents exist in environments with inadequate health care and housing and are at high risk for physical and mental health problems. Substance abuse, unintended pregnancy, malnutrition, history of sexual victimization, sexually transmitted diseases, and family conflict issues are examples of the multiple health problems that homeless adolescents face (Arnstein & Alperstein, 1987; Robertson, 1990).

Homeless adolescents seem to manage their vulnerability to the uncertainties of the homeless life-style by negotiating day-to-day survival using two phenomena valued by society, youth and mobility. The loosely structured homeless life-style makes therapeutic concepts in adolescent health, such as close observation, time out, room restriction, and school seem unrealistic to homeless adolescents living on the streets.

Nursing Intervention with Homeless Families

Professional nurses are playing increasingly significant roles in providing health care to homeless people. Psychiatric nurse clinicians assume seven essential roles in this regard, as follows:

1. Health educator: providing the homeless person with client teaching and community resource information necessary for managing and overcoming the health hazards of a homeless life-style
2. Interventionist: providing outreach and noninvasive emergency and supportive treatment for illness and injury to families experiencing homelessness
3. Advocate: negotiating for residential stability and providing access to needed health care services
4. Counselor: offering support within a therapeutic relationship to maximize the homeless person's coping abilities
5. Case manager: serving as a central facilitative

liaison between agencies, systematically coordinating and monitoring homeless clients' use of psychiatric, psychosocial, and medical services to assure continuity of care
6. Group leader: identifying and conducting medication, educational, support, self-help, and transition-focused groups for homeless people
7. Consultant: providing training and professional consultation to physicians, nurses, related disciplines, and volunteer people who develop and provide resources to homeless people

Nursing knowledge and interventions are essential to improve the health outcomes for homeless families, because using the nursing process can improve the quality of care for these families. In the assessment phase, baseline data about everyday challenges that homeless families face facilitate greater understanding of risk factors leading to homelessness and homeless families' needs. Developing appropriate nursing diagnoses and implementing psychiatric-mental health nursing strategies, including community health planning and comprehensive support services, promote nurses' understanding of the challenges facing homeless children and adolescents, improved client–nurse interactions, and greater access to and use of available health care services.

Whatever the composition of its members, homeless families have special needs that must be considered whether treating one member or the entire family. Table 13-3 lists examples of those special needs by major categories: housing, social services, education, and health care (Mead-Fox, 1990; Walsh, 1990; Weinreb & Bassuk, 1990).

It is important to understand the concept of encounter because of the transient nature of the homeless life-style. One-time only encounters, missed appointments, and dropping out of treatment are expected in the course of working with homeless people. Consequently, it is important to make client contact as comprehensive, educational, and meaningful as possible, without overwhelming the often physically exhausted client. Physical exhaustion is highlighted as a health hazard of the homeless life-style because it may go unnoticed by service providers.

Physical exhaustion influences individual motivation, behavior, and ability to learn new concepts. When working with homeless clients, it is important to remember that multiple problems require simultaneous multiple interventions paced in such a way that the client can adapt slowly and progressively. Small gains must be appreciated. It also is important to consider the length of time as homeless during the treatment phase of care; families who have experienced chronic homelessness may be less likely to adapt quickly and fully to treatment and services (Martin, 1988). Stable reentry to housing and community norms may be particularly difficult for families who have been homeless for 6 months or more.

The multiple problems faced by many homeless families would benefit from a nursing care plan that uses case management. According to Bassuk (1990), case management is a system that functions to coordinate housing, economic, social, educational, and health care services to ensure appropriateness of care and enhance continuity of care. Linking and coordinating services in the context of case management often are the responsibility of a designated individual who works with a team to support the client's treatment plan. Psychiatric-mental health nurses are in a unique position to function as case managers given their collaborative ability, educational background, and historical role as client advocates.

*H*olistic *a*ssessment, *r*eferral, *d*ocumentation, *m*onitoring, *a*dvocacy, and *t*reatment planning are essential skills that nurses and care managers use to provide comprehensive client care. The first letter of each skill component of case management spells out the word HARDMAT. This acronym can be used to remember the vital components of care planning for homeless families as a case manager: When life is hard, use the HARDMAT. Public policy initiatives aimed at improving the availability of affordable housing and economic opportunities can provide a safety net for homeless families.

In general, psychiatric-mental health nurses serve an increasingly important role in the mental health care delivery system as members of interdisciplinary public health teams (Aiken, 1987).

Summary

For some homeless families living in a world of residential instability and frequent relocation resulting in feelings of isolation, uncertainty, violence, and vulnerability, homelessness can be devastating. For others, homelessness is an extension of the turmoil they experienced at home. Homeless families need affordable housing, accessible physical and mental health care, community support, and special programs to meet their unique needs.

TABLE 13–3 Special Needs of Homeless Families

Category of Need	Short-Term Care	Long-Term Care	Preventive Care
Goals	Primary services Stabilization	Prevent reoccurence Empowerment	Health promotion Protection
Housing	Emergency/transitory housing	Low-cost, affordable permanent housing	Low-cost, affordable permanent housing
Social services	Intensive clinical case management Enriched child care or day care services Job training and employment Transportation Accessible entitlements Health family supports	Less intensive community case management Social service enriched housing Day care centers for children Crisis intervention counseling Community and family support center-based programs	Self-management Child care centers at the workplace Community service and social support centers Family support and counseling services Self-help group work
Education	Literacy programs Parent education, special education for children Social skill building Sex education	Health and nutrition education	Health and nutrition education Acquired immunodeficiency syndrome and drug abuse prevention Information and referral Healthy parenting styles
Health care	Food and nutrition Health and hygiene, clothes, dental health, podiatric care Mobile outreach and assessment services Psychosocial evaluation and rehabilitation Immunizations Substance abuse counseling and prevention	Developmental screening of preschool children After-school programs for school-age children Family planning services Health protection and promotion	Health screening Primary health care Health promotion Health management

Bassuk, E. L., & Harvey, M. R. (1990). Family homelessness: Recommendations for a comprehensive policy response. In E. L. Bassuk, R. W. Carman, L. F. Weinreb, & M. M. Herzig (Eds.), *Community care for homeless families* (pp. 13–16). Washington, DC: Interagency Council on the Homeless.

Nurses in general and advanced practice are accepting the challenge to provide comprehensive care to homeless and housed families coping with transition and turmoil.

Psychiatric-mental health nurses function in seven significant roles of providing services to homeless people, including homeless families. Nurses serve as health educators, interventionists, client advocates, counselors, case managers, groups leaders, and consultants while providing services to homeless families. Advanced practice nurses who work with homeless families are faced with the challenge of simultaneously establishing working relationships, responding to multiple problems, and using the nursing process in an interdisciplinary manner, while working within a community context. Professional nurses in general practice who encounter homeless family members can be most effective by facing personal assumptions about homeless people and becoming familiar with community resources available for homeless family members in the local and regional communities.

REFERENCES

Aiken, L. H. (1987). Unmet needs of the chronically mentally ill: Will nursing respond? *Image, 19*(3), 121–125.

Aldwin, D. M., & Revenson, T. A. (1986). Vulnerability to economic stress. *American Journal of Community Psychology, 14*(2), 161–173.

Arnstein, E., & Alperstein, G. (1987). *Health care for the homeless* (pp. 29–34). Public Health Currents. Time Saver Publication. Ross Laboratories.

Bachrach, L. (1981). Research on services for the homeless mentally ill: Some caveats. *Hospital and Community Psychiatry, 35*(9), 914–916.

Bachrach, L. L., & Nadelson, C. C. (Eds.). (1988). *Treating chronically mentally ill women.* Washington, D.C.: American Psychiatric Press.

Bassuk, E. L. (1990a). General principles of family-oriented care: Working effectively with clients. In E. L. Bassuk, R. W. Carman, L. F. Weinreb, & M. M. Herzig (Eds.), *Community care for homeless families* (pp. 25–31). Washington, D.C.: Interagency Council on the Homeless.

Bassuk, E. L. (1990b). The problem of family homelessness. In E. L. Bassuk, R. W. Carman, L. F. Weinreb, & M. M. Herzig (Eds.), *Community care for homeless families* (p. 7). Washington, D.C.: Interagency Council on the Homeless.

Bassuk, E. L., & Rosenberg, L. (1988). Why does family homelessness occur? A case control study. *American Journal of Public Health, 78*(7), 783–788.

Bassuk, E. L., & Rubin, L. (1987). Homeless children: A neglected population. *American Journal of Orthopsychiatry, 57*(2), 279–286.

Bassuk, E. L., Rubin, L., & Lauriat, A. S. (1986). Characteristics of sheltered homeless families. *American Journal of Public Health, 76*(9), 1097–1101.

Berne, A., Dato, C., Mason, D. & Rafferty, M. (1990). A nursing model for addressing the health needs of homeless families. *Image, 22*(1), 8–13.

Bingham, R. D., Green, R. E., & White, S. B. (Eds.) (1987). *The homeless in contemporary society.* Newbury Park, CA: Sage.

Brickner, P. W., Scanlan, B. C., & Conanan, B. (1986). Homeless persons and health care. *Annals of Internal Medicine, 104*(3), 405–409.

Brickner, P. W., Scharer, L. K., Conanan, B., Elvy, A., & Savarese, M. (1985). *Health care of the homeless people.* New York: Springer.

Cooper, M. A. (1987). The role of religious and nonprofit organizations in combating homelessness. In B. D. Bingham, B. E. Green, & S. B., White (Eds.), *The homeless in contemporary society* (pp. 130–149). Newbury Park, CA: Sage.

Feldstein, D. J. (1983). *Health care economics* (2nd ed.). New York: John Wiley & Sons.

Greer, N. B. (1985). The homeless: An urban crisis. *Architecture, 74*, 56–59.

Hays, A. (Ed.) (1987). *Working with homeless people: A guide for staff and volunteers.* New York: Columbia University Community Services.

Hopper, K. (1983). Homelessness: Producing the distance. *New England Journal of Human Services, 83*, 30–40.

Institute of Medicine (1988). *Homelessness, health and human needs.* Washington, DC: National Academy Press.

Jones, D. J. (1989). The almost homeless. *Practicing Anthropology, 11*(2), 11–12.

Martin, M. A. (1988). Homelessness among chronically mentally ill women. In: Bachrach, L. L., & Nadelsonn, C. C. *Treating chroncially mentally ill women* (pp. 125–140). New York: Macmillan.

McChesney, K. Y. (1987). *Women without: Homeless mothers and their children.* Unpublished Doctoral Dissertation, University of Southern California.

Mead-Fox, D. (1990). Supports to community and family: Family support centers. In E. L. Bassuk, R. W. Carman, L. F. Weinreb, & M. M. Herzig (Eds.), *Community care for the homeless families* (p. 83). Washington, D.C.: Interagency Council on the Homeless.

Mische-Berkey, K., & Hanson, S. (1989). Family health assessment and intervention. In P. J. Bomar (Ed.), *Nurses and family health promotion: Concepts, assessment, and interventions* (pp. 1115–156). Baltimore, MD: Williams & Wilkins.

Morrissey, J. P., & Dennis, D. L. (1990). *Homelessness and mental illness: Toward the next generation of research studies.* Proceedings of a NIMH-Sponsored Conference, Bethesda, MD, February 21–22, 1989.

Morrissey, J. P., & Dennis, D. L. (1986). *NIMH-funded research concerning homeless mentally ill persons: Implications for policy and practice.* Albany, NY: New York State Office of Mental Health.

Peroff, K. (1987). Who are the homeless and how many are there? In R. D. Bingham, R. E. Green, & S. B. White (Eds.), *The homeless in contemporary society* (pp. 33–45). Newbury Park, CA: Sage.

Robertson, J. M. (1988). Homeless adolescents: A hidden crisis. *Hospital and Community Psychiatry, 39*(5), 475.

Rossi, P. H., & Wright, J. D., (1987). The determinants of homelessness. *Health Affairs*, 19–32.

Roth, D., & Bean, J. (1986). New perspectives on homelessness: Findings from a statewide epidemiological study. *Hospital and Community Psychiatry, 37*(7), 712–716.

Sebastian, J. N. (1985). Homelessness: A state of vulnerability. *Family and Community Health, 8*(3), 11–24.

Taylor-Walton, C. (1988). Analysis of two concepts: Home and homelessness. Unpublished paper, Texas Woman's University, Denton, TX.

Taylor-Walton, C. (1989). Life is hard: A phenomelogical study of homeless women diagnosed as chronically mentally ill. Doctoral Dissertation, Texas Woman's University, 1989. *Dissertation Abstracts International.*

The McKinney Act (1989). *A Program Guide of the Interagency Council on the Homeless.* Washington, D.C.:

The National Resource Center on Homeless and Mental Illness. (1990). *Meeting the need for information about services for homeless mentally ill persons.* Delmar, NY: Policy Research Associate.

United States Department of Housing and Urban Development (1987). *Stewart B. McKinney Homeless Assistance Act of 1987, Public Law 11–77.* Washington, D.C.: Author.

Wagner, J., Melragon, B., & Menke, E. M. (1993). Homeless children: Interdisciplinary drug prevention intervention. *Journal of Children and Adolescent Psychiatric and Mental Health Nursing, 6*(1), 22–30.

Walsh, M. E. (1990). Developmental and socio-emotional needs of homeless infants and preschoolers. In E. L. Bassuk, R. W. Carman, L. F. Weinreb, & M. M. Herzig (Eds.),

Community care for homeless families (pp. 91–101). Washington, DC: Interagency Council on the Homeless.

Walsh, M. E. (1990). Educational and socio-emotional needs of homeless school aged children. In E. L. Bassuk, R. W. Carman, L. F. Weinreb, & M. M. Herzig (Eds.), *Community care for homeless families* (pp. 103–110). Washington, D.C.: Interagency Council on the Homeless.

Weinreb, L. F., & Bassuk, E.L. (1990). Health programs for homeless families. In E. L. Bassuk, R. W. Carman, L. F. Weinreb, & M. M. Herzig (Eds.), *Community care for homeless families* (pp. 67–77). Washington, DC: Interagency Council on the Homeless.

Weiss, M. (1985). *Study of homeless women: Health status, health practices and health services utilization.* Unpublished study. University of Washington, Seattle.

Wright, J. D. (1987). The national health care for the homeless program. In R. D. Bingham, R. E. Green, & S. B. White (Eds.), *The homeless in contemporary society* (pp. 150–169). Newbury Park, CA: Sage.

UNIT

IV

Mental Disorders

CHAPTER

14

Anxiety Disorders

Lynn M. Drost and Lisa Samenfeld Ross

Children and adolescents growing up in the 1990s must deal with the excessive demands of a changing world. Each one experiences a situation differently and reacts in an individualized manner. Some degree of anxiety often is unavoidable and can be useful in promoting growth, but anxiety that reaches overwhelming levels can result in a number of psychologic disorders. This chapter discusses anxiety disorders (including separation anxiety, school phobia, shy behaviors, overanxious disorder and phobia, panic attacks, post-traumatic stress disorder [PTSD], and obsessive–compulsive disorder [OCD]) that affect children, adolescents, and their families.

Anxiety Defined

Osol (1973) defines anxiety as a feeling of apprehension or tension derived from the anticipation of an imagined threat. Anxiety may be manifested by palpitations, diaphoresis, tachycardia, shortness of breath, or even paralysis.

Anxiety of the 1990s

The intensity of society's stressors places excessive demands on the family's integrity. This results in an increased incidence of anxiety in today's family systems.

The Changing Family System

The nontraditional family has become the rule, rather than the exception, in today's society. Many marriages result in divorce. As a result, more single parents rely on the help of extended family members or nonfamilial caretakers. In single-parent households, traditional roles may be altered in that the parent may rely on the child to provide the support that should ordinarily come from the spouse. With divorce comes a myriad of considerations. Children and adolescents often are caught in the middle of custody battles and parental discord. They attempt to adjust to the rules and expectations of two separate and changing households.

Dating and remarriage lead to new stages of adjustment for all family members. They renegotiate roles, boundaries, and expectations as new extended family members are introduced. Family members must adjust simultaneously to the new family system and to the loss of the old system. Each family member resolves his or her conflicts in a different way and at a different pace. Distance becomes an additional factor as the individual family units attempt to establish their own identities. Phones, cars, and airplanes are essential in maintaining relationships.

In many intact families, both parents find it necessary or choose to pursue careers. As a result, children are frequently expected to accept more responsibility in the home. Often the children or adolescents may not be developmentally ready to take on such increased demands.

There are more variations in today's nontraditional families. Lesbian and gay families are becoming more visible. Some women are choosing to raise children without a spouse. Inter-racial marriages and adoptions are more common. The incidence of alternative living situations, such as foster care and group homes, has increased. Each of these circumstances results in unique demands and adaptations.

Contemporary Childhood Experiences

Children today are faced with a multitude of complex stressors. Expectations from home, school, and society have produced these excess demands.

As described previously, changing family structures reflect many stressors. The school experience has taken on different characteristics with a focus on the early acquisition of skills. Learning may become a burden rather than a positive experience if a child is not developmentally ready. In crowded classrooms, teachers must attend to the group's progress rather than the needs of the individual. Therefore, the slower adjusting child may struggle to keep up with the class.

School staff and children's families place considerable attention on extracurricular activities. Competition and winning become the primary goals rather than the individual child's achievement. Parents may unwittingly place unnecessary stress on their children by requiring them to participate in a variety of after-school activities to provide supervision, which parents are unable to offer during their workday.

Advances in technology expose children to massive amounts of information from a variety of sources. Input is received at such a rapid pace that children cannot assimilate and process it adequately before new information arrives. Television, movies, and computerized systems inundate the child with vast and complex quantities of information. Violence, sex, and drug-related activities have become commonplace in a child's world. Cognitively, they may not be able to differentiate reality from fantasy. Additional factors to consider are environmental stressors, including floods, earthquakes, and environmental waste.

Contemporary Adolescent Culture

Along with the stressors that children face, adolescents take on the additional burden of an ever-changing subculture. Adolescents continue to deal with the peer pressures of sex and drugs, but today's youth must face the possibility of contracting communicable diseases, such as herpes and acquired immunodeficiency syndrome. Gang membership with its related violence has become a larger part of adolescents' school and social experience. Adolescents also must deal with expectations of high achievement in the academic and athletic arenas in preparation for future life plans.

Dysfunctional Family Systems

Because of society's stressors, an increasing number of family systems resort to dysfunctional ways of relieving stress and anxiety. Drugs and alcohol are easily obtained by family members, which may result in family violence or neglect. Dysfunctional families often force children to assume parental responsibilities. When children grow up in a violent or neglectful home, they have no exposure to effective ways of dealing with anxiety and tension. Dysfunctional patterns perpetuate other dysfunctional patterns. Children grow up lacking experience in common childhood pleasures and in role modeling of parenting skills. Without the knowledge of and experience with adequate parenting, they cannot pass these essential skills on to the next generation.

Separation Anxiety

DEFINITION AND SYMPTOMALOGY

Separation anxiety is defined in the *Diagnostic and Statistical Manual of Mental Disorders* 4th ed. (DSM-IV, 1994) as excessive anxiety resulting from the separation from home or from those to whom the person is attached. The child's response to the separation may be unexpected for his or her age level; the anxiety experienced is severe to the point of panic. This disorder develops before the age of 18 years. Children or adolescents with this disorder will become uncomfortable when they travel by themselves away from home or familiar environments. These children or adolescents may refuse to leave home to attend such activities as visiting at a friend's house, running errands, or going to camp or school. Some children may have difficulty remaining anywhere by themselves and will respond to being left alone by following the parent around or clinging to him or her whenever they are fearful of separation.

Children experiencing separation anxiety may demonstrate a variety of somatic complaints, such as headaches, stomach aches, and nausea and vomiting. These symptoms can occur when the child is separated from the parent or even when the child anticipates the separation. Although cardiovascular symptoms related to anxiety (i.e., vertigo, palpitations, and faintness) may occur in adolescents, these symptoms occur rarely in younger children (American Psychiatric Association [APA], 1994).

The child separated from a significant attachment figure may have morbid fears that an injury or illness will overtake the child or family members. Children with separation anxiety may be frightened of becoming lost and never seeing their parents again. Many children cannot identify a specific threat but relate generalized anxiety concerning danger or death. Younger children may not be aware of anticipated separations, but as they become older and can identify that a separation may be imminent, they may experience anticipatory distress. Children with separation anxiety exhibit anxieties and fears around various people and situations that they may perceive as threatening. They may be fearful of animals, monsters, burglars, or kidnappers. They have fears of accidents occurring in cars, planes, or other vehicles. The prevalent themes for these children or adolescents are fear of death and dying (APA, 1994).

Children also may have difficulty separating at bedtime. They may resist being left alone and seek out others to sleep with, such as siblings or parents. When they do finally fall asleep, they may be plagued with nightmares that contain their morbid fears. When these children or adolescents are away from home, they may become extremely homesick, uncomfortable to the point of panic, and preoccupied with returning home and rejoining their family. During periods of separation from their major attachment figure, these children may experience extreme sadness and apathy. They may have difficulty concentrating on any activities and may experience social withdrawal. Because they are needy of attention from significant others, children with separation anxiety may demand attention in an intrusive manner. They may feel unloved and uncared for and experience suicidal feelings. Some children, however, may respond in an opposite manner and exhibit compliant and conscientious behavior, hoping to please adults and avoid the separations. Adolescents with separation anxiety, especially boys, may deny any anxiety about separation from their mother, but this anxiety is reflected in their behavior (APA, 1994).

ETIOLOGY

Separation reactions occur in all normally developing children, described by Mahler, Pine, and Bergman (1975) as the rapprochement phase. Mahler describes these reactions as dependent on many variables in the mother–child relationship. When separation reactions are severe and long-lasting, the presence of separation anxiety should be considered. The DSM IV (1994) states that separation anxiety can occur after the child suffers a life stress, such as the death or loss of a family member or a pet. Other precipitants for this disorder could be a change in the child's environment, such as a move to a new neighborhood or attendance at a new school. Generally, families in which separation anxiety occurs are caring and close-knit. No differences have been noted in the incidence between male and female children. This disorder occurs more frequently in children whose mothers have been diagnosed with panic disorder (APA, 1994).

Freud addressed separation anxiety in a cursory manner until 1926, at which time he dealt with this disorder in a more specific manner (Bowlby, 1973). John Bowlby wrote three volumes on separation, attachment, and loss concerning the child and his or her major attachment figures. He addressed the importance of understanding the relationship between mother and child to understand why the child responds as he or she does to separation (Bowlby, 1969).

Margaret Mahler (1975) wrote about issues of separation and individuation as a part of the normal growth process that faces every child as he or she moves toward individuality. Mahler's work covered the separation process that occurs between mother and child, the phases facing every child in achieving individuation, and the expected stages of anxiety that children experience during the beginnings of autonomy.

Because the issues of separation anxiety are similar to those of school phobia, their therapeutic approaches are discussed together following the section on school phobia.

SCHOOL PHOBIA

School phobia is a syndrome of childhood characterized by severe anxiety concerning the attendance or absence at school (Last, Francis, Hessen,

Kazdin, & Strauss, 1987). The DSM IV (1994) states that school phobia may be a symptom of separation anxiety, but it does not need to be present to meet the criteria of separation anxiety.

A study comparing separation anxiety and school phobia by Last et al. (1987) found that children with the diagnosis of separation anxiety were generally prepubertal and female, and the families were from a lower socioeconomic background. When the diagnosis of school phobia was made, the children tended to be past puberty, male, and from a higher socioeconomic background. Children diagnosed with separation anxiety were more likely to have an additional DSM III-R diagnosis and were more disturbed than children with a school phobic disorder (Last et al., 1987).

Last et al. (1987) also found that mothers of children with separation anxiety were diagnosed with affective disorders, particularly major depression, four times more often than the mothers of children with school phobia. Last et al. (1987) concluded that the mothers of children diagnosed with separation anxiety were more disturbed than the mothers of school phobic children.

School refusal symptoms are prevalent in children and adolescents who are referred clinically for anxiety disorders. Failure to attend school results in negative consequences for the child or adolescent in academic and social areas. Absenteeism must be addressed verbally (Last & Strauss, 1990).

In families of school phobic children, the boundaries between the roles of parent and child may be poorly defined. The school phobic child or adolescent often exhibits hostility and defiance and maintains a controlling stance in the family dynamics. The parents are not effective in facilitating their child's return to the classroom (Bernsteen, Svingen, & Garfinkel, 1990).

THERAPEUTIC APPROACHES

The literature discusses the problems and treatment approaches for separation anxiety and school phobia together. Gittleman-Klein and Klein (1971) conducted a study of school phobic children and the use of the antidepressant azepine-5-propanamine (Imipramine). This medication was effective in relieving the anxiety school phobic children experienced, causing them to feel better when they returned to school. The investigators suggested that imipramine would be helpful in separation anxiety disorders (Gittleman-Klein & Klein, 1971). Once the initial anxiety is relieved, secondary symptoms are decreased and overall functioning improves.

Treatment approaches need to be individualized for each school phobic child or adolescent. Individual psychotherapy and behavior therapies should be addressed along with medications. Parents' involvement is significant in helping to facilitate and maintain progress. (See Clinical Example: Johnny Brown).

Shyness and Social Phobia

DEFINITIONS

Shyness is defined as the tendency to avoid social interaction and appropriate participation in social situations (Pilkonis, 1977). Shyness is a social phenomenon, expressed by behavior in relation to other human beings (Lewinsky, 1941). It is characterized by feeling anxious and uncomfortable in specific social situations, resulting in silence and withdrawal from the interaction (Crozier, 1979).

Shyness can range from being just somewhat bashful to the extreme of being fearful of contact with people. When an individual fears people in general, the problem becomes chronic. Children and adolescents who experience avoidant disorder exhibit a fear of strangers to such a degree that social functioning is impaired (Rapoport & Ismond, 1990).

SYMPTOMATOLOGY

Social phobia of childhood and adolescence and shyness may be seen in children as young as 2½ years, after normal stranger anxiety should disappear. A child with generalized social phobia shrinks away from contact with strangers for 6 months or more, which interferes with social functioning and peer relationships. This avoidance is coupled with the desire for affection and acceptance from family members and familiar significant others. Children with social phobia cling to their caretakers and become tearful and anxious when confronted with the contact of strangers. Lacking self-confidence, these children avoid social situations, are mute or inarticulate in social situations, and suffer from embarrassment and timidity, although they seem eager for social relationships (APA, 1994).

Children and adolescents who experience shyness or the more extreme social phobia experience the physical manifestations of anxiety and panic, such as stammering, blushing, perspiring, trembling, pallor, and increased urinary and fecal urges (Lewinsky, 1941). They may have tachycardia, palpitations, and a sensation of "butterflies" (Zimbardo, 1977).

CLINICAL EXAMPLE: JOHNNY BROWN

Johnny Brown was admitted to a child psychiatric inpatient unit after referral by the counselor at his school. Johnny, a 7-year-old anxious-looking child, was accompanied by his mother. During the intake interview, Johnny was clingy and relied on his mother to answer admission questions.

Mrs. Brown and her husband married shortly after high school; she became pregnant within the first year. Mrs. Brown's pregnancy and delivery were within normal limits. Mr. and Mrs. Brown experienced financial difficulties after Johnny's birth, and Mr. Brown began drinking heavily. When he became increasingly abusive toward his wife, she left him, returned to live with her mother, and filed for divorce. Since the finalization of the divorce, Mr. Brown has moved out of state and has had minimal contact with Johnny and his mother.

Mrs. Brown described Johnny as an anxious, fearful baby who became upset and tearful when separated from her. Developmental milestones were reached within normal limits. Mrs. Brown stated she has received professional help for episodes of anxiety in the past but is not presently seeing a therapist. Currently unemployed, Mrs. Brown has been caring for her mother whose health has deteriorated during the last year. Johnny attended kindergarten but was frequently absent due to his ongoing somatic complaints; his mother found it was "easier to keep him home." During first grade, even more absences from school occurred. Johnny has not been able to maintain peer relationships either at school or in the neighborhood.

The precipitant to the deterioration in Johnny's behavior was his grandmother's illness and death 2 months ago. Johnny has become increasingly resistant to leaving his mother. He has not attended school for the last 3 weeks and has been clingy with his mother and more withdrawn from his friends, preferring to stay at home. He has difficulty falling asleep and has frequent nightmares. His mother has allowed Johnny to sleep with her "to settle him."

During the intake procedure, the psychiatric staff set guidelines for visitations and phone calls. His mother could visit daily for 1 hour in the evenings and could call him in the mornings. Johnny could make one phone call a day in the afternoons. The nursing staff encouraged his mother to call and check on Johnny's progress as she needed. Separation was difficult for Johnny and his mother; both became tearful. Johnny was admitted to the inpatient unit with a diagnosis of separation anxiety.

Following a team conference the following care plan was implemented:

NURSING CARE PLAN

Nursing Diagnosis: Anxiety related to anticipated separation from mother

Goal: The client will demonstrate a decrease in the level of anxiety to a low level, as evidenced by his ability to tolerate separation from his mother.

Interventions:

1. Develop a therapeutic, trusting alliance with the client.
2. Label feelings for the child and encourage verbalization of those feelings.
3. Provide support for the client by addressing upcoming visits, and develop a plan for separation.
4. Provide support and reassurance to the client during times of anxiety and stress, especially during separation from the mother.
5. Assist the client in identifying alternative outlets for his anxiety, such as sports, running, climbing, and group games.
6. Initiate family therapy to address dynamics perpetuating the anxiety and adoption of alternative patterns of behavior.
7. Introduce the client to the teacher and classroom slowly to keep anxiety minimal and promote a positive school experience.

Nursing Diagnosis: Impaired Social Interaction related to minimal peer contacts and social skills

Goal: The client will be able to initiate social interactions with peers.

Interventions:

1. Introduce peer interactions slowly to the client to keep anxiety at a minimum.
2. Encourage the client to interact with one other child in an activity, with the assistance of the nurse.
3. Support the client initiating an interaction with one peer each day, when he is comfortable with his peers.
4. Provide support and reassurance to the client as he attempts to interact with peers.

Shy children and adolescents tend to avoid conversations and social functions and, when in these situations, they exhibit increasing anxiety. In the classroom they are obedient and are rarely troublesome. As Caspi, Bem, and Elder (1989) have identified, individuals actively seek out environments that are compatible with, reinforce, and sustain their dispositions.

Shy children and adolescents express their shyness verbally and nonverbally. The verbal indicators of shyness include a soft voice, infrequent speech, and hesitancy when speaking. The nonverbal signs include infrequent or no eye contact, a rigid body posture, inappropriate nervous smiles, and inappropriately fidgity hands (McClure, 1978).

Shy children and adolescents lack self-confidence and poise in social situations. They are at a loss as to what to do with their hands or how to sit or stand (Kaplan, 1972). Painfully apprehensive and lacking the ability to make small talk, they tend to engage in prolonged, vivid daydreams fantasizing personal achievements.

Caspi et al. (1989) and Caspi, Elder, and Bem (1988) describe the shy interactional style as one that moves the individual away from the world. Due to shy children's interactional style, they may not experience many of the role and rule negotiations necessary for the development of social knowledge and skills. Therefore, shy children and adolescents are not likely to initiate or respond appropriately to social overtures. They become increasingly isolated, even if they possess adequate social skills, because anxiety interferes with their initiating contacts with other people. The shy person's passivity may increase the risk of being ignored or overlooked.

Rubin, Hymel, and Mills (1989) studied children longitudinally from kindergarten to fifth grade. Their data suggested that social withdrawal in early childhood may predict internalizing difficulties in later childhood. Caspi et al. (1988; 1989) found that those who had been described as shy during childhood had difficulty as adults adjusting during major life transitions—times that would be ambiguous with regard to rules. Shy interactional styles were evident at times of critical decision making, such as marriage, family, and career choices.

THEORETICAL APPROACHES

Theorists have described a variety of explanations for the shy and anxious behaviors of children and adolescents. Zimbardo (1977) reported that 70% of the time parents and their children share the same shyness label. Shy children are not likely to be found in families with non-shy parents, whereas the incidence increases if at least one parent is labeled as shy.

Behaviorists view shyness as the result of failure to learn effective social skills (Zimbardo, 1977). Wassmer (1978) compared the shy response to that of a conditioned response; actions resulting in pain are avoided. The shy response may be based on one or two negative experiences that are generalized to a wide range of similar situations. The negative experience reinforces what the shy child believes to be true.

Wassmer (1978) stated that the roots of shyness lie in the negative thoughts a person has about himself or herself. Shy individuals interpret contacts with others as failures. The shy child enters a vicious cycle: The negative ideas about himself or herself result in a set of behaviors, which then cause the child to fail at contacts with other people, which, in turn, emphasizes and reinforces the shy child's negative self-image.

Social psychologists propose that the shy individual begins life with nothing more than a label of "shy" and that the label comes before the actual shyness. The shy child may adopt and accept the label without concrete evidence to support it (Zimbardo, 1977).

Psychoanalysts propose several approaches to explaining shy behaviors. One view describes shyness as the reaction to the unfulfilled primal wishes of the id. Among these wishes is the oedipal desire of the child to hold claim to the mother's total affection to the exclusion of all others (Zimbardo, 1977). Kaplan (1972) states that shyness results when there is conflict between the ego-ideal and the superego. Grandiose fantasies preoccupy the morbidly shy person and afford him or her enormous pleasure. Lewinsky (1941) conceptualized that shy people's behaviors are narcissistic, in that everything is directed toward the self with exclusion of the outside world. Constant guarding and watching tend to promote a rigid personality, which is inflexible to new situations and requirements.

TREATMENT APPROACHES

Adults must support the attempts of the shy person to grow and extend himself or herself. The anxious child or adolescent needs unconditional caring to learn to accept his or her own behavior while trying to increase his or her social repetoire. The focus should be on improving self-esteem through compliments and rewards. The child or adolescent should be encouraged to express feelings, knowledge, and talents freely (Zimbardo, 1977).

The shy child should be encouraged to take calculated risks while allowing for mistakes (Zimbardo, 1977). Practicing social and communication skills is essential. Role playing is useful to simulate anxiety-provoking situations. Masks, costumes, and puppet play can liberate inhibited or restrained behaviors (Zimbardo, 1977). The development of trust is imperative to alleviate the child's or adolescent's fear of rejection and ridicule.

Primary reinforcement can be used to increase wanted behaviors (i.e., to increase voice volume or the frequency of vocalizations). Meyer and Berg-Cross (1976) suggested using hierarchic levels when rewarding desired behaviors so that at each stage, the child or adolescent must make a more advanced response to be rewarded. The process should begin with a task that the child or adolescent can already accomplish successfully.

Several books about children and adolescents who have overcome their fears of social interactions are available at various grade levels. These texts can sensitize children and adolescents to their own rejecting behavior to help build their confidence and develop an awareness of problem-solving options (Meyer & Berg-Cross, 1976).

Any strategy should be designed to allow for natural progression through the stages of increasing social interaction. The goal of every intervention should be the intrinsic reward the child receives from behaving in a more assertive, successful, and self-satisfying manner (Meyer & Berg-Cross, 1976).

Generalized Anxiety

DEFINITION AND SYMPTOMATOLOGY

Children with generalized anxiety disorder exhibit excessive or unrealistic anxiety or worry. They worry about future events and past behaviors and spend a great deal of time inquiring about a variety of situations. Anxious children are self-conscious and need reassurance. They worry about being competent and what others will think of them (APA, 1994).

They demonstrate somatic complaints that can be manifested as gastrointestinal discomfort, shortness of breath, nausea, headaches, difficulty falling asleep, vertigo, or other various discomforts. These children usually look nervous or tense (APA, 1987).

Social and simple phobia also may be present in children with generalized anxiety disorder. These children seem older than their age because of their precocious concerns. They tend to strive toward perfection for fear of what others will think of them and may become obsessed with doubting themselves. Anxious children may exhibit excessive conformity, a desire to please others and win approval, restlessness, and nervous habits, such as hair pulling or nail biting (APA, 1994).

ETIOLOGY

Generalized anxiety disorder tends to occur more commonly in small families, in oldest children of families, and in upper socioeconomic level families. Parents exhibit concern about their child's achievement and success, even when the child is functioning at an adequate or superior level. Children 13 years or older are more likely to have the diagnosis of anxiety disorder. If the child has a diagnosis of separation anxiety, he or she usually is younger than 13 years of age. Parents of children with anxiety disorders are more likely to have anxiety disorders themselves.

Childhood Phobias

Every child experiences some fears or anxieties, particularly fears of doctors, strangers, the dark, or animals, during their development. Usually these fears are of a short duration and not extreme; when they are severe and continuous, however, they may be termed phobias. The APA (1994) describes a specific phobia as a persistent fear of a specific object or situation, which results in an immediate anxiety response. The child or adolescent avoids the phobic situation even though he or she realizes that the fear is excessive to the situation.

Children's phobias can impact the child and the family significantly. Children who are fearful of closed places, such as a classroom, may have difficulty concentrating on academic issues. Children who are fearful of dogs may have difficulty walking in the neighborhood, to the store, or to school, causing them to avoid stressful situations and remain at home or in the house most of the day.

Social phobia, usually beginning in late childhood or early adolescence, is a persistent fear of a situation in which a person is exposed to scrutiny by others and the fear that he or she may do something that would be embarrassing or humiliating. Exposure to the phobic stimulus provokes an anxiety response, and as in specific phobia, the child or adolescent begins to avoid social situations (APA, 1994).

Children may develop phobias as learned behaviors. Childhood phobias may result from traumatic or nontraumatic experiences. Phobic behavior may be maintained inadvertently or by deliberate reinforcement by parents or others (King, Hamilton, & Ollendick, 1988). It is important to involve the family in therapy to overcome conditioning by the parents.

THERAPEUTIC APPROACHES TO PHOBIAS

Preparing children for events that may be stressful or traumatic can encourage cooperative behavior and reduce the risk of fear reactions. For example, parents can work with their children to help prepare them for the stress of beginning school. Parents also can prepare children for any stressors, such as hospitalizations and upcoming surgeries, to help reduce anxiety.

Parents have a critical impact on childhood phobias and their treatment. In a negative sense, parents may reinforce the child's fear or phobia. In a positive sense, however, parents may be effective role models and help their child relearn new responses to fears. To foster a successful approach to phobias, parents must be supportive of the treatment and involved in behavioral approaches in the home (King et al., 1988).

Behavioral approaches effective with phobic children include systematic desensitization and modeling. Systematic desensitization consists of three steps: relaxation training, developing the hierarchy of anxiety, and systematic desensitization proper (King et al., 1988). The relaxation techniques serve to help the child to reduce anxiety when involved in imagery desensitization or in the real-life phobic situation.

To develop the anxiety hierarchy, the child or adolescent rates certain phobic situations according to the amount of anxiety provoked. An older child or adolescent can participate in this process without difficulty, but a parent or caretaker needs to provide this information for a younger child. After the child or adolescent achieves a state of relaxation, the therapist presents the least anxiety-provoking situation in the hierarchy. This procedure continues slowly until the child or adolescent can tolerate the most anxiety-provoking situation of the hierarchy without experiencing anxiety (King et al., 1988).

In the next step, systematic desensitization, the child or adolescent is exposed to the real-life phobic situation in a controlled setting. This procedure is more effective in decreasing anxiety than using imagery (King et al., 1988).

Modeling is another effective behavioral approach to treat phobic children. Modeling has three functions: It aids in the development of new response patterns for the child or adolescent; it strengthens or inhibits responses as needed; and the child or adolescent demonstrates an improvement in socially acceptable behavior. Learning appropriate skills for various situations reduces anxiety around the fear stimulus (King et al., 1988).

Psychotherapy is a useful therapeutic tool that can be used in conjunction with other therapies. It allows the child or adolescent to address any feelings and concerns about the anxiety.

Phobias also can respond to other psychotherapeutic approaches. A study of six children with phobic reactions to sleep was conducted by Connell, Persley, and Sturgess (1987). All the children experienced the recent death of an adult with whom they had had a close relationship, and they tended to equate sleep with death. Psychotherapy focused on clarifying each child's concept of death and sleep. The children were able to work through their feelings of death and their own mortality during this process (Connell, Persley, & Sturgess, 1987).

Phobic disorders in adults tend to respond to psychotherapy and behavioral training rather than pharmacologic interventions. In children, however, imipramine has been found to reduce the primary and secondary symptoms of anxiety in school phobias (Gittelman-Klein & Klein, 1971).

Panic Disorder

The APA (1994) describes panic attacks as periods of intense discomfort or fear. These attacks are usually unexpected and begin with a sudden onset of apprehension, fear, and terror. The individual may experience a feeling of impending doom. During a panic attack, a person suffers dyspnea, vertigo, faintness, palpitations, diaphoresis, depersonalization, or fear of dying.

Although panic disorder is described widely in adults, there is little information about panic attacks in children and adolescents. Nevertheless, adult and adolescent clients relate that their symptoms of panic disorder began in childhood (Klein, 1981). The literature identifies the occurrence of panic disorder in children as young as 5 years old. The children's symptoms are similar to those of adults presenting with panic disorder (Black & Robbins, 1990).

Children and adolescents with panic disorder have many somatic complaints and may be referred to pediatricians, at which time their condition may go undiagnosed. Adolescents with panic disorder frequently describe a recent loss, such as the death of a parent or rejection by a boyfriend or girlfriend. They may be anticipating the loss when symptoms appear (Black & Robbins, 1990).

Hayward, Killen, and Barr (1989) studied 106 ninth-grade students to determine the prevalence of panic attacks in young adolescents. At least one panic attack with four or more symptoms present was reported by 11.6% of the students. A significant number of children who had experienced panic attacks had parents who were either divorced or separated.

Klein (1981) has identified a relationship between panic disorder and separation anxiety of childhood. Depression and panic attacks overlap in adolescents. The finding that parents of adolescents with panic attacks are more likely divorced or separated suggests that the experience of early loss or a sensitivity to separations may be factors in the development of panic attacks later in life (Hayward et al., 1989).

THERAPEUTIC APPROACHES

Gittleman and Klein (1984) have found a significant familial overlap among panic disorder, separation anxiety, and depression. All three of these disorders respond to the same pharmacologic agents: tricyclic and monoamine oxidase inhibitor (MAOI) antidepressants (Klein & Gittleman-Klein, 1978).

Supportive and insight-oriented psychotherapy, pharmacologic intervention, and cognitive and behavioral psychotherapies are effective treatments for adult panic disorder. There has been no systematic evaluation of therapies for children with panic disorder (Black & Robbins, 1990).

We know very little about children and adolescents with panic disorders. Epidemiologic studies are needed to determine its prevalence, as well as studies of children and families at risk to identify early symptoms and etiology and treatment effectiveness studies.

Post-traumatic Stress Disorder

DEFINITION AND ETIOLOGY

PTSD often manifests itself with characteristic symptoms that are present after the occurrence of a traumatic event. This type of event would be psychologically traumatizing to anyone who experienced the same situation (APA, 1994).

The DSM IV identifies the causes of PTSD as a traumatic event usually involving a serious threat to the victim's integrity or life; a serious injury to the victim's spouse, children, or close family members or friends; a sudden loss of one's home or town; or the death or injury of a victim of physical violence or an accident. In some instances an individual may not need to observe the trauma but may instead receive information that a loved one could be seriously harmed. These traumas can occur to an individual when he or she is alone or with a group of people (APA, 1994) (Box 14-1).

The types of disasters that may lead to PTSD are natural disasters, accidental disasters, and man-made deliberate disasters. Natural disasters include earthquakes, tornadoes, and floods. Accidental disasters include car or airplane crashes, large fires, and collapsed structures that result in serious injury to people. Some man-made deliberate disasters are shootings, assaults, torture, war, and bombings. Disasters of man-made design result in a more severe and longer lasting traumatic stress disorder.

SYMPTOMATOLOGY

Children with PTSD are likely to experience the following:

- Reexperience the trauma through repetitive play that contains themes similar to the initial trauma
- Lose newly acquired developmental skills and regress to an earlier level of development
- Believe that the future is limited and no longer anticipate attaining some of life's goals (e.g., family, career, or even adulthood)
- Exhibit omen formation and the false belief that he or she can predict future events
- Present other psychologic symptoms, such as separation anxiety and general fearfulness (Brett, Spitzer & Williams, 1988)

The DSM IV identifies age-specific features of PTSD. The child initially may be reluctant to discuss the trauma, not because he or she cannot remember the experience, but because it may be too difficult to recall. The child also may become less interested in significant activities and have somatic complaints, such as headaches and stomach aches. The child's constricted affect may hinder his or her ability to relate and discuss the traumatic event. Mental health professionals should therefore evaluate information from several sources, including parents, teachers, and others close to the child.

BOX 14–1 • HISTORICAL NOTES ON POST-TRAUMATIC STRESS DISORDER IN CHILDREN

Sigmund Freud (1917; 1920) examined the effects of trauma during and after World War I. During World War II, Anna Freud and Dorothy Burlingham (1942) wrote about their experiences with the London children who were evacuated during wartime bombings. The study focused on the separation of the children from their parents more than the traumatic event (i.e., the bombings) (Freud & Burlingham, 1942).

The first peacetime study of children who had suffered traumas occurred in Vicksburg, Mississippi, when a tornado struck a movie theater in which a large number of children were watching a Saturday matinee (Block, 1956). The interviewers of this study worked only with the parents and never actually interviewed the children (Terr, 1987). After World War II, researchers studied children who had survived the Holocaust and Hiroshima. These studies of second-generation survivors of the Holocaust demonstrated that post-traumatic stress disorder (PTSD) incidence was higher in Israeli combat stress reaction casualties when the parents were Holocaust survivors (Solomon, Katler, & Mikulincer, 1988).

As mental health professionals learned more about PTSD and its impact on children, attention centered on the child's reactions and experiences after a traumatic event. Fredericks (1985) conducted a follow-up study of survivors of a tornado in Xenia, Ohio, 7 months after the incident. The researcher found that symptoms of PTSD were present in adults and children who survived the tornado. In school, children were required to share classrooms, so overcrowding resulted, and the truancy rate increased in the area. Some of the children developed conduct disorders and psychophysiologic problems.

In 1972, the Buffalo Creek Dam collapsed, causing a flood that killed 125 people, mostly women and children (Frederick, 1985). In interviews of 11 of the children who survived the disaster, the children's drawings and stories helped them identify their feelings surrounding the trauma. This method was a significant advance in obtaining relevant information from the children (Frederick, 1985).

Mental health professionals are acutely aware of the importance of follow-up for victims and their families and are responding promptly to those involved in catastrophic incidents. Research in the area of PTSD in children continues to identify the disorder's incidence and risk factors.

REFERENCES

Block,, D., Silber, E., & Perry, S. (1956). Some factors in the emotional reaction of children to disaster. *American Journal of Psychiatry, 113*, 416–422.

Frederick, C. J. (1985). Children traumatized by catastrophic situations. In S. Eth & R. Pynoos (Eds.), *Post-traumatic stress disorder in children* (pp. 71–99). Washington, D.C.: American Psychiatric Press.

Freud, A., & Burlingham, D. (1942). *Report 12, the writings of Anna Freud* (Vol. 3) (pp. 142–211). New York: International Universities Press.

Solomon, Z., Katler, M., & Mikulincer, M. (1987). Combat-related posttraumatic stress disorder among second generation holocaust survivors: Preliminary findings. *American Journal of Psychiatry, 145*(7), 865–869.

Terr, L. C. (1987). Childhood psychic trauma. In J. Noshpitz (Ed.), *Basic handbook of child psychiatry* (pp. 262–272). New York: Basic Books.

Lenore Terr worked with 26 children from Chowchilla, Texas, who were kidnapped on their school bus by three strangers and ultimately were placed in a buried truck-trailer. The children, ages 5 to 14 years, were missing for 27 hours but eventually were able to dig themselves out and returned to their families physically unharmed.

Terr's (1981) research into childhood psychic trauma noted that the children did not experience a period of amnesia after the traumatic event or a phase of denial (which adult victims of trauma frequently use as defenses). In addition, the children never had flashbacks; rather, they "played out" their traumas in a way similar to the repetitive dreams and reenactments that occur in children and adults. The children evidenced signs of ego dysfunction, as seen in cognitive malfunctions, overgeneralizations, and time distortions. These findings were relatively consistent across all three age groups (oedipal, latency, and adolescence) (Terr, 1981).

Martini, Ryan, Nakayama, and Ramenofsky (1990) interviewed five children and their families after a boating accident during the 1988 Pittsburgh Regatta. These children were from diverse psychosocial backgrounds, exhibited unique personality characteristics, and each experienced the trauma differently from the others. Some of the children with serious injuries did not experience the intense degree of trauma that other children with minor injuries did; the child who exhibited the greatest degree of PTSD also was the child who suffered the least physical trauma or changes in life-style after the accident. As a result of this study, Martini et al.

(1990) concluded that the following factors were critical to the development of PTSD in target populations:

- Level of family stress
- Client's and family's coping style
- Client's history of previous psychologic problems
- Client's effectiveness in dealing with past stressful situations

The degree of family stress is an important issue in evaluating the family's ability to support the traumatized child or adolescent. Family coping style indicates how family members will respond to a trauma; in dysfunctional families, members need to learn how to support each other.

Martini et al. (1990) discovered that the child with previous psychologic problems tended to develop a more severe level of PTSD and a possible recurrence of previously resolved symptoms. Families also are more likely to support their child or adolescent effectively following a traumatic event if they have dealt successfully with a stressful situation in the past. The child or adolescent who has received support from his or her family following traumas will be in a stronger position to tolerate and recover from its effects.

Martini et al. (1990) concluded that not only the severity of the trauma, but also the emotional makeup of the child and the family are considerations in the development of PTSD. As research continues to examine the effects of trauma, investigators must evaluate factors involving the client and the supportiveness of the family.

TREATMENT APPROACHES

PTSD is a relatively new diagnostic category, and the treatment approaches are still being developed and studied. Terr (1987) suggests that psychic trauma can be prevented by identifying areas in which natural disasters are likely to occur. The children in these areas would participate in classes to prepare them for a possible future disaster. However, regardless of preparation techniques, children may still be exposed to traumas. If they are exposed, the timeliness of medical intervention is crucial. The sooner victims of trauma receive aid, the less likely they are of suffering emotional disability (Terr, 1987).

Evaluating the family of the child victim also is important because siblings and parents can be traumatized by exposure to the child. Family members exhibit symptoms of PTSD. Parents can provide the needed history, which will lead to an accurate assessment. If the family has been exposed to the same traumatic event as the child, family members may need family therapy or individual therapy to address their separate reactions to the trauma. Parents who are involved in the therapy can work with their child to validate their own feelings about the experience. Involving the parents in therapy helps prevent symptoms being transferred to unexposed family members (Terr, 1987).

Some medications, such as the beta-blocking agents, tricyclic antidepressants, and MAOIs, are used for adults with panic attacks and phobias. Tranquilizers, propranolol (Inderal), and Imipramine have all been used to treat PTSD and accompanying symptoms in children and adolescents, but none of these medications are effective in treating the whole trauma syndrome itself (Terr, 1987).

The goal of treatment of PTSD is to regain some degree of control over the current life situation. Continual repetition or reliving the trauma, an unconscious process, may provide a temporary and transient sense of control. Feelings of helplessness and being out of control eventually return. Verbalization or playing out the trauma is essentially the purpose of individual therapy for the child or adolescent. The nurse therapist approaches the traumatic material in a controlled, slow manner to avoid an intensification of the symptoms of PTSD. Such intensification could cause an increase in the experience of reliving the trauma. Consciously addressing the traumatic event allows the child or adolescent to maintain some degree of control over reenacting the event. By maintaining a secure attachment to a parent or adult figure, children or adolescents are able to address their experiences with another person. This attachment process helps decrease the reenactment phenomena. When the child can experience the trauma as an event that occurred in the past, its impact can be controlled and diminished through present experiences. (See the Clinical Example for Mike Smythe.)

Obsessive-Compulsive Disorder

DEFINITION AND SYMPTOMOTOLOGY

Obsessions are recurrent and persistent thoughts, impulses, and images that are experienced, at some point, as intrusive and inappropriate and that cause marked anxiety and distress (APA, 1994). Compulsions are repetitive behaviors (eg, handwashing, checking, ordering) or mental acts

CLINICAL EXAMPLE: MIKE SMYTHE

Mike Smythe, 9 years old, was present during a boating accident 8 months ago in which his best friend drowned. Since that time, Mike's parents have become increasingly concerned about the deterioration in Mike's behavior at school and at home. Mike has become increasingly aggressive with his peers and his 7-year-old sister. His grades have dropped dramatically, and he has been engaging in more risk-taking behaviors. The Smythes decided to seek professional help after Mike was suspended from school for throwing a desk across the classroom.

The family was seen for intake sessions, including individual and family interviews. Mike presented as a well-groomed, well-nourished 9-year-old. He maintained a sad affect and did not smile during the interview. He became resistive to talking when asked why he thought he was being seen by the clinician. Throughout the interview, he denied the severity of his behaviors. He became tearful when the clinician asked him to share about the drowning incident. Mike was unable to label any of his feelings regarding the drowning incident or his behaviors at home or school. Mike also was experiencing some difficulty sleeping, and when he did fall asleep, had frequent nightmares. He gave no evidence of a thought disorder and denied suicidal ideation. Based on the assessment of post-traumatic stress disorder (PTSD), the nurse clinician planned to see Mike individually twice weekly and the family once a week.

NURSING DIAGNOSIS

Formulating the nursing diagnosis entails following the analysis of assessment data. Several nursing diagnoses are appropriate to the medical diagnosis of PTSD (Townsend, 1988). The clinician's diagnostic determination depends on the client's history and current status. Nursing diagnoses in this clinical example include:

1. Ineffective Individual Coping: Mike was unable to meet age-appropriate expectations due to his aggression with his peers and his sister. Mike also was unable to accept his behavior as being problematic. He couldn't follow the rules of school; he became aggressive and was suspended from classes.
2. High Risk for Violence: Self-Directed or Directed at Others. Mike's aggression could be related to his unresolved grief following the loss of his friend. Mike was aggressive with his peers and his sister, and he was involved in an increasing amount of risk taking. He has been unable to verbalize his feelings of anger and rage at his loss.
3. Sleep Pattern Disturbance: Mike related having sleep difficulties and nightmares since the drowning of his friend. These disturbances could be related to the drowning accident and fears for his friend and himself.
4. Powerlessness: Mike could feel powerless related to his inability to save his friend. His powerlessness could be caused by a dysfunctional grieving process. Mike was resistant to expressing his feelings concerning his loss.

PLANNING

The next step in the nursing process is to develop a plan of care and identify the goals and behaviors necessary for the client to meet those goals. Some of the goals formulated for a child with PTSD follow:

1. Mike will develop and use age-appropriate, socially acceptable coping skills, including verbalizing his feelings rather than acting them out.
2. Mike will not harm peers or family members.
3. Mike will sleep 6 to 7 hours at a time without interruption.
4. Mike will determine ways in which he can be in control of his life to reduce his feelings of powerlessness.

IMPLEMENTATION

Implementation of the treatment plan needs to be individualized for each patient. Involving the client in this process is imperative to achieving the stated goals successfully. Some of the interventions for Mike follow:

1. Mike will participate in individual and family therapy to help him address his anger and guilt about the traumatic experience. Play therapy will be a useful modality to help Mike re-enact the trauma and give some control over the event. Mike will need to explore alternative ways to handle his feelings and will need positive support and reassurance during the trials of new methods.
2. Mike needs to be observed for violent behavior. When he becomes angry, helping him identify his feelings will assist him to accept them. Role modeling how to discharge anger appropriately will help Mike handle feelings. He also will need positive feedback when he attempts to address his anger appropriately. Exploring alternative ways to handle anger will allow Mike to make choices for himself. It would be beneficial for the clinician to re-

(*continued*)

CLINICAL EXAMPLE: MIKE SMYTHE *(Continued)*

main with Mike when he is angry to provide support and reassurance.

3. The nurse must make a thorough assessment of Mike's sleep difficulties. Mike's parents should supply relevant data to the clinician. If Mike is too fearful to fall asleep, his mother or father should remain with him until he falls asleep. A set time for bedtime should be identified and adhered to as much as possible. Mike's parents should reassure him that they will be there if he awakens with a nightmare and that they will remain with him until he is settled again.
4. Mike needs to be able to take on age-appropriate responsibilities. It would be beneficial to involve Mike in the decision concerning which goals he would like to achieve in therapy. Mike will need positive reinforcement and feedback when he makes appropriate decisions. He will need assistance in identifying areas over which he does and does not have control. When Mike doesn't have control in an area, he needs to be helped to verbalize his feelings at that time. Mike should be encouraged to participate in areas in which he could excel.

EVALUATION

Evaluation is a continuous process that begins at the initiation of therapy. Initial goals must be examined periodically and interventions evaluated to determine progress. It is essential to include the family in establishing goals and evaluating the effectiveness of the interventions.

Weekly meetings with Mike's parents allowed them to participate in his treatment. These also offered opportunities for support and education. Mike and the nurse clinician were able to discuss progress made in individual therapy, and Mike's parents discussed changes in his behavior at home and at school. Because therapy is time-limited, Mike and his family established the goals needed to be achieved to terminate therapy. The nurse clinician was available for consultation on a follow-up basis.

(praying, counting, repeating words silently) that a person feels driven to perform in response to an obsession or according to rules that must be applied rigidly. Compulsions are aimed at preventing or reducing distress or preventing some dreaded event (APA, 1994). Children may not recognize that the obsessions or compulsions are excessive or unreasonable. The thoughts and behaviors of the client with obsessive-compulsive disorder (OCD) are time-consuming (more than one hour per day) and interfere significantly with a youth's normal routine. The effects of the symptoms can range from mild to incapacitating. The common themes for clients with OCD, often concerned with cleanliness, aggression, checking, and collecting, are that people cannot trust their judgment or believe their senses (Rapoport, 1989).

ETIOLOGY

OCD is not as rare as once believed. Estimates from recent community studies indicate a lifetime prevalence of 2.5% and a 1 year prevalence of 1.5%–2.1% (APA, 1994). OCD usually begins in adolescence and young adulthood, but may begin in childhood. More than 4 million people in the United States suffer from OCD (Rapoport, 1989), with approximately one-third to one-half of adult OCD patients having experienced their symptoms before age 15 (Wolff & Rapoport, 1988). Pitman (1987) found that clients with OCD frequently had accompanying panic and phobic disorders. The concordance rate for OCD is higher for monozygotic than for dizygotic twins. The rate of OCD in first-degree biological relatives of persons with OCD or with Tourette's disorder is higher than in the general population (APA, 1994). Differences in functioning in the caudate nucleus of the basal ganglia and parts of the frontal lobe of OCD clients have been demonstrated by means of PET (Rapoport, 1989).

TREATMENT APPROACHES

BEHAVIOR THERAPY. Behavioral treatment of OCD includes positive reinforcement, punishment, differential reinforcement of other behaviors, exposure therapy, satiation, modeling, cognitive restructuring, disruption of the behavioral chain, and relaxation delay, each of which has resulted in some success (Marks, 1986; Wolff & Rapoport, 1988).

MEDICATION. The antidepressants fluoxetine (Prozac) and clomipramine (Anafranil) have been useful in treating adults with OCD (Marks, 1986; Rapoport, 1989). These serotonin reuptake inhibitor medications and two newer and safer ones, sertraline hydrochloride (Zoloft) and paroxetine (Paxil), are the most useful pharmacologic treatments for children and adolescents with OCD.

Summary

Nurse clinicians are becoming more skilled at identifying children and adolescents experiencing anxiety disorders. Accurate nursing assessment and diagnosis promote the establishment of goals and interventions that will result in favorable outcomes for young clients and their families.

REFERENCES

American Psychiatric Association. (1994). *Diagnostic and statistical manual of mental disorders* (4th ed.). Washington, DC: Author.

Bernsteen, G. A., Svingen, P. H., & Garfinkel, B. D. (1990). School phobia: Patterns of family functioning. *Journal of the American Academy of Child and Adolescent Psychiatry, 29*(1), 24–30.

Black, B., & Robbins, D. R. (1990). Case study: Panic disorder in children and adolescents. *Journal of the American Academy of Child and Adolescent Psychiatry, 29*(1), 36–44.

Block, D., Silber, E., & Perry, S. (1956). Some factors in the emotional reaction of children to disaster. *American Journal of Psychiatry, 113*, 416–422.

Bowlby, J. (1969). *Attachment and loss (Vol. I): Attachment*. New York: Basic Books.

Bowlby, J. (1973) *Attachment and loss (Vol. II): Separation: Anxiety and anger*. New York: Basic Books.

Brett, E. A., Spitzer, R. L., & Williams, J. B. W. (1988). DSM-III-R criteria for posttaumatic stress disorder. *American Journal of Psychiatry, 145*, 1232–1236.

Caspi, A., Elder, G., & Bem D. (1988). Moving away from the world: Life-patterns of shy children. *Developmental Psychology, 24*(6) 824–831.

Caspi, A., Bem, D., & Elder, G. (1989) Continuities and consequences of interactional styles across the life course. *Journal of Personality, 57*(2), 375–406.

Connell, H. M., Persley, G. V., & Sturgess, J. L. (1987). Case report: Sleep phobia in middle childhood: A review of six cases. *Journal of the American Academy of Child and Adolescent Psychiatry, 26*(3), 449–452.

Crozier, W. R. (1979). Shyness as a dimension of personality. *British Journal of Social and Clinical Psychology, 18*, 121–128.

Gittleman-Klein, R., & Klein, D. F. (1971). Controlled imipramine treatment of school phobia. *Archives of General Psychiatry, 25*, 204–207.

Gittleman, R., & Klein, D. F. (1984). Relationship between separation anxiety and panic and agoraphobic disorders. *Psychopathology, 17*(1), 56–65.

Hayward, C., Killen, J., & Barr, T. (1989). Panic attacks in young adolescents. *American Journal of Psychiatry, 146*, 1061–1062.

Jenike, M. A., Baer, L., & Minichiello, W. E. (1987). Somatic treatments for Obsessive-Compulsive Disorders. *Comprehensive Psychiatry, 28*(3), 250–263.

Kaplan, D. M. (1972). On shyness. *International Journal of Psychoanalysis, 53*(4), 439–453.

King, N., Hamilton, D., & Ollendick, T. (1988). *Children's phobias: A behavioral perspective*. Chichester: John Wiley and Sons.

Klein, D. F., & Gittleman-Klein, R. (1978). Drug treatment of separation anxiety and depressive illness in children. *Advances in Biological Psychiatry, 2*, 50–60.

Klein, D. F. (1981). Anxiety reconceptualized. In D. F. Klein & J. Robkin (Eds.), *Anxiety: New research and changing concepts* (pp. 235–263). New York: Raven Press.

Last, C., Francis, G., Hessen, M., Kazdin, A., & Strauss, C. (1987). Separation anxiety and school phobia: A comparison using DSM-III criteria. *American Journal of Psychiatry, 144*(5), 653–657.

Last, C., & Strauss, C. (1990). School refusal in anxiety-disordered children and adolescents. *Journal of the American Academy of Child and Adolescent Psychiatry, 29*(1), 31–35.

Lewinsky, H. (1941–1942). The nature of shyness. *British Journal of Psychology, 32*, 105–113.

Mahler, M., Pine, F., & Bergman, A. (1975). *The psychological birth of the human infant*. New York: Basic Books.

Marks, I. (1986). Behavioural and drug treatments of phobic and Obsessive-Compulsive disorders. *Psychotherapy and Psychosomatics, 46*, 35–44.

Martini, D. R., Ryan, C., Nakayama, D., & Ramenofsky, M. (1990). Psychiatric sequelae after traumatic injury: The Pittsburg Regatta. *Journal of the American Academy of Child and Adolescent Psychiatry, 29*(1), 70–75.

McClure, W. J. (1978). Effectively counseling the shy minority client. *Journal of Employment Counseling, 15*(4), 150–156.

Meyer, M. E., & Berg-Cross, L. (1976). Helping the withdrawn child. *Theory Into Practice, 15*(5), 332–336.

Newman, C. J. (1976). Children of disaster: Clinical observations at Buffalo Creek. *American Journal of Psychiatry, 133*, 306–312.

Osol, A. (Ed). (1973). *Blakiston's pocket medical dictionary* (3rd ed.). New York: McGraw-Hill.

Pilkonis, P. A. (1977). The behavioral consequences of shyness. *Journal of Personality, 45*, 596–611.

Pitman, R. K., Green, R. C., Jenike, M. A., & Mesulam, M. M. (1987). Clinical comparison of Tourette's disorder and Obsessive-Compulsive disorder. *American Journal of Psychiatry, 144*(9), 1166–1171.

Rapoport, J. L. (1989). *The boy who couldn't stop washing*. New York: Penguin Books.

Rapoport, J. L., & Ismond, D. R. (1990). *DSM-III-R training guide for diagnosis of childhood disorders*. New York: Brunner/Mazel.

Rubin, K. H., Hymel, S., & Mills, R. (1989). Sociability and social withdrawal in childhood: Stability and outcomes. *Journal of Personality, 57*(2), 237–255.

Solomon, Z., Katler, M., & Mikulincer, M. (1987) Combat-related posttraumatic stress disorder among second generation holocaust survivors: Preliminary findings. *American Journal of Psychiatry, 145*(7), 865–869.

Terr, L. C. (1981). Psychic trauma in children: Observations following the Chowchilla school-bus kidnapping. *American Journal of Psychiatry, 138*(1), 14–19.

Terr, L. C. (1987). Childhood psychic trauma. In J. Noshpitz (Ed.), *Basic handbook of child psychiatry* (pp. 262–272). New York: Basic Books.

Terr, L.C. (1990). *Too scared to cry*. New York: Basic Books.

Wassmer, A. C. (1978). *Making contact*. New York: Fawcett Popular Library.

Wolff, R., & Rapoport, J. L. (1988). Behavioral treatment of childhood obsessive-compulsive disorder. *Behavior Modification, 12*(2), 252–266.

Zimbardo, P. G. (1977). *Shyness: What is it, what to do about it*. Reading, MA: Addison-Wesley.

Zimbardo, P. G., Pilkonis, P. A., & Norwood, R. M. (1975). The social disease called shyness. *Psychology Today, 8*(12), 68–72.

Parent: "He never listens to anything I say." "Nothing I do to discipline him works."

Teacher: "He never finishes anything he starts." "He won't sit still, and he talks out in class."

ADHD Child: "I can't do anything right. Maybe I *am* stupid." "They're always on my case. I wish they would just leave me alone." "Why does everyone pick on me?"

CHAPTER 15

Attention Disorders

Jane Baggett

The above statements reflect the perceptions of those affected by attention-deficit hyperactivity disorder (ADHD). Three to five percent of children in the United States have an attention deficit disorder (ADD), with or without hyperactivity. Boys with ADHD outnumber girls by as much as nine to one (American Psychiatric Association [APA], 1994). Teachers and parents frequently assume that any child who displays behavioral or academic problems has ADHD. As with any disorder, the diagnosis of an ADD requires a comprehensive evaluation that considers age, developmental level, and any coexisting disabling conditions.

ADHD is a developmental disorder. The symptoms change as the child develops. This disorder persists through childhood, often into adolescence, and into adulthood for perhaps one third of the patients (APA, 1994).

This chapter looks at the historic development of definitions and diagnostic criteria, the proposed etiologic theories, perspectives on behavioral problems, and associated conditions. The disorder of ADHD is examined in depth through the use of the nursing process.

Historic Review of Definitions and Diagnostic Criteria

The conceptualization of ADD has changed in the last 10 to 15 years as new data became available. Early theorists viewed ADD as a developmental or maturational lag, with the ADD child progressing along the same continuum as normal children but at a slower pace. The implication was that these children would eventually normalize, most likely during adolescence. As more studies were conducted, the evidence mounted that the developmental delay theory inadequately described a majority of children with ADD.

The "continual-display theory" arose, suggesting that the core symptoms of ADD remain, but are modified with age. A more extreme position, the "eventual-decay theory," suggested that children who manifest ADD are at risk for the development of severe psychopathology in adolescence and adult life. This severe psychopathology includes antisocial personality disorder, alcoholism, serious academic retardation, major affective disorder, other types of personality disorders, and even schizophrenia.

The diagnosis of ADHD is not made on the basis of a single symptom, but on the presence of a syndrome characterized by developmentally short attention span, impulsivity, and motor hyperactivity. Box 15-1 lists the *Diagnostic and Statistical Manual of Mental Disorders* criteria for diagnosis of ADHD.

Etiology of Attention-Deficit Hyperactivity Disorder

ADHD has a multifactorial etiology. The literature is filled with possible causes, including family genetic factors, biochemical factors, neurophysiologic fac-

BOX 15–1 • DSM IV DIAGNOSTIC CRITERIA FOR ATTENTION-DEFICIT HYPERACTIVITY DISORDER

A. Either 1 or 2:
   1. *Inattention:* Six (or more) of the following symptoms of inattention have persisted for at least 6 months to a degree that is maladaptive and inconsistent with developmental level:
      a. Often fails to give close attention to details or makes careless mistakes in schoolwork, work, and other activities
      b. Often has difficulty sustaining attention in tasks or play activities
      c. Often does not seem to listen when spoken to directly
      d. Often does not follow through on instructions and fails to finish schoolwork, chores, or duties in the workplace (not due to oppositional behavior or failure to understand instructions)
      e. Often has difficulty organizing tasks and activities
      f. Often avoids, dislikes, or is reluctant to engage in tasks that require sustained mental effort (such as schoolwork or homework)
      g. Often loses things necessary for tasks or activities (eg, toys, school assignments, pencils, books, or tools)
      h. Is often easily distracted by extraneous stimuli
      i. Is often forgetful in daily activities
   2. *Hyperactivity-impulsivity:* Six (or more) of the following symptoms of hyperactivity-impulsivity have persisted for at least 6 months to a degree that is maladaptive and inconsistent with developmental level:

      HYPERACTIVITY
      a. Often fidgets with hands or feet or squirms in seat
      b. Often leaves seat in classroom or in other situations in which remaining seated is expected
      c. Often runs about or climbs excessively in situations in which it is inappropriate (in adolescents or adults, may be limited to subjective feelings of restlessness)
      d. Often has difficulty playing or engaging quietly in leisure activities
      e. Often is "on the go" or often acts as if "driven by a motor"
      f. Often talks excessively

      IMPULSIVITY
      g. Often blurts out answers before questions have been completed
      h. Often has difficulty awaiting turn
      i. Often interrupts or intrudes on others (eg, butts into conversations or games)

B. Some hyperactive-impulsive or inattentive symptoms that caused impairment were present before age 7.
C. Some impairment from the symptoms is present in two or more settings (eg, at school [or work] and at home).
D. There must be clear evidence of clinically significant impairment in social, academic, or occupational functioning.
E. The symptoms do not occur exclusively during the course of a pervasive developmental disorder, schizophrenia, or other psychotic disorder and are not better accounted for by another mental disorder (eg, mood disorder, anxiety disorder, dissociative disorder, or a personality disorder).

American Psychiatric Association (1994). *Diagnostic and statistical manual of mental disorders* (4th ed.). Washington, DC: Author.

tors, gross brain damage, minimal brain dysfunction, environmental precipitants (e.g., lead poisoning), and dietary factors (e.g., food additives or coloring) (Cantwell, 1975; Ross & Ross, 1982; Barkley, 1981).

MINIMAL BRAIN DYSFUNCTION

This theory states that hyperactivity results from minimal brain damage that is too subtle to be expressed in more obvious neurologic symptoms. Minimal brain dysfunction syndrome includes behaviors associated with functional deviations of the central nervous system (CNS) (Holmberg, 1975).

HEREDITY

Genetic determinants may play a role in hyperkinesis. ADHD is more common in first-degree relatives than in the general population. Twenty to thirty percent of children with ADHD have a parent or family member with a similar history of short attention span, impulsivity, and hyperactivity.

BIOCHEMICAL FACTORS

A commonly accepted hypothesis is that disturbances in the brain neurotransmitter function, probably genetic in origin, produce the symptoms of ADHD (Myers et al., 1989). Children with ADHD may be deficient in the following neurotransmitters:

- Low epinephrine (CNS neurotransmitter) level —Stimulant drugs raise the norepinephrine level, thereby increasing CNS control over activity levels.
- Reticular activating system (RAS) dysfunction —The RAS filters out extraneous stimuli. Stimu-

lant medication corrects the dysfunction, which helps the individual to focus on one primary stimulus at a time.

DEVELOPMENTAL LAG THEORY

There has been discussion that ADHD represents a developmental lag. As children change, symptoms become less severe and eventually disappear with age. By puberty, 20% to 30% of ADHD children lose their symptoms. Though motor activity decreases with maturity, attention deficits and impulsivity often persist. The associated conduct and school or work performance difficulties may continue.

FEINGOLD'S THEORY OF FOOD ADDITIVES

The most widely publicized and controversial theory has been postulated by a California physician, Dr. Ben Feingold, who believes that many children develop ADD as a reaction to food dyes, artificial flavorings and preservatives, and salicylates that are found naturally in some fruits and vegetables. A diet that eliminates these chemicals is called a food additive-free or Feingold diet. Many favorite foods are forbidden on the diet (e.g., most packaged cereals; commercially baked goods; manufactured foods, such as ice cream, candy, soft drinks, pudding, and catsup; and processed foods, such as cheese, bologna, and hot dogs). In addition, the diet eliminates fruits, nuts, and vegetables with sodium salicylates. The Feingold diet appeals to parents who are opposed to the use of medication, but many studies, including those supported by the Food and Drug Administration and the Nutrition Foundation, have been unable to support the Feingold claims (Hadley, 1984). Because there is still some hope that the food additive-free diet may help some children, there is no harm in families trying this special diet as long as they pay attention to good nutrition and remain particularly alert to the need for vitamin C (Wender, 1987).

Associated Conditions

LEARNING DISABILITY

Fifty percent of children diagnosed with ADHD have a specific learning disability. Approximately three fourths of ADHD children are underachieving to some degree in the major academic subjects of reading, spelling, and mathematics. There is a strong relationship between early communication disorders, ADHD, and learning disorders. Children with learning disorders are likely to have a poorer outcome unless treatment focuses a direct attack on the learning problems and on the ADHD core symptoms (Cantwell & Baker, 1987).

CONDUCT DISORDER

The history of ADHD symptoms during early childhood helps to differentiate ADHD with conduct disorder from conduct disorder alone. Conduct disorders are characterized by a repetitive, persistent pattern of conduct that either violates the rights of others or violates major age-appropriate societal norms. Follow-up studies conducted in several settings suggest that one of the more common outcomes of untreated ADHD syndrome in childhood is adolescent and adult antisocial behavior (Morrison, 1979; Thorley, 1984).

DEPRESSIVE DISORDER

Several authors have noted an increased incidence of depressive symptoms in ADHD children when they reach adolescence. Cantwell's work (1985) has shown that 30% of depressed children had a preexisting history of ADHD. One could hypothesize that ADHD children who do poorly in the classroom, have poor peer relationships, and do poorly in leisure-time activities, such as sports, may perceive themselves as socially inadequate and consequently develop a depression disorder as a reaction to the core symptoms of the ADHD syndrome.

GILLES DE LA TOURETTE'S SYNDROME

Tourette's syndrome is characterized by recurrent, involuntary, repetitive, and rapid motor or vocal movements called tics. The peak onset of Tourette's syndrome is about 7 years of age, but onset may be anywhere from age 3 to 16 (see Chapter 20). The disorder involves a broad spectrum of dysfunction and tends to run in families. Studies of adults with Tourette's syndrome reveal a childhood history of ADHD in 30% to 40% of cases (Comings & Comings, 1987). Caution should be used in prescribing stimulant medication for ADHD to people with a personal or family history of tics.

ORGANIC BRAIN DAMAGE, MENTAL RETARDATION, AND PERVASIVE DEVELOPMENTAL DISORDERS

Many children with demonstrable brain damage have ADHD, but only a small minority (probably less than 5%) of children with ADHD have demonstrable brain damage.

Application of the Nursing Process to Attention Disorders

ASSESSMENT

In the diagnostic assessment of a child with suspected ADHD, the clinical nurse specialist plays an

BOX 15–2 • CHARACTERISTICS OF CHILDREN WITH ATTENTION-DEFICIT HYPERACTIVITY DISORDER

SYMPTOMS	EXAMPLES
Attention difficulties and distractability	Fails to finish tasks; does not listen; easily distracted; unable to concentrate or stick with play activities
Impulsivity Poor judgment/planning Problems with bowel and bladder control Social impulsivity (antisocial behavior)	Acts before thinking; shifts from activity to activity; disorganized; frequently calls out in class; has difficulty waiting turn
Motor hyperactivity	Runs or climbs excessively; fidgets and has difficulty sitting still or staying seated; moves during sleep; always "on the go" as if "driven by a motor"
Specific development disorders: Articulation disorder Language disorder Reading or other learning disorder Coordination disorder	"Perceptual" difficulties may be called specific developmental disorder (i.e., dyslexia, limited "fine motor control" [tying shoelaces, cutting, coloring, handwriting]). Mild problems with balance (learning how to ride bicycle); poor eye–hand coordination (throwing/catching ball)
Behavioral symptoms	Oppositional; stubborn; bossy or bullying with peers; temper tantrums; poor response to discipline
Emotional symptoms	Low frustration tolerance; increased lability of mood; low self-esteem; insatiability

essential role in the coordination of data collection and in the collection of data. Assessment is fundamental to planning effective interventions. The primary sources of clinical information are parents, school teachers, and a thorough interview with and observations of the child (Cantwell & Baker, 1987).

The diagnosis of ADHD essentially is based on a comprehensive evaluation that answers the following questions:

- Does this child have a psychiatric disorder?
- Does the clinical picture fit the symptom pattern of ADHD (Box 15-2)?
- Does the child have any other condition in addition to ADHD, such as depression, psychotic disorder, or learning disorder, which may complicate the clinical picture?
- In this case, what are the etiologic factors?
- What will be the likely history of the child's disorder if left untreated?
- Is intervention needed? (That is, does the disorder cause impairment in functioning in academic performance, behavior in school, peer relationships, family relationships, or use of leisure time?)
- Which types of therapeutic interactions are most likely to be effective for which aspects of the child's disorder?

Children with ADHD are generally referred for treatment because of school failure, poor peer relationships, or inability to abide by rules set by authorities. Parents usually are the most familiar with the child (e.g., his or her history and current problems); therefore, assessment often begins with an interview with the parents. It is strongly suggested that both mother and father participate in the interview because their perceptions of the child's behavior may be very different.

PARENT INTERVIEW. The following should be included in the parents' interview.

1. *Who referred the child for evaluation?* Frequently, it is the babysitter or teacher who is first aware that there might be a problem with the child. Early complaints about the child may be his or her inattention, poor peer relations (conflict with other children), nonresponsiveness to usual methods of discipline, and generalized impulsivity.
2. *Chief complaint.* Ask the parents to be as specific as possible. In preschoolers, the chief complaint generally is behavioral, whereas the school-age child will usually present with poor school performance and may or may not have behavioral problems.

3. *Description of present illness.* Obtain a thorough symptom inventory of recent behavior. (Mandatory data include recent examples of each symptom, frequency of symptom occurrence, severity of each symptom, and the context of its occurrence. What makes it better? What makes it worse? What have parents tried to deal with the particular symptom?)
4. *Premorbid history.* How do the parents describe their child's temperament and personality characteristics? Be alert to descriptions that vary from one parent to the other or between parents and teachers. The child may be reacting to environmental differences rather than having an internal problem with ADHD.
5. *Physical examination.* When did the child have his or her last physical examination? What were the results? What is the child's medical history? Children with impulse disorders often are described as accident-prone. Was a neurologic examination done, and if so, what were the results?
6. *Thorough developmental history.* The symptoms of hyperactivity, impulsivity, and inattention usually can be tracked back to infancy with children who have ADHD. Acute onset of these symptoms may be reactive to current stressors or may reflect other coping problems.
7. *Family history.* ADHD is seen more frequently in children who have a parent with this problem. Ask about maternal use of alcohol during pregnancy. Some recent research links ADHD with children who suffer from fetal alcohol syndrome.
8. *Detailed academic history.* When did the school problems begin? Are the problems pervasive (i.e., affecting all subjects)? How is the child dealt with in the classroom? What are the academic expectations of the parents and the teachers?

INTERVIEW AND OBSERVATION OF THE CHILD. The interview with the child will cover the same areas as were covered with the parents but from the child's perspective. Symptoms should be assessed by direct observation. In general, children older than 6 years can give accurate accounts of behavior that is observable to the parents. Children are better sources of certain types of information, such as internal experiences of mood, suicidal ideation, and delusional material. The child's developmental stage, intellectual level, language, and conceptual ability must be assessed to determine how reliable to consider his or her report of symptoms. Certain activities can help assess attention, impulsivity, and motor activity in the interview setting.

EVALUATION ACTIVITIES. The *sentence completion test* elicits responses to root sentences, such as the following:

The best thing that ever happened to me . . .
The worst thing that ever happened to me . . .
If I could have three wishes, I would wish for . . .
I am afraid of . . .
I get mad when . . .
School is . . .
I worry about . . .

The responses assist the interviewer to evaluate mental status and the emotional reactions to the current situation. The evaluator can monitor the child's ability to follow instructions, level of independence, ability to maintain attention, ability to read and write, and general level of understanding.

DRAWINGS. Ask the child to draw a *house,* a *tree,* and a *person* and to color the picture. Observe for colors used, size of the drawing, and obvious distortions. Ask the child to tell about the picture. Who lives in the house? What kind of tree? Is the tree healthy? Who takes care of the tree? Who is the person?

Ask the child to draw a *self-portrait.* Observe for obvious signs of distortion and the presence or absence of secondary sex characteristics.

Ask child to draw a *family portrait.* Note positioning of family members, who is included, and the size of members. The child's family portrait will provide information about alliances, generational boundaries (absence or presence), and how the child perceives his or her position in the family unit.

INFORMATION FROM TEACHERS. Teacher reports are an essential part of the clinical assessment. Standardized assessment measures for parents and teachers are useful in diagnosing ADHD and in monitoring treatment response. They provide a dimensional scoring system for a variety of common child and adolescent problem behaviors. Most frequently used assessment measures are those developed by Conners and Achenbach. Achenbach (1986) defines diagnosis as the identification of a specific diagnosis by a clinician. The symptoms of ADHD can be documented through use of a behavior rating scale; the signs of the disorder must be reported by adults (i.e., parents and teachers) in the child's environment.

In summary, the diagnosis of ADHD must be made on the basis of a comprehensive evaluation that includes data from parents, teachers, and the child. Failure to gather comprehensive information can result in ineffective treatment for the child and the family.

Nursing Diagnosis

After gathering data from the parents, child, and teachers, the nurse analyzes the information to formulate nursing diagnoses that will guide the therapeutic interventions. Some possible nursing diagnoses follow:

- Alteration in coping: Ineffective Individual Coping related to poor self-concept, poor social skills, and poor impulse control as evidenced by consistent rejection by peers at school, frequent fights on the playground, and reports that he or she has no friends
- Alteration in self-concept: Self-Esteem Disturbance related to repeated negative experiences, inadequate support system, and conflicted family relationships as evidenced by frustration level of parents with their inability to manage child's behavior, teachers' complaints about school performance, failing marks on papers, and inability to compete with peers of same age
- Compromised Family Coping related to lack of knowledge of parenting skills, chronic stress in the home, and lack of stable family unit as evidenced by parents' inability to set reasonable limits, inability to provide adequate structure for completion of assigned homework, and lack of knowledge about the child's limitations
- Altered Family Processes related to fears, guilt, lack of motivation, or suppressed anger as evidenced by parents' lack of concern about the child's behavior, denial of consequences of school failure, and projected blame for failure on outside authority
- Alteration in socialization processes: Impaired Social Interaction related to self-concept disturbance, poor attention and concentration, distractibility, and increased motor activity as evidenced by observed discomfort in social situations, observed inability to communicate a sense of belonging or shared interest, and dysfunctional interaction with peers and family

Planning

Any treatment plan must be instituted within the context of family-centered care. Successful treatment efforts recognize the inseparability of the child and family. During the planning process, information gained in the assessment process is shared with the parents. Together parents and mental

TABLE 15–1 Problem List for a Child with Attention-deficit Hyperactivity Disorder (ADHD)

Problem	Intervention	Desired Outcome
Hyperactivity Inattention Impulsivity	Medication	1. Child will complete assigned tasks in the classroom. 2. Child will sit in chair and not "blurt" out in class. 3. Child will follow directions.
Emotional disturbance	Psychotherapy Family therapy	1. Child will have understanding of ADHD and not see self as "dumb" or "bad" (improved self-esteem). 2. Parents will create a structure that supports successful experiences for child. 3. Parents will reinforce appropriate behavior. 4. Child will make friends.
Academic or school failure	Educational assessment or tutoring	1. Child will master basic skills. 2. Child will complete homework.
Poor social skills	Behavior modification program	1. Child's behavioral gains will be recognized and reinforced by parents and teachers. 2. Child will participate in small group activities with peers.

health nurse design a plan of care that best meets the needs of the child and family. The nurse uses this time to develop a therapeutic relationship with the parents, helping them to parent more effectively through an understanding of the child's illness and by exploring family dynamics. In treating ADHD, the most effective approach is a multimodal program, including the elements of parent involvement, environmental changes, academic or linguistic skill remediation, medication, behavior modification, social skills training, and psychotherapy. The clinical nurse specialist can play a major role in the management of the child with ADHD by planning and coordinating this multifaceted approach. Table 15-1 illustrates a typical problem list with interventions and desired outcomes.

Interventions

The treatment team selects interventions according to the needs and problems of the child and family. Treatment for the child with ADHD may include the following.

MEDICATIONS

The intervention most commonly prescribed by child psychiatrists for ADHD is the use of psychotropic medication, particularly stimulant drugs. These include methylphenidate (Ritalin), dextroamphetamine (Dexedrine), and pemoline (Cylert). These types of stimulants provide a positive response in 75% to 80% of ADHD children. For children who do not respond to the stimulants or with whom the side effects preclude usage, tricyclic antidepressants, particularly imipramine, are the next choice of medication.

The side effects of stimulants most frequently reported are insomnia, anorexia, weight loss, irritability, mood lability, abdominal pain, and headaches. Studies of suppression of weight and height are discrepant. Most conclude that there is no permanent effect on weight and height. Providing drug holidays, or periods of time when the child does not take the medication, diminishes the likelihood of growth delay.

There are reports of Tourette's disorder being precipitated by stimulants. When a family history of tics exists, stimulant medication should be used with caution.

Children may respond to one stimulant and not another. Dosage and schedule must be titrated for each client, considering maturation, changing life circumstances, and degree of severity of symptoms. Table 15-2 lists reasonable doses of dextroamphetamine, methylphenidate, and pemoline. With maturation or a decrease of environmental stress, it is sometimes possible to stop the medication permanently.

TABLE 15–2 Standard Dosages of Stimulant Medication for Children with Attention-deficit Hyperactivity Disorder (ADHD)

Drug	Starting Dose	Maximum Dose
Dextroamphetamine	5 mg once or twice daily (ages 6 years or older) 2.5 mg once daily (ages 3 to 5 years)	40 mg
Methylphenidate (Ritalin)	5 mg twice daily	60 mg
Pemoline	37.5 mg once daily	112.5 mg

Tricyclic antidepressants have been useful in treating ADHD. These are specifically indicated if the child presents with symptoms of depression. Tolerance to the tricyclic antidepressants and side effects limit their usefulness. Of particular concern is the potential cardiotoxic effects of the tricyclic antidepressants and the risk of death if there is an overdose. Baseline laboratory studies (complete blood count, electrocardiogram) are recommended prior to beginning medication.

The nurse assists in evaluating drug effects by documenting baseline function and monitoring the behaviors under medication. Questionnaires about side effects and behavior to parents and teachers are useful in quantifying and documenting medication effects.

Medication may increase the ability to concentrate and to some degree, decrease impulsive behavior and activity levels in settings where low levels of activity are required, such as the classroom. The medication should not interfere with high levels of activity when such activity is appropriate, such as on the playground.

Long-term effectiveness of medication alone to treat ADHD has not been demonstrated. Satterfield, Satterfield, and Schell (1987) demonstrated that patients receiving multimodal treatment (medication, individual or group counseling, family therapy, and individualized education program) did better than patients on medication alone.

FAMILY INVOLVEMENT

The clinical nurse specialist acts as an interface between the treatment team and family. This role includes documenting the treatment history, providing information about the disorder to the family, and suggesting reference material. Family education should include a description of the syndrome, the likely etiologic causes, the core and associated symptoms of the disorder, and the likely natural history for this particular child or adolescent without therapy.

Two recommended books are *The Hyperactive and Learning Disabled Child,* written for parents by Paul Wender, a child psychiatrist, and Esther Wender, a behavioral pediatrician (1978), and *Raising a Hyperactive Child,* by Stewart and Olds (1973).

In addition to information, parents of children with ADHD need support. Often they are frustrated that they have worked so hard, and their child is still having problems. They are tired of repeating themselves and are tired of feeling responsible every time the school calls to report on their child's misbehavior. Before they can learn to manage their child, they may need time to ventilate without being judged. Support groups have been started across the nation to provide a network of support for parents trying to manage children with ADHD.

ENVIRONMENTAL MANIPULATION

Research supports the contention that parents play a major role in the performance of "hyperactive children." Preventive measures should be emphasized so that the child can experience success. Simple guidelines for parents follow:

1. Set firm, responsible limits. Talking does not work with children with ADHD. Avoid lectures; simply state rules, and back them up. Use as few words as possible, and keep instructions simple, preferably focusing on one thing at a time. The goal is for the child to develop self-control and with it, self-respect.
2. Establish and maintain a predictable environment. Maintain regular routines of eating, sleeping, and playing. A united front of both parents, avoiding harsh criticism and disagreement with another in the child's view, helps maintain an emotional consistency within the household. Routines reduce stress for the parents and the child.
3. Maintain a calm and simple environment. Children with ADHD are unable to focus their attention when there are extraneous stimuli around them because they are unable to filter outside stimuli and therefore tend to react to all stimuli. A calm and simple environment promotes attention and subsequent learning. Examples include the following:
    - Establishing eye contact before giving instructions and asking child to repeat back what was understood
    - Allowing no television or radio while doing homework
    - Giving one assignment at a time (and a reward break after each completion)
    - Deciding on a place to do homework that is not in a traffic pattern nor heavily decorated
4. Create a positive environment. This is necessary to nurture the child's needs and abilities. Although limit setting and consistent discipline are needed to provide a predictable lifestyle, plans should include incremental gains in independence and freedom. The pride of accomplishment and the supportive approval of parents, siblings, and peers add to the child's self-esteem and desire to succeed. Box 15-3 outlines some principles for improving the play of children with ADHD.

EDUCATION INTERVENTION

Because children with ADHD frequently have associated developmental disorders, including communication disorders, learning disabilities, perceptual motor disorders, auditory processing disorders, and coordination disorders, an important aspect of intervention is skill remediation. The major goal is to build on the learning strengths while teaching ways to compensate for the areas of learning weakness.

Identifying specific learning disabilities and targeting the area of weakness preceeds the implementation of specific interventions. A multisensory teaching–learning approach supports skill building because it engages the whole child in the learning process.

PSYCHOTHERAPY

Psychotherapy is initiated primarily to treat secondary emotional problems relating to coping with the consequences of ADHD. In psychoanalytic theory, hyperactivity might be viewed as a child's defense to cope with anxiety. The hyperactive behavior becomes maladaptive during latency (age 6 to 10 years) because it interferes with learning, school performance, and socialization. School-age peers look down on overactive behavior. Repeatedly bombarded with negative responses and sneers, the child progressively loses self-esteem and to cope with mounting anxiety, may further isolate himself or herself. Therapy involves engaging the

BOX 15–3 • PRINCIPLES FOR IMPROVING THE PLAY OF CHILDREN WITH ATTENTION-DEFICIT HYPERACTIVITY DISORDER (ADHD)

Start with short periods of play time. The longer the activity, the greater the likelihood for loss of self-control. Select games or activities that can be completed in a short period of time, or end an activity just before the child starts to lose control.

Start with concrete games. The simpler the game, the easier it will be for the ADHD child to concentrate on the task at hand. Gradually increase the complexity of a game, or move on to a new game that requires slightly more patience and skill. Adult creativity is needed here in the area of game selections. Such standard childhood games as Pick-up Sticks, Jacks, Play Dough, Checkers, Connect Four, and Uno are all potentially "therapeutic" if they are used to gradually increase the attention span of the child.

Help a child learn to play appropriately in a variety of settings. The behavior of the ADHD child does not translate well from the office or living room to other settings. This is a major factor contributing to treatment failures for ADHD children. What the ADHD child is capable of accomplishing in a quiet setting may not carry over to settings with other distractions. If you believe that it is important for a child to learn to play in a specific setting (e.g., on a playground at recess), then you must spend time playing with or at least observing the child in that setting. Skills will eventually transfer to different settings but more slowly and under more controlled circumstances than with most children.

Move from one to many playmates. Almost any "caring" adult can help an ADHD child learn better play skills. It could be a psychotherapist, but with a little initial training it also could be a teacher, a parent, or a grandparent. If you have patience and provide a structured and systematic approach, you will have 90% of what is needed. Once an ADHD child has developed at least the rudimentary skills needed to play with another person, you should gradually introduce more people into the play activities. Begin with other family members who are already sympathetic and patient with the child. Then add the child's quieter and less demanding friends or acquaintances. Eventually the child will choose his or her own friends and playmates and hopefully will be able to enjoy more of the spontaneity associated with the world of childhood play. You'll know that the child has succeeded in learning to play in larger groups when everyone finishes the play activity with smiles and laughter.

Give immediate and constant feedback. The ADHD child cannot regulate moods or actions, largely because he or she is not aware of them. Adults working with these children need to provide ongoing and supportive feedback. When a child is learning a new skill (such as playing a board game), it is important to give a great-deal of positive reinforcement. "Behavior shaping" refers to gradually changing a person's behaviors by reinforcing even the smallest movement toward the desired goal, while ignoring inappropriate behaviors. Be specific in your praise, with phrases like "Now you're playing nicely. It's great that you can sit longer to finish this game!" As the child becomes more successful at learning the skills of playing, you can add other kinds of suggestive feedback: "I can see that you're being distracted. Should we take a break? Try to concentrate again. You were about to move your marker, remember?" Never lose your temper or harshly criticize a child during these play sessions. Be aware of your own inner controls, and stop playing before your patience runs out.

Ensure success. For many people, it might seem like a contradiction in terms to think of a child "failing" at play, but this is a common occurrence for the ADHD child. After the age of 3, play is largely a social experience, and this is an area that causes most ADHD problems. In this context, it becomes more understandable to assume that ADHD children must learn to play.

When it comes to learning, it is true that "nothing succeeds like success." When helping an ADHD child learn to play more appropriately, each play experience should be a successful one. Plan out each play activity so that it "fits" the style of each child. In addition to the various factors mentioned (i.e., choosing the right play medium, limiting and structuring the time involved in play, selecting the right number of players, choosing the right physical setting) the adult also should take into account the child's motor skills and specific interests. The more you can tailor the experience to the skills and needs of each child, the more likely you are to succeed. Also, remember that with ADHD children it is better to scale down your expectations to ensure a successful experience. A time that should be fun should never end in frustration and anger.

If you are serious about changing behavior, use behavioral charting. Professionals who work with ADHD children already know the importance of using behavioral charting. If you feel that learning to play appropriately is an important goal for a particular ADHD child, then charting a child's progress is the only way to know whether your effort is working. When a behavior is difficult to change (as most maladaptive behaviors are), it is important to target specific behaviors, and monitor them closely. Points are typically given when a child succeeds in modifying behavior, and these points can later be exchanged from a menu of small rewards. Behavioral charting can be performed by parents and professionals. The principles are easy to learn, and best of all, they *work!*

From Ziffer, R. (1990). Who wants to play with Jason? *Play, 1*(1), 10–12.

TABLE 15–3 An Outline for Multimodal Treatment of Attention-deficit Hyperactivity Disorder (ADHD) at Different Developmental Levels

	Medical Treatment	Psychologic Treatment	Educational Programming
Toddlerhood Through Preschool	Stimulant medication is generally not used unless symptoms are severe and incapacitating because of child's age and because children are generally not involved in formal academic instruction.	Parent education regarding the disorder Parent training in the use of behavior modification through modeling, rehearsal, and correction feedback Technical assistance and consultation with parents regarding specific problems Developmental play activities using behavior modification to target the symptoms of the disorder; parallel play with an adult describing appropriate behavior may be especially useful in children with language disorders. A structured daily routine with clearly defined rules of conduct	Direct teaching of skills necessary to be successful in school, such as sitting, listening, and following directions Direct teaching of social skills through parallel play Scheduling Social skill training by rehearsal Peabody Language Kits or Flannel Board to teach interaction or turn taking Games such as "Simon Says"
Kindergarten Through Third Grade	Give medication in low doses because higher doses may control hyperactivity but worsen attentional problems. Target specific symptom relative to academic success, and use data to define success. Record and chart data on the specific symptoms. Use periodic drug holidays to determine whether medication is still affecting specific symptoms, best done at end of school year.	Teacher education regarding the disorder Teacher training in the use of behavior modification through modeling, rehearsal, and cooperative feedback Periods of work interspersed with periods of activity Positive reinforcement targeted at task completion and elimination of task avoidance Supportive counseling if self-concept or interpersonal problems exist Training to aid in development and maintenance of peer relationships	Precision teaching strategies with emphasis on mastery of basic skills Shortened schoolwork assignments if task completion is otherwise not possible; make sure length of assignment is within child's true capability and not just the teacher's guess. Careful monitoring and remediation of any skill deficits that might develop Sight-word approach to reading if minor language problems are present Use of headphones or visual barriers not helpful and may be damaging to the child's self-concept Do not assign chores or tasks that one does not expect to be completed; encourage completion of tasks before allowing access to rewards
Fourth Grade Through Sixth Grade	Increase emphasis on decreasing the need for medication. Continue targeting and charting specific symptoms. Increase the duration of periods with decreased dosage or drug holidays. Children with well-developed compensatory skills may be weaned off medications.	Increased emphasis on development of compensatory skills through individual behavior therapy Self-monitoring of target behaviors Verbal mediation strategies Supportive counseling if self-concept or interpersonal problems exist	Increased emphasis on the development of individual work and study skills Use of teacher-provided outline and study guides

(continued)

TABLE 15–3 An Outline for Multimodal Treatment of Attention-deficit Hyperactivity Disorder (ADHD) at Different Developmental Levels *(Continued)*

	Medical Treatment	Psychologic Treatment	Educational Programming
Adolescence Through Adulthood	Contrary to common belief, risk for potential stimulant abuse is minimal. Individuals with severe symptoms may need continued treatment, but attempts at dose reduction should continue. Individuals with moderate to mild symptoms may benefit from occasional stimulant use for specific purposes (e.g., studying for and taking tests).	Emphasis on the development of self-reliance, good work habits, and interpersonal skills Use of daily work schedules with specific tasks to be completed at certain times Use of nonpunitive, corrective feedback and supportive counseling to improve interpersonal skills	Teaching in how to extract the important points from lecture and reading Having written material proofread by parent, peer, or teacher prior to handing it in for grading Use of memory techniques to help study for tests Use of study guides or study, question, read, recite, and review

Adapted from Fisher, W., Burd, L., Kuna, D. P., & Berg, D. (1985). Attention deficit disorders and the hyperactivities in multiply disabled children. *Rehabilitation Literature, 46*(9/10), 250–254.

child in a relationship that is nurturing, supportive, and safe. Within the context of the relationship, the child learns to understand and take responsibility for his or her own behavior, practice relationship skills (e.g., assertive vs. aggressive communication, sharing, taking turns, listening), and learn to express feelings in an appropriate manner.

BEHAVIOR MODIFICATION

ADHD children are frequently labeled "behavior problem" because of their increased activity level, short attention span, and impulsivity. Behavior therapy is a precise approach to bringing about behavioral change. The key in developing a behavior management plan is to reinforce appropriate behavior and be certain to provide a warning, and if necessary a consequence, for misbehavior. ADHD children need consistency and structure.

Parents and teachers must follow specific guidelines to promote change in behavior. Social learning theory and general knowledge support the notion that children respond better to praise than punishment. Often, because ADHD children display negative behavior repeatedly, this negative behavior gets the parents' attention and is the behavior that is reinforced. Positive behavior is taken for granted. Failure to recognize, praise, or reward the child often enough for doing the right thing is a common mistake that can lead to a weakening of appropriate behavior. Positive behavior followed by a reinforcer (e.g., verbal praise, a smile, a hug, or a reward of some sort) increases the chances of that behavior being repeated, but also it helps the child build self-confidence and self-esteem.

Before beginning a behavioral plan, the parents must be willing to invest the time and energy into carrying it out. Novice parents and therapists often develop complicated plans that must be abandoned because they are not workable. Some behavior plans do not work because parents are so angry and frustrated that they cannot praise the child. In effect, they ask, "why should I praise him now when he'll just act like a brat later?" Helping the parents deal with their own feelings, teaching them about ADHD, and providing them with support from other parents struggling with similar problems will set the stage for planning and implementing a successful behavioral management system.

Behavior therapy techniques help the child develop compensatory skills to cope with ADHD symptoms. Table 15-3 outlines comparative medical, psychologic, and educational intervention for progressive developmental ages.

Evaluation

Successful treatment of ADHD children requires a multimodal approach. Medication alone is not adequate for long-term benefit; medication in conjunction with academic and behavioral management offers the best long-term results (Hechtman, 1985).

Treatment programs must take into account the developmental level of the child. Table 15-3 shows how the focus changes as the child develops.

During preschool years, the focus is on parent and teacher education. During the first few years of school, the focus of treatment is on maximizing the generalized effects of stimulant medication and working with the teacher on using behavior mod-

CLINICAL EXAMPLE: SUSIE

Susie was a 10-year-old girl whose fourth grade teacher contacted her mother about her classroom behavior at the end of the first month of school. According to the teacher, Susie would not stay in her seat, often spoke out of turn, and was easily distracted. She would not complete assignments or would complete them and not turn them in. There was a wide variance in grades—some days making 100s and other days making 0s. Susie would draw other children into misbehaving by acting as class clown.

The teacher liked Susie ("She is a sweet child," she said) but found herself getting frustrated because nothing she did seemed to contain the behavior effectively. The teacher was concerned about the negative cycle that was being set up when her disciplinary measures were ineffective with Susie.

Susie's mother understood the teacher's concerns because Susie was difficult to manage at home as well. At home she required close monitoring to complete tasks. She did not follow verbal instructions without frequent repetition. She moved from one activity to another, never finishing or putting anything away. "She just wasn't organized." Her inattention and impulsivity had been a problem since she was a toddler. Her mother had responded by implementing a structure of continuous supervision to ensure her safety.

FAMILY HISTORY

Susie's mother was a good student throughout school with no evidence of learning problems. Her father described himself as "school phobic from first grade on." He said that he had trouble understanding directions but that he was not a behavioral problem because he was too afraid to get into trouble. Her father managed to finish college (which took 6 years) because he felt it was a family expectation.

MEDICAL HISTORY

Susie was the product of a full-term pregnancy. Her mother smoked cigarettes until the eighth month of pregnancy. No problems were noted during pregnancy and the labor and delivery were uneventful. Birth weight was 6 lb, 7 oz. Susie was a healthy, happy, active baby. She walked at 12 months. She wanted to be "busy" (entertained) all the time. Susie was into everything (e.g., she locked herself in the bathroom at 1 year and had to have the fire department come to get her out). Susie wanted "her own way" and would fight over what clothes to wear by the time she was 3 years old. She had little to no frustration tolerance. Both parents became aware that they were always yelling at her. Because the parents were educated, they tried to implement more positive behavioral plans. These were marginally effective. Of note was that Susie wet the bed at night until she was 8 years old.

SOCIAL HISTORY

Susie made friends easily, though she tended to be bossy and want everything to be "her way." She had had behavioral problems in school since kindergarten. She had been paddled frequently in school for running in the halls, getting out of line, chewing gum, cutting another child's bangs, and so forth.

ASSESSMENT

Susie's family took her to a behavioral pediatrician. Her history was presented and found to be consistent with the symptoms of attention-deficit hyperactivity disorder (ADHD), particularly the consistent report of inattention, impulsivity, and moderate hyperactivity. She was placed on Ritalin, 5 mg daily at 7:00 AM and noon.

NURSING DIAGNOSIS

The following nursing diagnoses were formulated for Susie and her family:

Anxiety related to threat to self-concept as evidenced by verbal expression of fear about ability to do academic assignments, self-derogatory statements (e.g., "I'm so stupid"), and emotional outbursts when frustrated

Self-Esteem Disturbance related to poor school performance, conflicted peer relationships, and conflicted family relationships

(Parent) Powerlessness related to perceived failure of parenting interventions to manage their child's behavior

PLAN

1. Provide information to the parents about Ritalin.
2. Teach Susie that the medicine will *help* her to control her behavior. She will still be able to run and play on the playground, but the medication may help her sit still in the classroom so that she can better understand what the teacher wants from her.
3. Work with parents to help them understand ADHD, learn more effective behavioral strategies, and refer them to a Parents of ADHD Children support group to help them cope with their own feelings (frustrations).

(*continued*)

CLINICAL EXAMPLE: SUSIE *(Continued)*

4. Work with the school teachers to develop a plan that will build on successful experiences and provide positive reinforcement.
5. Offer play therapy to provide an opportunity for Susie to work through her feelings and develop more adaptive coping skills that allow her to accept her limitations and build on her strengths.

OUTCOME CRITERIA

Susie will complete assignments, measured by daily reports from teacher to parent.

Susie's changes in behavior will be recognized and reinforced by the parents and teachers.

Family confusion and conflict will be decreased measured by parent report.

ification and teaching strategies that minimize the social and academic sequelae of ADHD. During the later primary school years, the emphasis moves toward having the child take increased responsibility for compensating for the symptoms of ADHD. The child is taught self-directed behavior techniques and given more responsibility for self-control and self-direction.

The process of increasing the child's self-control and self-direction continues into adolescence and adulthood with the tasks and settings changing from the home and school to more occupation-related skills (Fisher, Burd, Kuna, & Berg, 1985).

Summary

The former notion that ADHD was a benign condition limited to childhood no longer holds scientific merit. The likelihood is that left untreated, ADHD children will do rather poorly, and the syndrome may predispose them to a wide variety of psychopathologic outcomes in adolescence and adult life. For example, these children may be at significant risk for school failure, social and interpersonal dysfunction with peers and teachers, disruption of family functioning, and problems with self-concept (Weiss, 1985).

A total management plan should include a multimodal approach. Mediction, if warranted and effective; parental counseling; therapeutic communication; intervention with school personnel; and above all, support for the child make up a comprehensive treatment approach for the child with ADHD. (See the Clinical Example of Susie.)

REFERENCES

Achenbach, T. M. (1986). How is a parent rating scale used in the diagnosis of attention deficit disorder? *Journal of Children in Contemporary Society, 19*(½), 19–31.

American Psychiatric Association (1994). *Diagnostic and statistical manual of mental disorders* (4th ed.). Washington, D.C.: Author.

Barkley, R. A. (1981). *Hyperactive children.* New York: Guilford Press.

Bloomingdale, M. (1984). *Attention deficit disorder: Diagnostic, cognitive and therapeutic understanding.* New York: Medical and Scientific Books, Spectrum Publications.

Cantwell, D. P. (1975). *The hyperactive child: Diagnosis, management and current research.* New York: Spectrum Publications.

Cantwell, D. P. (1986). How are DSM-III and DSM-III-R used to make the diagnosis of attention deficit disorder? *Journal of Children in Contemporary Society, 19*(½), 5–17.

Cantwell, D. P., & Baker, L. (1987). Attention-deficit disorder in children: The Role of the Nurse practitioner. *Nurse Practitioner, 12*(7), 38–54.

Carlson, G. A., & Cantwell, D. P. (1979). A survey of depressive symptoms in a child and adolescent psychiatric population: Interview. *Journal of American Academy of Child Psychiatry, 8*, 587–599.

Comings, D. E., & Comings, B. G. (1987). A controlled study of Tourette Syndrome. *American Journal of Human Genetics, 41*, 701–741.

Connors, C. (1986). How is a teacher rating scale used in the diagnosis of attention deficit disorder? *Journal of Children in Contemporary Society, 19*(½), 32–52.

Donnelly, M., & Rapoport, J. L. (1985). Attention-Deficit Disorders. In J. M. Weiner (Ed.), *Diagnosis and psychopharmacology of childhood and adolescent disorders* (pp. 179–197). New York: Wiley and Sons.

Feingold, B. F. (1975). *Why your child is hyperactive.* New York: Random House.

Fisher, W., Burd, L., Kuna, D. P., & Berg, D. (1985). Attention deficit disorders and the hyperactivities in multiply disabled children. *Rehabilitation Literature, 46*(9/10), 250–254.

Hadley, J. (1984). Hyperactivity. *Children Today*, July–August, *13*(4), 8–13.

Hechtman, L. (1985). Adolescent outcome of hyperactive children treated with stimulants in childhood: A review. *Psychopharmacology Bulletin, 21*, 178–191.

Holmberg, N. J. (1975). Serving the child with MBD and his family in health maintenance organizations. *Nursing Clinics of North America, 10*(2), 381–392.

Morrison, J. (1979). Adult psychiatric disorders in parents of hyperactive children. *American Journal of Psychiatry, 136*, 13–17.

Munoz-Millan, R. J., & Casteel, C. R. (1989). Attention-deficit hyperactivity disorder: Recent Literature. *Hospital and Community Psychiatry, 40*(7), 699–707.

Myers, D. A., Claman, L., Oldham, D. G., et al. (1989). The hyperactive child: An update. *Texas Medicine, 85*(3), 25–31.

Porter, L. S. (1988). The what, why, and how of hyperkinesis: Implications for nursing. *Journal of Advanced Nursing, 13*, 229–236.

Ross, D. M., & Ross, S. A. (1982). *Hyperactivity* (2nd ed.). New York: John Wiley and Sons.

Satterfield, J. H., Satterfield, B. T., & Schell, A. M. (1987). Therapeutic interventions to prevent delinquency in hyperactive boys. *Journal of the American Academy of Child and Adolescent Psychiatry, 26*, 56–64.

Stewart, M. A., & Olds, S. W. (1973). *Raising a hyperactive child.* New York: Harper and Row.

Thorley, G. (1984). Review of follow-up and follow-back studies of childhood hyperactivity. *Psychiatric Bulletin, 96*(1), 116–132.

Weiss, G. (1985). Follow-up studies on outcome of hyperactive children. *Psychopharmacology Bulletin, 21*, 169–177.

Wender, P., & Wender, E. (1978). *The hyperactive and learning disabled child.* New York: Crown Press.

Wender, P. (1987). *The hyperactive child, adolescent, and adult: Attention deficit disorder through the lifespan.* New York: Oxford University Press.

CHAPTER

16

Conduct Disorders

John Conley

Chapter Preview

They lie even when there is nothing to be gained by lying. They steal even when the stolen items are not needed. They taunt and bully their peers even when they desperately need friends. Conduct disorders defy values and violate rules. The conduct disordered youth is a uniquely disturbed individual for whom there are many focal problems and too few reliable treatments.

Antisocial behavior is not uncommon in the course of normal growth and development. Many children violate rules and test limits to varying degrees on their way to developing a sense of trust in their environment. Lying, stealing, fighting, and noncompliance are relatively common occurrences along the developmental continuum (Achenbach & Edelbrock, 1981). As children develop an internalized set of rules and values, many of these antisocial behaviors diminish over time. For most children, interpersonal relationships remain intact, prosocial skills are developed, and few residual consequences continue into adulthood. A small percentage of children younger than age 18 (approximately 11% of boys and 5% of girls) continue to demonstrate a severe enough pattern of antisocial activity to meet *Diagnostic and Statistical Manual of Mental Disorders* 4th ed. (DSM IV) criteria for conduct disorder (American Psychiatric Association [APA], 1994). Many of these children or adolescents come to the attention of the criminal justice system and are adjudicated delinquent. Others are referred to the mental health system and presented for evaluation and treatment.

Indeed, conduct disorder is the most common reason for referral for psychiatric evaluation (O'Donnell, 1985). Most psychiatric nurses working with a child or adolescent population have encountered a conduct disorder client and have faced the challenges of engaging in a therapeutic relationship with him or her. The potential for power struggles and failed attempts to gain the child's compliance can be draining and demoralizing. Often, the nurse's own negative beliefs, attitudes, and feelings toward children and adolescents in this group can become a block to a therapeutic outcome.

This chapter examines models for understanding antisocial behavior in children and adolescents and applies the nursing process to their treatment.

Definition of Conduct Disorder

Conduct disorder is an imprecise and controversial term used to describe a wide range of antisocial acts (Harnett, 1989). These diverse behaviors include aggressive acts, lying, stealing, fire setting, truancy, and cruelty. Antisocial behaviors exist on a continuum of overt to covert acts and in isolation are not pathognomonic of any particular psychiatric disorder. Overt acts, such as fighting, and covert acts, such as embezzling, are displayed by people with and without any psychiatric disorder.

Because conduct disorder is an imprecise term, attempts have been made to define clearly criteria for diagnosing the disorder. Under the DSM IV taxonomy, the child or adolescent must demonstrate a "persistent pattern of conduct in which the basic rights of others and major age-appropriate societal norms or rules are violated" (APA, 1994). The DSM IV further specifies the types of behavior that may indicate conduct disorder. To meet diagnostic criteria according to the DSM IV for conduct disorder, the child or adolescent must demonstrate at least three of the following behaviors in the past 12 months and at least one in the past 6 months:

- Bullies, threatens, or intimidates others
- Stealing, with or without confrontation, on more than one occasion
- Running away or staying out at night
- Lying
- Fire setting;
- Being truant from school
- Breaking into someone else's home, building, or car
- Deliberately destroying others' property
- Being physically cruel to animals
- Being physically cruel to people
- Forcing someone into sexual activity
- Using a weapon in a fight
- Initiating physical fights (APA, 1994)

The following subtypes of conduct disorder also are delineated in the DSM IV based on the age at onset of the disorder. The childhood-onset type is characterized by at least one criterion prior to age 10. These youth are usually male, display physical aggression and poor peer relationships, may have had oppositional defiant disorder in childhood, and may have persistent conduct disorder. Adolescent-onset type is defined by the absences of any criteria characteristic of conduct disorder prior to age 10. These adolescents are less likely to be aggressive and more likely to have normative peer relationships, although they often display conduct problems in the company of others (APA, 1994).

Implicit in these criteria is a marked and obvious impairment in interpersonal functioning. The severity of the disorder increases as the number of conduct problems increases, and there is an inverse relationship between the severity of the disorder and the subsequent prognosis for recovery (Kazdin, 1990). Children and adolescents with a conduct disorder often are unmanageable at home and disruptive in the community.

Complicating Factors

As stated previously, conduct disorder is an imprecise term with many untoward implications. Despite more rigid criteria for diagnosing a conduct disorder, none of the inclusion criteria alone are specific to the disorder. Isolated antisocial acts are increasingly common and may not have any connection to a psychiatric disorder. These antisocial acts must occur in combination with other similar acts for a sustained period and across situations to meet diagnostic criteria. As such, conduct disorder is more aptly described as a syndrome with many overlapping diagnostic features.

Indeed, conduct disorder often occurs comorbidly with other psychiatric disorders, such as depression or attention deficit disorder (Shapiro & Garfinkle, 1986; Szatmari, Boyle, & Offord, 1989). Some researchers have found that the degree of diagnostic overlap between conduct disorder and other psychiatric disorders is so great as to make them indistinguishable from one another (Shanok et al., 1983).

Another factor contributing to the imprecision of the conduct disorder label is its frequent interchangeability with the legal designation of delinquency. Children and adolescents exhibiting antisocial behavior are frequently brought to the attention of the criminal justice system. The courts may adjudicate a youth as delinquent, yet he or she may not meet diagnostic criteria for a conduct disorder. Conversely, a youth may meet or exceed criteria for a conduct disorder but never have been apprehended by the police and subsequently avoid the label of delinquency. More than a matter of semantics, this lack of clarity may have negative implications for the child or adolescent.

A third complicating factor relates to patterns of payment by third-party payers for the treatment of conduct disorders. It is arguably more common for managed care companies and other third-party payers to influence indirectly diagnostic decisions by limiting coverage for conduct disorders. Clinicians may feel some external pressure to overlook the conduct disorder diagnosis to qualify for continued treatment funding.

Etiologic Theories

Conduct disorders are multidetermined and complex in their origin. Despite being widely researched, conduct disorder remains a poorly understood disorder for which no clear etiologic factors or agents have been identified.

While no clear pathways lead to the development of a conduct disorder, risk factors associated with increased vulnerability and models for understanding aspects of antisocial behavior have been extensively studied.

RISK FACTORS

To be at risk for a particular disorder means that an individual has a greater likelihood over base rates to develop that disorder. The risk factors associated with vulnerability for conduct disorder are fairly well known. The occurrence of an isolated risk factor in a child's life probably has little or no significance in the future development of the disorder. A cluster of risk factors in a susceptible individual, however, may predispose that person to demonstrate the disorder at some point.

One of the earliest risk factors for conduct disorder is the child's temperament. The degree to which an infant or child is perceived by the primary caretaker as difficult or easy affects the establishment and maintenance of interpersonal rhythms and attachment (Thomas & Chess, 1977). Children identified as difficult often exhibit behavior disturbances, such as conduct disorder or attention deficit disorder later in childhood or adolescence (Szatmari et al., 1989). Parental psychopathology, particularly related to physically abusive, antisocial, or coercive parenting styles, also has been shown to increase the risk of developing a conduct disorder (Pollock et al., 1990). Aggressive behavior, poor impulse control, and antiauthority behavior are strongly linked to these parenting styles and are core features of a conduct disorder (Rutter, 1975). The presence of an attention deficit disorder or learning disability also is thought to be associated with the development of a conduct disorder and often exists comorbidly with one (Szatmari et al., 1989). Many children with a learning disorder or an attention deficit disorder display global deficits in impulse control, problem solving, and prosocial skill development (Shapiro & Garfinkle, 1986). It often is difficult for these children to establish a stable prosocial peer group with these deficits; many are either alienated or gravitate toward children with similar deficits. Not all children with a learning disorder are at risk for conduct disorder, and this is certainly not a unidirectional risk factor. Truancy, school disruption, and substance abuse all interfere with learning, and academic difficulties often are the outcome of antisocial behavior.

Other risk factors, such as intrauterine insults, substance abuse, or neurologic impairment, are less understood and are associated with a wide variety of psychiatric disorders.

PROTECTIVE FACTORS

The factors that inhibit the formation of a conduct disorder in vulnerable children are poorly understood. Why one child perseveres and resists an antisocial response while another in an identical situation exhibits floridly antisocial behavior is a mystery. The presence of protective factors to mediate the antisocial response is hypothesized (Kazdin, 1990). Anxiety is thought to be one such protective factor. Fear of being caught and facing punishment is generally thought to show superego strength, and the resultant anxiety interferes with the completed antisocial act. The absence of anxiety has been associated with aggressive behavior (Pfeffer, Plutchik, & Mizurchi, 1987). However, conduct disordered boys with a comorbid anxiety disorder have been found to be much less impaired than their strictly conduct disordered peers (Windle, 1989).

The presence of a supportive, cohesive family unit to help the child or adolescent cope with transitions is another protective factor (Tolan, 1988). The family's ability to rally at times of crisis and remain integrated and structured helps the at-risk child or adolescent maintain sufficient ego strength through a vulnerable period. The identification of other protective factors will be an important part of preventing conduct disorder.

Contributing Theories

Conduct disorder in vulnerable individuals is caused by many determinants. While there are no clear etiologic pathways to the development of a conduct disorder, these contributing determinants often affect the severity of disorder and response to treatment an individual may experience. For the nurse working with an adolescent with conduct disorder, an understanding of these contributing theories may be helpful in guiding assessment and planning intervention.

BIOLOGIC THEORIES

Recent studies have suggested that there are basic biologic substrates to the expression of aggressive and conduct disorder behavior. Based in the biobehavioral assumption that thought, feeling, and behavior are neurologically derived, these studies illustrate the role of brain structures and neurotransmitters in the development of normal and abnormal variants of behavior.

The roles of two balanced neurologic systems, known as the behavioral inhibition system (BIS) and the behavioral activation system (BAS), have been studied in adolescents experiencing conduct disorder (Gray, 1982; McBurnett et al., 1991; Shapiro & Garfinkle, 1986). The BIS is thought to be located in the septal–hippocampal system, the Papez loop, and the prefrontal, cingulate, and entorhinal cortical areas of the brain. In addition, the BIS is thought to produce symptoms of anxiety when given cues of impending punishment. These anxiety symptoms inhibit behavior in normal subjects. The BAS is thought to be located in the medial forebrain bundle and the lateral hypothalamus. The BAS becomes activated when given cues of impending reward or escape from punishment. Walker et al. (1991) and McBurnett et al. (1991) applied the BIS/BAS model to conduct disorder boys and found an inverse relationship between anxiety and conduct disorder symptoms. Other studies also examining the role of these two neurologic systems have yielded results suggesting an imbalance in the BIS/BAS systems. Thus, antisocial behavior is thought to be the result of a domination of reward seeking (BAS) over inhibition and anxiety (BIS) (Gray, 1982; McBurnett et al., 1991; Little & Kendall, 1979).

The role of the neurotransmitter system in the expression of aggressive behavior is not fully understood and is predominantly based on animal studies. Similar mechanisms mediating aggressive behavior in humans are thought to exist as well. The three major neurotransmitter systems in animal and human brains (GABAergic, noradrenergic, and serotonergic systems) have all been implicated in mediating aggressive behavior. The GABAergic and the serotonergic systems are both thought to inhibit aggressive behavior, while the noradrenergic system is thought to enhance aggressive behavior. The basis of many pharmacotherapeutic interventions with aggressive adolescents is postulated to be in the regulation of central nervous system neurotransmitters.

COGNITIVE THEORIES

Childhood and adolescence are clearly periods of great leaps in cognitive development. The transition from concrete cognitive operations to formal cognitive operations is a normal developmental task for most adolescents. There is tremendous variability in the transitional schedule for adolescents within and among sociocultural subgroups. For most adolescents, however, cognitive development proceeds in a fairly linear fashion, and problem-solving skills build on themselves. For many normal adolescents, cognitive development involves acquiring problem-solving skills, role-taking skills, and self-control. For the conduct disorder adolescent, these aspects of cognitive development are poorly developed or developed in ways considered antisocial (Box 16-1).

For the conduct disorder adolescent, an inadequately developed problem-solving repertoire polarizes choices into extremes and prevents the adolescent from considering options from a variety of alternatives. This all-or-nothing dichotomy often presents itself as "splitting," the fragmentation of an object or a situation into an all-good or all-bad, win-or-lose outcome.

For most children, the acquisition of role-taking skills is fully developed by age 9 or 10. This shift away from egocentric thought is a necessary condition for future interpersonal relations. The conduct disorder adolescent often demonstrates a persistent inability to take another person's perspective (Bandura, 1973). The inability to develop interpersonal empathy decreases the conduct disorder adolescent's social sensitivity and elicits peer disapproval, conflict, and further opportunities to distort interactions and interpret them as hostile. This sequence often leads to the interruption of the third cognitive skill, self-control.

Self-control is the individual's ability to govern one's own behavior through a process of evaluating alternatives (problem solving) and inhibiting a response that does not consider another's perspective. Self-control requires the application of language skills involved in "self-talk" and is largely a function of age (Bandura, 1973). The conduct disorder adolescent often demonstrates difficulty inhibiting aggressive impulses and consequently fails to develop a repertoire of responses, including this critical element of self-control.

BEHAVIORAL THEORIES

Behavioral theory suggests that an individual's behavior is shaped over time in response to environmental reinforcers. It is thought that an individual increases the rate that a particular behavior occurs when provided with positive reinforcement and decreases a behavior in response to a negative reinforcer, that is, the withholding of a desired object, activity, or status.

BOX 16–1 • COGNITIVE DISTORTIONS: ERRORS IN THINKING

DISTORTION	CLIENT ACTION/RESPONSE	NURSE'S RESPONSE
Victim stance	Generally attempts to blame others: "I couldn't help it." "He started it."	Accept no excuses; bring the focus back to the individual.
"I can't" attitude	Makes a statement of inability, which is actually a statement of refusal.	Realize that "I can't" means "I won't" and usually refers to that which the client does not feel like doing.
Lack of concept of injury to others	Does not stop to think how his actions harm others (except physically); no concept of hurting another's feelings.	Point out how he or she is injuring others.
Failure to put himself or herself in another's place	Shows little or no empathy unless it is to deceive someone; does not consider the impact of behavior on others.	Ask client to stop and take another's perspective.
Lack of effort	Unwilling to do anything that he or she finds boring or disagreeable; engages in self-pity and looks for excuses, including psychosomatic aches and pains to avoid effort.	Advise client of the consequences if no effort is exerted; remind him or her that he or she has energy for that which he or she wants to do.
Refusal to accept obligation	Does what he or she wants and ignores the obligatory; does not view something as an obligation in any case; "forgets."	Advise client of the consequences for not attending to obligations; point out that he or she remembers what he or she wants.
Attitude of ownership	Treats others' property as if it were his or hers; steals or "borrows" without permission.	Inform the client of the consequences of theft.
No concept of trust	Blames the nurse for not trusting; says that he or she cannot trust the nurse.	Insist that trust must be earned. Do not allow betrayals of trust to go unnoticed; point out when and how the client betrayed your trust.
Unrealistic expectations	Believes that because he or she thinks something will happen, it must happen (magical thinking).	Try to get the client to specify expectations. Advise that he or she is expecting too much; point out what might happen, and prepare the client for disappointment.
Irresponsible decision making	Does not find facts or suspend judgement; makes assumptions, and blames others when things go wrong.	Help client to discern the facts, examine assumptions, and understand that decisions may have to be deferred.
Pride	Refuses to back down, even on little points. Insists on own point of view, clings to initial position, even when proved wrong.	Role model appropriate admission of errors.

(*continued*)

BOX 16–1 • COGNITIVE DISTORTIONS: ERRORS IN THINKING *(Continued)*

DISTORTION	CLIENT ACTION/RESPONSE	NURSE'S RESPONSE
Failure to plan ahead	Does not consider the future unless it is to accomplish something illicit or to create a fantasy of tremendous success.	Assist the client to think ahead at every step; point out how thinking ahead could have avoided an unpleasant situation.
Flawed definition of success	Defines success as being "number one" immediately and failure as being anything less than "number one."	Help the client see things in stages; remind him or her that one learns from mistakes.
Fear of being put down	Does not receive criticism without flaring up; feels put down when unrealistic expectations are not met.	Remind the client that he or she can learn from criticism if it is merited.
Refusal to acknowledge fear	Denies feeling afraid; views fear as weakness.	Reassure client about some fears, and help examine others.
Uses anger to control people	May become abusive, aggressive, or threatening.	Realize that anger often is a defense against fear; explore what the client fears.
Power tactics	Enjoys fighting for power for its own sake (the issue may be secondary); constantly attempts to overcome authority.	Call attention to the client's attempts to exert power over others: "I don't like your trying to manipulate me." Help him or her differentiate between power legitimately acquired through achievement and manipulation to be "number one."

Adapted from conference handout, "Errors in Thinking," by Stanton E. Samenow, PhD, Alexandria, VA. Used with permission.

Reinforcement for the conduct disorder individual comes in many forms. Material gain or an improved status among peers offers positive reinforcement, while the avoidance of school is negative reinforcement to the academically disinterested. Substance abuse, chemical dependency, and addiction are the result of a basic reinforcement process that habituates the individual to persistently abuse intoxicants.

The impact of antisocial role models in the conduct disorder adolescent's life is poorly understood. On a primary level, Bandura (1973) demonstrated the effect of direct modeling of aggressive behavior as children acted out an observed beating on an inflatable doll. On a secondary level, chronic exposure to aggressive role models engaged in conflicted relationships at home is among the most robust predictors of future antisocial and aggressive behavior in children (Pollock et al., 1990; Deutsch & Erickson, 1989; Puig-Antich, Perel, & Lupatkin, 1987). The roles of surrogate families, such as gangs or cults, in the exacerbation of conduct disordered behavior continue to be studied.

Application of the Nursing Process to the Client with a Conduct Disorder

ASSESSMENT

The conduct disorder client may have a variety of clinical presentations. The client may be hostile, sarcastic, defensive, and provocative. Paradoxically, the client also may appear calm, social, and engaging. Seldom are individuals with conduct disorders self-referred. Often they are coerced into treatment or enter a hospital as a result of an accident, toxic ingestion, or suicide attempt. In any setting or under any circumstance, the assessment of a client with a conduct disorder is complex. Deficits in several areas of biopsychosocial functioning often exist and complicate the assessment process. For example, an adolescent may have an attention deficit disorder, a learning disability, and a chemical dependency in addition to criminal charges pending against him or her. Comorbid personality disorders and Axis I psychiatric disorders often exist simultaneously in an individual referred for conduct disordered behavior. The nurse may feel overwhelmed at the complexity of the presenting problem and may feel anger and hopelessness as the adolescent attempts to lie, manipulate, and misrepresent the circumstances of the referral. The conduct disorder adolescent frequently uses denial, projection, and anger as defense mechanisms when asked for self-disclosure.

The assessment of a conduct disorder adolescent is best accomplished using a structured assessment tool to decrease the likelihood of being manipulated away from inquiring about sensitive areas, such as sexuality or substance abuse. Additionally, it is helpful to adopt a nonjudgmental approach to the assessment while being cautious to avoid giving the adolescent any opportunities to lie. Asking the adolescent *when* a particular behavior occurred, rather than asking *if* that behavior occurred, is more likely to elicit an honest reply.

With any assessment of children and adolescents, it is usually helpful to obtain a history from more than one source. Parents and immediate family should always be interviewed to contribute to the assessment and help the nurse build rapport with the family. Future compliance with therapeutic interventions may depend on how well rapport was established during this critical phase of assessment.

It is not uncommon for the family of a conduct disorder adolescent to be experiencing a great deal of conflict and chaos within the family unit. Marital conflicts, substance abuse, physical or sexual abuse, antisocial adult behavior, or other "secrets" may lie just beneath the surface, and the family may mobilize to prevent disclosure. The conduct disorder adolescent's symptoms may serve to provide homeostasis for the family system, and it may be a challenge for the nurse to gather an accurate assessment.

Additionally, client histories from the school, peers, criminal justice system, and employers are helpful in formulating a balanced and comprehensive assessment. Often issues of client confidentiality risk compromise, and families may be reluctant to authorize further inquiry into these areas. The family's and client's report on these areas may suffice.

Because there is a tremendous amount of overlap between the symptoms of conduct disorder and other psychiatric disorders, it is essential that the assessment contain inquiry into the client's affective domain (predominant moods and feelings), the behavioral domain (actions, reactions, and general behavior), and the cognitive domain (thoughts, self-talk, and perceptions). This assessment can be completed during the mental status examination and may reveal evidence of an associated depression, thought disorder, or other comorbid psychiatric disorder.

A final area of assessment is a physical assessment. Many conduct disorder adolescents are at high risk for physical injury or infection as a result of fighting, pregnancy, parasites, or sexually transmitted diseases as a result of sexual acting out or chemical toxicity as a result of ingestion or suicide attempts.

The nurse's role in the assessment process is not to "play detective" and ferret out the truth of a history given. Inconsistencies, distortions, and lies are common in the assessment of an individual with conduct disorder. Assessment is a continuous process that is built with each successive interaction. Some of the reported history may remain unclear and inconsistent with other pieces of the history. The assessment is a dynamic tool, which need not be flawless to be used.

PLANNING

Treatment planning involves using assessment data to construct an organized series of interventions targeting the client's identified problems. For the nurse working with a conduct disorder adolescent, this process may be formidable.

Five primary goals in the treatment planning process are as follows:

1. The maintenance of client, family, and milieu safety
2. The development of a healthy set of internal limits
3. The development of an expanded problem-solving repertoire
4. An increase in awareness of interpersonal responsibilities
5. The application of cognitive techniques to increase positive self-talk and decrease impulsivity

A treatment plan designed in collaboration with the client and family and addressing these goals will help the client develop some internal sense of limits.

INTERVENTION

To assist the client in meeting these goals, the nurse must establish a trusting relationship with the client. However, the nature of conduct disorder makes this a very difficult task. Therapeutic progress often is slow and marked by repeated acting out by the client. Because inpatient treatment lengths of stay are rapidly becoming shorter, the most realistic interventions are those aimed at establishing safety so that the assessment may be completed.

Be consistent and firm in the expectations of the client's behavior. Consistency does not mean that all of the client's behavior is met by the same staff response every time it occurs. Consistency implies that limits will be set so that growth and learning occur. The nurse must understand what and why limits need to be set. In most cases the nurse sets limits on excessive dependence and aggression in its destructive forms. The purpose of limit setting is not to control the client, but to provide a set of consistent expectations for him or her and to provide guidance toward self-control.

Encourage the client to examine his or her behavior and the reactions of peers within the context of the therapeutic community. The peer group can act as a potent reinforcer of prosocial behavior and assist in modeling appropriate interactions.

Communicate expectations and goals to the client and staff so that all have a clear understanding of what is to be done. Let the client know the consequences for appropriate and inappropriate behavior.

Be reasonably aware of the feelings the client's behavior arouses in you, and evaluate your responses to him or her in reaction to these feelings.

Be alert to the client's attempts to manipulate you. This will be an ongoing therapeutic issue as the individual with Conduct Disorder attempts to intimidate you and raise your anxiety. Let him or her know that you are aware of the attempts to manipulate and intimidate you. Help the client examine this device and the reasons he or she is using it.

The following intervention modalities are useful in gaining compliance and training parents to manage oppositional and acting-out behavior of children and adolescents.

PARENT TRAINING. Behavioral parent training involves helping parents change some aspect of their relationship with their child by teaching parents to rearrange the antecedents and consequences for their child's behavior. The parents are taught to use contingency management programs (for younger children) or contingency contracting (for older children and adolescents). Contingency refers to an object, status, or situation desired by the child. There are three approaches to parent training:

1. Consultation between the nurse and the parent
2. Role-playing and guided interaction with the nurse serving as a coach
3. Educational parent group meetings

The goal of behavioral parent training is to help change the pattern of parent–child interactions and not simply eliminate discrete problem behaviors. Parents of conduct disorder children and adolescents often develop behavioral responses to their child's behavior that serves to reinforce the undesired behavior. These "parent traps" are as follows:

- Parents use persistent yelling and arguing. This serves to reinforce the child's argumentativeness. Additionally, this serves to role model arguing as an acceptable way of communicating.
- Parents make nagging and repetitive requests. This teaches the child that consequences rarely occur when they do not comply. Parents usually find themselves using more and more coercive techniques to gain compliance.
- Parents display anger. Anger may serve as a powerful reinforcer for the child's provocative behavior.
- Parents engage in long discussions about the child's lack of compliance with rules. This may serve to reinforce undesirable behavior with parental attention.

Sometimes it is helpful with adolescents to negotiate a contingency contract. A contingency contract is a written agreement between parents and an adolescent in which the troublesome aspects of their relationship are specified in terms of behavior and consequences. It is a formal means of stating explicitly "who does what to whom and when" so that parents and children give and receive more positive reinforcement and engage in fewer aversive interactions. Critical to contingency contracts is that they are based on reciprocity among all relevant family members. For a contingency contract to be effective, the following is needed:

- Behaviors to be changed need to be written in clearly defined, objective terms.
- The behaviors must be able to be monitored.
- Parents must have control over relevant consequences.

- Consequences must be delivered at appropriate times.

CONTINGENCY MANAGEMENT STRATEGIES IN THE SCHOOL FOR YOUNGER CHILDREN. These strategies target appropriate behavior that is incompatible with disruptive behavior. For example, the teacher praises a child for sitting still or completing an assignment.

VIOLENCE AND AGGRESSION. Violence and aggression are heterogeneous occurrences that are not unique to the conduct disorder client. However, because the conduct disorder client often demonstrates poor problem-solving and impulsive behavior, violence and aggression are not uncommon.

Aggressive behavior often is used to intimidate and manipulate others and may be tacitly supported, encouraged, and exacerbated by others on a unit. When such behavior occurs, it may be helpful for the nurse to facilitate a community meeting to explore the antecedents, consequences, and feelings raised, after the client is given an opportunity to recover from his or her aggressive behavior.

Because violence threatens a sense of safety and self-esteem, it also is necessary for nurses to lend support to one another and actively encourage a debriefing period after the violent incident to share feelings and observations.

MEDICATION. The use of medication to treat symptoms of aggression in conduct disorder is gaining widespread acceptance. Aggression is a heterogeneous phenomenon that is not limited to conduct disorder. However, most of the diagnostic criteria for conduct disorder relate to various forms of aggression. As part of a comprehensive treatment plan for conduct disorder, medication may be useful in managing episodes of aggression.

Depression is known to exist comorbidly with conduct disorder in many cases. The use of antidepressants has been shown to decrease conduct disorder symptoms in children diagnosed with a comorbid depression (Puig-Antich et al., 1987). Lithium and haloperidol have been helpful in decreasing symptoms of aggression and impulsivity in conduct disorder boys (Campbell, Small, & Green, 1984). More research is needed to help further define the parameters of pharmacologic treatment in conduct disorder.

Evaluation

Evaluation of a conduct disorder adolescent's progress toward the goals of intervention will be difficult to establish. Many conduct disorder adolescents are adept at becoming socialized to the milieu and appearing more prosocial than they really are. These adolescents may show rapid "improvement" and offer a great deal of self-disclosure and compliance. Because of shortened hospital stays related to restricted reimbursement schedules, it may be impossible for the nurse to evaluate the attainment of intermediate and long-term goals. Evaluation may best be accomplished in the context of short-term goals and treatment team consensus about the client's progress toward those goals.

Summary

This chapter discusses the complex syndrome of conduct disorder. A controversial diagnosis given to children and adolescents who exhibit a persistent pattern of antisocial behavior, conduct disorder is an imprecise term for which there are no clear etiologic pathways nor reliable treatments.

Conduct disorder is one of the most frequent reasons for psychiatric referral of children and adolescents. It has multiple determinants, but the most significant appears to be the realm of parent–child interactions that potentiate the expression of the disorder in vulnerable populations.

Conduct disorder often appears comorbidly with other psychiatric disorders common in childhood and adolescence. Attention-deficit hyperactivity disorder and depression are the two most common psychiatric disorders associated with conduct disorder.

Treatment of the conduct disorder child or adolescent is difficult and marked by slow progress and regression. Insight-oriented therapies tend to be insufficient in the treatment of conduct disorder. Intensive behavioral therapies with significant parent training components seem to hold the most promise.

The evaluation of nursing interventions is difficult and sometimes impossible when clients are not in a controlled environment. Conduct disorder is a stable disorder that lingers into adulthood in many cases.

Nurses working with conduct disorder children, adolescents, and their families often experience conflict, negative cognitions, and signs of "burnout" The frequent manipulation, intimidation, aggression, and milieu disruption take their toll on even the most experienced and educated nurse. Peer support and supervision are critical for the nurse to remain effective with this subpopulation of adolescents.

CLINICAL EXAMPLE: DAVID

Sixteen-year-old David was admitted to an adolescent inpatient psychiatric unit following the nonlethal ingestion of a substance he claimed was a floor cleaner while he was awaiting a court hearing in juvenile hall. David reported feeling depressed and hopeless after being arrested for receiving stolen property from an older acquaintance. He admitted having frequent thoughts of suicide but had never acted on those thoughts until his incarceration.

David's family history revealed that his parents divorced when he was 3 years old, after several years of a violent and abusive marriage. David, an only child, lived with his father until 2 years ago, when he moved in with his mother because his father was sentenced to jail for assault. David's relationship with his mother was conflicted, and he avoided staying at home for more than several days at a time. David often stayed out all night with friends, consuming alcohol and committing small acts of vandalism or theft.

David had been arrested twice for stealing but was never charged. Both times he was sent home with a parent. He was not currently enrolled in school and had not attended school consistently since the sixth grade.

David's peer group consisted of older adolescents and young adults who engaged in similar activities. David denied any gang memberships. David denied having any stable heterosexual relationships and was visibly angry when asked about any homosexual experiences.

The nurse who interviewed David on admission was struck by his small size and cooperative demeanor. He appeared mildly anxious, smiling frequently and clearing his throat, and reported difficulty sleeping in the youth detention center. He expressed a great deal of worry about being charged with this crime. There were no neurovegetative signs of depression nor evidence of a thought disorder. He admitted to alcohol abuse on weekends but denied any drug or other substance abuse. The nurse set the following treatment goals with David:

1. David will become aware of his feelings of isolation and loneliness and discuss strategies for establishing a prosocial, supportive social network.
2. David will engage in family therapy with his mother to facilitate healthy individuation.
3. David will take responsibility for his feelings and behavior through a guided process of rational problem solving and decision making.

The first week of hospitalization was uneventful for David. He attended all treatment modalities and was appropriately verbal in community meeting. His group therapist observed and commented on David's subtle anger and defensiveness in group therapy. David denied being angry or defensive and became quiet in group therapy. Several days later, a hospital maintenance worker discovered a razor blade, several linen sheets, and two bottles of "liquid paper" in a removable air conditioning duct beside David's bed during a routine filter replacement. When confronted, David denied knowing anything about these items and proposed that they belonged to another client. When the issue of an unsafe milieu was raised in a community meeting that evening, David remained silent while the other clients glared at him. When the nurse suggested that off-unit activities be canceled the next day in the interest of regaining unit safety, another client spoke up angrily and confronted David about their mutual plan to use those items to "get high" and escape from the unit. David remained silent and averted his gaze.

While his peers confronted David about the violation of trust and the creation of an unsafe therapeutic environment, he remained depressed and withdrawn. He admitted to the return of suicidal thoughts and asked to be placed on suicide precautions.

This pattern of compliance and therapeutic "progress" marked with regression continued on and off for several weeks. Nursing staff spoke openly about the difficulty they were experiencing in trusting David and viewing his work as sincere. Progress in family therapy was slow as well. David's mother was extremely ambivalent about parenting David, because he reminded her of her ex-husband.

After 8 weeks of hospitalization marked by David's repeated efforts to sabotage trust with the staff and the staff willing to distrust him, he was discharged back to juvenile hall with a schedule of weekly therapy appointments to keep.

Progress with David was difficult to evaluate. The nursing staff identified David's inability to establish and maintain a trusting therapeutic relationship as the most important block to therapy. His discharge at the request of the insurance company was secured by frustration and a lack of tangible progress.

QUESTIONS FOR DISCUSSION

1. What factors in David's history suggest high risk for conduct disorder?
2. What other assessment information would have been helpful in planning intervention?

(continued)

CLINICAL EXAMPLE: DAVID *(Continued)*

3. Do you agree with the nurses' goals for David? What other goals would you select?
4. What are some strategies for establishing a trusting therapeutic relationship?
5. Describe specific interventions you would use to work with David.
6. How would you evaluate the outcomes of your plan?

REFERENCES

Achenbach, T. M., & Edelbrock, C. S. (1981). Behavioral problems and competencies reported by parents of normal and disturbed children aged four through sixteen. *Monographs of the Society for Research in Child Development, 46,* 188.

American Psychiatric Association (1994). *Diagnostic and statistical manual of mental disorders* (4th ed.). Washington, DC: Author.

Bandura, A. (1973). *Aggression: A social learning analysis.* Englewood Cliffs, N.J.: Prentice-Hall.

Campbell, M., Small, A. M., & Green, W. H. (1984). A comparison of haloperidol and lithium in hospitalized aggressive conduct disordered children. *Archives of General Psychiatry, 41,* 650–656.

Deutsch, L. J., & Erickson, M. T. (1989). Early life events as discriminators of socialized and undersocialized delinquents. *Journal of Abnormal Child Psychology, 17*(5), 541–551.

Gardner, F. E. M. (1989). Inconsistent parenting: Is there evidence for a link with children's conduct problems? *Journal of Abnormal Child Psychology, 17*(2), 223–233.

Gray, J. A. (1982). The neuropsychology of anxiety: An inquiry into the functions of the septo-hippocampal system. Oxford: Oxford University Press.

Harnett, N. E. (1989). Conduct disorder in childhood and adolescence: An update. *Journal of Child and Adolescent Psychiatric Nursing, 2*(2), 74–77.

Kazdin, A. E. (1987). Treatment of antisocial behavior in children: Current status and future directions. *Psychological Bulletin, 102,* 187–203.

Kazdin, A. E. (1990). *Prevention of conduct disorder.* Paper presented at the National Conference on Prevention Research, National Institute of Mental health, Bethesda, MD.

Little, V. L., & Kendall, P. C. (1979). Cognitive-behavioral interventions with delinquents: Problem solving, role-taking and self-control. In P. C. Kendall & S. D. Hollon (Eds.), *Cognitive behavioral interventions: Theory, research, and procedures.* New York: Academic Press.

Loeber, R. (1991). Antisocial behavior: More enduring than changeable? *Journal of the American Academy of Child and Adolescent Psychiatry, 30*(3), 393–397.

McBurnett, K., Lahey, B. B., Frick, P. J., Risch, C., Loeber, R., Hart, E. L., Christ, M. G., Hanson, K. (1991). Anxiety, inhibition, and conduct disorder in children: II: Relation to salivary cortisol. *Journal of the American Academy of Child and Adolescent Psychiatry, 30*(2), 192–196.

O'Donnell, D. J. (1985). Conduct disorders. In J. M. Wiener (Ed.), *Diagnosis and psychopharmacology of childhood and adolescent disorders* (pp. 251–287). New York: John Wiley & Sons.

Pfeffer, C. R., Plutchik, R., & Mizurchi, M. S. (1983). Predictors of assaultiveness in latency age children. *American Journal of Psychiatry, 140,* 31–35.

Pfeffer, C. R., Plutchik, R., Mizurchi, M. S., & Lipkins, R. (1987). Assaultive behavior in child psychiatric inpatients, outpatients, and nonpatients. *Journal of the American Academy of Child and Adolescent Psychiatry, 26*(2), 256–261.

Pollock, V. E., Briere, J., Schneider, L., Knop, J., Mednick, S. A., & Goodwin, D. W. (1990). Childhood antecedents of antisocial behavior: Parental alcoholism and physical abusiveness. *American Journal of Psychiatry, 147*(10), 1290–1293.

Puig-Antich, J., Perel, J., & Lupatkin, W., (1987). Imipramine in prepubertal major depressive disorders *Archives of General Psychiatry, 44,* 81–89

Rutter, M. (1975). *Aggression, overactivity, and delinquency: Helping troubled children* (pp. 241–167). New York: Plenum.

Shanok, S. S., Malani, S. C., Ninan, O. P., Guggenheim, P., Weinstein, H., & Lewis, D. O. (1983). A comparison of delinquent and nondelinquent adolescent psychiatric inpatients. *American Journal of Psychiatry, 140*(5), 582–585.

Shapiro, S. K., & Garfinkle, B. D. (1986). The occurrence of behavior disorders in children: The interdependence of attention deficit disorder and Conduct Disorder. *Journal of the American Academy of Child Psychiatry, 25*(6), 809–819.

Szatmari, P., Boyle, M., & Offord, D. R. (1989). ADHD and conduct disorder: Degree of diagnostic overlap and differences among correlates. *Journal of the American Academy of Child and Adolescent Psychiatry, 28*(6), 865–872.

Thomas, A., & Chess, S. (1977). *Temperament and development.* New York: Brunner/Mazel.

Tolan, P. (1988). Socioeconomic, family, and social stress correlates of adolescent antisocial and delinquent behavior. *Journal of Abnormal Child Psychology, 16*(3), 317–331.

Walker, J. L., Lahey, B. B., Russo, M. F., Frick, P. J., Christ, J. G., McBurnett, K., Loeber, R., Stouthamer-Loeber, M., & Green, S. (1991). Anxiety, inhibition, and conduct disorder in children: I: Relation to social impairment. *Journal of the American Academy of Child and Adolescent Psychiatry, 30,* 187–191.

Windle, M. (1989). *Adolescent temperament: Childhood problem precursors and problem behavior correlates.* Paper presented at the Annual Meeting of the American Academy of Child and Adolescent Psychiatry, New York.

CHAPTER

17

Personality Disorders

Brenda Wagner

Personality is defined as the composite of the physical, mental, emotional, and social characteristics of an individual. The personality is believed to develop as the individual learns to adapt to the environment. However, genetic tendencies, temperament, and life events are all believed to affect this development. This chapter discusses theories of personality development, personality traits versus personality disorders, and literature relating to specific personality disorders believed to be manifested in children and adolescents. Following each disorder are highlights of nursing care plans typically used in treatment.

Personality Theories

Most of the theories developed to explain the origin and development of personality are psychoanalytic. The theories are Freudian, ego psychology, object relations, and biosocial.

FREUD'S CONCEPT OF PERSONALITY

Sigmund Freud believed that the driving forces motivating personality are sex and aggression. He believed that these dynamic forces are instinctual and require immediate gratification, which results in conflict with social rules that require controlling sexual and aggressive urges. To keep sexual and aggressive impulses under control, the individual develops defense mechanisms that serve to keep the individual out of danger from rules of social order. These defense mechanisms also help to keep the individual from experiencing the anxiety and guilt that would be elicited by desires to break social rules. These defense mechanisms operate on an unconscious level, outside of the knowledge of the individual, keeping the sexual and aggressive urges out of the individual's awareness.

Freud presents four stages in the individual's ability to avoid active and forbidden expression of sexual and aggressive impulses. The first is the oral stage, evidenced by satisfaction at sucking at the breast. The urge is intense and urgent. The way in which the parent(s) respond to this urge is believed to greatly influence the infant's personality. If the need is ignored or overly indulged, the infant may fixate on this stage to continue to meet the unmet need or to recreate and repeat the intensely gratifying condition. Personality traits often associated with fixation at this stage include polarized traits, such as optimism–pessimism, gullibility–suspiciousness, cockiness–self-belittlement, manipulativeness–passivity, and admiration–envy (Abraham, 1927; Glover, 1925). Individuals with these personality traits often are considered by others as immature rather than pathologic.

The second stage in Freud's theory, the anal stage, is perhaps the most intensely conflictual for the individual. Social reactions are intense and rejecting toward fecal discharge and fecal smells; displaying one's bottom is considered a serious social offense. Individuals who become fixated at this stage also can be polarized on one extreme or the other, resulting from intense denial or indulgence of these anal functions. The traits, articulated by Freud (1925) and Fenichel (1945), include stinginess–overgenerosity, stubbornness–acquiescence, orderliness–messiness, meticulousness–dirtiness, punctuality–tardiness, and precision–vagueness. If the individual is not required to "hold on" to the sexual–aggressive urges during this stage, the individual develops traits of wastefulness, explosiveness, or lackadaisical behavior. If too much emphasis is placed on the anal urges and little regard given for the individual's willingness to "give," the individual develops traits such as stinginess, constriction of feelings, and stubbornness. It is as if the individual refuses to give again.

The third phase is called the phallic stage, named with reference to Freud's belief that girls envy boys' penises. This stage seems somewhat dependent on the child's relationship to the opposite sex parent. If the parent is overly rejecting, the child is likely to develop qualities of self-rejection, extremes in social isolation or social gregariousness, or excessive humility. If the opposite sex parent is overindulgent or sexually inappropriate, the child may become vain, focus on outward appearances, and be viewed as superficial in relationships.

The final stage in Freud's personality theory is the genital stage, considered the most mature. Freud believed no one approached this stage without conflicts in earlier stages, with traits typically related to that stage. Thus, at the genital stage, the personality is represented as the culmination of traits developed out of earlier conflicts. Stressful life events may cause the individual to regress to these earlier stages or the traits representing earlier stages to be more evident when environmental demands are too great. If the traits become dysfunctional, the individual is viewed as psychopathologic.

EGO CONCEPTS OF PERSONALITY

Some theorists have moved from Freud's theory of development to what is known as ego theories of personality development (Erikson, 1950; Rapaport, 1958). These theories focus on the function of the ego, rather than the id and the impulse conflict, in the individual's adaptation to reality and mastery of the environment. This adaptation requires the development of judgment and moral reasonings and skills, such as communication and cooperation, which render the individual able to function as a member of society. Ego theorists do not limit themselves to early development in the formation of personality but also are concerned with later development, such as the development of industry, identity processes, and issues of intimacy. The ego is believed to be an innate part of the personality that has several functions when maturely developed, including the following:

- Reality testing: distinguishing between one's own experience and that which is actually occurring
- Judgment: locating alternatives and selecting options that offer the most desired consequences
- Sense of self: absence of depersonalization within the environment
- Regulation of drives, affect, and impulses: ability to modulate impulses and affect without over- or under-restricting
- Object relations: perceiving self as a complete person related to the larger environment and able to participate in mature relationships
- Thought processes: ability to think in a manner that reflects reality and can be viewed as purposeful
- Defensive functioning: ability to use defense mechanisms to function with the least amount of distortion of reality
- Stimulus barrier: ability to cope adequately among fluctuations in levels of stimulation
- Autonomous functioning: ability to maintain autonomous functioning, such as memory and learning, which are critical for successful coping
- Mastery/competence: drive to master the environment beyond the level of surviving and ability to use available resources to adapt

Ego psychology is helpful in identifying inadequacies in the specific ego components in the development toward maturity. Through assessment of the level of functioning for each ego task, the clinician is better prepared to construct specific treatment plans that help to promote healthy personality traits.

OBJECT RELATIONS THEORY OF PERSONALITY

The third major theory related to personality development is object relations theory, which was generated by ego psychologists and has developed into a theoretical framework of its own merit. According to this theory, object relations are affected by early interpersonal relationships and affect later interpersonal relationships. However, the structures of object relations are intrapsychic rather than interpersonal. Object relations theorists, such as Mahler, Pine, and Bergman (1975); Kernberg (1975, 1976); and Kohut (1977), emphasize relationships between the self and objects as the major organizing principle in people's lives. These theorists are developmentalists in their exploration of personality but focus on attachment and separation as the primary force determining perceptions and trait development. Mahler (1970), a major contributor to object relations theory, traces the significant events from birth through various separation individuation stages. The first stage is referred to as the normal autistic stage and exists for the first 4 weeks after birth. During this time, the infant is unaware that there is another separate individual responding to expressed needs. This stage is followed by the symbiotic stage, in which the infant is minimally aware of limitations in meeting self-needs and the necessity of a significant other to meet needs. These two stages are the forerunners of the psychologic birth of the infant known as the separation–individuation process. The process involves

> the establishment of a sense of separation from, and relation to, a world of reality, particularly with regard to the experiences of one's own body and to the principal representative of the world as the infant experiences it, the primary love object (Mahler et al., 1975, p. 3).

The process evolves from the fourth month through the 36th month of the infant's life but is evident throughout the life cycle.

The separation–individuation phase is marked by four subphases: differentiation, practicing, rapprochement, and object constancy. During the differentiation subphase, the individual's perceptual activity becomes outwardly focused. The child becomes aware that there are "good" and "bad" experiences and that the "bad" experiences cannot be alleviated by the child. The expectation of maternal omnipotence is maintained because she is expected to relieve the infant of all "bad" experiences. Practicing refers to the toddler's attempts to move away from the maternal object to explore the environment, a necessary precursor to self-sufficiency. Rapprochement is the phase of rediscovery of the mother as a separate individual from the toddler. The awareness of separateness is acute for many toddlers, and ambivalence may become intense. The mother's emotional availability during the rapprochement subphase allows the toddler to struggle with the fear of losing either the love object (mother) or the newly found autonomy. If too much of the child's energy is spent in mediating self-needs, the ego is unable to continue, and fixation can occur.

Kohut (1977) offers a picture of the autonomous self who is characterized by self-esteem, the ability to not be overly dependent on others, and the ability to sustain relationships. His work with narcissistic personalities reflects his belief that without having their needs mirrored and idealized early in childhood by parents who have accepted their own struggle in identity, the individual believes that only people who are perfect and admired are valuable. These individuals move from relationship to relationship in search of someone to admire or from performance to performance to have others admire them.

BIOSOCIAL CONCEPT OF PERSONALITY

The biosocial approach to personality development focuses on the heritable, or genetic traits that are influenced by environmental forces in the shaping of the personality. Personality in the biosocial approach is defined in terms of the differences between individuals in the way they receive, process, and store information about the environment. Personality disorders can develop from inconsistent or inappropriate social learning. The most recent and more fully developed biosocial model has been proposed by Cloninger (1986; 1987). He offers the brain system as the base of determining an individual's reaction to situational cues and events; in other words, individuals have a genetic predisposition to respond to the environment based on the neurobiologic chemicals most active in the brain. Cloninger's model delineates three dimensions of personality. The origins of these dimensions are genetically separate from each other and consist of a central behavior pattern with a primary neurotransmitter as the neurochemical base.

The first central behavior pattern of Cloninger's (1986) model is called novelty seeking, in which the individual seeks frequent exploratory activity and intense excitement in response to novel stimuli. The principal monoamine neuromodulator for this behavior pattern is dopamine. The second of the behavior patterns is called harm avoidance and is due to a heritable tendency to respond in-

TABLE 17-1 Three Major Brain Systems and Their Associated Learning and Personality Characteristics

Brain System (Related Personality Dimension)	Learning Characteristics		Personality Characteristics	
	Relevant Stimuli	*Behavioral or Learned Response*	*High Scorer*	*Low Scorer*
Behavioral activation (novelty seeking)	Novelty (potential reward)	Exploratory pursuit	Curious, exploratory	Content, quiet
	Monotony (potential nonreward)	Active avoidance	Fickle, easily bored	Rigid, patient
	Complexity	Collative approach	Impressionistic Impulsive	Methodic, reflective
	Cues to reward	Appetitive approach	Extravagant Enthusiastic	Frugal, reserved
	Conditioned signals of punishment or frustrative nonreward	Active avoidance	Disorderly Unconventional	Orderly, regimented
	Punishment or frustrative nonreward	Fight or flight	Quick tempered Excitable, evasive, deceptive	Slow-tempered, stoical, forthright, honest
Behavioral inhibition (harm avoidance)	Conditioned signals of punishment	Passive avoidance	Cautious Worrying	Confident Carefree
	Conditioned signals of frustrative nonreward	Extinction	Pessimistic, restrained	Optimistic, risk taking
	Novelty (potential danger)	Slow habituation Passive avoidance	Fearful, shy	Bold, outgoing
	Inescapable or unpredictable punishment	Sensitization Helpless inactivity	Fatigable, asthenic	Energetic, vigorous
Behavioral maintenance (reward dependence)	Pairing of collative (novel) stimuli with rewards or relief from punishment	Classic appetitive conditioning	Sentimental, socially sensitive	Practical, insensitive
	Frustrative nonreward or punishment of previously rewarded behavior (after opportunity to form conditioned signals of reward)	Resistance to extinction Fighting and flight	Persistent Tender-hearted Dedicated	Irresolute Cold-blooded Detached

Reprinted from Cloninger, C. R. (1988b). (p. 87.) Used with permission.

tensely to reward and succor and to learn to maintain rewarded behavior. The principal monoamine neuromodulator for this behavior pattern is serotonin. The last central behavior pattern is reward dependence, in which the individual has a genetic tendency to respond to conditioned signals for reward or relief of punishment. Table 17-1 highlights the three major brain systems and their associated learning and personality characteristics.

Cloninger's work has had a mixed review among researchers and psychologists but is becoming a more widely accepted approach to understanding personality development and the disorders frequently viewed. Combinations of these three central patterns are used as the basis for understanding many of the somatic and anxiety disorders, as well as personality types. Figure 17-1 reflects the approach used by Cloninger in exploring the more

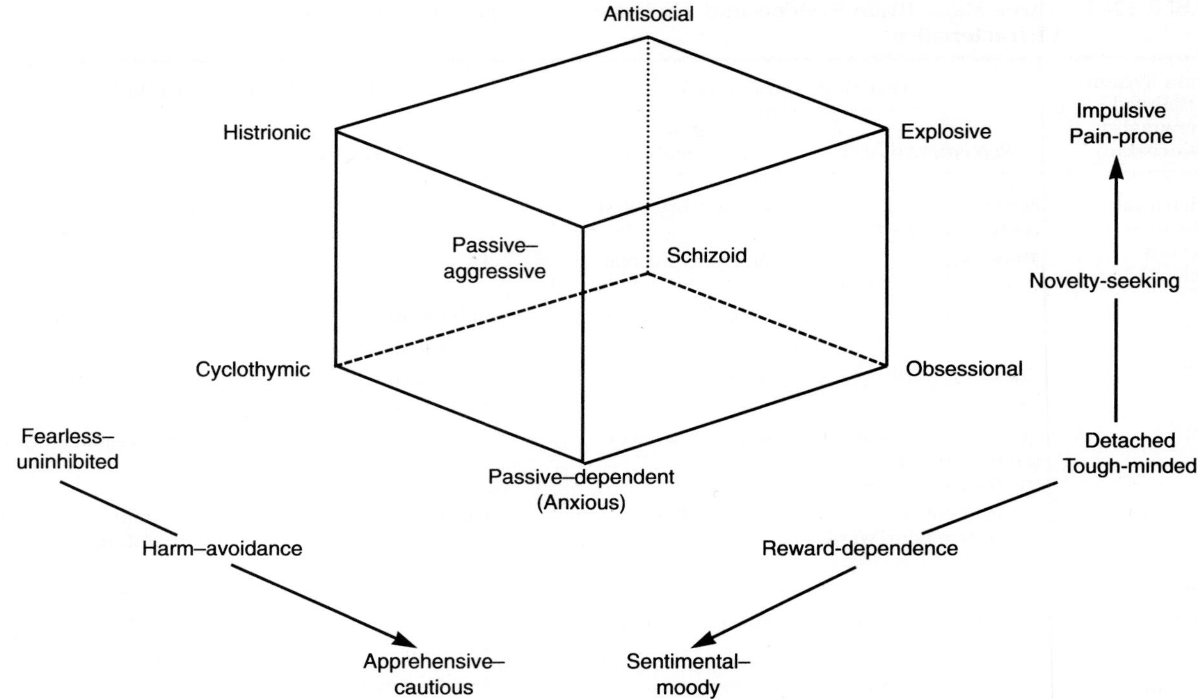

FIGURE 17–1 • Traditional personality disorders related to the three personality dimensions of novelty-seeking, harm–avoidance, and reward–dependence. (Reprinted [with permission] from Cloninger, C. R. [1988a], [p. 14].)

common personality types. His work has provoked much interest recently in the area of personality development because it offers an integrated model of genetic and environmental forces impacting development.

From the previous discussion of personality theory, it is clear that relationships in the life of young children are significant in the development of traits that either support or defeat later mature adult living. However, studies of temperament in children reveal genetic predispositions to the development of personality traits regardless of the life experiences. After examining life events in psychiatric illnesses, Paykel (1978) concludes that some combination of several factors interact for life events to precipitate psychiatric illness. Anthony and Cohler's (1987) work exploring children who are less vulnerable for emotional illness in spite of life events also supports the notion that children are not alike in their responses to life events. It appears that some personality traits, such as neuroticism, increase the likelihood of negative life events (Brown, Harris, & Petro, 1973). Clearly there is an interactive effect between life events and personality traits, but it is unclear which is more significant in the development of personality disorders (Tyrer, 1988).

Assessing Personality

How can a clinician evaluate traits and vulnerability to later personality disorders or make judgments relative to the emotional competency in children and adolescents? Very little in the literature assesses specific traits in children or determines the level of dysfunction of traits. Table 17-2 lists several instruments that might be useful in assessing traits and the level of functioning in children and adolescents. None of the instruments require formal training; however, clinicians will most likely need to confer with individuals typically involved in formal testing to validate interpretation of results.

These assessment tools are somewhat helpful in assessing progression of behaviors and in describing temperament. However, the greatest criterion for personality assessment is endurance of traits. As children are exposed to more varied situations and are required to accommodate greater numbers of relationships, personality traits and patterns unfold and become easier to view across life events. It is in accommodating to more complex and interactive situations that the individual develops persistent approaches to situations that can be examined. Deciding the degree of accommodation and the healthiness of the accommodation also is difficult to assess.

It is not clear to parents and professionals which activities or specific environmental characteristics are required for developing adaptive, healthy personality traits. There is, perhaps, some general agreement as to what characterizes psychologic maturity, but the specific psychologic skills that delineate adaptation and functions have not been clearly articulated. Strayhorn (1988), in his approach to developing competency in children, offers nine groups of skills that are helpful in assessing the child's or adolescent's degree of adaptive interaction. However, these skills do not address specific personality traits that limit accomplishing the particular skills addressed in each group. Strayhorn includes the following:

- Group 1: Experiencing closeness, trusting, relationship building
- Group 2: Handling separation and independence
- Group 3: Handling joint decisions and interpersonal conflict
- Group 4: Dealing with frustration and unfavorable events
- Group 5: Celebrating good things, feeling pleasure

TABLE 17–2 Comparison of Personality Scales for Children and Adolescents

Scale	Positive Features of Scale	Negative Features of Scale
Children's Personality Scale (1973)	Good reliability Includes positive and negative traits in assessment profile Designed to be used with companion tool (parents' report)	Seems less appropriate for older children and adolescents
Personality Inventory for Children-Revised (1984)	Covers wide age range (3–16) Offers multidimensional assessment Well validated	Lengthy Completed solely by parent Tedious to hand score
Child Assessment Schedule (1989)	High internal consistency Includes traits, behaviors, and interaction of these	
Semistructured Clinical Interview for Children Aged 6–11 (1990)	Designed to mesh with Children's Behavior Checklist Allows probing while maintaining orderly review Acceptable reliability	Limited age range Takes 1½–2 hours

Achenbach, T. M., & McConaughy, S. H. (1989). *Semistructured clinical interview for children aged 6–11 (SCID).* Burlington, VT: University of Vermont.

Hodges, K., & Saunders, W. (1989). Internal consistency of a diagnostic interview for children: The child assessment schedule. *Journal of Abnormal Child Psychology, 17*(6), 691–701.

Wirt, R. D., Lachar, D., Klinedinst, J. K., & Seat, P. D. (1984). *Multidimensional description of child personality: A manual for the personality inventory for children.* Los Angeles: Western Psychological Services.

- Group 6: Working for delayed gratification
- Group 7: Relaxing, playing
- Group 8: Cognitive processing through words, symbols, and images
- Group 9: Developing an adaptive sense of direction and purpose

Strayhorn's work is particularly helpful in isolating particular skills necessary for healthy interpersonal relationships. Clinicians or parents might use this framework when selecting activities for individuals or groups of children in attempts to support healthy personality development. Obviously, activities that encourage self-reflection, self-management, and self-enjoyment are necessary in promoting healthy ego or adaptive functions. This may include allowing the infant periods of time alone in the crib or playpen to explore the surroundings or his or her body. For the toddler, this might be accomplished by providing time for solitary play activities. For the school-age child, offering some activities that can begin to require self-questioning would be helpful. For the young adolescent, this self-reflection will occur as the teenager makes self comparisons with other peers, is challenged by successes and failures, and competes with his or her former abilities or the abilities of others. These are all necessary for the development of self-assessment and self-adjustment. Interaction skills, such as communication, negotiation, and sharing, are developed as the child is placed in situations with siblings and peers that require working out differences. For the isolated child, these skills may be less developed, and the personality trait of inflexibility may be seen as the child is faced with more social demands. Generally, a balance of solitary tasks or reflection time with interactive, social activities is best for healthy personality development. Finally, the child and adolescent must be challenged to reason and problem solve and test cognitive and physical skills in a safe, trusting environment. Being encouraged to develop and pursue personal interests also is crucial to personality development.

Personality Traits Versus Personality Disorders

Even when assessing adults, it is difficult to determine when a personality trait is detrimental to the extent that the individual is dysfunctional. The decision to "label" a child with a particular personality disorder is even more difficult, because the very definition of personality relates to the persistence of patterns of perceiving and relating over time and situations. Children develop and acquire new approaches to coping and interacting within the environment, and the extent to which a trait may be characteristically displayed depends on several factors, including cognitive problem-solving skills, mood, fatigue, and frequency of exposure to similar situations. There is limited agreement among clinicians, but distinguishing personality traits from disorders depends on the extent to which the personality traits become inflexible, maladaptive, and chronic. In addition, the traits must result in significant function impairment, reflect sudden or unpredictable shifts, or cause extreme subjective distress.

Personality Disorders

There are two commonly used systems of classifying personality disorders. Both are used in psychiatric settings because funding agencies differ in which system of classification they require for reimbursement. Table 17-3 shows the similarities and differences in these two classification systems.

In this chapter, the personality disorders are examined using the *Diagnostic and Statistical Manual of Mental Disorders* (DSM IV) classification and criteria. Most of the personality disorders are recognizable at least by adolescence and continue through most of adult life. However, personality disorders are not typically coded for children or adolescents unless stability of pattern can be assessed with certainty.

- Cluster A: paranoid, schizoid, schizotypal (odd and eccentric)
- Cluster B: antisocial, borderline, histrionic, narcissistic (dramatic, emotional, erratic)
- Cluster C: avoidant, dependent, obsessive–compulsive, passive–aggressive (anxious or fearful)

According to the DSM IV, the personality disorders typically evident in infancy, childhood, or adolescence are limited to antisocial personality disorder, avoidant personality disorder, and borderline.

PERSONALITY DISORDER

Each of these is presented with a focus on traits and characteristic patterns of perceiving experiences and relating to self and others. In addition,

TABLE 17–3 Comparison of Current Classifications of Personality Disorders

Code	International Classification of Disorders—10	Diagnostic and Statistical Manual of Mental Disorders III-Revised	Code
F60.0	Paranoid—excessive sensitivity, suspiciousness, preoccupation with conspiratorial explanation of events, with a persistent tendency to self-reference	Paranoid—interpretation of people's actions as deliberately demeaning or threatening	301.00
F60.1	Schizoid—emotional coldness, detachment, lack of interest in other people, eccentricity, and introspective fantasy	Schizoid—indifference to social relationships and restricted range of emotional experience and expression	301.20
	No equivalent	Schizotypal—deficit in interpersonal relatedness with peculiarities of ideation, appearance, and behavior	301.22
F60.5	Anakastic—indecisiveness, doubt, excessive caution, pedantry, rigidity, and need to plan in immaculate detail	Obsessive–compulsive—pervasive perfectionism and inflexibility	301.40
F60.4	Histrionic—self-dramatization, shallow mood, egocentricity, and craving for excitement with persistent manipulative behavior	Histrionic—excessive emotionality and attention seeking	301.50
F60.7	Dependent—failure to take responsibility for actions, with subordination of personal needs to those of others, excessive dependence with need for constant reassurance and feelings of helplessness when a close relationship ends	Dependent—persistent dependent and submissive behavior	301.60
F60.2	Dyssocial—callous unconcern for others, with irresponsibility, irritability, and aggression and incapacity to maintain enduring relationships	Antisocial—evidence of repeated conduct disorder before the age of 15 years	301.70
	No equivalent	Narcissistic—pervasive grandiosity, lack of empathy, and hypersensitivity to the evaluation of others	301.81
F60.6	Anxious—persistent tension, self-consciousness, exaggeration of risk and dangers, hypersensitivity to rejection, and restricted life-style because of insecurity	Avoidant—pervasive social discomfort, fear of negative evaluation, and timidity	301.82
F60.3	Impulsive—inability to control anger, to plan ahead, or to think before acts, with unpredictable mood and quarrelsome behavior	Borderline—pervasive instability of mood, interpersonal relationships, and self-image	301.83
	No equivalent	Passive–aggressive—pervasive passive resistance to demands for adequate social and occupational performance	301.84

Adapted from *Tyrer, P. (1988). Personality disorders.* (p. 21.) Boston: Wright. Permission requested.

some recent literature on narcissistic personality disorder in children is presented because there is adequate evidence that this personality disorder can be distinguished in childhood. Following the presentation of disorders, typical nursing diagnoses used are explored with appropriate interventions for hospitalized children and adolescents. For a more thorough exploration of the genesis of multiple personality disorder, the reader is referred to Chapter 10.

Nursing Care for Patients with Personality Disorders

When developing the care plan for the child or adolescent with a personality disorder, the nurse must keep in mind the specific traits or behaviors that are considered maladaptive. However, the nurse also must have an understanding of the underlying needs these traits or behaviors represent and the normative, developmental abilities of the client. Most frequently, the nurse will use nursing diagnoses related to alterations in self-concept, disturbances of mood, or disruptions in relatedness. The evaluation of the nursing care plan also must consider normal developmental capabilities based on the individual's age, cognitive abilities, and opportunities for growth.

NURSING ASSESSMENT

Assessing ego and super-ego functions are reliable ways the nurse can determine the degree of psychopathology, keeping in mind developmental cognitive and affective milestones. For example, prior to latency, children are consistently able to support only one view of others and cannot articulate "good" *and* "bad" features. People are seen as "good" *or* "bad." Likewise, they process information in a concrete fashion, ignoring incongruencies they cannot easily justify. Goldstein (1984) uses ego theory to offer questions that can be used for overall assessment of functioning:

1. To what extent is the client's problem a function of stresses imposed by his or her current life roles or developmental tasks?
2. To what extent is the client's problem a function of situational stress or of a traumatic event?
3. To what extent is the client's problem a function of impairment in his ego capacities or of developmental difficulties or dynamics?
4. To what extent is the client's problem a function of the lack of fit between inner capacities and external circumstances?
5. What inner capacities and environmental resources does the client have that can be mobilized to improve his or her functioning?

NURSING GOALS

The overall goals of nursing care with individuals with personality disorders include preventing injury to client and others; providing a supportive, consistent model of mature behavior; increasing problem-solving skills; mobilizing anxiety; reducing acting-out behaviors; identifying and supporting strengths; and promoting clear communication.

NURSING PROPERTIES FOR EFFECTIVE CARE OF CLIENTS WITH PERSONALITY DISORDERS

Generally, the nurse must maintain an open and accepting approach with children or adolescents exhibiting maladaptive personality traits. Being empathetic and supportive is essential. However, the nurse also must offer realistic, truthful information and affect in working with these clients. To accept maladaptive behavior as reasonable or acceptable will lessen the likelihood that the child will try to learn more functionally healthy behaviors.

The nurse has the responsibility to be approachable and nondefensive while maintaining clear judgment in working with clients with personality disorders. The need for modeling mature behavior and offering a trusting relationship is important. Often, the nurse must be able to tolerate verbal abuse when enforcing limits and accept the child's feelings without agreeing to the modes of behavior. Manipulative behavior is one of the most common behavioral manifestations of personality disorders. General characteristics of manipulative behaviors include the following:

- Using bargains, threats, demands, or intimidation to get his or her own way
- Having the ability to identify and use other people's weaknesses for his or her own benefit
- Making continuous, unrealistic demands
- Putting one individual against another (e.g., clients against staff)
- Pretending to be helpless and sorry for behavior
- Lying to gain sympathy of staff or other clients
- Setting up situations that will be detrimental to others (e.g., selling drugs, alcohol)
- Acting out even when given acceptable behavioral alternatives
- Keeping all relationships on a superficial level
- Using flattery, charm, and excessive compliments with or without self-degradation
- Using fear of physical violence to control others
- Exploiting the generosity of others
- Appearing unconcerned or detached when confronted with maladaptive behavior
- Identifying with staff or authority figure and acting as if he or she is not incarcerated
- Finding a way around the unit rules and expectations
- Using sexuality to gain control over others; also may approach the staff sexually
- Showing history of encounters (major or minor) with the law

BOX 17–1 • DIAGNOSTIC CRITERIA FOR 301.70 ANTISOCIAL PERSONALITY DISORDER

A. There is a pervasive pattern of disregard for and violation of the rights of others since age 15, as indicated by three (or more) of the following:
   1. Failure to conform to social norms with respect to lawful behaviors as indicated by repeatedly performing acts that are grounds for arrest
   2. Deceitfulness, as indicated by repeated lying, use of aliases, or conning others for personal profit or pleasure
   3. Impulsivity or failure to plan ahead
   4. Irritability and aggressiveness, as indicated by repeated physical fights or assaults
   5. Reckless disregard for safety of self or others
   6. Consistent irresponsibility, as indicated by repeated failure to sustain consistent work behavior or honor financial obligations
   7. Lack of remorse, as indicated by being indifferent to or rationalizing having hurt, mistreated, or stolen from another

B. The individual is at least 18.

C. There is evidence of conduct disorder (see p. 90) with onset before age 15.

D. The occurrence of antisocial behavior is not exclusively during the course of schizophrenia or manic episode

ANTISOCIAL PERSONALITY DISORDER

This classification is not given to adolescents younger than 18 years of age. However, the irresponsible and antisocial behaviors must have occurred before the age of 15. The DSM IV lists the traits typically seen in this disorder as irresponsible, irritable, aggressive, often promiscuous, remorseless for wrongdoing, and self-justifying for wrong deeds. Associated traits include subjective distress such as tension, boredom, depression, and interpersonal dissatisfaction. Relationships are typically transient and conflictual. This disorder is found within 3% of American males and 1% of females. Genetic predisposition may be present because the disorder is five times more common among first-degree biologic relatives of males with the disorder than among the general population; for females the risk increases to nearly 10 times that of the general population. Concurrent disorders include somatization disorder and psychoactive substance use disorder. For a more complete profile, see Chapter 16. The diagnostic criteria listed in the DSM IV are provided in Box 17-1.

The nursing assessment of clients with antisocial personality traits must focus strongly on strengths and ways in which the client can use these strengths in a socially appropriate manner. Inappropriate social relations and an inability to have a moral commitment to the community are the cornerstones for antisocial personality disorders. Generally, these clients are manipulative, deceitful, and antagonistic.

The nursing approaches for individuals identified with antisocial personality disorder generally include setting reasonable social limits, acknowledging strengths without incorporating acceptance of misconduct toward others, and reinforcing appropriate behaviors. The prognosis for this disorder is low, and the client is not generally seen in the hospital setting. More frequently, individuals with this disorder are seen in prison or long-term residential facilities because the antisocial behaviors have been persistent and often include criminal activities.

In formulating the interventions most helpful for altering the behavior pattern, the nurse must focus on the child's or adolescent's skills. For example, if the client has leadership abilities, using these skills to make decisions that benefit the group would be especially helpful. If the behavior can be shown to have specific and personal benefit, cooperation is more likely. With several successful experiences in a community environment, the client may see some benefits of social limits that not only constrain members of the community, but also benefit members. Conveying a willingness to listen and establishing a mutually respectful relationship is crucial if the individual is to benefit from the nurse–client relationship. This particular personality disorder is not likely to benefit from brief therapy or a punitive environment. The interventions of choice typically include pairing the client consistently with the same staff, setting consistent and firm limits, and encouraging adoption of socially appropriate behaviors within the treatment setting.

In evaluating the changes made by the client, the nurse will need to examine not only the behavioral

CLINICAL EXAMPLE: ALEX

Alex is a 19-year-old youth referred to the mental health clinic for therapy after his discharge from a youth correctional institution. He was adopted at 3 months of age, and little is known about his biologic parents. His behavior in elementary school was unremarkable except for frequent fights with peers and one incident where he cursed a teacher for reprimanding him. His parents report his behaviors became noticeably worse at age 11 when he refused to participate in scouts and was expelled from a football team for giving cigarettes to teammates and cursing at the coach. His grades in school declined in junior high, and by age 15, he was referred for counseling by his school counselor for truancy, belligerent behavior, stealing from peers' lockers, and fighting on school grounds. His attendance in counseling was poor; he stated he "hated talking to adults since they never understood [him] anyway."

At age 17, he was picked up for reckless driving and lost his driver's license. Two months later, he was again picked up for reckless driving without a license and placed on probation. After breaking his probation with a third violation, he was sent for 6 months to a Young Offenders Correctional Program. The report provided by the correctional institution stated he seemed uninterested in any specific career but had skills in mechanics and drafting. He had improved in his ability to get along with other males in his dorm but had no relationships with counselors. He was consistently involved in "conning" other inmates for cigarettes or personal hygiene items. He reported having a girlfriend but no one except family had visited him since his arrival at the institution.

changes, but also his or her attitudinal changes. Accurate self-appraisal reflects a dramatic improvement in the client. One of the outcomes that would reflect client success is if he or she is able to recognize and acknowledge the effects of behaviors on the community. (See Clinical Example: Alex and Table 17-4.)

The treatment of individuals diagnosed with antisocial personality disorder includes psychopharmacologics and residential placement with a focus on behavioral and interpersonal alterations in functioning. Unfortunately, simplistic approaches are frequently adopted because of court expectations, and treatment may be difficult within a "corrective rather than restorative" model. Forensic assessment is typically all that is afforded because of the person's involvement in criminal, assaultive behaviors.

NARCISSISTIC PERSONALITY DISORDER

There are marked similarities between narcissistic personality disorder and borderline personality disorder both in the acceptance of the diagnostic category for nonadults and in the believed developmental genesis of the disorder. Narcissistic personality disorder is controversial as an appropriate label for children because of the normalcy of narcissistic behaviors at specific stages in the child's development of personality. In general, normal narcissism reflects the integration of libidinally and aggressively determined object and self-representations into a cohesive self-concept. The individual can view actual behaviors from desired or ideal. In pathologic narcissism, the individual cannot distinguish between the real and ideal self, nor can he or she clearly distinguish between feelings and behaviors of self and significant others.

Some theorists agree that borderline personality disorder and narcissistic personality disorder are merely points on the same continuum, with narcissistic personality being more functionally healthy and developmentally advanced (Rinsley, 1989). Narcissistic personality also needs to be differentiated from obsessional personality and hysterical personality disorders. The primary distinction is the absence of a deeply traumatic early childhood and evidence of a more adequate separation–individuation process in obsessional and hysterical personality disorders. However, on a behavioral, superficial level, there are many similarities.

The narcissistic individual has a fragile sense of self, resulting from a constant emotional hunger, a sense of frustration, and a sense of frustration and rage. The child takes admired qualities and develops these into a self-image. When the image cannot be maintained, a sense of failure follows. This child requires constant "refueling." The need to be admired constantly promotes some of the devaluing of others and excessive demands for attention. For narcissistic individuals, interest in others is fleeting, achievement is only good as long as it is recognized by others, and reliance on social norms for mirroring appropriate relationships is nearly impossible. Everything in the life of this individual is important only in the context that it relates to the mirroring of achievement in the self.

The DSM IV criteria for adult diagnosis of narcissistic personality disorder (Box 17-2) require some modification if applied to children and adolescents. Kernberg (1989) outlines some of the common indicators of narcissistic personality traits seen in children. These include severe learning disabilities despite high intelligence; erratic school performance; attitude reflecting haughtiness, arrogance, or self-idealization; frequent gaze aversion; marked disinhibition in play; impaired social and peer interactions; separation anxiety; need for constant attention; preoccupation with self-image; superego functioning coupled with antisocial traits; and paranoid anxieties expressed through somatic and hypochondriac symptoms.

Kernberg (1989) identifies several groups of children at risk for the development of a narcissistic personality disorder:

- *Children of narcissistic parents.* These children

TABLE 17–4 Highlights from Nursing Care Plan for Antisocial Personality Disorder

Nursing Diagnosis	Client Outcome	Interventions
Alterations in self-concept R/T lack of sense of responsibility for wrongdoing, using others for selfish gain, overevaluated self-importance.	Expanded self-awareness Increased accuracy in self-appraisal Increased sense of responsibility for actions	Establish a respectful and trusting relationship through active listening and nonjudgmental responding. Identify ego strengths by first confirming identity. Accept and clarify verbal and nonverbal communication. Set limits on unacceptable behavior in a kind yet firm manner. Define consequences for failure to observe rules. Reinforce appropriate behavior, and enforce limits when violations occur. Convey that he or she is a responsible individual, and clarify his or her responsibility for behavior. Offer opportunities for successes for which he or she can assume responsibility. Avoid challenges to self-esteem. Be alert to impending tension, and offer alternatives to violent behavior. Support effective coping mechanisms.
Alteration in social relations R/T manipulative behaviors and repeated lying.	Expanded reality testing in social situations Improved interactions and meaning in social relations	Describe behaviors interfering with social relations. Explore social consequences to manipulative behaviors. Offer alternative ways to meet needs. Set consistent limits for manipulative behaviors. Restrict social circle to a small, manageable group. Encourage peer feedback for positive and negative consequences of behaviors. Offer social situations that allow appropriate interactions with peers.

BOX 17–2 • DIAGNOSTIC CRITERIA FOR 301.81 NARCISSISTIC PERSONALITY DISORDER

A pervasive pattern of grandiosity (in fantasy or behavior), need for admiration, and lack of empathy, beginning by early adulthood and present in a variety of contexts, as indicated by five (or more) of the following:

1. Has a grandiose sense of self-importance (eg, exaggerates achievements and talents, expects to be recognized as superior without commensurate achievements)
2. Is preoccupied with fantasies of unlimited success, power, brilliance, beauty, or ideal love
3. Believes that he or she is "special" and unique and can be understood by only, or should associate with, other special or high-status people (or institutions)
4. Requires excessive admiration
5. Has a sense of entitlement (ie, unreasonable expectations of especially favorable treatment or automatic compliance with his or her expectations)
6. Is interpersonally exploitative, (ie, takes advantage of others to achieve his or her own ends)
7. Lacks empathy: is unwilling to recognize or identify with the feelings and needs of others
8. Is often envious of others or believes that others are envious of him or her
9. Shows arrogant, haughty behaviors or attitudes

remain projections of the parents and are not allowed to develop an individualized sense of self.

- *Adopted children.* Adopted children struggle to accommodate being "chosen" because of their specialness with fear of having been "unchosen." This struggle is compounded if the adoptive parents experience difficulty in attaching to "someone else's" child or in accepting their own inability to have a child. The child may sense their grief or disappointment and externalize to ward off fear that he or she is not satisfactory.
- *Abused children.* The grandiose self may be produced as a result of the need to fuse with an idealized parent image in an attempt to protect themselves from actual abuse.
- *Overindulged or wealthy children.* These children are at risk for narcissistic personality disorder if they have had no opportunity to experience frustration, exercise tolerance, or become aware of reality limitations.
- *Children of divorced parents.* These children can develop a narcissistic personality in one of two ways. If the child becomes a substitute for the missing parent, the result is an opportunity to fulfill the oedipal wish and blurred generational lines; the child feels powerful and equal to the parent, rather than small and needy. On the other hand, the child who is denied access to the missing "bad" parent is cut off from his or her past and can experience a loss of identity when the custodial parent will not accept the child's traits that are like those of the "bad parent." To ward off feelings of depersonalization, these children may develop a grandiose self and devalue the custodial parent, whom the child views as an underlying enemy.
- *Children who have experienced the death of a parent.* To escape the sense of loss, the child may develop a grandiose self with permission to satisfy any desire through manipulation and compliant behavior.

These children are not typically admitted to the hospital for narcissistic behaviors. However, narcissistic traits may be presented by clients admitted with other disorders, including conduct disorder, oppositional disorder, depression, or anxiety disorders.

The nursing assessment of the individual identified with narcissistic personality disorder includes a careful assessment of the family system. Narcissistic personality traits generally stem from a dysfunctional family system with structural and systemic incongruencies. For example, the parent may expect the child to take on nurturing responsibilities toward the parent, exchanging the normal relationships available in families. The family system may not acknowledge differences between members and ignore individualized needs. These relational problems lay a foundation on which the child cannot form a clear sense of identity. Relationships are maintained with little understanding of mutual sharing.

Nursing diagnoses typically seen in these clients are those pertaining to impaired relationships or family dysfunction. Because of the underlying family dysfunction, family therapy is crucial in altering the improper coalition and interaction patterns. Some clinicians suggest alternating family with individual therapy because the child must accommodate self separate from the parental system. Interventions with the child and the parents are designed to acknowledge the child's separateness and feelings of aggression. Offering opportunities for the child to express the anger and despair in a socially appropriate manner is important. These clients are very vulnerable, and it is important to recognize this vulnerability when the child is demonstrating grandiose behaviors. The grandiose behavior must be interpreted in terms the child can understand. Providing the parents with support for their own needs and separating their needs from those of their child often are required throughout the course of therapy.

In evaluating progress, the nurse must consider the child's normal stage of development. Acknowledgement of others' autonomy or separateness indicates major adjustment, and tolerance for triadic or group relations clearly is a positive stride toward psychologic health. (See Clinical Example: Neal and Table 17-5.)

BORDERLINE PERSONALITY DISORDER OR BORDERLINE SYNDROME

This disorder was labeled in adults in the 1950s and has generated much controversy and exploration. The controversy involves whether there is a single disorder with subtypes and where the disorder ranges on the continuum between neurosis and psychosis (Pine, 1986; Goldstein, 1983; Kernberg, 1976). In child and adolescent psychiatry, it has been even more difficult to accept the terminology of borderline personality disorder because many of the characteristic traits can be seen normally at various developmental stages. As a result, some in psychiatry have adapted the term borderline syndrome to describe a cluster of characteristics that seem to precipitate a borderline personality disorder in adulthood. Kernberg (1990) believes that these characteristics define the "hidden" personality disorder, generating behaviors and conditions typically categorized on Axis I. Among children and adolescents, these conditions include conduct disorder, severe separation anxiety, identity disorders, eating disorders, elective mutism, attention-deficit hyperactivity disorder, and various developmental disorders. Most adults diagnosed in adulthood as borderline have been in treatment since childhood or report their symptoms started in childhood. However, the DSM IV offers only adult diagnostic criteria for borderline personality disorder without comparable criteria for this disorder in children or adolescents.

In children and adolescents with borderline characteristics, symptoms pervade thinking, feeling, and behavior domains. These individuals seem unable to cope with anxiety and instead use neurotic defenses or psychotic distortions. In terms of diagnostic assessment, no children's scale is as well developed as Gunderson's Adult Diagnostic Interview for Borderline Patients (Gunderson, Kolb, & Austin, 1981).

In play and conversation, these children display anxiety about mutilation, disintegration, or death. The ability to distinguish fantasy from reality is im-

CLINICAL EXAMPLE: NEAL

Neal, 15 years old, came to the Mental Health Outpatient Clinic with his mother for treatment. His family background is middle class; both parents work to provide for the family. His relationship with both parents is poor, and he frequently describes his mother as "that lady." When he is disciplined, he becomes aggressive and blames others for "getting" him into trouble. His parents feel they are unable to change this pattern. In school he is frequently in trouble for being the "class clown," not completing assignments, blaming others for this failure, and breaking classroom rules. His intellectual functioning is normal, but he gets C's and D's. He views teachers and principals as ignorant and useless.

He played soccer for 2 weeks but stopped playing because his "teammates would not let him have the ball." He reports having a lot of friends, but these seem short term and limited to peers with antisocial traits. He focuses on quantity of friends but does not acknowledge any particular behaviors in them he admires. He appears to have no remorse for wrongdoing and denies any need for changes in his behavior.

TABLE 17–5 Highlights from Nursing Care Plan for Narcissistic Personality

Nursing Diagnosis	Client Outcome	Interventions
Ineffective Family Coping	Parents will regain status in family as structural limit setters and authority figures.	Explore how family system operates, focusing on structural and systemic incongruencies. Reduce parents' anxiety in communicating with son. Instruct and support parents in regaining control in family system. Offer strategies for supporting the other parent when dealing with son's outbursts.
Ineffective Individual Coping	Improved coping with grief and loss of identity and opportunities.	Establish a trusting relationship that allows open communication. Support grieving statements as genuine and significant. Acknowledge anger and envy of others when expressed. Offer reconstruction of grandiose self-statements with realistic self-statements.

paired well past developmental expectations. Peculiar thought intrusions coupled with fantasy result in misunderstanding of common experiences or presentation of inappropriate content in conversations. Behavior patterns may be dull, monotonous, and repetitive or agitated and vacillating between calm and excited with little environmental alteration. Anxiety may quickly turn into panic, aggression, or self-destructive behaviors. Intellectually, these children may function well below their potential. Delayed gratification is difficult, if not impossible, for these individuals. Relationships are often problematic because of the individual's unpredictable behaviors or because they are viewed as superficial or uninteresting. As a result of social rejection, the individual's behavior and range of affect may become even more erratic.

Children with borderline characteristics commonly experience school problems. The school system is focused on compliance and pleasing others, delaying gratification, group cooperation, and self-management. Each of these requirements is oppositional to typical borderline patterns, reinforcing a negative view of self and the external environment (Schimmer, 1983).

The etiology of borderline disorders is unknown but is believed to include neurologic factors, possible genetic predisposition, and chaotic families (Egan, 1986; Gunderson & Englund, 1981; Masterson & Rinsley, 1975). Neurologic problems may include hyperactivity, poor motor coordination, perceptual–motor deficits, and abnormal electroencephalograms (Bemporad & Smith, 1985; Lewis & Miller, 1990). Genetic factors are difficult to determine because of the interaction between genetic and familial environment. However, the existence of mood and affective disorders in family members and coexisting disorders leads some to credit genetics as a contributing influence (Stone, 1980). Ego psychology theories are most commonly used to explain the origin and development of borderline personality disorders. Explanations range from premature oedipal conflicts (Kernberg, 1967) to disturbances in rapprochement phase (Pine, 1986) to arrest in affective or cognitive development (Adler & Buie, 1979).

Families of borderline individuals have only recently been studied. Generally, these families typically have unclear boundaries, inappropriate coalitions, and inappropriate roles. Gunderson and Englund (1981) describe four patterns of family relationships frequently seen in borderline individuals. The first pattern is intense parental overinvolvement with rejection whenever separation or individuation behaviors are attempted by the child. In the second pattern, the individual has no self-identity but is viewed by the parents as an object through which they can meet their own needs. In this pattern the child is a "transferential object," and the parents project positive or negative views of themselves onto the child to maintain their own narcissistic equilibrium. The child is viewed typically in a polarized fashion as if "all good" or "all bad." The third pattern is characterized by neglect and rejection. Externalization may be the only defense available against the anxiety and despair of the parent's nonacceptance. The fourth pattern is characterized by family isolation and ineffective family role modeling. Without appropriate and strong role models, the individual is unable to complete the task of identity formation. Typically, these individuals develop either a reactive identity that negates parental beliefs and behaviors or a malignant identity that overly conforms to the parents' limited or negative view of the child or adolescent.

Pine (1986) integrates psychodynamic theory, object relations theory, and attachment theory in a model for describing the development of the "Borderline child-to-be." He includes three steps in the model: 1) the experience of early trauma; 2) the evolution of early developmental deficits; and 3) the construction of survival coping mechanisms to which the child adheres desperately and which become pathologic defenses. His model is based on Mahler's theory of separation–individuation and the development of object constancy. Pine's steps, however, are broad and could easily account for several other personality disorders, including narcissistic personality disorder or multiple personality disorder.

In individuals with borderline personality traits, normal repression fails to develop, and primitive defense mechanisms of splitting, projecting, introjection, regression, and denial persist. The ego's synthesizing function is impaired, and there is failure to sublimate the raw instinctual impulses. Ego boundaries are fluid; reality perception and impulse control are poor. There is a lack of basic trust. The need for affection and approval to build ego structure continues, and rage and frustration at deprivation are so great that the child fears these feelings may destroy himself or herself or the mother.

Follow-up studies are limited primarily to borderline patients identified during childhood in Scandinavia. Wergeland (1979) examined the outcomes of 29 children hospitalized with borderline psychosis and found no significant differences between treated and untreated cases of borderline personality disorders with symptomatology ranging from psychotic to symptom-free. Dahl (1976) examined six borderline children 20 years after hospitalization and found three of these children had been rehospitalized. Of these, two were diagnosed as borderline, and one was labeled schizoid character disorder. Although methodologic shortcomings preclude specific prognosis, clearly no evidence supports optimism in the present treatment of borderline personality disorder patients.

Nursing assessment of borderline personality includes assessment of cognitive, attitudinal, and behavioral patterns. The interrelatedness of these components makes the assessment complex. The assessment must incorporate specific patterns of engaging social relations and distancing or alienating these same social relations. The nursing diagnoses typically seen in care plans are those for relatedness and disturbance in mood.

It is difficult to characterize a model treatment plan for borderline children and adolescents because of the extreme changeability of symptoms and the wide range in severity. Insight-oriented approaches are appropriate for older and only moderately disturbed adolescents. Supportive therapy is not helpful if it reinforces pathologic defenses, but insight therapy coupled with reality therapy has been used with moderate success. Psychoanalytic approaches include interpreting negative transferences and the need to "act out" (Egan, 1986; Kernberg, 1979).

The overall approaches of therapy include establishing a trust relationship between the therapist and client, focusing on relating behaviors to feelings in the here and now, and limiting polarization of views to the extremely negative or positive. Establishing a trust relationship includes the therapist's ability to withstand oppositional behaviors, set appropriate limits without rejection, and recognize competencies and failures.

The interventions used with these clients include developing a supportive relationship and being willing to listen. However, the nurse also must be clear in the expectations of the client and be able to set limits in a kind, yet firm, manner. The nurse must recognize the client's tendency to misinterpret environmental cues and must evaluate the client's interpretation carefully and offer alternative explanations in a supportive manner.

Individual psychotherapy is essential for clients with borderline personality, even though emotional fluctuations make this difficult (Bemporad & Smith, 1985). Tolerating emotional outbursts is necessary and intervening in management of these outbursts requires understanding and limit setting. Defensive reactions by the therapist or staff are detrimental, because they may result in fear and more exaggerated responses by the child. Likewise, therapists must avoid reacting with shock

CLINICAL EXAMPLE: BETH

Fifteen-year-old Beth was brought to the mental health clinic after she locked herself in the bathroom at school and threatened to kill herself. She had not been involved in any type of therapy prior to this situation. However, teachers reported her as uninterested in classwork, having no lasting friendships, and often giving responses to questions that were tangential or even irrelevant. Her parents describe her as moody, immature, and selfish. They reported she had run away the previous year, and they believed she was sexually active. They reported no serious concerns about Beth's behavior but frustration, and only after rather intense probing did they report several suicidal statements and one suicidal gesture the preceding year. On one occasion, she reportedly cut up all of her clothing and demolished her bedroom. On another occasion, she cut off her hair and threw it at her mother following an argument over a missed curfew. Beth stated that this behavior was instead of cutting her wrists. As Beth continued in therapy, her behavior varied from compliant to resistive. She would frequently call the counselor seeking information to seemingly insignificant questions. At times, she refused to speak during the session but would make another appointment before the scheduled appointment time, stating it was an emergency. When confronted about the inappropriateness of any action by the counselor or teachers, she would react with intense anger, loud cursing, and threatening behaviors.

when psychotic-like behaviors are exhibited (Rosenfeld & Sprince, 1963)

Evaluation of the client's progress generally revolves around the accuracy of cognitive interpretations and the ability to form significant and trusting relationships. The degree to which the individual can accommodate others' views yet differentiate self-views in interpreting situations often is a good-indicator of progress. (See Clinical Example: Beth and Table 17-6.)

Because of the self-mutilating behaviors, psychotic or psychotic-like behaviors, and poor parental support, hospitalization or residential care frequently is required. Therefore, some comments about staff involvement in treatment are warranted. Most of the literature about treating borderline children and adolescents focus on the role of the primary therapist. The therapist's role remains central even during hospitalization, while the staff role is best described as reality based. Staff training is essential to understand the disorder and to avoid typical difficulties in treating these patients. Staff members need to be trained to recognize countertransference responses and ways to avoid participation in "splitting behaviors" where some staff members are perceived by the client as "all good," while others are "all bad." Staff members should consistently offer a realistic view of events occurring on the unit. Responding in an accepting manner when setting limits is essential, especially when setting limits to prevent self-injury by the client. On the unit, working with the borderline client in small groups is preferable. Approaching the client as a team member rather than as an individual often lessens splitting within the team. The issue of client safety is paramount in all nursing interventions. These youth need to be observed discretely but consistently; harmful objects need to be used with supervision.

Psychopharmacologic treatment depends on the symptomatology. Minor and major tranquilizers frequently are prescribed for anxiety symptoms. Major tranquilizers (neuroleptics) are prescribed for psychotic reactions. Imipramine often is used for treating depression. Methylphenidate and dextroamphetamine often are prescribed for attention-deficit hyperactivity disorder. There is some concern about the misconceptions that may be possible in borderline children about medications. Bemporad et al. (1982) warns that borderline children and their families often have "extreme and magical fantasies about drugs and their effect on the body" (p. 250).

AVOIDANT PERSONALITY DISORDER

Avoidant personality disorders are generally preceded by a long history of shyness, limited positive experiences in social situations, and family tolerance for isolation. These children often present for treatment only when the avoidant behaviors begin to interfere with school performance. These children report no friends and may express no interest in making friends. They are overly sensitive and often infer negative connotations to neutral

TABLE 17–6 Highlights from Nursing Care Plan for Borderline Personality Disorder

Nursing Diagnosis	Client Outcome	Interventions
Altered emotional processes R/T inappropriate rage.	Expression of anger will be within acceptable limits.	Accept anger as a normal human emotion without condoning excessive angry actions. Assume a calm and direct manner. Convey concern and interest in his or her issues. Initially listen rather than attack defenses. Offer alternatives to rage experiences.
Powerless R/T inability to control impulses and urges.	Self-expressions will reflect increase in emotional self-regulation.	Verbally recognize and support self-regulation attempts (cut hair instead of body, reduced telephone calls to therapist). Explore ambivalent feelings that generate excessive anxiety. Offer anxiety-reducing strategies. Model mature responses to anxiety or anger-producing events in the therapeutic relationship. Set limits on phone calls to therapist in a kind yet firm manner.

environmental events. As adults, they may report social phobia and even panic attacks in social situations. Symptomatology may result in an Axis I diagnosis of social phobia, generalized anxiety disorder, depressive episode, or separation anxiety disorder (Box 17-3).

Nursing assessment of these children or adolescents must include a thorough family assessment for social adaptation and relationships. This assessment often is difficult because the family may share the child's trait of avoiding disclosure. However, understanding the family system of allegiances and coalitions is necessary to form interventions that focus on reinforcing healthy relationships.

The nursing interventions are designed to reduce social anxiety and reinforce a healthy self-concept that can tolerate social exposure. Systematic desensitization of social stimuli is a common intervention. Family interventions that focus on strengthening positive self-evaluations and competencies often are useful. For example, the family

BOX 17–3 • DIAGNOSTIC CRITERIA FOR 301.82 AVOIDANT PERSONALITY DISORDER

A pervasive pattern of social inhibition, feelings of inadequacy, and hypersensitivity to negative evaluation, beginning by early adulthood and present in a variety of contexts, as indicated by four (or more) of the following:

1. Avoids occupational activities that involve significant interpersonal contact, because of fears of criticism, disapproval, or rejection
2. Is unwilling to get involved with people unless certain of being liked
3. Shows restraint within intimate relationships because of the fear of being shamed or ridiculed
4. Is preoccupied with being criticized or rejected in social situations
5. Is inhibited in new interpersonal situations because of feelings of inadequacy
6. Views self as socially inept, personally unappealing, or inferior to others
7. Is usually reluctant to take personal risks or to engage in any new activities because they may prove embarrassing

CLINICAL EXAMPLE: VICKI

Vicki is a 14-year-old who was brought to the school mental health clinic following a "breakdown" in the classroom. Because of her difficulty in discussing the event, her teacher sent another student with her. Vicki was crying and kept her head down. Her mother reports that Vicki has always been shy and often chooses to remain home rather than go shopping or out to eat with the family. She has never spent the night with a friend. She has gone to camp twice but always ended up returning home on the first day. She visited her brother and his family for a week last summer but reported difficulty eating and sleeping; her brother stated she spoke very little and seemed withdrawn and lonely.

The parents report having difficulty since preschool in getting Vicki to accept new situations or to interact with peers. She would observe other children but not participate in play.

may be enouraged to provide positive feedback when the child is able to initiate interactions with a close relative or neighborhood peer. The family might be encouraged to have family celebrations or events that include another child to offer opportunities for the client's confidence to increase in social situations. The nurse may want to work with the family in exploring the underlying concerns of the child when in social situations and how the family can modify future social events to be more tolerable.

The evaluation of the client's progress tends to be more behavioral than attitudinal. The evaluation should be designed to determine if the child is able to engage in social interactions and tolerate greater self-disclosure. Family progress can be based on their willingness to support the child in social situations while requiring some level of par-

TABLE 17–7 Highlights from Nursing Care Plan for Avoidant Personality Disorder

Nursing Diagnosis	Client Outcome	Interventions
Social isolation R/T anxiety in social situations.	Reduction of anxiety in social situations.	Provide a climate of acceptance by providing basic physiologic care. Offer support for initiating conversation in the therapy session. Offer instruction and practice in relaxation and anxiety reduction techniques. Provide feedback and social rewards when social behaviors are approached. Set up desensitization program for social involvement. Do not emphasize or provide undue attention to noninteractive behaviors. Offer small group and one-to-one opportunities for social skill practice. Initially, these interactions should require minimal verbalization.
Disturbance in self-concept R/T poor self-image, excessive fear of failure.	Realistic self-assessment.	Explore self-perceptions in an environment of trust acceptance. Reframe excessive self-devaluing statements into more realistic statements. Offer opportunities for success in a semicontrolled environment, and explore skills. Role play positive self-statements she can use for self-talk outside the session.

ticipation in these social settings. (See Clinical Example: Vicki and Table 17-7.)

Summary

The treatment of personality disorders in children is controversial. The treatment is less likely to be conducted in a hospital setting and generally requires long-term treatment rather than brief interventions. The assessment of the family and inclusion of the family in treatment are crucial. Nursing interventions generally center on increasing relational skills and accurate self-evaluation in the client. The approaches used within the treatment process require an understanding of his or her cognitive, attitudinal, and overt behavioral patterns. The underlying needs of the client represented by the behaviors must be considered carefully and the client approached in a supportive yet firm manner.

REFERENCES

Abraham, K. (1927). The influence of oral eroticism on character formation. In K. Abraham (Ed.), *Selected papers*. London: Institute for Psychoanalyses and Hogarth Press.

Adler, G., & Buie, D. (1979). Aloneness and borderline psychopathology: The possible relevance of child developmental issues. *International Journal of Psychoanalysis, 60*, 83–96.

American Psychiatric Association (1994). *Diagnostic and statistical manual of mental disorders* (4th ed.). Washington, DC: Author.

Anthony, E. J., & Cohler, B. S. (1987). *The invulnerable child.* New York: Guilford Press.

Bemporad, J. R., Smith, H. F., Hanson, G., & Ciccheti, D. (1982). Borderline syndromes in children: Criteria for diagnosis. *American Journal of Psychiatry, 139*, 596–602.

Brown, G. W., Harris, T. D., & Petro, J. (1973). Life events and psychiatric disorders: Part 2: Nature of causal link. *Psychological Medicine, 3*, 159–176.

Cloninger, C. R. (1986). A unified biosocial theory of personality and its role in the development of anxiety states. *Psychiatric Developments, 3*, 167–226.

Cloninger, C. R. (1987). A systematic method for clinical description and classification of personality variants: A proposal. *Archives of General Psychiatry, 44*, 573–588.

Dahl, V. A. (1976). A follow-up study of a child psychiatric clientele with special regard to the diagnosis of psychosis. *Acta Psychiatric Scandanavica, 54*, 106–112.

Egan, J. (1986). Etiology and treatment of borderline personality disorder in adolescents. *Hospital and Community Psychiatry, 37*(6), 613–618.

Erikson, E. H. (1950). *Childhood and society.* New York: W.W. Norton.

Fenichel, O. (1945). The psychoanalytic theory of neurosis. New York: W.W. Norton.

Freud, S. (1925). Character and eroticism. In S. Freud (Ed.), *Collected papers.* London: Institute for Psychoanalyses and Hogarth Press.

Glover, E. (1925). Notes on oral character formation. *International Journal of Psychoanalysis, 6*, 131–154.

Goldstein, W. M. (1983). DSM III and the diagnosis of borderline. *American Journal of Psychotherapy, 37*(3), 312–327.

Goldstein, E. G. (1984). *Ego psychology and social work practice.* New York: Free Press.

Gunderson, J. G., & Englund, O. W. (1981). Characterizing the family of borderlines. *Psychiatric Clinics of North America, 4*(1), 159–168.

Gunderson, J. G. (1984). *Borderline personality disorder.* Washington, D.C.: American Psychiatric Press.

Gunderson, J. G., Kolb, J., & Austin, V. (1981). The diagnostic interview for borderline patients. *American Journal of Psychiatry, 138*, 896–903.

Kernberg, O. (1967). Borderline personality organization. *Journal of the American Psychoanalytic Association, 15*, 641–685.

Kernberg, O. (1975). *Borderline conditions and pathological narcissism.* New York: Jason Aronsen.

Kernberg, O. (1976). *Object-relations theory and clinical psychoanalysis.* New York: Jason Aronsen.

Kernberg, O. F. (1979). *Psychoanalytic psychotherapy with borderline adolescents.* Chicago: The University of Chicago Press.

Kernberg, P. (1989). Narcissistic personality disorder in children. *Pediatric Clinics of North America, 12*(3), 671–694.

Kernberg, P. F., & Shapiro, T. (1990). Resolved: Borderline personality exists in children under twelve. *American Academy of Child and Adolescent Psychiatry, 29*(3), 478–483.

Kohut, H. (1977). *The restoration of the self.* New York: International Universities Press.

Lewis, M., & Miller, S. M. (1990). *Handbook of developmental psychopathology.* New York: Plenum Press.

Mahler, M. S. (1970). *A study of the separation-individual process.* Paper presented as the Twentieth Freud Anniversary Lecture Series of the New York Psychoanalytic Institute. New York: International Universities Press.

Mahler, M. S., Pine, F., & Bergman, A. (1975). *The psychological birth of the human infant.* New York: Basic Books.

Masterson, J. F. (1972). Treatment of the adolescent with borderline syndrome: A problem in separation-individuation. *Bulletin of the Menninger Clinic, 35*, 5–18.

Masterson, J. F., & Rinsley, D. B. (1975). The borderline syndrome: The role of the mother in genesis and psychic structure of the borderline personality. *British Journal of Psychoanalysis, 56*, 163–177.

Paykel, E. S. (1978). Contributions of life events to causation of psychiatric illness. *Psychological Medicine, 8*, 245–253.

Pine, F. (1986). On the development of the borderline-child-to-be. *American Journal of Orthopsychiatry, 56*, 450–457.

Rapaport, O. (1958). The theory of ego autonomy: A generalization. *Bulletin of Menninger Clinic, 22*, 13–35.

Rinsley, D. B. (1989). Notes on the developmental pathogenesis of narcissistic personality disorder. *Psychiatric Clinics of North America, 12*(3), 695–707.

Rosenfeld, S. K., & Sprince, M. P. (1963). An attempt to formulate the meaning of the concept “borderline.” *The Psychoanalytic Study of the Child, 18*, 603–635.

Schimmer, R. (1983). The borderline personality organization in elementary school: Conflict and treatment. In K. S. Robson (Ed.), *The borderline child: Approaches to etiology, diagnosis, and treatment* (pp. 277–293). New York: McGraw-Hill.

Stone, M. H. (1980). *The borderline syndromes: Constitution, adaptation and personality.* New York: McGraw-Hill.

Stone, M. H. (1981). Borderline syndromes: A consideration of subtypes and an overview, directions for research. *Psychiatric Clinics of North America, 4*(1), 3–24.

Strayhorn, J. M. (1988). *The competent child: An approach to psychotherapy and preventive mental health.* New York: The Guilford Press.

Tyrer, P. (1988). *Personality disorders.* Boston: Wright Publishing.

Wergeland, H. (1979). A follow-up study of 29 borderline psychotic children 5 to 20 years of after discharge. *Acta Psychiatrica Scandanavica, 60,* 465–476.

CHAPTER

18

Mood Disorders

Geraldine S. Pearson

The concept of mood disorders in children and adolescents has undergone a radical transformation in the last 20 years. While previously unrecognized as a psychiatric syndrome of childhood, mood disorders, particularly childhood depression, have become some of the most researched and documented disorders in child psychiatry.

Nurses who treat children in outpatient and inpatient settings are familiar with mood disorders. While rare in the general population of children and youth, mood disorders often coexist with other diagnoses, such as conduct disorder or anxiety disorder. It has been suggested that impoverished children suffer most from depression or dysthymic conditions. Economic stress may increase the incidence of depression as families become less able to meet the physical and emotional needs of their children.

The long-term effects of mood disorders are well documented. They negatively influence the normal development of children and adolescents who are unable to complete age-appropriate tasks of latency or adolescence. Academic progress and peer relationships often are compromised in the depressed child. Mood disorders put adolescents at risk for suicide. While treatment has been shown to ameliorate the effects of depression, relapse during later adolescence and adulthood is common (Kovacs, Feinbert, & Crouse-Novak, 1984).

Treatment methodology for mood disorders includes cognitive–behavioral therapy, models of family therapy, psychoanalytic therapy, and pharmacotherapy. No single treatment model has proven completely successful in treating mood disorders, which reflects the complexity of etiology, manifestation, and effects on the developing individual.

Historic Perspectives

In 1946 Spitz coined the term anaclitic depression to describe a condition pertinent to babies and young children in which the withdrawal of parental attention and affective caring resulted in crying, despair, and a failure to thrive. Erikson later noted that the withdrawal of "mother love without proper substitution" could lead to acute infantile depression or a milder, more chronic state of mourning that would continue throughout life (1950, p. 80).

In the late 1950s and early 1960s a number of writers suggested that children could not become depressed because their psychologic development was not complete (Rie, 1966; Rochlin, 1959). Glaser (1968) noted the presence of a masked depression in which the depressed feelings are concealed by other behaviors. These included conduct disorders, school phobias, and difficulties with learning.

The most recent literature supports the notion

of child and adolescent mood disorders that are congruent with adult forms of the disorder (Lewis & Volkmar, 1990). Although depression may appear differently at various developmental stages, the use of the same criteria to diagnose mood disorders (the Research Diagnostic Criteria and *Diagnostic and Statistical Manual of Mental Disorders*, IV) has furthered the view of depression in children as analagous to adult manifestations of the disorder (Spitzer, Endicott, & Robins, 1978; American Psychiatric Association [APA], 1994).

Puig-Antich later noted the high rate of "coexisting disorders" in children and adolescents identified as depressed (1982). Depressive and nondepressive disorders show a high comorbidity with overlap, particularly with anxiety and behavior disorders (Fleming & Offord, 1990). There was also speculation that the more severe the depression, the more likely the presence of co-morbidity with another disorder. It is unclear how level of depression affects the presence of other psychiatric disorders (Fleming, Offord, & Boyle, 1989; Kashani et al., 1987).

Nurses are likely to see depressed children and adolescents in their inpatient and outpatient populations. Kashani and Sherman (1988) report that in the United States, 0.9% of preschoolers, 1.9% of school-age children, and 4.7% of adolescents meet criteria for depression. These statistics do not reflect the numbers of children who meet the full criteria for depression but may manifest dysthymia, which in its chronicity can be detrimental to the accomplishment of essential developmental tasks.

Depression is equally common among young boys and girls, more common in boys just prior to puberty, but more prevalent in girls from puberty until adulthood. Children whose parents have a mood disorder, are young, or have any psychiatric illness are more at risk for a mood disorder. If one parent has a mood disorder, there is a 30% chance that their offspring will develop a mood disorder. If both parents are afflicted with a mood disorder, the chance of their children developing this disorder rises to 50% to 70% (Weissman, Gershon, & Kidd, 1984a).

Theories of Etiology

Theories of etiology tend to be complex and overlapping. They generally fall under biologic and psychosocial models and are categorized accordingly in this discussion.

BIOLOGIC MODELS

Research has generally supported the view of depression as biologic. Biochemical agents implicated in causality include neurotransmitters and monoamines, including catecholamines and indolamine (Zis & Goodwin, 1982). Affective disorders are thought to result from a lack or excess of one or more neurotransmitters or by an imbalance of these agents.

Neuroendocrine abnormalities involving noradrenaline, serotonin, and acetylcholine also have been implicated in biologic theories of depression (Sachar, 1982).

Genetic influences on depression have been accepted for some time. Depression in adult first-degree relatives may preclude an increased risk of the disorder occurring in offspring (Nurnberger & Gershon, 1982). Monozygotic twins showed 65% concordance for affective disorders when compared to dizygotic twins, with 14% concordance (Gershon, Targum, Kessler, Mazure, & Bunney, 1977). "Research has also explored biological markers, i.e., genetic, biochemical, or related characteristics that permit identification of who is at risk for affective disorders" (Kazdin, 1990, p. 140).

PSYCHOSOCIAL THEORIES

Psychosocial theories emphasize the "intrapsychic, behavioral, cognitive, and interpersonal underpinnings of depression" (Kazdin, 1990, p. 140). They include psychoanalytic, cognitive, learning, and object loss theories.

PSYCHOANALYTIC THEORY. This theory has postulated that a dysfunctional or flawed mother–child relationship puts an individual at risk for depression. As the infant's needs are unfulfilled, the unsatisfied libidinal strivings translate into a loss (Mendelson, 1982).

Psychoanalytic theory notes that self-rejection and criticism are the result of the ego and superego striving to meet parental ideals and values. Freud (1917) believed that internal conflict and self-criticism reflected anger and hostility toward parents. After Freud's early interpretations, other psychoanalytic theories expanded on explanations of depression and included oral stage fixation, loss of self-esteem, helplessness, and anger turned inward.

COGNITIVE THEORY. This theory proposes that depression occurs as a result of impaired cognition. Beck (1987) postulated the cognitive triad of depression (i.e., negative views of self, the world, and the future), which accounts for an individual's affective, behavioral, and motivational symptoms of depression.

LEARNING THEORY. The learned helplessness model of depression, proposed by Seligman (1975), viewed depression as resulting from an individual's sense that they had limited influence over their lives. Passivity, sense of failure (real or imagined), social impairment, and depression stem from the feeling of helplessness. The individual abandons trying to succeed and becomes depressed. Abramson, Metalsky, and Alloy (1989) further defined this as the hopelessness theory of depression.

BEHAVIORAL THEORY. Behavioral explanations for depression focus on learning, environmental consequences, skill acquisition, and deficits (Clarizio, 1985). Depression results from an interactional problem in the environment, generally one of positive reinforcement. Passivity, withdrawal, and depression result when the environment is perceived negatively.

Social skill deficits, impaired family interactions, and deficient processes of self-regulation have been postulated by behaviorists as behavioral explanations for depression.

PARENT–CHILD RELATIONSHIP MODEL

This model suggests that depression results from a poor parent–child relationship that jeopardizes the child's sense of well-being. Children of depressed parents have shown higher rates of perinatal complications and cognitive or emotional delays, as well as difficulties separating from parents. As latency-age children, they showed depression, school problems, excessive rivalry with peers for attention, and hyperactivity. As teenagers, they tended to be defiant, rebellious, withdrawn, and conflicted with parental authority (Beardslee et al., 1983).

Weissman et al. (1984b) noted that children of depressed adults were three times as likely to manifest a DSM III-R diagnosis. Severity and chronicity of parental depression are likely to have an impact on the level of maladaptive behavior in the child, including depression. Maternal depression is more strongly associated with psychopathology in children (Keller et al., 1986).

There is considerable overlap in all theoretical explanations of depression. Many authors contend that depression results from a combination of circumstances and events that converge to precipitate depression. Many models of depression admit that life events and stressors are significant factors in the individual who manifests a mood disorder.

BIOBEHAVIORAL MODEL

While there has been minimal effort to integrate the different models, Whybrow, Akiskal, and McKinney (1984) proposed a biobehavioral model that looked at predispositions to depression, such as genetics, temperament, age, sex, physical illness, attachment disorders, and experiences with loss. Whybrow suggests that these factors alter the central nervous system to produce biologic responses that receive further support from the environment. Kazdin (1990) notes the attractiveness of this integrated model because it acknowledges the presence of various explanations and theories.

The biobehavioral model is particularly useful to nurses as a view of depression and the converging factors that precipitate its development. The overlay of genetic vulnerability and environmental stress is a more logical predictor of those at risk for mood disorder. The presence of mood disorder in parents and first-degree relatives, while providing markers of risk, does not automatically predict that children or adolescents will develop mood disorders. Family stress, parental level of physical and mental health, and presence or absence or crisis events, in conjunction with predisposition, are more likely to influence the development of the disorder.

Definition

Mood disorders can be divided into two general categories, unipolar depressive disorders and bipolar disorders. Both types of depression are thought to exist across age spans with some differences across developmental lines. The DSM IV notes that mood disorders generally are accompanied by a full or partial manic or depressive syndrome that is not attributed to any other physical or mental disorder (APA, 1994).

UNIPOLAR DEPRESSIVE DISORDERS

Also known as depressive disorder, unipolar depressive disorders are characterized by dysfunction that has lasted at least 2 weeks and includes at least five of the following symptoms:

- Depressed mood
- Diminished interest or loss of pleasure in almost all activities

- Sleep disturbance
- Weight change or appetite disturbance (failure to achieve expected gain in children or greater than 5% loss of body weight in 1 month)
- Decreased concentration or indecisiveness
- Suicidal ideation or thoughts of death
- Psychomotor agitation or retardation
- Fatigue or loss of energy
- Feelings of worthlessness or inappropriate guilt

Depressed mood or diminished interest or loss of pleasure must be present to diagnose depression (APA, 1994).

Unipolar depressions can be rated as mild, moderate, severe, and with or without psychotic symptoms that may or may not be mood congruent. Depressions also can be in full or partial remission; when the episode has lasted 2 consecutive years without at least 2 months of improved functioning, the disorder is considered chronic (Weller & Weller, 1991).

Although more difficult to diagnose in children and thought to be less common, depressions also can be of the melancholic subtype. One of the DSM IV criteria is the presence of one or more previous depressive episodes with complete or near-complete recovery. Children are less likely to have had previous episodes of major depression accompanied by full recovery.

Seasonal mood disorders also might affect children and adolescents. Diagnosis must occur after "a regular temporal relationship between depression, mania, and a particular 60-day period of the year. A full remission or switching from depression to mania should occur within a 60-day period of the year" (Weller & Weller, 1991, p. 653). Three distinct episodes of mood disturbance must be documented seasonally for 3 years.

Dysthymia often begins in childhood or adolescence and is characterized by a depressed or irritable mood that lasts at least 1 year. At least two of the following must be present:

- Appetite change
- Sleep change
- Decreased energy
- Low self-esteem
- Difficulty making decisions or poor concentration
- Feelings of hopelessness

The individual is not symptom-free for more than 2 months (APA, 1994).

Dysthymia is chronic and can exist with a variety of other disorders, including attention-deficit/hyperactivity disorder, conduct disorder, specific developmental disorders, and chronic illness. Nurses are likely to see children with dysthymia in school or clinic settings where their symptoms are not as debilitating as those of a major depression. They may not be receiving treatment for their dysthymia, even though the disorder compromises daily functioning and developmental mastery.

BIPOLAR DISORDERS

Bipolar disorders also are referred to as manic disorders or manic depressions and are characterized by the following:

- Inflated self-esteem or grandiosity
- Decreased need for sleep
- Increased talkativeness or pressure to keep talking
- Racing thought or flight of ideas
- Distractibility
- Increased activity or psychomotor agitation
- Excessive involvement in pleasurable activities that have high potential for painful consequences (APA, 1994)

Bipolar disorders generally impair the individual's functioning in school or work and with friends and family members. Inpatient hospitalization often is necessary to prevent the individual from harming self or others.

As with depressive episodes, manic episodes can be rated as mild, moderate, or severe. Psychotic symptoms may or may not be present; several other subclassifications also exist and include bipolar disorder mixed episode, bipolar disorder depressed, cyclothymia, and bipolar disorder not otherwise specified (APA, 1994).

While bipolar disorder has been diagnosed in prepubertal children (Carlson & Strober, 1978; Weinberg & Brumback, 1976), its presence in this age group has been questioned. The presence of bipolar illness in adolescents more closely resembles the adult course of the illness and presents similar symptoms of grandiosity, sleeplessness, bizarre speech or behavior, and flight of ideas (see Clinical Example: Linda). Children younger than age 9 are more likely to appear with irritability and affective lability, while older children may be more euphoric, elated, paranoid, or grandiose (Carlson, 1983).

Other psychiatric disorders must be ruled out before diagnosing bipolar disorder. Children with attention-deficit hyperactivity disorder may present with similiar symptoms of distractibility and hyperactivity; the symptoms and affects of mania are much more acute and include irritability and

CLINICAL EXAMPLE: LINDA

Linda, a 15-year-old, became increasingly hyperactive at home and school. Historically, her peers considered her somewhat odd, but she had a small group of supportive friends with whom she regularly interacted in and out of school. She had great difficulty sitting still in school and at times, paced the halls. Her parents, a somewhat intellectually limited couple with many interpersonal problems of their own, reported she had difficulty sleeping at night. Her speech became pressured and difficult to understand, and she reported racing thoughts. Her own explanation for the change in behavior was "that the world had become clearer, and I have the energy to deal with it."

She was brought to the emergency room of a local hospital after she pushed her way into the principal's office at her junior high, locked the door to his office, and began using the intercom system to the entire school. Before being restrained by staff and removed by ambulance, she announced that she was tired of people talking about her; she was a new, reborn person and would be the most popular student in the school. Her speech gradually became more garbled, and she finished her diatribe with hysterical laughter.

euphoria. Conduct disorder children, with difficult to manage, antisocial behavior, may exhibit behaviors easily confused with mania. However, they do not tend to show the paranoid thinking or grandiose thinking that characterizes mania.

In addition, it may be difficult to differentiate between schizophrenia and bipolar disorder because both are characterized by bizarre, delusional, and paranoid behaviors. Schizophrenia usually appears gradually, while mania has a more acute onset. Assessment of premorbid history and onset of symptoms is essential in the differentiation of the two disorders (Weller & Weller, 1991). Underdiagnosis of mania has historically occurred for children and adolescents.

Suicide

In recent years, the incidence of suicide, especially among adolescents with affective disorders, has risen dramatically and caused great concern. While affective illness in adolescents is associated with completed suicide, suicide attempts, and ideation (Pfeffer et al., 1988), most adolescents with affective illness do not attempt or complete suicide. However, suicidal behaviors have been linked consistently with depressive symptoms or disorders. Conduct and substance use disorders also have been considered psychiatric risk factors because they are often associated with behavioral impulsivity (Kovacs, Goldston, & Gatsonis, 1993).

Suicide attempts in children younger than age 12 are relatively rare. The rate of completed suicide attempts in these children is thought to be associated with developmental, cognitive levels of maturity. Some investigators suggest that formal operational levels of cognitive maturation must be present to experience the hopelessness and despair that precludes suicidal ideation or attempts (Carlson, Asarnow, & Orbach, 1987). Similarly, children between the ages of 5 and 10 years may not have a clear understanding of death and may become confused by the concept. It is only between the ages of 10 and 15 years that the youngster begins to form an understanding of mortality that is influenced more by emotional issues rather than cognitive capacity (Lewis & Volkmar, 1990). It is unclear whether children in this age group completely understand the finality of dying and believe that they can have control over the process of suicide (Box 18-1).

Suicide attempts rise sharply at age 13 to 14 years (Rutter & Garmezy, 1983). For youth age 15 to 24 years, suicide is the third leading cause of death (Shaffer & Fisher, 1981). The highest suicide rates occur in white males, with the next highest rates occurring in nonwhite males. Nonwhite and white adolescent females have significantly lower rates of suicide than their male counterparts (Pfeffer, 1988).

The literature notes that adolescent thoughts of suicide increase with age. As they age, adolescents attempt suicide more frequently and more often complete these attempts (Pfeffer, 1986; Shaffer, Garland, Gould, Fisher, & Trautman, 1988;). Myers, McCauley, Calderon, and Treder (1991) hypothesize that "these changes with age may represent a developmental proclivity for older youths to think self-destructively or to act on their depressive or impulsive feelings" (p. 804). Risk factors are thought to include affective illness, parental divorce rates, and the use of firearms as a suicide method (Boyd & Moscicki, 1986) (Box 18-2).

Adolescents who attempt suicide have been found to experience more turmoil in their family, beginning in childhood and continuing into adolescence. They may be sexually abused during adoles-

BOX 18–1 • SUICIDE ASSESSMENT OF THE PREPUBERTAL CHILD

QUESTIONS FOR PARENTS

1. What behavior has the child recently exhibited that would make you worry he or she might hurt self?
2. Describe recent changes in behavior, life stresses of past year, and the child's current functioning.
3. Has the child been exposed to death or suicide of a friend or relative?
4. Does the child have access to dangerous objects, such as guns or knives? How do parents plan to safeguard these items?
5. Is there a family history of suicide or depression?

QUESTIONS FOR CHILD

1. What does it mean to die?
2. Have you ever seen or known anyone who has died?
3. Do you ever think about hurting yourself?
4. Have you ever tried to hurt yourself? How did you do this?
5. Did you ever tell anyone about trying to hurt yourself?
6. How do you feel right now?

cence and experience further stresses, such as changes in residence or failure in school (de Wilde, Kienhorst, Diekstra, & Wolters, 1992).

Suicide attempts and completions are related to mood disorders in several ways. First, a diagnosis of early-onset bipolar disorder was the most common diagnosis in a group of individuals who completed suicide. (Welner, Welner, & Fishman, 1979). Second, suicidal ideation and behaviors in adolescents present a risk for completed suicide. When these behaviors are combined with a mood disorder, the quality of life experienced by these youngsters is markedly compromised (Myers et al., 1991).

Shaffer et al. (1988) point out that many individuals with mood disorders are not suicidal. The specificity of a mood disorder is not a predictor to later suicide attempts (Shaffer et al., 1988).

Although the literature attempts to understand the causes and antecedents of suicide, no systematic studies have demonstrated the exact developmental risk and protective factors (Borst, Noam, & Bartok, 1991). Some researchers have suggested a developmental link to cognitive functioning that allows an individual to feel the despair, self-hate, and hopelessness necessary for suicide risk (Carlson et al., 1987). Others have noted the need to move beyond age as a singular risk factor in predicting suicide and to look at multiple risk factors, such as alcohol use, problematic interpersonal relationships, or immediate interpersonal crises. Shaffer (1974) suggested that disciplinary crises, a dispute with a peer or boyfriend or girlfriend, an argument with parents, or another stressful event contributed to completed suicides. Shafii et al. (1985) noted other environmental factors influencing youth suicide as exposure to parental, peer, or relative suicidal ideas or acts; parental emotional problems or absence; and evidence of physical abuse.

Suicides can occur in clusters (Gould, Wallenstein, & Kleinman, 1990). Imitation, exposure to fictional suicide in the media (Gould & Shaffer, 1986), or exposure to completed suicide in a school system (Brent et al., 1989) are all thought to preclude the clustering phenomenon. Hazell and Lewin (1993) explored the friends of those who have attempted or completed suicide and found them to show a greater degree of disturbance than comparison groups. They suggest that friendship with someone who has attempted suicide may be a marker of preexisting vulnerability to suicidal behavior. Interven-

BOX 18–2 • ADOLESCENT SUICIDAL ASSESSMENT

1. Have you ever thought about trying to hurt yourself? If yes, how would you do this?
2. Have you ever thought about killing yourself? If yes, how would you do this?
3. Have you ever attempted to kill yourself? When did this occur? How many times have you tried this? What method did you use to try to commit suicide?
4. Have you known anyone who attempted suicide? Have you known anyone who killed themselves? When did this occur?
5. Do you engage in risky behaviors that might put your life in danger (i.e., driving when drunk, doing drugs and not knowing what they are, playing chicken with cars, playing Russian roulette with a gun)?
6. Do you have access to a firearm?
7. Have you ever been hospitalized for suicidal behavior?
8. Have you ever told anyone about wishing to kill yourself?
9. How do you feel right now?

tions are recommended for friends of those who have attempted or completed suicide.

Clinical Management

All threats or gestures to hurt oneself must be taken seriously regardless of the individual's developmental age. Clinical strategies must be aimed at assisting the child or adolescent in staying safe, while maintaining the least restrictive environment needed to accomplish this.

Specific treatment strategies used by the nurse vary depending on the child's living situation, psychiatric history, and social and family supports available in the community. If the child is hospitalized, the milieu will have specific strategies in place for addressing suicidal behaviors or ideation. This might involve invoking a "special watch" or "precautions" status that restricts the child's movement in and out of the living environment. All dangerous objects or potentially harmful pieces of clothing, such as shoelaces or belts, must be removed to facilitate safety.

If the child or adolescent is living at home and involved with a mental health provider in the community, interventions could include behavioral contracts to "keep safe." Parents, friends, and school personnel can assist in this process and should be brought in as supports to potentially suicidal individuals. Pfeffer (1991) emphasizes that treatment should be aimed at focusing on the motivations of the suicidal youngster. Exploration of the feelings and identification of the impetus behind the suicide attempt are essential to clinical management.

The issue of confidentiality must always be superceded by the need for safety. Therapists are discouraged from singularly dealing with suicidal clients without community support. Suicidal threats and ideation signal a crisis that requires a network of care. Prevention of suicide involves identifying this network and strengthening the communication between treating clinician, the youngster, the family, and others involved in the crisis (Pfeffer, 1988). Hospitalization should occur when the child or adolescent is no longer safe in a less restrictive environment, even if they protest and attempt to refuse the intervention.

Pfeffer (1988) suggests that clinicians should take the role of "network coordinator" for the support system, working with the involved youngster and the community linkages necessary to prevent suicide. Nurses are particularly adept at assuming this role on the clinical treatment team. Careful identification of the specific risk factors that put the individual in jeopardy of suicide becomes another part of the network coordinator's role. This involves noting exposure to suicide gestures or completions among peers, family members, or in the media. Affective illness should automatically alert the clinician that suicide risk is present whether or not the youngster raises it as an issue in treatment.

Nurses also may be involved in school-based crisis teams that provide mental health services to large numbers of youth after a death or suicide has occurred in a school (see Clinical Example). This intervention might involve individuals or groups. It is most often short term and immediate to the crisis.

TREATMENT: PRIMARY PREVENTION

At primary or preventive levels of care, nurses can offer educational programs for children and parents that deal with parenting, development of coping skills, normal growth and development, and risk factors. Nurses are most likely to encounter at-risk children and families in primary health care settings, battered women's shelters, and school-based clinics.

Helping parents and other adults closely involved with children and adolescents identify risk factors and symptoms of depression, especially when coupled with other psychiatric disorders, is essential to early treatment. Identifying suicidal risk factors and particular populations at risk is vital to prevention of suicide in adolescents. The nurse provides primary prevention services to families and other non–health care professionals, such as teachers and social workers. Their services often are indirect and consultative to others who work with children and youth.

Finn (1986) has cited affective education as an important factor in strengthening children's awareness of inner states, while increasing self-esteem. This becomes a source of primary prevention of anxiety, depression, and suicidal behavior in school-age children. School nurses and school-based nurse therapists can initiate and facilitate these school-based interventions.

Primary prevention also must be aimed at strengthening the family unit, especially in underprivileged communities where hopelessness and poverty erode parents' ability to care for their children. Head Start and other early intervention programs aimed at preschoolers are particularly useful in identifying at-risk youngsters and their parents and providing family support services needed to shore up the vulnerable family.

CLINICAL EXAMPLE

A school-based day treatment program for 10 males was run by a staff that included a clinical nurse specialist, a special education teacher, and several teacher assistants. Two of the students were kidnapped by a gunman as they walked home from being dropped off by a van in their neighborhood. The kidnapper drove both boys through the community, followed by police. The kidnapper was eventually shot and killed in front of the students. Both students suffered gunshot wounds and were hospitalized.

The crisis team mobilized for the next day of school and included the classroom staff, the school nurse, the industrial arts teacher familiar and supportive to the class, the educational administrator of the program, and the clinical nurse consultant to the program. The initial intervention involved a group between these individuals, all students, and their family members. Subsequent groups occurred twice daily for the remainder of the week as the crisis passed, the students progressed out of physical danger, and the usual therapeutic interventions of the program resumed. The youngsters injured in the kidnapping eventually recovered and rejoined the class.

Other populations at risk for mood disorders include chronically physically ill children and their families. Kashani and Hakami (1982) found that children and adolescents with cancer had a significantly higher rate of major depression when compared with normal, physically healthy populations. Nelms (1986) noted that parental recognition of depression in their chronically ill children was illness related, rather than psychiatrically related, to a mood disorder. Nurses working in settings that treat chronic physical illness can be instrumental in identifying early symptoms of depression and assisting the child and family in receiving treatment.

TREATMENT: SECONDARY INTERVENTIONS

When a mood disorder has been identified in a child or adolescent, the nurse begins providing a secondary level of care to the individual and family (Box 18-3). Planning the degree of psychiatric care required to maximize safety involves asking the following questions during a thorough evaluation:

1. How debilitating is the mood disorder? What spheres of the child are most affected by the dysfunction? Note functioning in family, school, and neighborhood.

   A number of self-report measures are available for assessing depression in children and adolescents. Self-report measures are especially useful in assessing symptoms such as sadness, feelings of worthlessness, and loss of interest in everyday activities. These symptoms particulary reflect self-perceptions and subjective reactions. The most widely used measure is the Children's Depression Inventory (Kovacs, 1981), which has normative data on same gender and age peers (Kazdin, 1990). A number of other self-report, peer-report, and significant other-report measures are available for use by clinicians of various disciplines.
2. Is individual physical safety compromised through suicide risk? Are others at risk for physical harm because of the individual's high level of impulsivity toward dangerous activity?
3. What is the family or primary caretaker's ability or willingness to seek outside interventions to treat the mood disorder? What levels of disturbance are present in the adult caretaker?
4. What resources are available within the community that can provide the least restrictive environment while maintaining safety? Can the school or other community resources be mobilized to provide increased support to the child or adolescent experiencing a debilitating mood disorder so that treatment can proceed in an outpatient rather than inpatient setting?
5. Is medication available or indicated for the individual with a mood disorder? Are family and treatment resources adaquate for maintaining a safe environment while a medication trial is attempted?

The most important question the nurse must examine in planning care for a depressed child or adolescent involves physical safety. The family's ability to join the nurse in planning care, to provide a safe environment for their offspring, and to comply with treatment recommendations will influence the decision to treat in an outpatient versus inpatient setting.

Models of Care

The three predominant modes of care for mood disorders are pharmacotherapy, milieu management, and outpatient or community management. The three overlap in many ways. For example, use of medication is appropriate in inpatient or outpatient settings. Similarly, individual, family, and group treatment can occur in the hospital and the community treatment setting.

PHARMACOTHERAPY

While antidepressant medication has been used for years with children and adolescents with mood disorders, there is little research to support the efficacy of such treatment (Ambrosini, Bianchi, Rabinovich, & Elia, 1993). Antidepressants are used successfully to treat adult patients with mood disorders; the same rate of success is less clear in developmentally younger patients.

Many reasons for the lack of documented efficacy of medication treatment in child clients have been postulated. These include a difference in the biologic nature of depression in children and youth (Ambrosini et al., 1993), an earlier onset disorder characterized as a more virulent illness not as easily responsive to medication (Geller, Cooper, Graham, Marsteller, & Bryant, 1990), and the heterogeneity of depressed children and youth compared with a more homogeneous population of depressed adults (Strober, Freeman, & Rigani, 1990). Ambro-

BOX 18–3 • NURSING DIAGNOSES AND CLINICAL EXAMPLES RELATED TO MOOD DISORDERS

NURSING DIAGNOSIS	EXAMPLE
Ineffective Individual Coping	The individual is unable to cope with tasks of daily living or stresses of life.
Disturbance in Self-Concept and Self-Esteem	The individual's view of himself or herself is distorted to negative proportions, resulting in negative self-esteem.
Altered Thought Processes	Individuals experiencing an episode of major depression or an acute manic episode as part of bipolar illness may exhibit a thought disorder that impairs judgment.
High Risk for Self-Harm	The individual expresses suicidal ideation, threats, or attempts.
Self-Care Deficit	The individual may be unable to care adequately for himself or herself (bathing, dressing, other activities of daily living) if mood disorder is acute.
Altered Nutrition	Individuals with major depression may experience a sudden weight gain or loss.
Altered Activity and Rest	Individuals with an acute episode of depression may be slowed down or sleep disordered; similarly, those with bipolar illness may be hypomanic and unable to sleep because of excessive activity.
Altered Sexuality	In adolescents, a lack of interest in sexual issues may be part of the anhedonia characteristic of a major depression.

sini et al. (1993) note that while the phenomenology of depression is characterized similarly across developmental lines, the responses to pharmacologic management suggest that differences between children, adolescents, and adult responses to medication differ greatly and should be explored further.

Nurses practice in settings in which antidepressant medications are used with youthful populations and should be aware of the management issues inherent in their use. Nursing management is influenced by the type of practice setting, the care system's philosophy around pharmacotherapy, and the length of time the nurse provides care to the client.

Inpatient settings have been most influenced by the managed care system, which often dictates length of stay in days rather than weeks and forces the milieu to treat disorders quickly and after expedient evaluation. Children may be placed on antidepressant medication and discharged before the full effects of the medication can be noted. This necessitates a clear understanding of family commitment to follow-up and ability to maintain safe management of the medication.

Careful outpatient management of antidepressant medication is especially crucial if the child or adolescent is suicidal. Parents or caretakers must thoroughly understand the responsibilities inherent in managing their child's antidepressant medication. For suicidal children and youth, outpatient management might involve dispensing a few days of medication at a time with frequent contact and renewals to lessen the chance of overdose. These medications are notably lethal when injested in large quantities.

Sudden discontinuation may produce withdrawal effects that include nausea, vomiting, diarrhea, abdominal pain, or flu-like symptoms. Medication should be gradually decreased when pharmacotherapy has ended.

Children differ in the ways they biologically metabolize antidepressants. Given their faster metabolic rate, increased relative liver mass, and lower adipose tissue mass, there is a shorter half-life with most antidepressants. Children are more susceptible to the cardiotoxic effects of tricyclic antidepressants, which can include a rare risk of sudden death (Riddle et al., 1991). The most common changes in electrocardiogram (EKG) involve a slight increase in resting heart rate (to no greater than 130 beats per minute), lengthening of the PR interval (to no more than 0.22 second), and widening of the QRS (to no more than 30% increase over baseline). The PR interval and the QRS complex of waves represent the rhythmic excitation process of the heart reflected in the EKG. A baseline EKG is essential for any child or adolescent beginning a course of treatment with antidepressant medication.

The most common side effects include dizziness, usually caused by hypotension; blurred vision; dry mouth; constipation; tachycardia; sensitivity to sunlight; and allergic skin reactions. Other side effects can include palpitations, tremors, jaundice, and blood disorders.

Lithium alters the sodium transport in nerve and muscle cells, causes a shift toward intraneuronal metabolism of catecholamines, and is used to treat bipolar disorders and other types of depression in children and adolescents. Delong and Aldershof (1987) demonstrated that lithium treatment could be beneficial in the long-term management of bipolar affective disorder and explosive aggressive disorders in children. They noted that accurate diagnosis should be followed by a lithium trial to assess the development of side effects.

Medication should never be substituted for careful psychotherapy, family counseling, and special education planning if warranted. Antidepressants should be used after other methods of treatment have been unsuccessful. This is especially true given the lack of efficacy of this form of treatment for depression.

MILIEU MANAGEMENT

The need for psychiatric hospitalization can be assessed after reviewing several factors. Hendren (1991) notes the following as important guidelines when considering hospitalization. The guidelines have been adapted for children and adolescents with mood disorders:

1. Nature of the presenting psychiatric disorder
   - Severity and duration of the mood disorder
   - Degree of impairment
   - Coping abilities of the child or adolescent and family
   - Social and cultural supports
2. Capacity to relate to others
   - How available is the child or adolescent to a therapeutic interpersonal relationship?
   - Will a trial of antidepressant medication make the child or adolescent more available to therapeutic resources?
3. Capacity to benefit from treatment
   - Might the mood disordered individual benefit from a period of inpatient hospitalization?
4. Appropriateness of less restrictive settings
   - Can the child or adolescent be managed safely in a less restrictive setting, such as

outpatient, day treatment, or residential treatment setting?

Are community resources available that will facilitate the discharge of the individual to a less restrictive setting?

Psychiatric hospitalization is the most restrictive type of psychiatric care and usually occurs after the individual is determined to be any of the following:

- A danger to self, others, or property
- Exhibiting bizarre behavior
- In need of high-dose, unusual medication that requires careful management at initial administration
- In need of 24-hour skilled observation

Once the child or adolescent is admitted to the inpatient setting, nursing goals involve orienting the individual to the treatment setting, the staff, fellow clients, and the existing unit routine. Assessment of suicide potential will result in "special watch" or "precautions" status that is reviewed on a regular basis. In most milieus, unit privileges may be related to special watch status and the suicidal status of the client.

When the individual is suffering from a major depression, activities of daily living skills must be assessed. The goal of nursing interventions at this time is to return the individual to the same or a higher level of functioning.

Social interactions with peers and staff should be encouraged, and isolation on the living unit should be discouraged. Use of a time-out room or bedroom for seclusion might necessitate one-to-one observation, depending on the individual's suicide risk. Unit consequences for inappropriate or unsafe behavior might be initially altered to accommodate a child's period of adjustment to the unit. However, rules and consequences should be integrated into the structure and boundaries of the unit as quickly as possible (Pearson, 1992).

The managed care system of psychiatric treatment with its concomitant shortened length of stay has forced inpatient nursing staff to be creative in their interventions and management of children and adolescents with mood disorders. Stabilization of depressive symptomatology, initiation of antidepressant medication, and return to the community become the primary goals of the brief time in the hospital.

PSYCHOTHERAPY FOR MOOD DISORDERS

Clinical management of the child or adolescent with a mood disorder will depend on the following:

- Severity of the mood disorder: Acute episodes of mania in the individual with bipolar illness will be difficult to manage with outpatient care and may require at least a short hospitalization. Similarly, a major depression may require hospitalization to ensure the individual's safety and maximize treatment interventions. In both situations, the individual must experience some stabilization of mood and be able to interpersonally engage before other types of therapy, such as individual, family, or group, will be most effective.
- Availability of treatment resources: Planning outpatient care will depend, in part, on the availability of community resources. Many clinic settings provide one mode of treatment at a time, and the clinician will be forced to decide on the best intervention at that point in the child's life.
- Willingness of the family to participate in treatment: Family style of coping and level of dysfunction will influence and predict the course of illness in a child or adolescent with a mood disorder. Increasingly, the family's role in mental health issues is recognized. Measures of family environment have been found to predict the course of some psychiatric disorders; family treatment interventions may provide more efficacy than patient-centered models of care.

Because of its genetic origins, children and youth with depression often have parents with mood disorders that influence their style of parenting and ability to cope with a disturbed child. The children of disturbed parents frequently show a higher rate of dysfunction that those from emotionally healthy parents.

Asarnow and Horton (1990) found that most parents of children hospitalized with severe depressive and schizophrenia spectrum disorders noted "disruption in their family lives, personal relationships, social and leisure activities, and work functioning" (p. 154). They also noted the importance of seeking community support and resources as assistance to their child and family.

Children become depressed for obvious and not-so-obvious reasons. The death of a pet or close family relative may precipitate a depressive episode in a child or adolescent. This varies from the dysthymia, or chronic depressed mood, that comes from living with dysfunctional parents, living in poverty, or living in a violent environment where safety is uncertain.

While level of depression and degree of suicide risk influence the decision to psychiatrically hospitalize, the level of organization in the family system and the ability to keep the individual safe also can influence the nurse's care decisions.

Therapy Models

INDIVIDUAL PSYCHOTHERAPY

The therapist's theoretical framework will influence the type of treatment. A major goal of individual psychotherapy is to examine the child's self-perception of competence (Weller & Weller, 1991). Ascertaining how much the child's perception reflects reality will affect the intervention. Interventions may focus on social skills training or resolution or acceptance of life stressors leading to the depression, or they may involve play therapy to help the younger child discharge stress through motoric activities and use of toys.

Cognitive therapy models assume that depression is the result of irrational beliefs and distorted cognitions. The role of the therapist is to challenge these distorted cognitions while encouraging the child or adolescent to see and practice alternative behaviors. Cognitive therapy models are flexible and particularly useful for mildly depressed individuals.

GROUP PSYCHOTHERAPY

Nurses have historically used groups in inpatient and outpatient settings to provide health teaching and as a therapeutic tool to influence change. These might involve community groups in the milieu, activity groups or social skill development groups in school settings, or psychotherapy groups for a specific developmental cohort of children. Individuals hospitalized because of a manic episode may need a period of stabilization before joining a milieu community or therapy group. Integration should occur as soon as the client is able to safely handle the experience.

Children and adolescents with chronic mood disorders function best when integrated with a variety of individuals from other diagnostic realms. The depressed individual may tend to be quiet and uninvolved while experiencing difficulties in communicating. Engagement of a group composed entirely of these individuals may be problematic. Socialization may be enhanced by exposure to other, more communicative individuals.

Adolescents will especially make use of group therapy that focuses on interpersonal learning, affective identification, communication skills, and expression of affect. Role playing and therapeutic games may assist this process.

FAMILY THERAPY

As with other forms of treatment, the clinician's theoretical framework will influence the type of family treatment used when a child or adolescent has a mood disorder. Specific literature about family treatment with affective disorder individuals is scarce. Pofnanski and Krull (1970) noted that families in which offspring were depressed tended to have a lack of generational boundaries, severe marital conflict, projection of parental feelings to the child or adolescent, rigid or chaotic rules, and disengaged or enmeshed relationships.

The importance of family interventions in the treatment of depressed youngsters is unquestioned. Regardless of one's clinical view of mood disorders, their genesis, or their treatment, one must recognize the importance of the family system in influencing outcome and recovery.

Family attitudes about the affected individual, the family view of medication, and the family's willingness to engage in a treatment process will influence outcome. The younger the child, the more dependent the clinician is on family cooperation and involvement in treatment. The emancipated adolescent might warrant an individual approach to their disorder; children must have active parental consent and commitment to the treatment.

Choosing an intense family therapy model of care versus family counseling that focuses more on parenting techniques and management will depend on the willingness and ability of the family to self-reflect, understand, and benefit from more intense interventions.

The movement towards more biopsychosocial models of care influences a more holistic, systems perspective. With this perspective, the family therapist treating an affective disorder integrates the body and brain, mind and person, family and community, medical science and art, and research subject and researcher. With this model, the family therapist continues using the basic principles of family therapy while integrating the individual's vulnerability or dysfunction. The biopsychosocial interactional model broadens the role of the therapist to include medical management of the individual's difficulties.

Implications for Nursing Research and Practice

Nurses are in a key position to provide primary, secondary, and tertiary levels of care to individuals with mood disorders. Opie and Slater (1988) discuss the mental health needs of children in

CLINICAL EXAMPLE: JENNY

Jenny was a 12-year-old female who revealed to her outpatient therapist during a weekly session that she had overdosed on her insulin the previous day. Diagnosed with insulin-dependent diabetes mellitus 2 years previously, she had always been responsible for her own insulin injections, diet, and glucose testing.

She had begun outpatient therapy after she stopped attending school the previous September. Juvenile authorities had become involved and ordered her and her mother to obtain therapy services. The family complied with this, and Jenny and her mother were each seen weekly for therapy.

Jenny initially presented to her therapist as an odd girl who seemed unrelated and distant. Jenny had slowly become attached to her outpatient therapist and, with her assistance, had begun to confront some of the behaviors that made her peer relationships difficult. She had begun attending school the previous spring with much therapeutic and academic support. Now, in the summertime, Jenny's therapist had announced that she was leaving the agency and would no longer be treating Jenny or her mother.

Other losses included the untimely death of Jenny's grandmother 1 year prior to the overdose and her father's death from heart failure when Jenny was 7 years old. Jenny was the youngest of four children. The three oldest children were in their late 20s and early 30s; Jenny had been born when her parents were in their mid-40s.

Jenny's mother presented as a depressed, overwhelmed woman who was not employed and lived in public-assistance housing. The family was financially supported by social security and a small pension. While Jenny's mother seemed concerned about her daughter's suicide attempt, she admitted to the nurse evaluator that she had tried suicide a "couple of times," and nothing came of it. She also admitted that she had been depressed much of her life, especially after her husband died. She had experienced one trial of antidepressant medication after his death and had found this helpful.

Jenny's diabetes had been diagnosed 2 years previously after she presented with symptoms of polyuria and polydipsia. She was hospitalized for 9 days for stabilization of diabetes and began following an insulin regimen that involved injections three times a day. Her therapist believed that she viewed herself as permanently damaged and "bad" because of the diabetes. As the therapist announced the need for termination, Jenny had just begun talking about her diabetes being punishment for being a "bad person."

She arrived on the milieu neatly dressed, with one suitcase. She presented as an obese youngster with black hair and dark eyes. Her affect was constricted, and she made infrequent eye contact. She spoke only when asked direct questions and cried openly when her mother left the unit. She curled up on her bed and refused supper her first evening on the unit.

The three predominant nursing diagnoses in her initial nursing care plan follow.

1. High Risk for Self-Directed Violence related to hopelessness, depressed mood, a chronic physical condition, loss of a beloved therapist, and recent death of a grandmother as evidenced by self-destructive behavior with insulin, talking of committing suicide, and thoughts of being "bad."

SHORT-TERM GOAL

Client will seek out staff when feelings of self-harm occur. The client will make short-term contracts around keeping safe.

LONG-TERM GOAL

Client will not attempt to harm herself during the hospitalization.

NURSING INTERVENTIONS

1. Place Jenny on a level 1 precautions, which would restrict her to the unit and require checks by staff every 5 minutes.
2. Avoid isolation in her room, and require that she stay in the dayroom and by nurses' station during wakening hours. Keep the door to her bedroom open when she is asleep
3. Carefully supervise all glucose testing and insulin administration. Allow Jenny to draw up insulin into the syringe, with the nurse checking the dose before administration.
4. Involve Jenny in daily routine of unit program, including daily community group, classroom instruction on the unit, and family group twice a week.

2. Altered Nutrition, Less than Body Requirements related to depressed mood, lack of appetite, ideas of self-injury as evidenced by irregular eating patterns, recent loss of weight, instability of insulin requirements.

SHORT-TERM GOAL

The client will maintain stable eating habits and begin to eat in a regular, planned way that assists in regulation of diabetes.

LONG-TERM GOAL

The client will maintain a healthy weight status while covering insulin needs with diet, medication, and exercise.

(*continued*)

CLINICAL EXAMPLE: JENNY *(Continued)*

NURSING INTERVENTIONS

1. In collaboration with pediatrician and nutritionist, nursing staff will develop a diet plan that balances nutritional and metabolic needs of client.
2. Involve Jenny in planning diet and exercise strategies that help regulate insulin needs.
3. Assess knowledge gaps in management of diabetes and diet and provide education as needed.

3. Social Isolation/Impaired Interaction related to absence of peer relationships, unresolved grief over grandmother's death, distorted view of self as defective person as evidenced by sad, dull affect; social withdrawal; dysfunctional interactions with peers.

SHORT-TERM GOAL

The client will develop a trusting relationship with a staff member within 5 days and will seek that person out when they are on the milieu.

LONG-TERM GOAL

The client will begin to have social relationships with peers by discharge and will appear less socially odd.

NURSING INTERVENTIONS

1. One staff member will talk individually with Jenny each shift, attempting to encourage trust and positive regard.
2. The client will be encouraged to attend group activities on the unit, at her own pace and with staff support.
3. Staff will begin to provide direct feedback to client about her behavior and the effect if has on peers.
4. Assist the client in planning structured activities that include school, regular meals, and rest periods while living in the milieu.
5. Staff will provide positive reinforcement for client behaviors that are adaptive and more health promoting (i.e., eating in healthy ways, remembering regular glucose testing, eating regular and carefully planned meals).

Jenny made enormous gains during her hospitalization and developed a close relationship with her nurse therapist on the unit. She had no more episodes of trying to overdose with insulin, managed to develop a more stable diet and exercise routine, and was eventually discharged home to her mother with a referral to outpatient mental health services. She began regularly attending school and at a 6-month follow-up was doing well in the community.

school systems and nurses' key roles in providing preventive mental health care. Affective education and a system of early identification of emotional disturbance similar to early identification of physical health problems are encouraged. Head Start programs provide a particularly good arena for mental health promotion. Nursing interventions can help families minimize stress and maximize social supports (Killeen, Smith, & Killinger, 1990). This is one of many arenas in which nursing interventions prevent development of mood disorders or provide multidimensional interventions at early stages of illness.

School-based early intervention programs promote collaboration between parent, teacher, and mental health nurse. Treatment is facilitated in a "mutually familiar and accepted environment" (Opie & Slater, 1988). Children at risk for depression and their parents should be supported at early signs of the disorder, reducing the need for hospitalization and other more intensive forms of treatment.

Gross and Semprevivo (1988) studied charts of psychiatrically hospitalized women with children younger than age 6. They found a notable lack of information assessing the quality of the mother–child relationship or the mother's ability to resume her parenting role post-hospitalization. Given that maternal absence can preclude a child's depression, nurses must consider the parent–child dyad whenever psychiatric hospitalization occurs. This is especially true if the reason for parental inpatient care involves a mood disorder and thus increases the child's genetic vulnerability.

Nursing research should focus on the efficacy of creative treatment strategies that emphasize the child and family rather than the mood disorder. Given the questionable efficacy of antidepressants in treating childhood depression and the lack of research documenting treatment success, aggressive interventions that improve functioning must be proposed and researched. Nursing theories can provide the framework of such interventions.

Perhaps the most important role nurses can take in preventing, treating, and researching mood disorders is one of advocacy. Depression in childhood and adolescence results from a complex interplay of factors, including parental dysfunction, marital stress, and most importantly, poverty. The fewer economic and emotional resources available to families, the more the risk for psychiatric disorder, especially mood disorders.

This nursing advocacy must extend to the state and federal legislative efforts aimed at strengthening children and families. Welfare reforms that support families, early intervention programs, school-based treatment resources, and parent advocacy represent arenas where the proactive role taken by nurses may prevent the development of psychiatric disorders. Genetic vulnerability alone does not account for the development of a mood disorder, but rather the layering with interpersonal and societal stressors precipitating the illness. Nurses are challenged to ameliorate societal stressors at multiple levels of care and advocacy (see Clinical Example: Jenny).

Summary

Mood disorders in children and adolescents are some of the most documented and researched disorders in child psychiatric care. The historic perspectives of mood disorders are discussed. The biologic theories of depression and mood disorders include neurotransmitter, monoamine, neuroendocrine, and genetic abnormalities; psychosocial theories encompass intrapsychic, cognitive, learning, behavioral, parent–child relationship, and biobehavioral models. Manifestations of depressive and bipolar syndromes and primary prevention have been described. Clinical management of the child or adolescent with mood disorders include attention to safety issues, confidentiality, coordination of support systems, crisis intervention, pharmacotherapy, milieu management, and psychotherapy for the client and family.

REFERENCES

Abramson, L. Y., Metalsky, G. I., & Alloy, L. B. (1989). Hopelessness depression: A theory-based subtype of depression. *Psychological Review, 96,* 358–372.

Ambrosini, P. J., Bianchi, M.D., Rabinovich, H., & Elia, J. (1993). Antidepressant treatments in children and adolescents: I: Affective disorders. *Journal of the American Academy of Child and Adolescent Psychiatry, 32*(1), 1–6.

American Psychiatric Association (1994). *Diagnostic and statistical manual* (4th ed.). Washington, D C: Author.

Asarnow, J. R., & Horton, A. A. (1990). Coping and stress in families of child psychiatric inpatients: Parents of children with depressive and schizophrenia spectrum disorders. *Child Psychiatry and Human Development, 21*(2), 145–157.

Beardslee, W. R., Bemporad, J., Keller, M. B., & Klerman, G. (1983). Children of parents with major affective disorders: A review. *American Journal of Psychiatry, 140,* 825–832.

Beck, A. T. (1987). Cognitive models of depression. *Journal of Cognitive Psychotherapy, An International Quarterly, 1,* 5–37.

Borst, S. R., Noam, G. G., & Bartok, J. A. (1991). Adolescent suicidality: A clinical-developmental approach. *Journal of the American Academy of Child and Adolescent Psychiatry, 30,* 796–803.

Boyd, J. H., & Moscicki, E. K. (1986). Firearms and youth suicide. *American Journal of Public Health, 76,* 1240–1242.

Brent, D. A., Kerr, M. M., Goldstein, C., Bozigar, J., Wartella, M., & Allan, M. J. (1989). An outbreak of suicide and suicidal behavior in a high school. *Journal of the American Academy of Child and Adolescent Psychiatry, 28,* 918–924.

Carlson, G. A. (1982). Suicidal behavior and depression in children and adolescents. *Journal of the American Academy of Child and Adolescent Psychiatry, 21,* 361–368.

Carlson, G. A. (1983). Bipolar affective disorders in childhood and adolescence. In D. P. Cantwell & G. A. Carlson (Eds.), *Affective disorders in childhood and adolescence—an update.* New York, Spectrum, 1986, pp. 61–84.

Carlson, G. A., Asarnow, J. R., & Orbach, I. (1987). Developmental aspects aspects of suicidal behavior in children: I. *Journal of the American Academy of Child and Adolescent Psychiatry, 26,* 186–192.

Carlson, G. A., & Strober, M. (1978). Manic-depressive illness in early adolescence. *Journal of the American Academy of Child Psychiatry, 17,* 138–153.

Clarizio, H. F. (1985). Cognitive-behavioral treatment of childhood depression. *Psychology in Schools, 22,* 308–322.

Delong, G. R., & Aldershof, A. L. (1987). Long-term experience with lithium treatment in childhood: Correlation with clinical diagnosis. *Journal of the American Academy of Child and Adolescent Psychiatry, 26,* 389–394.

de Wilde, E. J., Kienhorst, I. C. W. M., Diekstra, R. F. W., & Wolters, W. H. G. (1992). The relationship between adolescent suicidal behavior and life events of childhood and adolescence. *American Journal of Psychiatry, 149,* 45–51.

Erikson, E. H. (1963). *Childhood and society* (2nd ed.). New York: W. W. Norton.

Finn, P. (1986). Self-destructive behavior in school-aged children: A hidden problem? *Pediatric Nursing, 12,* 198.

Fleming, J. E., & Offord, D. R. (1990). Epidemiology of childhood depressive disorders: A critical review. *Journal of the American Academy of Child and Adolescent Psychiatry, 29*(4), 571–580.

Fleming, J. E., Offord, D. R., & Boyle, M. H. (1989). The Ontario child health study: Prevalence of childhood and adolescent depression in the community. *British Journal of Psychiatry, 155,* 647–654.

Freud, S. (1917). *Mourning and melancholia* (standard ed., Vol. 14) (pp. 243–258). London: Hogarth Press.

Geller, B., Cooper, T. B., Graham, D.L., Marsteller, F. A., & Bryant, D. M. (1990). Double-blind placebo-controlled study of nortriptyline in depressed adolescents using a "fixed plasma level": Design. *Psychopharmacology Bulletin, 26,* 85–90.

Gershon, E. S., Targum, S. D., Kessler, L. R., Mazure, C. M., & Bunney, Jr., W. E. (1977). Genetic studies and biological strategies in the affective disorders. *Progress in Medical Genetics, 2,* 101–164.

Glaser, K. (1968). Masked depression in children and adolescents. *Annual Progress in Child Psychiatry and Child Development, 1,* 345–355.

Gould, M. S., & Shaffer, D. (1986). The impact of suicide in television movies: Evidence of imitation. *New England Journal of Medicine, 315,* 1257–1261.

Gould, M. S., Wallenstein, S., & Kleinman, M. (1990). Time-clustering of teenage suicide. *American Journal of Epidemiology*, *131*, 71–78.

Gross, D., & Semprevivo, D. (1989). Mentally ill mothers of young children. *Journal of Child and Adolescent Psychiatric and Mental Health Nursing*, *2*, 105–109.

Hazell, P., & Lewin, T. (1993). Friends of adolescent suicide attempters and completers. *Journal of the American Academy of Child and Adolescent Psychiatry*, *32*, 76–81.

Hendren, R. L. (1991). Determining the need for inpatient treatment. In R. L. Hendren & I. N. Berlin (Eds.), *Psychiatric inpatient care of children and adolescents: A multicultural approach* (pp. 38–65). New York: John Wiley & Sons.

Jacobson, J. M. (1991). The relationship between social support and depression in adolescents. *Journal of Child and Adolescent Psychiatric and Mental Health Nursing*, *4*(1), 20–24.

Kashani, J. H., Carlson, G. A., Beck, N. C., Hoeper, E. W., Corcoran, M. A., McAllister, J. A., Fallani, C., Rosenberg, T. K., & Reid, J. C. (1987). Depression, depressive symptoms, and depressed mood among a community sample of adolescents. *American Journal of Psychiatry*, *144*, 931–933.

Kashani, J., & Hakami, N. (1982). Depression in children and adolescents with malignancy. *Canadian Journal of Psychiatry*, *27*, 474.

Kashani, J. H., & Sherman, D. D. (1988). Childhood depression: Epidemiology, etiological models, and treatment implications. *Integrative Psychiatry*, *6*, 1–8.

Kazdin, A. E. (1990). Childhood depression. *Journal of Child Psychology and Psychiatry*, *31*, 121–160.

Keller, M. B., Beardslee, W. R., Dorer, D. J. Lavori, P. W., Samuelson, H. & Klerman, G. R. (1986). Impact of severity and chronicity of parental affective illness on adaptive functioning and psychopathology in children. *Archives of General Psychiatry*, *43*, 930–93.

Killeen, M. R., Smith, C. A., & Killinger, P. A. (1990). Using head start centers for teaching mental health promotion. *Journal of Child and Adolescent Psychiatric and Mental Health Nursing*, *3*, 79–84.

Kovacs, M. (1981). Rating scales to assess depression in school aged children. *Acta Paedopsychiatrica*, *46*, 305–315.

Kovacs, M., Feinbert, T. L., & Crouse-Novak, M. (1984). Depressive disorders in childhood. II: A longitudinal study of the risk for subsequent major depression. *Archives of General Psychiatry*, *41*, 643–649.

Kovacs, M., Goldston, D., & Gatsonis, C. (1993). Suicidal behaviors and childhood-onset depressive disorders: A longitudinal investigation. *Journal of the American Academy of Child and Adolescent Psychiatry*, *32*, 8–20.

Lewis, M., & Volkmar, F. (1990). *Clinical aspects of child and adolescent development.* Philadelphia: Lea & Febiger.

Mendelson, M. (1982). Psychodynamics of depression. In E. S. Paykel (Ed.), *Handbook of affective disorders* (pp. 162–174). New York: Guilford.

Myers, K., McCauley, E., Calderon, R., & Treder, R. (1991). The 3-year longitudinal course of suicidality and predictive factors for subsequent suicidality in youths with major depressive disorder. *Journal of the American Academy of Child and Adolescent Psychiatry*, *30*, 804–810.

Nelms, B. C. (1985). Stress during childhood: Long-lasting effects? *Pediatric Nursing*, *11*, 95–98.

Nurnberger, J. I., & Gershon, E. S. (1982). Genetics. In E. S. Paykel (Ed.), *Handbook of affective disorders* (pp. 109–125). New York: Guilford.

Opie, N. D., & Slater, P. (1988). Mental health needs of children in school: Role of the child psychiatric mental health nurse. *Journal of Child and Adolescent Psychiatric and Mental Health Nursing*, *1*, 31–35.

Pearson, G. S. (1992). Nursing interventions with children and adolescents experiencing thought disorders. In P. West & C. L. S. Evans (Eds.), *Psychiatric and mental health nursing with children and adolescents* (pp. 329–342). Gaithersburg, MD: Aspen Publications.

Pfeffer, C. R. (1991). Attempted suicide in children and adolescents: causes and management. In M. Lewis (Ed.), *Child and adolescent psychiatry: A comprehensive textbook* (pp. 664–672). Baltimore: Williams and Wilkins.

Pfeffer, C. R. (1986). *The suicidal child.* New York: The Guilford Press.

Pfeffer, C. R. (1988). Risk factors associated with youth suicide: A clinical perspective. *Psychiatric Annals*, *18*, 652–656.

Pfeffer, C. R., Newcorn, J., Kaplan, G. Mifruchi, M. S., & Plutchik, R. (1988). Suicidal behavior in adolescent psychiatric inpatients. *Journal of the American Academy of Child and Adolescent Psychiatry*, *27*, 357–361.

Pofnanski, E. O. & Krull, J. P. (1970). Childhood depression: Clinical characteristics of overtly depressed children. *Archives of General Psychiatry*, *23*, 8–15.

Puig-Antich, J. (1982). Major depression and conduct disorder in prepuberty. *Journal of the American Academy of Child Psychiatry*, *21*, 118–128.

Riddle, M. A., Nelson, J. C., Kleinman, C. S., Rasmusson, A., Leckman, J. F., King, R. A., & Cohen, D. J. (1991). Sudden death in children receiving Norpramin: A review of three reported cases and commentary. *Journal of the American Academy of Child and Adolescent Psychiatry*, *30*, 104–108.

Rie, H. E. (1966). Depression in childhood: A survey of some pertinent contributions. *Journal of the American Academy of Child Psychiatry*, *5*, 653–685.

Rochlin, G. (1959). The loss complex. *Journal of the American Psychoanalytic Association*, *7*, 299–316.

Rutter, M., & Garmezy, N. (1983). Developmental psychopathology. In E. M. Hetherington (Ed.), *Socialization, personality and social development. Mussen's handbook of child psychology* (Vol. 4). New York: John Wiley and Sons.

Sachar, E. J. (1982). Endocrine abnormalities in depression. In E. S. Paykel (Ed.), *Handbook of affective disorders* (pp. 191–201). New York: Guilford.

Seligman, M. E. P. (1975). *Helplessness: On depression, development and death.* San Francisco: Freeman.

Shaffer, D. (1974). Suicide in childhood and early adolescence. *Journal of Child Psychology and Psychiatry*, *15*, 275–291.

Shaffer, D., & Fisher, P. (1981). The epidemiology of suicide in children and adolescents. *Journal of the American Academy of Child and Adolescent Psychiatry*, *20*, 545–565.

Shaffer, D., Garland, A., Gould, M., Fisher, P., & Trautman, P. (1988). Preventing adolescent suicide. *Journal of the American Academy of Child and Adolescent Psychiatry*, *27*, 675–687.

Shafii, M., Carrigan, S., Whittinghill, J. R. & Derrick, A. (1985). Psychological autopsy of completed suicide in children and adolescents. *American Journal of Psychiatry*, *142*, 1061–1064.

Spitz, R. A. (1946). Anaclitic depression. *Psychoanalytic Study of the Child*, *2*, 213–241.

Spitzer, R. L., Endicott, J., & Robins, E. (1978). Research diagnostic criteria. *Archives of General Psychiatry*, *35*, 773–782.

Strober, M., Freeman, R., & Rigani, J. (1990). The pharmacotherapy of depressive illness in adolescence: I: An open label trial of imipramine. *Psychopharmacology Bulletin*, *26*, 80–84.

Weinberg, W. A., & Brumback, R. P. (1976). Mania in childhood. *American Journal of Diseases of Children, 130*, 380–385.

Weissman, M. M., Gershon, E. S., & Kidd, K. K. (1984a). Psychiatric disorders in the relatives of probands with affective disorders: The Yale-NIMH collaborative family study. *Archives of General Psychiatry, 41*, 13.

Weissman, M. M., Prusoff, B. A., Gammon, G. D. Merikangas, K. R., Leckman, J. F., & Kidd, K. H. (1984b). Psychopathology in the children (age 6–18) of depressed and normal parents. *Journal of the American Academy of Child Psychiatry, 23*, 78–84.

Welner, A., Welner, Z., & Fishman, R. (1979). Psychiatric inpatient: Eight to ten year follow-up. *Archives of General Psychiatry, 36*, 698–700.

Whybrow, P. C., Akiskal, H. S., & McKinney, W. T. (1984). *Mood disorders: Toward a new psychobiology.* New York: Plenum.

Zis, A. P., & Goodwin, F. K. (1982). The amine hypothesis. In E. S. Paykel (Ed.), *Handbook of affective disorders* (pp. 175–190). New York: Guilford.

CHAPTER

19

Pervasive Developmental Disorders

Geraldine S. Pearson

The term pervasive developmental disorders (PDD) has historically applied to a spectrum of psychiatric disorders in children characterized by the most serious deficits in cognitive, social, and emotional functioning. This has included diagnoses such as infantile autism or Kanner's autism (Kanner, 1943), childhood schizophrenia (Fish, 1977), and borderline syndrome of childhood (Pine, 1983).

In DSM IV (APA, 1994) PDD is characterized on Axis T and includes autistic, Rhett's, childhood disintegrative, and Asperger's disorders and pervasive developmental disorder not otherwise specified (PDD, NOS) (American Psychiatric Association [APA], 1994). Autism has been well researched and defined; this is not the case for variants of this diagnosis. Children who present with the social dysfunction of autism but without the severity and compromised functioning in other developmental realms are less understood and defined.

The PDD, NOS diagnosis is used when criteria are not met for a specific PDD. While each disorder has idiosyncratic characteristics, PDD usually is defined as a disorder with a qualitative impairment in social relatedness and interaction or in the development of verbal and nonverbal communication skills. As stated in DSM IV, "the qualitative impairments that define these conditions (PDD) are distinctly deviant relative to the individual's developmental level or mental age" (APA, p. 65). DSM-IV has addressed the need for a more descriptive diagnostic schema than that which previously existed. This chapter reviews the disorders encompassed by a PDD diagnosis.

These children present complicated challenges to nurses providing care in psychiatric and nonpsychiatric settings. While many are successfully managed at home with special school services, they often require inpatient or residential placement for stabilization and medication management. Self-help skills generally are delayed; normal socialization skills may be absent.

The chronicity of the disorder coupled with unclear etiology stresses normal family resources. Family dysfunction creates another dimension of disorder requiring intervention. These children usually challenge the most functional families, especially at points of developmental change, such as beginning school or early adolescence.

Barbara Schoen Johnson: CHILD, ADOLESCENT AND FAMILY PSYCHIATRIC NURSING, © 1994 J.B. Lippincott Company

Childhood Autism

Kanner (1943) first defined the spectrum of behaviors that became known as early infantile autism. While he noted the early biologic origins of the disorder, subsequent researchers tended to attribute a psychogenic cause to the disorder that blamed parental, or more specifically maternal, dysfunction, for the child's development of autism.

This attribution of childhood autism to parental dysfunction has been discounted; it became evident that parents of autistic children were not deficient in their childrearing abilities (McAdoo & DeMyer, 1978) and did not differ with matched controls of normal parents in areas of warmth or caretaking (DeMyer, Hingtgen, & Jackson, 1981). Infantile autism has become known as a disorder of early child development characterized by autistic social dysfunction, gross deficits in language, and impairments in communication. Associated features can include a resistance to environmental change, oddities of movement, self-mutilation, self-stimulation, excessive fascination with or attachment to inanimate objects, and an absence of imaginative play (Cohen, Paul, & Volkmar, 1987).

Autism becomes evident before 36 months of age (APA, 1994). While many parents will report a period of normal interaction between their infant and others, the quality of the relationships between the autistic infant and others seems compromised. These infants often are unresponsive to touch and difficult to comfort.

The young autistic child may engage in predominantly solitary activities, with little or no response to familiar adults. There is a striking lack of interest in the social environment but extreme sensitivity to the animate environment. For example, children may become quite distressed if the furniture arrangement is changed in the household (Volkmar, 1987) (see Clinical Example: Jon and Clinical Example: Diane).

While always compromised in their developmental gains, the major behavior problems that children with autism present in the early preschool years tend to lessen, especially with structured, intensive educational or treatment interventions. Some children become somewhat independent in their functioning as adults, although they most always retain some form of the impairment in social relationships (Wing, 1980).

Other individuals face increasingly difficult problems in adolescence and young adulthood and exhibit behavior characterized by temper tantrums and aggression (Gillberg & Schaumann, 1981). Prognosis can be related to intelligence (DeMyer et al., 1973). While other psychiatric diagnoses may be imposed on individuals with autism as they move into young adulthood, the relationship between autism and schizophrenia remains unproven. Although the presenting symptoms are similar (i.e., impaired social interactions), verbal and nonverbal communication, the clinical history, and progression of the disorder are markedly different (Wing & Attwood, 1987).

Asperger's Syndrome

This syndrome has been used to describe some individuals who vary in their autistic symptomatology. They make spontaneous approaches to others that are characterized as peculiar, one-sided, or naive. Speech may be better than that of autistic individuals, but nonverbal communication remains impaired. Individuals with Asperger's syndrome have been characterized as "active but odd" (Wing & Attwood, 1987).

Some clinicians have used Asperger's syndrome to describe individuals with unusual social relatedness accompanied by good language abilities (Wing, (1981). Asperger has acknowledged many similarities between his syndrome and Kanner's infantile autism. The predominant difference involves Asperger's view that autism is a psychotic process, while his syndrome represents a stable personality trait (Kilman & Negri-Shoultz, 1987). Most researchers agree that Asperger's syndrome is a slightly different manifestation of the same problems that typify autism. It is often not differentiated in discussions involving infantile autism.

Fragile X Syndrome

Fragile X syndrome is defined as part of a constellation of developmental disorders encompassed by PDD because of its overlap with infantile autism. Identified in 1969 by Lubs, it represents a chromosomal disorder in which a pinched or constricted end on the X chromosome is present in mentally retarded males.

The disorder follows an X-linked mendelian inheritance pattern in which an unaffected female carrier has a 50% chance of transmitting the affected X chromosome to her daughters. They then become carriers and have a 50% chance of transmitting the affected X chromosome to their sons,

CLINICAL EXAMPLE: JON

When the nurse evaluator for a university-affiliated center for developmental disorders visited the family requesting an evaluation for their 3½-year-old son Jon, she found the child running aimlessly through the house. He muttered repetitive words and made no eye contact with the nurse or his mother. He did not verbally or visually acknowledge the nurse's presence and brushed by her as if she were a piece of furniture.

His mother appeared exhausted and depressed, cradling her newborn son on her arm. When she escorted the nurse to the barren living room, she gestured to the kitchen where the table top sat on its side and the legs and screws lay in pieces on the floor. As Jon passed, he began screaming and flapping his hands. His mother wearily offered the nurse a chair and began nursing her baby.

She began describing the extreme difficulty she and her husband had in managing Jon. He was frequently sleepless, and his parents had resorted to locking him in his barren room at night to prevent his wanderings. She shared that they had sought the evaluation in desperation at the advice of their pediatrician who believed Jon was autistic.

who are affected with the disorder (Dykens & Leckman, 1990).

Unlike other recessive X-linked disorders, approximately one third to one half of the women with the fragile X marker will exhibit some aspect of the disorder, albeit mild. This includes learning disabilities, historically poor school performance, and mild to moderate retardation (Fishburn, Turner, Daniel, & Brookwell, 1983; Hagerman & Smith, 1983). These affected mothers are likely to have 50% of their daughters as carriers and all sons affected by fragile X syndrome. This contrasts with asymptomatic female carriers; their sons who inherit the affected chromosome have a 75% rate of clinical impairment, and 30% of the daughters are affected.

Males with fragile X syndrome tend to exhibit characteristic physical features that include an elongated face, high forehead, and enlarged ears. Other symptoms have included connective tissue dysplasia and macroorchidism or enlarged testes (Bregman, Dykens, Watson, Ort, and Leckman, 1987).

Fragile X syndrome is the most common inherited form of mental retardation in males. It may account for 2% to 7% of all cases of mental retardation in males (Webb, Bundey, Thake, and Todd, 1986). Intellectual impairments can range from borderline to profound although affected males with average or near average IQs have been noted (Daker, Chidiac, Fear, and Berry, 1981). Dykens, Hodapp, and Leckman (1987) found relative weakness in sequential processing skills coupled with significant strength in simultaneous processing abilities. Also, fragile X males exhibit some linguistic impairment with particular problems in auditory memory, reception, and articulation (Howard-Peebles, Stoddard, and Mims, 1979).

Fragile X males may exhibit a spectrum of behavioral difficulties, including aggressive outbursts, hyperactivity, attention deficits, and self-injurious behavior (Bregman et al., 1987). The estimated presence of infantile autism in this population has ranged from 7% (Bregman, Leckman, and Ort, 1988) to 14% (Fryns, Jacobs, Kleczkowska, and Van den Berghe, 1984) to 47% (Hagerman, Jackson, Levitas, Rimland, and Braden, 1986). While the numbers of fragile X males with autism may be low, many of these individuals exhibit significant difficulties with impulsivity, hyperactivity, and attention (Hagerman, Murphy, and Wittenberger, 1987). Many (29%) meet DSM IV criteria for attention-deficit hyperactivity disorder. Both disorders have significant effects on the social adaptability and appropriateness of these individuals.

There have been attempts to identify the presence of autism in individuals with fragile X syndrome. Research showed that the fragile X syndrome accounted for the developmental problems in some patients with infantile autism. However, the frequency of the disorder in autistic males was not significantly greater than that seen in other retarded, nonautistic males (Watson et al., 1984).

Childhood Schizophrenia

Under the current DSM IV schema, the term childhood schizophrenia was omitted and there was a reaffirmation of the classification of infantile autism as a valid diagnostic schema. Most investigators believe that the term childhood schizophrenia has been excessively used (Rutter, 1972). For many, this term has been the object of controversy and debate.

Currently, childhood schizophrenia is defined

under the same diagnostic criteria as that used for adults. This involves characteristic symptoms, deficits in adaptive functioning, and a duration of at least 6 months (APA, 1994). Psychotic symptoms include delusions, hallucinations, loose associations or incoherence, catatonia, and inappropriate or flattened affect; symptoms must be present for most of 1 month. Failure to achieve expected levels of social development define the deficits in adaptive functioning. The 6 months' duration can include a prodromal and residual phase, and the disorder cannot be diagnosed in the presence of organic factors. Stringent application of the diagnosis of childhood schizophrenia is urged given the difficulty documenting a period of disorganization or defining the presence of delusions of hallucinations in younger children (Volkmar, 1991a).

Historically, Kanner (1943) noted that his proposed disorder of infantile autism differed from schizophrenia. Volkmar (1991a) notes, "In retrospect it appears that a central aspect of this controversy related to an assumption of continuity based on severity; that is, since autism is a severe psychiatric disorder with a very early onset, must it not be the case that it represents the earliest manifestation of a similarly severe psychiatric disorder in adults?" (pp. 622–623).

Other works (Kolvin, 1971; Rutter, 1982) suggest that differentiations between autism and childhood schizophrenia can be made on the basis of age of onset, clinical characteristics, family history, and presence of central nervous system dysfunction. Most notably, an early age of onset within the first year seems to indicate a disorder closely resembling autism. Later onset of symptoms seemed more aligned with a diagnosis of childhood schizophrenia. The delusions, hallucinations, and other symptomatology associated with schizophrenia are more prominent in the later-onset age group characterized with childhood schizophrenia (Kolvin, 1971). Current thought indicates that autism and childhood schizophrenia are two distinct disorders; this viewpoint is reflected in the current edition of DSM IV (APA, 1994).

Childhood schizophrenia is rarely diagnosed before the age of 5 years. Onset usually follows a gradual period of deterioration in functioning. Occasionally, the onset is acute with few premorbid warnings in behavior. Males are more likely to have an early onset of the disorder (Green et al., 1984).

In the current diagnostic schema, a child given the diagnosis of schizophrenia must meet the DSM IV criteria established for adults. Clinicians must exercise caution in labeling a child with schizophrenia. While appropriate in rare situations, it should follow intensive evaluation that has ruled out differential diagnoses, such as mental retardation, language disorders, or deafness. This diagnosis has negative connotations and may serve to bias others against the child who carries this diagnosis. Similarly, it is important to use this diagnosis accurately if it describes the disorder affecting the child. Unfortunately, it is easier to justify an increased number of needed inpatient days to third-party payers when the child carries a diagnosis of schizophrenia.

Multiple Complex Developmental Disorders

The term multiple complex developmental disorders (MCDD) first emerged in the literature as a way of differentiating a group of children and adults from those with autism and nonautistic PDD (Cohen et al., 1987). These individuals were initially noted to have early-onset, long-lasting serious disturbances in development affecting social relationships, emotional development, and cognitive processing. While some areas of development may be more impaired than others, the individuals are thought to fall within a spectrum between the PDD

CLINICAL EXAMPLE: DIANE

Diane, when first brought to the child guidance clinic by her mother, was an attractive, dark-haired 5-year-old who stared vacantly at objects and walls but made no eye contact with people. She flapped and twirled her hands and ran aimlessly around the playroom, first touching objects, then obsessively sniffing her fingers. Her only verbal comments were single word "echoes" of words spoken by her mother and the nurse. When her mother pulled her into her lap, she stiffened, then squirmed free to sit in a corner rocking. Her mother believed Diane became "unresponsive" at 16 months at the birth of a younger sister. At that time, she stopped talking and seemed to withdraw into herself. She had managed her at home but was now faced with the need to decide about special school placement.

CLINICAL EXAMPLE: TIM

Tim attended a small private church school with a low pupil-to-teacher ratio during grades one through four. During his fifth-grade year the family moved to a larger, more urban community where Tim began public school. While his bizarre behavior and difficulties communicating with teachers and peers had been previously tolerated with understanding and compassion, Tim's new classroom teacher and peers saw his behavior as much more deviant. With the culture of his environment altered, his strange behaviors were less tolerated and he was scapegoated. As the environment became less supportive, he became more thought disordered and was eventually hospitalized. Tim's functioning within the social system of his new school deteriorated when the system could not tolerate his deviance from the cultural norms. Without the support, his behavior worsened.

and specific developmental disorders (Cohen et al., 1987). Clinicians may see these children as falling out of any specific DSM IV diagnoses and may instead give them a number of diagnoses that describe one aspect of their behavior but inaccurately portray the variance or severity of their symptoms.

More recently, this disorder has been recharacterized as MCDD. Specifically, it is characterized by impairments in affective state and anxiety, social behavior and social sensitivity, and cognitive processing and the presence of thought disorder. Inconsistency and fluctuations in the expression of each of these features is considered key to the disorder (Towbin, Dykens, & Pearson, 1991).

Recent research compared psychiatrically hospitalized children characterized with MCDD to control groups of children with DSM III-R diagnoses of dysthymia and conduct disorder. Analyses of variance determined that MCDD subjects were significantly younger than controls when they first had psychiatric contact. They showed significantly lower peer relation scores than peers, lower Children's Global Assessment Scale (CGAS) ratings, and higher Child Behavior Checklist scores in the internalizing, externalizing, and severity scales. Also, MCDD subjects were hospitalized significantly longer than controls and had lower CGAS ratings at discharge (p values for all of these comparisons were $<.001$). IQ was the only variable that did not significantly differ across groups. Rorschach analyses indicated that MCDD subjects manifested significantly more indices of cognitive slippage than controls. These children were more vulnerable to emotional lability and illustrated, at times, peculiar communication styles, neologisms, circumstantial thinking, and poor judgment and emotional control. Although MCDD subjects had earlier psychiatric hospitalization and treatment than controls, they seemed less responsive to treatment (Towbin et al., 1991).

Although it is in its early stages, this research begins to define a subcategory of children with PDDs who present intense challenges to their caregivers. Their vulnerability to environmental stress and change, the wide fluctuations in functioning, and the variance in symptom manifestation require sophisticated treatment planning in the community and the psychiatric milieu (see Clinical Example: Tim).

Borderline Syndrome of Childhood

The term borderline syndrome of childhood has generated much controversy and discussion in the literature and in clinical settings where children receive psychiatric care. The term borderline often is used carelessly by mental health professionals. Although most would like to think the term has uniform applicability and meaning, its unspoken meanings include conjectures about untreatable, difficult children, and comparisons to adult borderline psychopathology. Nurses often are brought into diagnostic discussions and should maintain awareness of potential difficulties in labeling a child as borderline. Consensus agreement about meaning does not yet exist (Shapiro, 1983). The term has numerous and controversial meanings and is at best inexact in describing a child's difficulties.

The term borderline was originally coined to describe children whose behavior "bordered" between neurotic and psychotic in its origins (Frijling-Schreuder, 1969). Detailed definitions, which have emerged in the literature, often are confusing and mix concepts from developmental psychology, psychoanalytic thought, and descriptive psychopathology (Pine, 1974; Rosenfeld & Sprince, 1963).

In the early 1950s when literature began to emerge, these children were seen as healthier variants of children with what was formerly called childhood schizophrenia or psychosis. They were seen as pleasant and intelligent when alone with an adult but showed uncontrolled aggression or extreme withdrawal in groups with other children. When they became frustrated they exhibited severe temper tantrums and were paranoid-like and panicky. They seemed to experience a brief loss of contact with reality, especially when agitated or presented with environmental stress. Originally, as with many childhood psychiatric disorders, it was postulated that the mother–child relationship was disturbed. Later, Mahler noted the presence of a less serious case of childhood psychosis with neurotic-like defense mechanisms (Mahler, Ross, & DeFries, 1949).

In 1953, Weil saw fantasies of omnipotence, magical thinking, impaired reality testing, and rapid alteration of symptoms in the face of severe and diffuse anxiety or a need satisfying interpersonal relationship. This was further termed faulty ego development.

Ekstein and Wallerstein (1956) diagnosed borderline children and noted a particular vulnerability to regression, especially in response to therapists' inadvertent failure to empathize. Freud (1956) saw these children as exhibiting extreme levels of regression and massive developmental arrests. There was a withdrawal of libido from the object world and displacement of this onto the self or body. These children were unable to receive comfort from others and showed numerous ego defects and poor reality testing. Most notable was the poor development of age-appropriate defenses. Finally, Engel (1963) in a classic paper on psychologic testing with borderline children described an excess of primary process fantasy on projective testing.

Regardless, most theorists agree that the borderline syndrome represents a primary developmental failure in ego function and object relations. Pine (1986) conceptualizes that children develop a level of pathology between neurosis and psychosis because of early experiences of being overwhelmed (trauma), the evolution of developmental deficits, and desperate reliance on maladaptive survival mechanisms for coping. He notes the presence of "profound developmental deficits of certain kinds and by adaptive modes that are pathological, rendering the maturation of object contact, drive expression, and defense style unsuccessful" (p. 456). The borderline child exhibits degrees of disturbance in nearly all areas of functioning, resulting in a profound failure to master the developmental tasks of latency. These included areas of peer relationships, stabilization of defenses, and expansion of cognitive abilities.

Bemporad, Smith, and Hanson (1982) saw six factors as characteristic areas of general pathology in the borderline syndrome of childhood. These include a fluctuation of functioning, the nature and extent of anxiety, relationships to others, lack of control, and associated symptoms. Under stress, children shift to a psychotic-like world of fantasy and have difficulty distancing from stressful material. They are defenseless against anxiety and decompensate in the face of escalating feelings of anxiety. They experience excessive fluidity of thought and lack the proper demarcations between fantasy and reality. Themes flow from neutral topics to those of mutilation and death. Relationships are fixated at a symbiotic stage, and others are sought as need-fulfilling objects. There is an extreme need for reassurance, support, and internal organization. These children assume an "as if" quality in choosing a supplier of emotional needs. Much of their functioning is centered around assuming a role, and their own identity is unclear. When experiencing a lack of control, these youngsters escalate their feelings of frustration in tantrums or aimless hyperactivity. Behaviorally, they might hurt themselves or others or destroy objects in their environment.

Associated symptoms include poor social functioning, relative failure to learn from experience, lack of personal grooming and self-concern, inconsistent ability to adapt to new situations, and a fluctuation in development.

The current DSM IV classification system does not acknowledge Borderline Syndrome of childhood as a distinct symptom cluster. Instead, the children who appear with the aforementioned symptoms are subsumed under the PDD, NOS classification. There continue to be problems with uniformity in classification, confusion with the adult borderline personality syndrome, and a lack of systematic research to define this population clearly.

Treatment

INDIVIDUAL PSYCHOTHERAPY (PLAY THERAPY)

It is difficult to generalize specific individual treatment techniques given the wide range of problems presented by children with PDD. Generally, individual psychotherapy for these children is based on the child's developmental stage, degree of active thought disorder, level of object relatedness, and ability to tolerate intimacy. Play can be the learning modality in which the acquisition of cognitive, communicative, and social or emotional skills are promoted (Rogers & Lewis, 1989). Individual therapy is generally recognized as a valuable intervention within the constellation of other services, including family treatment, extended day services, special education, and psychopharmacology. Treatment usually occurs within an outpatient clinic, school program, at the patient's home, or within a private psychotherapy practice.

As in any individual play therapy with a child, an equipped play space will facilitate treatment. When working with psychotic children, it is imperative that the physical space and range of available toys remain constant. Regressive techniques, such as finger painting or water play, must be carefully considered in the context of the child's need for ego organization. Therapists usually are advised to begin with a small number of play choices geared to the child's developmental level versus a confusing array of toys aimed at all age groups. Chronologic age often will not coincide with play interests. For example, an 11-year-old may shun board games to play with a doll house.

The degree of thought disorder may determine the therapy style adopted by the clinician. Escalona (1964) notes two specific therapy styles that either encourage suppression or expression of disturbed affect. Expressive therapy techniques tend to encourage the expression of feelings with the goal of understanding affect and behavior. Suppression techniques assist the child in containing affect and discourage the acting-out play behaviors that might normally be seen with neurotic children who have intact ego functioning. Both techniques rely on the developed relationship between child and therapist for short- and long-term improvements in behavior.

If the goal of individual treatment is to assist the child in managing feelings and understanding behaviors, it is imperative that the therapist maintain and encourage reality. Allowing children to denigrate into a floridly psychotic process during the course of a therapy hour may not help when they leave the clinician's office and return to family or school. While the clinician may choose to explore the nature of the child's psychosis, this must be done carefully and with an awareness of the treatment goal, which is usually to facilitate the child's reality testing.

When considering the child's level of psychosis or thought disorder, the nurse must consider the child's degree of impulsiveness in behaviors that could be injurious to self or others. Personal safety of the child and therapist must be maintained at all times. Treatment strategies might include meeting in a more open public place, keeping the office door open, or shortening sessions.

When choosing an individual model of treatment, the nurse must respect the child's emotional fragility and need for continuity and predictability. Proper termination and conclusion of treatment is essential to the child whose relationships tend to be shaky and uncertain, given their own internal struggles with reality.

Escalona (1964) further notes that even the most psychotic and disturbed child can, with time, form a positive dependent relationship with a therapist. This is counter to the accepted notion that children with this level of disturbance are incapable of forming strong attachments to caregivers. When choosing long-term versus short-term models of care, the nurse must avoid underestimating the importance of the relationship to the child.

The case manager role is essential in coordinating care needs beyond individual therapy. The nurse individually treating the child may or may not fulfill this role. Providing case management and individual therapy requires a sense of boundaries, need prioritization, and awareness of competing system demands. The frequent lack of resources makes holding dual or more roles in the child's care a practical necessity. A high level of family dysfunction may necessitate a shared or cotherapy treatment model. In most situations it is advantageous to share treatment with a colleague. Clinical supervision is imperative when treating children with this level of disturbance.

Specific outcomes and improvement in functioning from individual therapy with severely disturbed youngsters have been difficult to ascertain. Most sources note that the poor long-term prognosis and chronicity of PDD will undermine the age-appropriate gains in social relating that may be observed within the context of a long-term therapy relationship.

MILIEU MANAGEMENT OF CHILDREN WITH PDD

Children with PDD may be psychiatrically hospitalized for initial assessment and diagnosis, management of symptom exacerbation, and pharmacologic intervention. Milieu management involves management of the child within the context of the other adults and children in the milieu. It involves the child's functioning, the individual's influence on the patient group, and management of staff reactions to children with a chronic disorder.

Predominant treatment goals in the milieu involve facilitating the child's highest level of functioning. The first nursing goal is to assess the child's emotional, cognitive, and activities of daily living skills. From this evolves the encouragement of age-appropriate skills, realizing that the child's developmental presentation may be uneven and may shift with emotional stability to instability.

It is essential to maintain consistency and predictability in all milieu environments involving the child. This necessitates cohesive treatment planning between therapist, family, living unit, and school. It involves keeping a predictable routine to therapy hours, mealtimes, and bedtimes. Children with PDD are acutely aware of changes and tend to become disorganized in response to environmental or affective change.

It is critical to develop strategies that repeatedly assist the child to regain emotional equilibrium. Staff should encourage the child to assist in planning these strategies at a point of higher functioning. Working with parents or other caretakers to ascertain what strategy they use to calm the child maintains consistency between home and milieu.

Medication should be considered a treatment strategy that also can assist the child in averting a complete escalation of behavior. Conversely, nursing staff may choose to capitalize on and foster the child's ability to use internal resources to become calm.

The milieu staff must avoid isolation unless absolutely necessary for the safety of the child and the living unit. The poor social relating that characterizes children with PDD makes it imperative that they remain in the therapeutic community as much as possible. While the quiet room is often the only alternative to aggressive or assaultive behaviors, time in isolation should be as limited as possible. As soon as possible, the child should be returned to the unit program and integrated into the rest of the patient population.

The treatment staff should facilitate reality testing, which can be accomplished in many ways. Staff should continually help the child make distinctions between what is real and what is pretend or imagined. Children with PDD may have difficulty understanding or appreciating the nuances of nonverbal communication. Clear, concrete, simple directions, given as part of a predictable routine are most effective.

Holidays such as halloween can be particularly disorganizing, especially if costumes blur the line between reality and fantasy. Scary movies, even scary television commercials, are disturbing and difficult. Management of staff issues involves one of the most difficult parts of milieu management. It becomes a challenge to gear the staff's expectations of the child to his or her actual capabilities. This becomes especially difficult with children whose autistic symptoms approach but do not replicate the full syndrome of infantile autism. Periods of higher or near normal functioning may lead staff to believe that a child is manipulating or "choosing" not to behave. In fact, the opposite usually is true, and the child desperately wants to understand what the staff wants.

The staff needs assistance in understanding unpredictable behavior. While the child's tantrums and behavioral disorganization may be viewed by some as a personal failure, this attitude is not useful to the child. Children with PDD cannot be "outpunished" and may need repetitive directions and prompts about what their behavior should be. Their periods of higher functioning make staff believe that they are capable of a more normal learning curve. This simply does not work. Teaching models must be geared to the child's capabilities at the moment, as illustrated by the Clinical Examples for Janine and Mel.

These children tend to be the most chronically disturbed individuals on the unit and are emotionally draining for the staff who care for them. Measurable change often is difficult to see. Lack of community resources for the most disturbed child makes discharge planning frustrating.

Children with PDD may provide minimal emotional gratification for the staff who work with them. The most important intervention is helping understand what this behavior means to the child, to depersonalize the negatives, and to gear their expectations to what is realistically possible for that child.

These children may return over and over to the hospital. Their chronic disorder poses lifelong issues that will stress their developmental gains. They will, in all likelihood, not be considered "normal," and depending on their family supports, intelligence, level of thought disorder, and level of aggression, they may or may not be productive adults. Long-term follow-up of these children will help shed more light on prognosis and the treatment strategies that best help them develop and achieve near normal milestones.

PHARMACOLOGY IN PERVASIVE DEVELOPMENTAL DISORDERS

None of the pharmacologic agents that exist have proven effective in curing autism and other PDD. However, certain medications, specifically major tranquilizers, have had a role in symptom management and often are the drug of choice in treating these disorders (Campbell & Spencer, 1988). Haloperidol has been shown to enhance learning and improve behavior. "The major tranquilizers may act to decrease activity levels, increase relatedness and task involvement, and increase accessibility to remediation programs" (Volkmar, 1991, p. 505).

Caution is indicated when children with autistic or related disorders are treated with neuroleptic medications. Evidence has shown that medication is less effective with childhood-onset versus adolescent- or adult-onset schizophrenia or psychotic disorder (Green, 1989).

The risk of side effects is significant when neuroleptics are used in treatment; this has particular implications for nurses observing and treating these children. Although subtle, the side effects can have serious implications for later functioning. Neuroleptic-induced dyskinesias in children have reportedly ranged from 8% to 51% and constitute a serious health risk (Campbell, Grega, Green, & Bennett, 1983).

Baldessarini (1990) has defined six types of extrapyramidal syndromes associated with the use of neuroleptic medications. They include the following early-onset reactions:

- Acute dystonic reactions: Maximum risk is within 5 days of initial administration and at dose increases.
- Parkinsonism: Maximum risk is 5 to 30 days after beginning neuroleptics.
- Akathisia (motor restlessness): Maximum risk 5 to 60 days after initiation of neuroleptic therapy.
- Neuroleptic malignant syndrome: Potentially fatal and characterized by severe muscular rigidity, stupor, catatonia, hyperpyrexia, and labile pulse and blood pressure.

Later-onset syndromes (after months or years of neuroleptic therapy) include the following:

- Tardive dyskinesia: no adequate treatment
- Rabbit syndrome (perioral tremor)

A 4-week trial of medication usually is recommended (Campbell & Spencer, 1988). After a treatment period of 4 to 6 months, Campbell et al. (1985) recommend discontinuing neuroleptic medication to ascertain if additional treatment is warranted.

Green (1991) notes that medication treatment of children with autism and PDD should be approached with conservatism and instituted only when other less invasive treatment options have been exhausted. The lowest possible dose should be used for the shortest amount of time (Volkmar, 1991).

The newest medication for use with thought disorder individuals appears to be clozapine, a medication as effective as available neuroleptics without the extrapyramidal side effects. While this drug was discovered nearly 25 years ago, the high risk of agranulocytosis resulted in serious restrictions throughout the United States and other countries (Marder, 1988).

While not approved by the Food & Drug Administration for use with children and adolescents, this medication is most effective for individuals with treatment-resistant schizophrenia that severely compromises functioning. This may have future im-

CLINICAL EXAMPLE: JANINE

Janine, a 7-year-old, was admitted to the milieu after refusing to speak and exhibiting other unusual autistic-like behaviors. She presented with psychomotor retardation and notably deteriorated self-care skills. After ascertaining from her parents that she had previously been able to wash her face independently, the nursing staff began working with her to restore that skill.

When nurses realized she was fearful of seeing herself in the mirror, they began a washing routine in her bedroom with cloth and basin. At first the nurse and Janine washed her face together with the nurse gradually encouraging her to take on the activity herself. Verbal praise and bonus points (that could be traded in at the unit bonus store) were given as rewards. Gradually, Janine regained this skill, especially when allowed to avoid a mirror, which frightened her.

Careful assessment of Janine's responses to the environment (e.g., the mirror) resulted in a revised plan of care that helped her regain a previously lost skill. Rather than force the child to confront immediately the frightening delusion, nursing staff adjusted the environment to give some measure of success in regaining a skill. While the intervention might have appeared subtle, it gave a powerful message of acceptance to this confused, regressed child who was retreating into her own world.

CLINICAL EXAMPLE: MEL

Mel, a 13-year-old white boy, was admitted to a 12-bed unit of 11- to 14-year-olds. He presented with oddities in speech and behavior that quickly targeted him for scapegoating from peers. The nursing staff enlisted the "leader" of the youngsters, a young man with difficulties controlling his aggression, to orient and assist Mel in understanding the unit. This boy was able to help his peers understand that Mel could not contain all of his bizarre behaviors, and it soon became a unit ethic to ignore Mel or, when indicated, to call for staff assistance. Similarly, his peers began praising his appropriate behaviors and including him in structured activities where he could succeed, such as board games or art activities.

Mel was fortunate that the milieu was populated by a higher functioning group of peers who could tolerate his behaviors. The same type of peer pressure might not have occurred with a lower functioning population.

plications for that small group of children and adolescents who develop serious tardive dyskinesia from long-term use of neuroleptics or who have a treatment-resistant thought disorder. Clozapine is being described as a useful therapeutic advance for even the small number of patients who respond positively and go on to more productive lives (Kane, Honigfeld, Singer, & Meltzer, 1988).

Effects of Pervasive Developmental Disorders on the Family

Most families of children diagnosed with PDD report that their children appeared normal at birth and during the early neonatal months. Autism is not diagnosed at birth, and the symptoms generally emerge into parental awareness after the child's first year. Fragile X syndrome may be diagnosed prenatally or soon after birth, but only if the family is aware of the mother as a genetic carrier. For mothers who are asymptomatic carriers, the knowledge that their sons may have fragile X comes after birth and genetic testing when there are developmental problems.

Families cannot prepare for the emotional, financial, and physical burdens imposed by a child with PDD. The burdens become gradually evident when the child's failure to negotiate each developmental milestone occurs. Parents of children with severe psychiatric disturbance report feeling guilty, wondering if they could have prevented their children's disorder, and feeling that mental health professionals blame them for their children's dysfunction (Asarnow & Horton, 1990). It was once postulated that a child's autism was directly related to the presence of severe family dysfunction. The current view, that PDD is the result of an organic brain dysfunction, relieves some of the parental blame prominent in the past.

As the child's behavioral adaptation to his or her environment becomes more conflicted, parents are faced with the need to define their child's behaviors and search out an etiology. They also may engage in increasing self-blame and retribution, particularly if the medical community is unable to help diagnose and plan treatment for the child.

Lettick (1987) notes the pain and despair experienced by families when they learn that their child is diagnosed with PDD or autism. The difficulties integrating a severely delayed individual with regressed behaviors into a family system becomes challenging, and for some parents, impossible. Problems with siblings and the wider community, a lack of school or day treatment services, and a paucity of various support services may force families to pursue residential care. Lettick further notes the difficulties of mainstreaming PDD children within the broader community of normal individuals. She notes that the profoundly involved individual rarely benefits simply from being with people without impairment. For children with less severe impairments than classic autism, this mainstreaming must be carefully evaluated. Children may receive valuable benefits from careful exposure to less impaired individuals. Each situation must be evaluated carefully (see Clinical Example: Sara).

Recent research indicates that some parents perceive themselves as victims of their children's psychiatric disorder and require extensive support to function in a parenting role. The most chronically disturbed children seem to produce the most disruption in their parents lives. Similarly, the presence of a close relationship for mothers seemed to serve a protective function in buffering family stress. This pointed to the need for community support for any family dealing with a seriously disturbed child, especially ones with chronic disorders such as PDD (Asarnow & Horton, 1990).

CLINICAL EXAMPLE: SARA

Sara, the third child of Ted and Maria, appeared normal at birth. Described as a happy, placid baby, Sara accomplished her physical milestones at the same age as her siblings. Her language consisted of babbling and two to three words. At 14 months she appeared to become more lethargic and withdrawn and would sit in her playpen for long periods of time watching the sunlight on the windowsill or playing with her fingers. Her mother, who had taken a part-time job, was relieved that she could occupy herself so well, even though she realized that at the same age, her other two children were loathe to spend any time in the playpen.

At her 18 month check-up, Sara was alarmingly passive and had stopped all speech. Her pediatrician, who had done hearing tests and a battery of blood work, was concerned about her developmental slippage and referred the family to a university-based developmental clinic in a nearby city for evaluation.

The evaluation occurred over a 2-month period and involved numerous appointments. Maria took a leave of absence from her part-time secretarial job to complete the evaluation. Her babysitter for the other two children, ages 6 and 4, was "afraid" to care for Sara as she appeared "possessed" and "strange." Maria felt overwhelmed and terrified about the outcome of the evaluation. Ted became more and more withdrawn from the family system, preferring to work long hours of overtime in his factory job, which he justified was needed to pay for the expensive evaluation not covered by insurance. Maria became increasingly frustrated at his withdrawal, and they began verbally arguing more than usual. Their 6-year-old began wetting the bed after nearly 3 years of nighttime dryness. By the conclusion of the evaluation, Maria and Ted admitted that they felt their family was "falling apart."

Case Management of the Child with PDD

The lack of services available to children with chronic psychiatric disorders is reportedly due not to the number of available facilities, but to the collaborative relationships essential to coordination of care (Tuma, 1989). It has been consistently documented that children receive fragmented psychiatric services because of poor communication between treatment and community systems responsible for care. This is especially true for children with a chronic disorder such as PDD.

The Federal Child and Adolescent Service System Program was developed in 1984 to assist state mental health systems to coordinate care for seriously emotionally disturbed children. Funding was directed to states to conduct interagency planning and needs-assessment activities and to attempt to develop a more effective system of service (Friedman, 1986).

Case management is a concept applicable to chronically disturbed adults and children. It involves assessment, coordination, advocacy, referral, teaching, outreach to home, crisis intervention, and medication monitoring (Baier, 1987). Nurses are well equipped to assume this multidimensional role with the chronically disturbed child.

Case management is essential to avoid the disruption of hospitalization, assist parents' learning management skills in their home, and coordinate the school's role in providing special education or day treatment services to the child with PDD. Case management ultimately improves the quality of care children and their families receive from a myriad of services.

Implication for Nursing Research

While children with PDD represent a small number of those with psychiatric disorders (10 to 15 in 10,000), they represent the most seriously disturbed and those most in need of services (Tuma, 1989). The implications for nursing research are many. Nurses have not traditionally done research on children with psychiatric disturbances. While biologic research has focused on identifying these children and the nature of their disorder, it is time to look more carefully at treatment strategies that successfully help the child regain equilibrium and potentiate developmental gains.

Research is needed on the efficacy of treatment programs that occur in nontraditional settings, such as schools or home-based care systems. Data on the success of case management, conducted over several years, are not yet available. It is unclear what milieu techniques are most successful with a child presenting with PDD.

Strategies to help families cope, effects of these children on families, and the role of community supports are all areas in which systematic research

CLINICAL EXAMPLE: JANE

Jane was the product of a brief marriage between her psychotic father and developmentally handicapped mother. Her early life was characterized by frequent moves, unstable parenting, and a gang rape by her father and his friends when she was 3. She first came to the attention of mental health professionals around the age of 4, while enrolled in a Head Start Program. At that time, she was noted to be severely regressed in her behavior and language. She had almost no social skills and limited self-help skills and seemed to be hallucinating at intervals about creatures on the walls and in the faces of the adults around her. Her mother was oblivious to her daughter's obvious problems, and Jane was soon withdrawn from the program as the family made yet another move.

Mother's involvement with boyfriend Tim marked a 2-year period in which Jane and she were held hostage in an inner city apartment. During that time, it was rumored that Tim involved Jane in satanic worship, and she experienced the ritualistic sacrifice of animals and continual physical and sexual abuse and torture. Her first psychiatric hospitalization occurred around the age of 8 when her mother left Tim, and Jane became involved with the public school system.

At that time, she presented with violent outbursts directed toward others, periods of psychosis, and an inability to deal with peers. She had no reading or math skills and had spent no prolonged time within a school setting.

From a nursing perspective, she exhibited the following human response patterns (Loomis, et al., 1987) when admitted to the inpatient milieu:

ACTIVITY PROCESSES

1. *Altered motor behavior:* characterized by bizarre hand movements, ataxia, and difficulty coordinating gross motor movements
2. *Self-care deficit:* Jane had difficulty accomplishing even the most simple of daily tasks and required frequent prompting and direction before completing self-care.
3. *Sleep pattern disturbance:* characterized by frequent nightmares in which she imagined seeing Tim on the walls of her bedroom. She also experienced the transition from evening routine to sleep as stressful and frequently avoided bedtimes.

COGNITION PROCESSES

1. *Knowledge deficit:* Jane was functioning far below developmental norms for children her age. She showed a significant knowledge deficit, and her mental status seemed to prohibit making gains in the classroom.
2. *Altered memory:* Jane's memories seemed distorted and delusional, although it was difficult to ascertain if the violent information she shared was truth or part of an elaborate delusional system.
3. *Altered orientation:* At her most thought-disordered points, Jane appeared confused and uncertain about her environment and the people around her. She saw Tim's face in those around her and became more aggressive at these points.
4. *Altered thought processes:* Jane showed no ability to participate in abstract thinking or problem solving and had little ability to concentrate on a task whether in school or in the milieu.

EMOTIONAL PROCESSES

1. *Abuse response pattern:* Jane exhibited symptoms of a rape trauma syndrome and seemed to experience flashbacks in which she relieved the trauma of the sexual abuse. This most often occurred when she required physical restraint to prevent her from hurting herself or others in the environment.
2. *Altered feeling patterns:* Jane would frequently become out of control with little provocation and would exhibit extreme affects of anger and fear. At her highest level of functioning, she seemed continually wary and fearful of adults in the environment, especially males.

INTERPERSONAL PROCESSES

1. *Impaired verbal communication:* Verbally, Jane often had difficulty expressing her thoughts in a clear way. Nonverbally, she would make hand gestures and face grimaces that her peers found odd.
2. *Altered conduct/impulse processes:* Jane was prone to violent and unpredictable outbursts in which she would strike out against the environment and peers with little provocation. She would turn over chairs, kick furniture, and hit peers.

   She also displayed a variety of dysfunction behaviors that included diurnal eneuresis, bizarre conversations about imaginary friends, and graphic stories of torture and sexual abuse that were told at socially inappropriate times. She required frequent prompts about completing activities of daily living and around using table manners.
3. *Impaired social interaction:* Jane was fre-

(continued)

CLINICAL EXAMPLE: JANE *(Continued)*

quently isolative from peers and staff in the milieu and required prompts to join others.

PERCEPTION PROCESSES

1. *Altered self-concept:* Jane saw herself as ugly and worthless and took little care of her personal self and grooming.
2. *Sensory-perceptual alterations:* Jane frequently experienced auditory and visual hallucinations in which she imagined a person in the walls talking with her. When out of control, she imagined seeing the perpetrator of her abuse in the faces of staff who were trying to help her regain control of her behavior.

Nursing staff chose several of the previous nursing diagnoses on which to focus during the first month of the hospitalization. The following is an example of the nursing care planning that occurred with this child. Each problem was addressed similarly to the following prototype.

Problem 1: Difficulty controlling aggressive impulses.

Plan: Nursing staff will monitor pattern of aggressive behavior to ascertain if certain times of day present more difficulty for Jane.

Outcome: Staff found after 1 week of assessment that times of transition were most difficult and began providing one-to-one support for Jane during these times. They intervened more quickly with peer difficulty and separated Jane from difficult situations. Two nurses on first and second shifts were assigned as primary caregivers so that Jane experienced minimal changes in caregivers but had consistent staff dealing with her at all times in the week.

Plan: Nursing staff will set up a system of rewards for each day that Jane is able to avoid an aggressive confrontation.

Outcome: Jane chose one of three special activities, such as being read to, baking with staff, or taking a walk on the grounds, as a reward for avoidance of assaultive behavior. At first the reward occurred every 3 days and then was lengthened to weekly. Gradually, the assaultive behavior decreased.

Plan: Nursing staff will monitor changes in psychotropic medication and will document Jane's response to this regarding thinking and aggressive behaviors.

Outcome: Jane's dose of haloperidol was gradually increased to 2 mg h.s., and she was observed to have no side effects while coming under better behavioral control.

The degree of disorder presented by this child was, at times, overwhelming to nursing staff. Identifying goals and planning care around prioritized problems assisted staff in implementing a care plan that best met Jane's needs, facilitated her functioning in the milieu, and ensured some measurable success for the staff dealing with her on a daily basis.

could contribute to better understanding practical management of the chronically disturbed child.

Nurses work with these children in medical and nonmedical settings. They are in excellent positions to conduct outcome studies and to examine the care models that most facilitate functioning. It is a nursing responsibility to monitor care, improve care, and write about findings. The historic thrust of research with this population has focused on biologic issues. Nursing can contribute to the fund of knowledge about management and care of children with PDD (see Clinical Example: Jane).

SUMMARY

This chapter describes the disorders of childhood autism, Asperger's syndrome, fragile X syndrome, childhood schizophrenia, MCDD, and borderline syndrome of childhood. Treatment of children with PDD and their families includes individual psychotherapy, such as play therapy, family approaches, milieu management, and the administration of pharmacologic agents. The burdens and challenges experienced by families of children with PDD and their case management needs are considerable. Nursing research should focus on treatment approaches that help the child gain developmental and social skills and help families effectively accomplish their childrearing tasks.

REFERENCES

American Psychiatric Association. (1994). *Diagnostic and statistical manual of mental disorders* (4th ed.). Washington, D.C.: Author.

Asarnow, J. R., & Horton, A. A. (1990). Coping and stress in families of child psychiatric inpatients: Parents of children with depressive and schizophrenia spectrum disorders. *Child Psychiatry and Human Development, 21,* 145–157.

Baier, M. (1987). Case management with chronically mentally ill. *Journal of Psychosocial Nursing, 25,* 17–20.

Baldessarini, R. J. (1990). Drugs and the treatment of psychiatric disorders. In A. F. Gilman, R. W. Rall, & A. S. Nies. (Eds.), *Goodman and Gilman's the pharmacological basis of therapeutics* (8th ed.). (pp. 383–435). New York: Pergamon Press.

Bemporad, J. R., Smith, H. F., & Hanson, G. (1982). Borderline syndromes in childhood: Criteria for diagnosis. *American Journal of Psychiatry, 139,* 596.

Bregman, J., Dykens, E., Watson, M., Ort, S., & Leckman, J. (1987). Fragile X syndrome: Variability in phenotypic expression. *Journal of the American Academy of Child and Adolescent Psychiatry, 26,* 463–471.

Bregman, J., Leckman, J., & Ort, S. (1988). Fragile X syndrome: Genetic predisposition to psychopathology. *Journal of Autism and Developmental Disorders, 18,* 343–354.

Campbell, M., Grega, D. M., Green, W. H., & Bennett, W. G. (1983). Neuroleptic-induced dyskinesias in children. *Clinical Neuropharmacology, 6,* 207–222.

Campbell, M., & Spencer, E. K. (1988). Psychopharmacology in child and adolescent psychiatry: A review of the past five years. *Journal of the American Academy of Child and Adolescent Psychiatry, 27,* 269–279.

Campbell, M., Green, W. H., & Deutsch, S. I. (1985). *Child and adolescent psychopharmacology.* Beverly Hills: Sage Publications.

Cohen, D. J., Paul, R., & Volkmar, F. R. (1986). Issues in the classification of pervasive and other developmental disorders: Toward DSM-IV. *Journal of the American Academy of Child Psychiatry, 25,* 213–220.

Cohen, D. J., Paul, R., & Volkmar, F. R. (1987). Issues in the classification of pervasive developmental disorders and associated symptoms. In D. J. Cohen & A. M. Donellan (Eds.), *Handbook of autism and pervasive developmental disorders.* New York: John Wiley & Sons.

Daker, M., Chidiac, P., Fear, L., & Berry, A. (1981). Fragile X in a normal male: A cautionary note. *Lancet, 1,* 780.

DeMyer, M. K., Barton, S., DeMyer, W. E., Norton, J. A., Allen, J., & Steel, R. (1973). Prognosis in autism: A follow-up study. *Journal of Autism and Childhood Schizophrenia, 3,* 199–246.

DeMyer, M. K., Alpern, G. D., Barton, S., DeMeyer, W. E., Churchill, D. W., Hingtgen, J. N., Bryson, C. Q., Pontius, W., & Kimberlin, C. (1972). Imitation in autistic early schizophrenic, and non-psychotic subnormal children. *Journal of Autism and Childhood Schizophrenia, 2,* 263–287.

DeMyer, M. K., Hingtgen, J. N., & Jackson, R. K. (1981). Infantile autism reviewed: A decade of research. *Schizophrenia Bulletin, 7,* 388–451.

Dykens, E., Hodapp, R., & Leckman, J. (1987). Strengths and weaknesses in the intellectual functioning of males with fragile X syndrome. *American Journal of Mental Deficiency, 92,* 234–236.

Dykens, E., & Leckman, J. (1990). Developmental issues in fragile X syndrome. In R. Hodapp, J. Burack, & E. Zigler (Eds.), *Issues in the developmental approach to mental retardation* (pp. 226–245). New York: Cambridge University Press.

Ekstein, R., & Wallerstein, J. (1956). Observations on the psychology of borderline and psychotic children. *The Psychoanalytic Study of the Child, 11,* 303–311.

Engel, M. (1963). Psychological testing of borderline children. *Archives of General Psychiatry, 8,* 426–434.

Escalona, S. (1964). Some considerations regarding psychotherapy with psychotic children. In M. R. Haworth (Ed.), *Child psychotherapy* (pp. 50–58). New York: Basic Books.

Fish, B. (1977). Neurobiological antecedents of schizophrenia in children: Evidence for an inherited congenital neurointegrative defect. *Archives of General Psychiatry, 34,* 1297–1313.

Fishburn, J., Turner, G., Daniel, A., & Brookwell, R. (1983). The diagnosis and frequency of X-linked conditions in a cohort of moderately retarded males with affected brothers. *American Journal of Medical Genetics, 14,* 713–724.

Freud, A. (1956). The assessment of borderline cases. In *The Writings of Anna Freud* (Vol. 4). New York: International Universities Press.

Friedman, R. M. (1986). *Major issues in mental health services for children.* Paper presented at the meeting of the American College of Mental Health Administration, San Diego, CA.

Frijling-Schreuder, E. (1969). Borderline states in children. *The Psychoanalytic Study of the Child, 24,* 307–327.

Fryns, J., Jacobs, P., Kleczkowska, A., & Van den Berghe, J. (1984). The psychological profile of the fragile X syndrome. *Clinical Genetics, 25,* 131–134.

Gillberg, C., & Schaumann, H. (1981). Infantile autism and puberty. *Journal of Autism and Developmental Disorders, 11,* 365–371.

Green, W. H. (1991). Principles of psychopharmacotherapy and specific drug treatments. In M. Lewis (Ed.), *Child and adolescent psychiatry: A comprehensive textbook* (pp. 770–795). Baltimore: Williams & Wilkins.

Green, W. H. (1989). Schizophrenia with childhood onset. In H. I. Kaplan & B. J. Sadock (Eds.), *Comprehensive textbook of psychiatry* (5th ed.). (pp. 1775–1781). Baltimore: Williams & Wilkins.

Green, W. H., Campbell, J., Hardesty, A. S., Grega, D. M., Padron-Gayol, M., Shell, J., & Erlenmeyer-Kimling. L. (1984). A comparison of schizophrenic and autistic children. *Journal of the American Academy of Child Psychiatry, 23,* 399–409.

Hagerman, R., Jackson, A., Levitas, A., Rimland, B., & Braden, M. (1986). An analysis of autism in 50 males with fragile X syndrome. *American Journal of Medical Genetics, 23,* 359–374.

Hagerman, R., Murphy, M., & Wittenberger, M. (1987). *A controlled trial of stimulant medication in children with the fragile X syndrome.* Paper presented to the First national Fragile X Conference, Denver CO.

Hagerman, F., & Smith, A. (1983). The heterozygous female. In R. Hagerman & P. McBogg (Eds.), *The fragile X syndrome: Diagnosis, biochemistry, and intervention.* Dillon, CO: Spectra Publishing.

Howard-Peebles, O., Stoddard, G., & Mims, M. (1979). Familial X-linked mental retardation, verbal disability, and marker X chromosomes. *American Journal of Medical Genetics, 31,* 214–222.

Kane, J., Honigfeld, G., Singer, J., & Meltzer, H. (1988). Clozapine for the treatment-resistant schizophrenic. *Archives of General Psychiatry, 45,* 789–796.

Kanner, L. (1943). Autistic disturbances of affective contact. *Nervous Child, 2,* 217–250.

Kilman, B., & Negri-Shoultz, N. (1987). Developing educational programs for working with students with Kanner's autism. In D. J. Cohen & A. M. Donnellan (Eds.), *Handbook of autism and pervasive developmental disorders* (pp. 440–451). New York: John Wiley & Sons.

Kolvin, I. (1971). Studies in childhood psychoses: I: Diagnostic criteria and classification. *British Journal of Psychiatry, 118,* 381–384.

Lettick, A. L. (1987). Educational and residential placement: Difficulties, decisions, and issues. In D. J. Cohen & A. M. Donnellan (Eds.), *Handbook of Autism and Pervasive Developmental Disorders* (pp. 722–734). New York: John Wiley & Sons.

Lubs, H. (1969). A marker-X chromosome. *American Journal of Mecical Genetics, 21,* 231–244.

McAdoo, W., & DeMeyer, M. (1978). Personality characteristics of parents. In M. Rutter & E. Schopier (Eds.), *Autism: A reappraisal of concepts and treatment.* New York: Plenum.

Mahler, M., Ross, Jr., J. R., & DeFries, Z. (1949). Clinical studies in benign and malignant cases of childhood psychosis. *American Journal of Orthopsychiatry, 19,* 295–305.

Marder, S. R. (1988). Who should receive clozapine? *Archives of General Psychiatry, 45,* 865–867.

Pine, F. (1974). On the concept "borderline" in children: A clinical essay. *The Psychoanalytic Study of the Child, 29,* 341–368.

Pine, F. (1986). On the development of the "borderline-child-to-be." *American Journal of Orthopsychiatry, 56,* 450–457.

Rogers, S. J., & Lewis, H. (1989). An effective day treatment model for young children with pervasive developmental disorders. *Journal of the American Academy of Child and Adolescent Psychiatry, 28,* 207–214.

Rosenfeld, S. K., & Sprince, M. P. (1963). An attempt to formulate the meaning of the concept "borderline." *The Psychoanalytic Study of the Child, 18,* 603–635.

Rutter, M. (1972). Childhood schizophrenia reconsidered. *Journal of Autism and Childhood Schizophrenia, 2,* 315–338.

Schepp, K. G. (1992). A symptom management program for adolescents with psychotic illnesses: Theoretical basis. *Journal of Child and Adolescent Psychiatric and Mental Health Nursing, 5*(4), 7–12.

Shapiro, T. (1983). The borderline syndrome in children: A critique. In K. S. Robson (Ed.), *The borderline child: Approaches to etiology, diagnosis, and treatment* (pp. 12–29). New York: McGraw-Hill.

Towbin, K. E., Dykens, E., & Pearson, G. S. (1991). *Progress in characterizing multiple complex developmental disorder.* Unpublished manuscript.

Tuma, J. M. (1989). Mental health services for children: The state of the art. *American Psychologist, 44,* 188–199.

Volkmar, F. R. (1987). Social development. In D. J. Cohen & A. M. Donnellan (Eds.), *Handbook of autism and pervasive developmental disorders* (pp. 41–60). New York: John Wiley & Sons.

Volkmar, F. R. (1991a). Childhood schizophrenia. In M. Lewis (Ed.), *Child and adolescent psychiatry: A comprehensive textbook* (pp. 621–628). Baltimore: Williams & Wilkins.

Volkmar, F. R. (1991b). Autism and the pervasive developmental disorders. In M. Lewis (Ed.), *Child and adolescent psychiatry: A comprehensive textbook* (pp. 499–508). Baltimore: Williams & Wilkins.

Watson, M. S., Leckman, J. F., Annex, B., Breg, W. R., Boles, D., Volkmar, F. R., & Cohen, D. J. (1984). Fragile X survey of 75 autistic males. *New England Journal of Medicine, 310,* 1462.

Webb, T., Bundey, S., Thake, A., & Todd, J. (1986). Population incidence and segregation ratios in the Martin-Bell syndrome. *American Journal of Medical Genetics, 23,* 573–580.

Weil, A. (1953). Certain severe disturbances of ego development in childhood. *The Psychoanalytic Study of the Child, 8,* 271–287.

Wing, L. (1980). *Autistic children: A guide for parents.* London: Constable.

Wing, L. (1981). Language, social, and cognitive impairments in autism and severe mental retardation. *Journal of Autism and Developmental Disorder, 11,* 31–44.

Wing, L., & Attwood, A. (1987). Syndromes of autism and atypical development. In D. J. Cohen & A. M. Donnellan (Eds.), *Handbook of autism and pervasive developmental disorders* (pp. 3–19). New York: John Wiley & Sons.

CHAPTER

20

Tic Disorders

Maureen T. McSwiggan-Hardin

The growth and advances in basic neurobiology and neurochemistry have provided a better means of understanding the function of the brain and thus a more comprehensive knowledge of the mechanisms that are associated with the neuropsychiatric disorders. Understanding the etiology of neuropsychiatric disorders provides for new approaches to early detection or prevention. Childhood neuropsychiatric disorders imply a biologic or genetic etiology and include the disorders of autism, attention-deficit/hyperactivity disorder (ADHD), the tic disorders, and obsessive–compulsive disorder (OCD).

This chapter discusses the tic disorders, which include Tourette's disorder syndrome (or TS), chronic motor or vocal tic disorder (CMT), and transient tic disorder. TS and CMT have been the focus of recent neurobiologic research, which has demonstrated the importance of bringing together scientific understanding of pathology, clinical assessment, and clinical treatment. Implicit in this chapter is the attention not only to the neurobiologic mechanisms, but to the developmental and psychodynamic understanding of the child or adolescent within the context of a family and social environment.

History

Historically, tic symptoms were first described systematically by Itard in 1825. Sixty years later, Gilles de la Tourette described a group of nine patients with "motor incoordination or tics" and "inarticulate shouts, accompanied by articulated words with echolalia and coprolalia." In his description, Tourette also noted the appearance of obsessive–compulsive features and the high incidence of a familial transmission of symptoms (Goetz & Klawans, 1982).

Awareness and interest on the part of the lay public and scientific community concerning the tic disorders has increased dramatically over the last 2 decades. Tic disorders have become the focus of neurochemical, genetic, and nongenetic research. Tics, once thought to be associated with anxiety or emotional conflict, are now understood as involuntary phenomena with a neurobiologic basis and probable genetic etiology.

TS exemplifies specifically a childhood neuropsychiatric disorder that encompasses multiple dimensions, including neurobiologic and neurochemical mechanisms; developmental and psychodynamic mechanisms; family relationships and dynamics; the impact of social systems outside the family, such as schools; and other associated features, such as ADHD and OCD.

Definition

A *tic* is a sudden, repetitive movement, gesture, or utterance. Tics are of brief duration, usually not more than a second long, and frequently occur in

Barbara Schoen Johnson: CHILD, ADOLESCENT AND FAMILY PSYCHIATRIC NURSING, © 1994 J.B. Lippincott Company

bouts. At times the bouts can resemble paroxysms or can appear as orchestrated movements or sounds. They can be characterized by number, frequency, intensity, complexity, and interference (Leckman, Towbin, Ort, & Cohen, 1988). Though tics are defined as involuntary, many individuals describe a premonitory urge or sensation. Tics can usually be suppressed for brief periods and in general, have a waxing and waning course over days or weeks. Tics usually increase during times of stress, fatigue, and excitement; and are less frequent and intense when the individual is asleep, engaged in an absorbing activity, or in a highly structured situation. Some tics may be stimulated by certain experiences, such as hearing a person cough. Over time tics commonly change in anatomic location and repertoire, some may disappear entirely, and others remain constant with a waxing and waning course.

In children the ability to suppress tics is often confusing to parents and teachers who may mistake the expression of symptoms as more controlled. Long periods of consciously or unconsciously suppressing symptoms is invariably followed by a need to release the tension built up by "holding the tics in." A common example is children who hold in their tics in front of classmates only to have a flurry of tics as soon as they get off the school bus.

MOTOR TICS

Motor tics usually begin with simple, brief bouts of transient movements, such as eye blinking, head jerks, or shoulder shrugs in children, beginning in kindergarten or early school grades. The symptoms may remain for several months then disappear for an extended period. Frequently within 1 to 2 years, the tic occurrences are no longer transient. The progression of motor tics has frequently been described as rostral–caudal, with tics of the eyes, face, head, and shoulders appearing before motor tics of the lower extremities. Examples include eye blinking, facial grimacing, head jerking, abdominal tensing, or rapid darting movement of any part of the body. Simple motor tics are rapid, sudden, meaningless movements. Complex movements rarely occur in the absence of simple tics. They are more purposeful in appearance and include such examples as spinning, touching, facial gestures, and obscene gestures (copropraxia) or an array of several different muscle groups that occur together, such as a movement that includes spinning, touching, and head jerking. Copropraxia or self-abusing behaviors (biting or hitting) are much less common and usually occur in the more severe cases of tic disorders.

VOCAL TICS

Vocal or phonic tics usually occur after the appearance of motor tics. They generally follow the same progression of transient to more sustained vocalizations, beginning with simple vocal utterances, such as throat clearing, high-pitched squeaking noises, or coughing. The range of possible phonic tics is also limitless. Complex phonic tics occur less and are characterized by appearing more purposive and of longer duration. Such examples include uttering words ("honey," "wow," "see ya"), echolalia (repeating what others say), or palilalia (repeating one's own speech). Phonic tics, as with motor tics, can be characterized by number, frequency, intensity, and disruption. Intensity refers to the volume, while complexity refers to simple noises versus syllables, words, and phrases.

Classification of tic disorders in Diagnostic and Statistical Manual of Mental Disorders, 4th ed. (DSM IV) includes TS, chronic multiple motor or vocal tic disorder, transient tic disorder, and tic disorder not otherwise specified (American Psychiatric Association, 1994). The criteria that distinguish the three major tic disorders include duration and types of tics (Table 20-1). These criteria assist in establishing assessment guidelines for the clinician and in differentiating the less severe disorder (transient tic disorder) from the more complex and usually more severe disorder, TS.

Epidemiology

Prevalence refers to the frequency of cases reported in a population at a given time. When considering the prevalence of TS and tic disorders it is important to distinguish TS from CMT and transient tics. Transient tics are relatively common, with estimates running as high as 13 per 100 boys and 11 per 100 girls (Zahner, Clubb, Leckman, & Pauls, 1988).

Chronic multiple (motor or vocal) tic disorder is presumably less common. However, an accurate estimate of prevalence is difficult to obtain because there have been few well-designed epidemiologic surveys.

The prevalence of TS in the United States has not been firmly established. A survey of physicians and mental health centers conducted in North Dakota found 9.3 and 1.0 per 10,000 for boys and girls, respectively. In the same survey the prevalence was much lower for adults, with estimates of 0.77 and 0.22 per 10,000 for men and women, respectively. The male-to-female ratio of TS for children below the age of 18 years in the North Dakota

TABLE 20–1 Diagnostic Criteria for Tic Disorders

Tic Disorder	Symptoms	Course of Time
Transient tic disorder	Either motor or vocal tics may be present	< 12 months
Chronic multiple (motor or vocal) tic disorder	Either motor or vocal, not both	> 12 months
Tourette's syndrome	Both motor and vocal tics (may include history of vocal tics)	> 12 months

survey was 9:1; for adults the ratio decreased to 3:1 (Burd, Kerbeshian, Wilkenheiser, & Fisher, 1986a; 1986b). In a recent study of 28,000 draftees into the Israeli Army, ages 16 and 17 years old, a lifetime prevalence for TS of approximately five cases in 10,000 in males and three cases in 10,000 females was determined (Apter et al., 1993).

Clinical Description

Transient Tic Disorder

DSM IV diagnostic criteria describe this disorder as characterized by symptom presentation of less than 12 months. Tics may disappear for months only to reappear episodically for several years. Transient tics are most commonly seen in the upper extremities and are frequently associated with a stressful event, such as starting school. Nonetheless, it would be incorrect to associate the tic(s) with nervousness in the child or a habit that the child can control with effort.

CHRONIC MULTIPLE (MOTOR OR PHONIC) TIC DISORDER

DSM III-R diagnostic criteria characterize this disorder as symptoms that exceed 12 months, with the expression of motor or phonic tics but not both. Motor tics of the upper extremities are the most common presentation, with chronic vocal tics seen less frequently. The symptoms most often develop in childhood, between the ages of 6 and 10 years, and have a waxing and waning course. The periods of greatest severity occur in early to middle childhood and in many cases, subside in intensity and frequency after adolescence. Family genetic studies have recently supported a probable etiologic relationship between CMT and TS, yet this is still being investigated (Pauls, Kruger, Leckman, Cohen, & Kidd, 1984; Pauls & Leckman, 1986).

TOURETTE'S SYNDROME (OR DISORDER)

TS is the most severe tic disorder. The typical presentation is transient bouts of simple motor tics starting at age 3 to 6 years that eventually become chronic and include motor and vocal tics. The progression is most commonly simple motor to simple vocal to complex motor and phonic tics for some, but not all, affected individuals. The array of symptoms is limitless, and the expression of the disorder varies in each child from mild to severe. Typically the period of greatest difficulty is mid-childhood, with symptoms decreasing in intensity and frequency during late adolescence. Motor and vocal tics can occur in bouts and as single, isolated events. At times, the child may present with an orchestrated pattern of symptoms involving several muscle groups and multiple sounds. An example is eye blinking

CLINICAL EXAMPLE: TONY

Tony is a 7-year-old, second-grade student, who first presented with tics in the fall of first grade. His initial symptoms included frequent eye blinking, which prompted his parents to have his eyes checked. The examination was normal, and the ophthalmologist suggested that Tony had a "nervous habit." Tony's parents became concerned once again when his eye blinking returned in the fall of second grade. His teacher who had experience with other children with tics suggested that the parents consult their pediatrician and consider that the blinking might be a tic. No one in Tony's family had ever heard of tics, and there was no family history of a tic disorder. The pediatrician provided the parents with information about tics and explained that the eye blinking was not something Tony could control. This movement did not necessarily indicate that he would go on to develop more tics, but the parents were told to notify the pediatrician if the eye blinking caused problems or other tics appeared. Not calling attention to the tics by asking him to stop also would be less stressful. The tic was determined to be, most likely, a transient movement that would disappear during the next few months, possibly reappearing periodically over the next few years; the tic was considered unlikely, given a lack of family history, to develop into a more severe, chronic tic disorder.

CLINICAL EXAMPLE: SARAH

Sarah was 7 years old when her parents noticed a repetitive facial movement that seemed most intense and frequent when she was watching television or when she first came home from school. Over the next year, the movement changed in frequency and intensity but never disappeared completely. When Sarah was 8 years old, her facial twitching was accompanied by a mild shoulder shrug and a neck jerk. Sarah's pediatrician was familiar with tic disorders and referred her to a pediatric neurologist for consultation.

Sarah's developmental and medical history were normal, except for an exposure to decongestants starting at age 7 years because of allergies and chronic rhinitis. The family history revealed that Sarah's father had mouth and shoulder movements since childhood. His movements have been mild and have never caused any significant problems. In addition, a paternal uncle has a history of motor and phonic tics, and the paternal grandmother has a lifelong history of facial movements. The pediatric neurologist gave a provisional diagnosis of CMT Disorder and recommended that Sarah's allergy symptoms be treated with medications that do not contain sympathomimetic decongestants, which may exacerbate tics.

accompanied by shoulder shrugging and a high pitched sound, all occurring in such rapid succession that it is difficult to determine when one begins and the other ends. Frequency can vary from seldom to nearly constant.

The intensity, or the forcefulness of motor tics and the volume of vocal tics, also can vary from an abdominal tensing or guttural noise that can hardly be perceived by others to an upper body jerk or shouting sound that is physically uncomfortable and disturbing to the child and others.

Premonitory urges or sensations, commonly reported in adolescent and adult patients, are more difficult to elicit from younger children. It is unclear if this is due to a maturational stage in the child's ability to perceive the urge or sensation or if it does not exist. Nonetheless, some very young children may be able to describe their tics, both motor and phonic, as "an itchy feeling that builds up, and the tic makes the feeling go away briefly."

The symptoms that have made TS well known, coprolalia, copropraxia, and self-abusive behavior, are not common. When they do occur, they may be a hallmark of a more severe disorder.

Children and adolescents may present with associated features or secondary difficulties, which at times may be more disruptive and impairing than the tics themselves. Such associated phenomena may include disinhibited speech or conduct, impulsivity, distractibility, motoric hyperactivity, mood lability, and obsessive–compulsive symptoms. Secondary difficulties may include depression, school failure, or behavior problems.

NATURAL HISTORY

The average age of onset of tics is about 7 years. Symptoms may develop gradually over several years, or a child may present with a more dramatic onset. The repertoire of tics usually changes over time with certain tics remaining more constant. The course is generally described as one that has periods of intensity and frequency following by a period of quiescence (Scahill, Ort, & Hardin, 1993; Singer & Walkup, 1991).

At the onset, the child may not notice the tics if they are mild. For some children, the course of the disorder will remain mild with symptoms that are perceived as part of the child's natural expression. For others, the intensity, frequency, and complexity of some or all of their symptoms will be moderate to severe.

ASSOCIATED FEATURES

Associated features and secondary emotional difficulties complicate TS. The child with multiple motor and vocal tics and problems with attention and motoric hyperactivity may be more severely affected and difficult to treat than the child with tics alone. Occasionally, a child will have TS, problems with distractibility, impulsivity, a learning disorder, obsessive worries, and compulsive behaviors. Having one neurologic or neuropsychiatric disorder does not exclude the possibility of having others. Also, children can have a diagnosis of TS without other complicating features.

Debate continues about the relationship between impulsiveness, inattention, low frustration tolerance, and restlessness with TS. Are these manifestations of a separate neurologic disorder, ADHD, or intrinsic to TS (Pauls & Leckman, 1986; Comings & Comings, 1984)?

Family studies, using questionnaires and direct interviews of extended family members, have indicated strong evidence for a relationship with obsessive–compulsive symptoms. At times, it becomes difficult to distinguish complex motor tics from compulsive behaviors, and at other times, a child may initially present with motor and vocal tics and later develop OCD. As indicated in the family studies, obsessive–compulsive symptoms or OCD may be an alternative expression of the same underlying genetic disorder (Pauls, Raymond, Stevenson, & Leckman, 1991).

Learning difficulties in children with TS may present as a specific learning deficit or academic and classroom difficulty related to the description of the tics. Neuropsychoeducational studies have not revealed any basic cognitive impairment, yet they have indicated specific learning deficits, including impaired visual perceptual performance, reduced visual motor skills, and discrepancies between verbal and performance IQ (Bornstein, Carroll, & King, 1985; Erenberg, Cruse, & Rothner, 1986; Ferrari, Mathews, & Barbas, 1984). Some postulate that some neuropsychologic difficulties in TS may be "deficits in the executive domain," or rather the "capability to plan and sequence complex behaviors and to organize and sustain goal directed activities" (Singer & Walkup, 1991).

Behavioral problems in TS can be a primary reason for a child's referral for help. The basis for the difficulties, such as argumentativeness, aggressiveness, rebelliousness, or irritability, may be a secondary consequence of having a disorder that is stigmatizing or may be related to symptoms of ADHD.

Etiology

Despite rapid changes in our understanding of the mechanisms of neurobiology and the success of certain pharmacologic agents in reducing tics, the underlying etiology of tic disorders is unknown. It

CLINICAL EXAMPLE: MARK

The onset of Mark's difficulties began when he was 7 years old, shortly after starting second grade. Mark's teacher noted that he was somewhat less mature than his peers, was easily distracted, and had a more difficult time with reading than most of his classmates. His athletic skills and eagerness to make friends diminished the impact of these difficulties. Looking back to kindergarten, his teacher was aware of his difficulty with concentration and fidgetiness and felt that he needed more time to mature. By second grade, his teacher and parents also noticed that for weeks at a time he would have a head jerking movement but that at other times it appeared to be totally absent. Mark did not seem bothered by this until some of his peers started asking him why he did it. Mark was embarrassed and never answered their questions. At home, his parents asked him to stop the head movement, which seemed most evident as Mark tried to do his homework or when he was eating a meal with the family. Their requests seemed useless, which made the parents feel even more frustrated.

Mark was the third child. His oldest sister, age 17, had been in treatment during adolescence because of obsessive worries and numerous washing compulsions, which caused much stress for the sister and the entire family. In addition, the maternal grandmother and a maternal aunt had obsessive–compulsive symptoms.

Mark's own developmental history was generally unremarkable. There was no history of prenatal or postnatal complications. His medical history was noteworthy for chronic otitis media from the age of 18 months to 6 years, for which he was treated with decongestants and antibiotics. Otherwise his medical history was normal.

Mark was referred to a child psychiatrist late in the winter of his second grade because of the increasing difficulties he was having at school and the concern about his head movement. During the assessment, Mark had numerous movements and repetitive sounds. None were as disturbing as the head jerk and thus had been overlooked previously. They included facial twitching, throat clearing, small humming noises, and the need to even-up. For example, if Mark bumped the wall with his right shoulder, he would feel the urge to turn and bump it with his left shoulder. If he touched an object with his right hand, he would need to touch it with his left hand. A neurologic assessment was otherwise normal, and because there were no outstanding neurologic questions, Mark was not referred for an electroencephalogram or other neurologic tests. The problems with concentration and fidgetiness were causing increasing difficulties for Mark in school. Were these problems related to the tic disorder (the effort to suppress the head jerks or the break in concentration during a bout of head jerks) or a separate neurologic disorder, ADHD? In addition, it was evident that Mark also was a child who had numerous worries that included unreasonable fears that something terrible might happen to his parents or himself if he did not do certain things in "just the right way." An initial diagnosis was make of mild to moderate TS, possible ADHD, and possible OCD.

has been 30 years since the initial successful clinical trials by Seignot, using the dopaminergic blocking agent haloperidol (Shapiro, Shapiro, & Young, 1988). This was a turning point in the understanding of TS. It led to a greater appreciation of a neurobiologic cause for the disorder, as opposed to an association with hysterias or "nervous habits." The last 30 years of research have focused largely on the dopaminergic system. Various investigators have hypothesized that TS is a disorder in which postsynaptic dopaminergic D_2 receptors are hypersensitive (Leckman & Cohen, 1991). However, investigations to date have not supported this theory, nor have they disproven it (Leckman & Cohen, 1991). It is noteworthy that dopamine blocking agents, such as the neuroleptics (haloperidol and pimozide) only partially alleviate symptoms. They do not stop symptoms totally, nor do they change the course of the disorder. In contrast, tics are usually exacerbated by exposure to central nervous system stimulants, such as amphetamine and L-dopa, both of which increase central dopaminergic activity.

Precise neuroanatomic localization of the pathobiology of TS remains unknown. Substantial data imply significant roles of the basal ganglia and related cortical and thalamic structures (Chappel et al., 1990). Dysfunction in the basal ganglia has been indicated because of its established implication in other movement disorders, for example, Huntington's chorea, Parkinson's disease, and encephalitis lethargica (Singer & Walkup, 1991).

Brain neuroimaging studies in adults, including the more advanced techniques of magnetic resonance and computer image analysis and positron emission tomography, have recently yielded interesting preliminary findings, especially when TS individuals have been compared with individuals with OCD or a combination of TS and OCD. Development of safer techniques for brain imaging in children, especially children who have not been exposed to high doses of neuroleptics, is an area of current, yet underdeveloped, interest.

Dysfunction within the central neurotransmitter systems is the primary focus of biochemical investigation. This relates to several factors, including the response of symptoms to specific medications, results of studies of neurotransmitter metabolites in cerebrospinal fluid, and beginning studies of postmortem brain tissue. As such, the dopaminergic, serotonergic, noradrenergic, cholinergic, τ-aminobutyric acid-ergic, and opioid systems have each shown abnormalities in TS patients, but as yet there is no clear indication of a primary biochemical substrate. Singer and Walkup (1991) suggest the possibility of an abnormality involving a second messenger system, such as adenylate cyclase "acting to unify findings of alterations within multiple transmitter systems." A similar proposal by Leckman et al. (1992) hypothesizes that because the basal ganglia are composed of pathways that contribute to multiple and parallel circuits serving a variety of sensorimotor, motor, oculomotor, cognitive, and limbic activities, TS is associated with a failure to inhibit subsets of these neurotransmitter circuits.

Genetic family and twin studies have recently provided evidence that the vulnerability for TS and related disorders (chronic motor and phonic tic disorder and OCD) may be inherited as an autosomal dominant trait. Price, Kidd, Cohen, Pauls, and Leckman (1986) demonstrated that the concordance rate for TS among monozygotic twin pairs was greater than 50% compared with the concordance rate among dizygotic twins, which approaches 10%. When CMT was included as a diagnosis, the concordance rate increased to 77% for monozygotic twins and 30% for dizygotic twins.

Genetic family history studies have demonstrated that first-degree family members of individuals with TS are at significantly increased risk for TS, CMT, and OCD when compared with either the population prevalence or a control group (Pauls & Leckman, 1986). The risk to first-degree male family members is approximately 50%, with an 18% risk for TS, a 31% risk for chronic motor or phonic tic disorder, and a 7% risk for OCD. The risk to first-degree female family members is much less, with 5% for TS, 9% for chronic motor and phonic tic disorder, and 17% for OCD (for a complete review see Scahill et al., 1991).

Differential Diagnosis

Motor tics are defined as abnormal involuntary movements. The differential diagnosis includes movements associated with other movement disorders, including dystonias, akathisia, paroxysmal dyskinesias, stereotypies, athetosis, chorea, myoclonus, and ballism. Involuntary phonations are rare except when associated with either TS or chronic ic vocal tic disorder. The other abnormal movements listed above are associated with Huntington's chorea, Wilson's disease, or hemiballismus. Myoclonic movements occur in epilepsy. Complications of infectious diseases may produce choreiform movements, as in Sydenham's chorea. Finally, the use of pharmacologic agents, such as neuroleptics, may cause akathisias, acute dystonias, or withdrawal dyskinesias (Fahn & Erenberg, 1988).

Assessment

The goals of an initial assessment are the following:

- To understand the specific problems that the parents and child want answered
- To identify the presenting symptoms and associated features
- To assess the frequency, intensity, complexity, and interference of the tic symptoms and their impact on functioning
- To assess the severity of the associated features, if present, and their impact on functioning
- To determine the highest adaptive functioning level of the child and family
- To understand the child's strengths and areas of weakness in general and in school, both academically and socially
- To identify the supports available to the child at home, in the school, and through other outside resources

Clinical rating instruments, parent questionnaires, and self, teacher, and parent rating instruments are helpful adjuncts in the assessment of children with tic disorders. A parent questionnaire, such as the Tourette's Syndrome Questionnaire (Jagger et al., 1982), completed by the parents and child initially, is an important source of background information about developmental history, history of relevant symptoms, medical history, medication history, and family history of tics. Clinical ratings have been developed to quantify the number, anatomic location, frequency, intensity, interference, and overall impairment of tic disorders. The Yale Global Tic Severity Scale (Leckman et al., 1989) and the Tourette's Syndrome Severity Scale (Shapiro et al., 1988) are examples of valid and reliable clinical rating instruments that can be used during the assessment to document symptoms and ascertain severity at baseline.

During the assessment, it is essential to understand the impact the symptoms have on the child and family currently and when symptoms were at their worst. For some children and families, one or two tics can be devastating, resulting in embarrassment and social withdrawal; for others, the same degree of symptoms may not greatly interfere with their daily lives. Also important is the presence or absence of comorbid diagnoses in the child. The presence and level of severity of associated difficulties, such as obsessive–compulsive symptoms, inattention or impulsiveness, and less frequently, learning difficulties, need to be considered. As suggested previously, in many situations, the associated difficulties outweigh the tics in terms of overall importance.

Treatment

The treatment issues discussed in this section are relevant to TS and CMT. Transient tic disorder generally does not require intervention, except possibly education and support for the parents.

Because tic disorders usually involve many aspects of a child's and family's life and are usually chronic, treatment intervention can necessitate approaches in multiple areas:

- Education and supportive intervention with the child and family
- School intervention
- Individual counseling or psychotherapy
- Family or parent counseling or therapy
- Pharmacotherapy

EDUCATION AND SUPPORTIVE INTERVENTION

The goal of education is to help provide the most positive and supportive environment at home and at school. Frequently this is the only treatment intervention necessary and involves helping the child, parents, and educators understand what it means to have a tic disorder. It also means helping parents become supportive to their child and to other family members. Parents often benefit from information about the involuntary nature of tics, the natural history of the disorder, the fact that the child does not have a "mental disorder," and that the widely publicized and socially inappropriate symptoms (coprolalia, copropraxia, and self-abusive symptoms) are very rare. The national Tourette's Syndrome Association (TSA), a national lay organization, can provide important information and support to parents. There are regional chapters in most states, with the national headquarters in Bayside, New York.

SCHOOL INTERVENTION

School and learning difficulties can present in various ways. The chronic nature of the disorder may cause the child to lose motivation and develop low self-esteem or occasionally to become depressed. The tics themselves may interfere with learning by their forceful nature or by the child's attempts to suppress them. For children with associated difficulties, such as obsessions and compulsions, the

CLINICAL EXAMPLE: THERESA

Theresa is a 15-year-old high school student who was referred for evaluation of a possible tic disorder with an onset of motor tics at age 7 years. By 9 years of age, she had persistent but mild motor and phonic tics that did not interfere with her social life or school work. At age 14, Theresa started repeating behaviors, such as going through a doorway twice, rereading paragraphs in books, and closing and opening the door to her room. These behaviors started shortly after Theresa started a new school, in ninth grade. They progressed to needing to repeat certain behaviors until it felt right to her to avoid the thought of something bad happening. Theresa could not explain what would happen if she did not perform the behaviors but she sensed a vague feeling of distress. During this time, the motor and phonic tics continued.

The purpose for this referral was to obtain treatment for a loud throat clearing noise that annoyed her family. The family was not fully aware of Theresa's obsessive–compulsive symptoms because she did them in private. For Theresa, the worst feeling was that she was "crazy" and that no one would understand her.

The assessment consisted of meeting initially with Theresa and her parents to listen to what concerned everyone. Individual time for evaluation with Theresa would ensure her sense of "adolescent privacy" and allow the clinician an opportunity to complete a mental status assessment and current and past history of tics and associated symptoms. Interviewing the parents together for the developmental, social, and family history and their own understanding of the history of the presenting problems is also important. A diagnosis of TS and OCD is made by history. No laboratory tests or structured psychologic tests aid in such diagnoses. Information about other aspects of social, emotional, and cognitive development also will provide important information necessary in establishing realistic treatment goals. In addition, it is important to understand if the child is struggling in school and if so, why. Discussion with teachers may be very helpful in understanding school difficulties. The use of questionnaires, which are discussed later in this chapter, is a helpful adjunct to the clinical interview.

The assessment resulted in a diagnosis of OCD of moderate severity and TS of mild severity. The treatment plan included education and reassurance for Theresa and her parents, with the possible addition of psychotherapy if Theresa's distress was not relieved. In addition, medication intervention could be considered if the obsessive–compulsive symptoms began to interfere with her progress academically or socially. Initially, the therapist thought that the vocal tic might be less problematic once Theresa and her parents were able to understand more about her symptoms and the natural history of TS and OCD. Education and reassurance considerably decreased the anxiety that Theresa experienced by not knowing what was happening to her.

symptoms may interfere in ways that are not obvious to the teacher. The child may appear to have poor concentration or to "daydream," when in fact, he or she may have frequent involuntary obsessional thoughts or compulsive behaviors. It may be very difficult for other children with inattention, distractibility, and hyperactivity to stay on task and to learn. Consultation with teachers can lead to interventions for the child's specific needs. For example, children with attentional difficulties may perform better if learning tasks are brief and can be checked frequently or if the child is seated away from unnecessary distractions. The child experiencing a disturbing bout of tics may find it helpful to take a brief break.

Children with impulse control difficulties, caused either by the tic disorder or ADHD, frequently find themselves getting into trouble with teachers. Such children may not be able to handle unstructured parts of the school day, such as recess time. They may not have the same abilities to regulate behavior, follow the rules of games, or even modulate aggressive instincts.

Defining the difficulties that impact on the child's school adjustment or performance is the first step in school intervention. Consultation with teachers before problems develop or after problems have been identified will help parents and teachers devise a specific plan to help the child with a tic disorder.

INDIVIDUAL COUNSELING OR PSYCHOTHERAPY

Children and adolescents confronted with a chronic disorder marked by confusing behaviors and sounds they cannot control frequently need more attention from a clinician than a simple explanation and a prescription for medication. Treatment intervention therefore needs to address the whole child, not just the child with motor and phonic tics. Children should have the opportunity to explore the meaning of having a chronic disorder characterized by involuntary movements and sounds, behavioral disinhibition, and for some children, obsessive thoughts and compulsive behaviors. The course of the disorder may be influenced by how well children function in their daily life, how they feel about themselves, and how the world around them accepts or rejects them. Individual treatment often is focused on all these factors. In short, attention needs to be given to the impact of the disorder on development and how the child can be assisted in returning to an optimal level of functioning.

Although the family is critically important in treatment, working with the family as a whole or with the school need not be a substitute for addressing the individual child. The treatment approach depends on the developmental level and the specific needs of the child. Children, ages 5 to 7 years, can benefit from a combination of talking and interactive therapy, which is helpful in allowing the child to resolve feelings and ideas that might be confusing to them about having movements or making sounds they cannot control. For the preadolescent, similarly a combination of talking and activity might be a useful approach to individual therapy.

The adolescent with a tic disorder is attempting to come to terms with independence and personal identification, while trying to find his or her place in the adult world. Years of having to live with a tic disorder and possibly having to struggle with issues of self-control and ridicule from peers and adults who do not understand the symptoms make individual treatment of the adolescent unique and challenging. Respecting adolescents' privacy and individual rights, while at the same time addressing their primary difficulties, are the guiding principles of individual therapy with this age group. Adolescents may have very strong ideas or fears about medication, or some may have already experienced difficulties of unpleasant side effects. They also may have experienced several years of teasing and social difficulties.

For children of all ages, the ideas and emotions generated by having a chronic tic disorder can be confusing, disorganizing, and frightening. The children may wonder whether they are "crazy" or "damaged," if they will ever be "normal" like their peers, or if they will ever be successful at dating. Their feelings might include anger, fear, or frustration at not being able to control their body. Such feelings may be expressed by acting out against those individuals they love the most, such as their mother, father, or siblings. Thus, for some children the primary reason they are brought for treatment is related to their emotional adjustment difficulties in response to their chronic illness. As with all childhood psychiatric disorders, an important principle for individual therapy would be to approach the child at his or her current level of maturity and to focus on the emotional difficulties or struggles.

FAMILY THERAPY AND PARENT GUIDANCE

The method of family or parent intervention with a child varies depending on the strengths and difficulties that each family experiences uniquely. Treatment approaches based on goals that help the child with TS attain a maximum level of functioning, return to successful development, and achieve a healthy self-esteem are the most likely to be successful. Family treatment addresses these same issues. As with other chronic illnesses, the family's response to a child with TS will impact on the child's adjustment. When developing a treatment strategy, the therapist should be mindful of the family's ability to be supportive. The extent and method of family intervention depends in part on the clinician's assessment of the family's needs.

Family intervention begins with the initial assessment. The clinician begins to learn not only about the primary questions that bring the family for treatment, but also how the family works together, what strategies are used for coping, how parenting roles are expressed and understood, how siblings relate, how these relationships affect the functioning of the family, and how the family relates to the larger social group. In the treatment of a child with TS, other issues that become important include the impact of the child's symptoms on family relationships and parenting skills. Areas of consideration often include the chronicity of the disorder, the siblings' reactions to the nature of the tics that can be socially unattractive, and the confusion of parents and siblings about the waxing and waning and uncontrollable nature of tics. Parents also may struggle with feelings of guilt related to misconceptions and attributions about tics prior to diagnosis, failed treatment, or medication side effects.

Clinicians may recommend more than one treatment intervention to the family; in addition, the kind of treatment appropriate at one time may not be the best approach at other times. For example, a clinician and family may decide that family therapy is indicated, but as the family sessions progress, it becomes clear that the child is experiencing difficulty with adolescent issues and increasing feelings of depression. The goal of working with families is to assess progress and adjust intervention goals continually, depending on the needs of the child and family within the context of their social environment.

The concept of the nurse as case manager can be important as one considers the multiple systems involved when a child has TS. Coordination of other services from the school and community with the need to develop an overall plan of intervention is often a role that advanced practice nurses or clinical nurse specialists have the skills to accomplish.

PHARMACOTHERAPY

Medication is the most widely used treatment for TS. The goal of treatment for most children and adolescents is to decrease tics. Hence, clinicians frequently turn to pharmacotherapy. Most cases of TS are mild and do not require medication, yet some children with TS may have periods in their development in which symptoms are severe enough to warrant medication. Pharmacotherapy is most effective when combined with the other treatment interventions discussed previously.

At times, the choice of medication is determined by the associated difficulties, rather than the tics. For example, it is not uncommon for a child who has had multiple motor and phonic tics since early childhood to have these symptoms decrease only to have obsessions and compulsions become prominent in adolescence. The decision to use pharmacotherapy requires several steps, including assessment of the following:

- The symptoms that are currently most distressing to the child and family
- Whether these symptoms can be handled by means other than medication
- The meaning to the child and family of starting medication

In addition, as with all psychopharmacotherapy, the following should be assessed prior to starting and before choosing the specific medication:

- Conduct a thorough medical history (obtain pediatric records, and make sure the pediatrician or family physician is aware of medication).
- Depending on the medication chosen, obtain baseline medical assessment: standard laboratory tests, electrocardiogram (EKG), height and weight, blood pressure, and pulse.
- Obtain baseline rating of severity using a clinical rating instrument if possible to compare changes during treatment.
- Discuss all options openly with parents and child.

The goal of treatment is to help the child return to an optimal developmental level of functioning. Pharmacotherapy should be reserved for situations in which symptoms are impeding the child's continued development or causing significant disruption.

Starting the child on the lowest dose possible and increasing the dose gradually can decrease the incidence of side effects or adverse reactions. Adequate trials of a medication allow the clinician to judge optimal efficacy of the specific medication. If the dose is too small, it is difficult to measure the true effect on the child. The goal of treatment need not be to eliminate all tics, but rather to decrease frequency and intensity to the degree that the child can return to optimal functioning without disabling side effects. Therefore, the dose should be the lowest possible to obtain a tolerable level of symptoms. The use of more than one medication to treat symptoms is usually complicated, especially in assessing efficacy and side effects. It is difficult to know which agent is responsible for changes or unpleasant reactions and therefore which medication dose to adjust. However, in complicated cases of TS, it may be necessary to use small doses of more than one agent. Changing a medication dose, altering the time at which it is given, or stopping one medication or starting a new one should be done in definitive stages. This prevents confusion on the part of the clinician in assessing the impact of the change.

Although the clinical nurse specialist may not be the clinician who prescribes medication, this does not decrease the amount of involvement in the management of care. Children with TS have medication prescribed by pediatricians, pediatric neurologists, family practitioners, and child psychiatrists. The clinical nurse specialist's role varies according to the setting in which he or she sees the child and what part he or she assumes on a treatment team. On an inpatient unit, this role may involve milieu management, individual therapy, or family therapy. In an outpatient setting, this role may include clinician for the individual or family or being part of a larger treatment team. Regardless of the setting or treatment role of the clinical nurse specialist, when a child is started on medication, or comes to treatment on medication, the clinical nurse specialist uses a background in psychopharmacology to assist in the assessment of efficacy, side effects, and adverse reactions and the impact this has on the whole child.

CLINICAL RATING INSTRUMENTS USED IN ASSESSMENT

Assessment of medication efficacy is best achieved by using clinical rating instruments. A baseline rating documents a description of symptoms and a rating of severity. Weekly, monthly, or periodic clinical assessments are made using the same instrument(s). Several clinician rating instruments are available for assessment of TS. In particular, one that works well for children, adolescents, and adults is the Yale Global Tic Severity Scale (YGTSS) (Leckman et al., 1989). This scale is a valid and reliable measurement of tic severity and looks at various dimensions, including the number of tics, anatomic location, frequency, intensity, complexity of the tics, direct interference caused by the tics, and overall impairment caused by this chronic disorder. This is a structured, clinical interview involving the child and a parent, because severity of tics is often difficult to judge by the child alone. Clinical ratings are difficult because of the waxing and waning nature of tics, so to avoid some of this difficulty, it is best to focus on the past week and rate an average of all the tics, not specific symptoms alone. Some indication of the primary and most prominent tics is helpful to document and review in subsequent assessments.

The Children's Yale-Brown Obsessive Compulsive Scale (CY-BOCS) is a valid and reliable clinical rating instrument used to rate the severity of OCD symptoms (Riddle et al., submitted). As with the YGTSS, this is a structured, clinical interview involving the child and a parent. Some children prefer to be interviewed alone because of the difficult nature of some of their obsessions or compulsions. One or both parents may be interviewed separately, with the child's understanding that they are sharing their observations of the symptoms during the past week. The CY-BOCS rates obsessions and compulsions separately, assessing frequency, interference, distress associated with symptoms, resistance against symptoms, and degree of control with an overall severity score. The children's version of the Leyton Obsessive Compulsive Inventory, used for individuals up to age 16 years, or the adult version, used for adolescents older than 16 years, is a self-report that also can be useful in assessing treatment changes (Berg, Rapoport, & Flament, 1986; Cooper, 1970)

Rating instruments designed to assess attentional, impulsivity, and hyperactivity symptoms are usually more accurate if completed by parents and the classroom teacher(s). The most widely used parent and teacher rating instruments are the Connors Parent Questionnaire, the Connors Teachers Questionnaire (Connors, 1970), and the Child Behavior Checklist with versions for parents, teachers, and a self-questionnaire for children 11 years and older (Achenbach & Edelbrock, 1981).

MEDICATIONS USED TO TREAT TS AND ASSOCIATED FEATURES

A vast number of agents have been used to treat TS in children. The results of valid double-blind clinical trials have only demonstrated that D_2 receptor agonists, specifically haloperidol and pimozide, have been effective in reducing tics. An alternative agent used to treat TS is clonidine, an alpha-adrenergic agonist, which, though not as dramatically effective as a neuroleptic, is helpful in reducing tics in approximately 40% of individuals who use it and has fewer side effects overall.

HALOPERIDOL. The butyrophenone, haloperidol (Haldol), is a powerful dopaminergic receptor blocking agent at the D_2 receptor site and is the most widely used medication to treat children and adolescents with TS. Shapiro and Shapiro (1988) have conducted several studies and have reviewed the literature concerning the efficacy and side effects of haloperidol in all age individuals with TS. Their results indicate that 25% of individuals have at least a 70% reduction of their tics, without developing significant side effects. Fifty percent develop side effects that can be managed successfully and still achieve therapeutic benefit. Another 25% develop side effects that are significant enough to negate the positive effects and can be considered treatment failures.

No long-term clinical studies have examined the effect of using haloperidol for extended periods in children.

A recommended treatment regimen is to start the child with 0.25 mg of haloperidol before bedtime and increase by 0.25 mg every 5 to 7 days, until symptoms decrease 50% to 70% or up to a 2- to 4-mg total dose. The doses used to treat TS are much lower than those commonly used in other psychiatric disorders. Older adolescents may require a more rapid dose increase, such as 0.5 mg every 4 to 5 days. In young children and many adolescents, a 0.5 to 1.5 mg total daily dose is enough to control symptoms. More extreme cases may require and respond to higher doses, from 8 to 10 mg/day.

Side effects of haloperidol include parkinsonian effects, akathisia, akinesia, sedation, weight gain, decreased concentration, social or school phobia, decreased memory, anergia, dysphoria, personality changes, sexual dysfunction, loss of libido, and tardive dyskinesia (TD). Acute dystonia, which occurs in less than 10% of individuals, usually develops within the first 72 hours of treatment. It involves sustained or occasionally intermittent contraction of unilateral or bilateral muscles, most commonly of the upper torso, with the potential for mandibular and oculogyric spasms, speech and swallowing difficulties, torticollis, hyperextension of the neck and upper torso, and torsion spasm. It is not related to dose and is treated with administration of benztropine. Haloperidol does not have to be stopped and the acute dystonia rarely returns. There is some variation among clinicians about the introduction of antiparkinsonian medication to prevent or decrease side effects. Some clinicians advise starting both the haloperidol and an antiparkinsonian agent simultaneously to prevent the development of side effects. Other clinicians suggest waiting until the dose of haloperidol has reached 2 to 3 mg/day before starting an antiparkinsonian agent, and a third group of clinicians suggests waiting until side effects appear. Frequently, children do not require the addition of antiparkinsonian agents.

It is important to educate parents and children about the potential side effects, adverse reactions, and the potential for developing TD. Careful monitoring of children while on a neuroleptic is imperative. Children should be assessed frequently (every 4–6 weeks) while they are starting medication and as the dose is increased. After a maintenance dose is reached, children should be monitored for efficacy and side effects every 3 to 6 months during the first year. Dyskinetic movements are assessed through the use of the Abnormal Involuntary Movement Scale.

The severity of potential side effects associated with haloperidol and other neuroleptic medications indicates that these agents should be reserved for children with severe symptoms or with symptoms that greatly impede their ability to function either in school, socially, or within their family setting. Generally, families can learn to become more tolerant of tics; thus, the home can be a place where the child with TS can feel more at ease. It is not uncommon to see children with TS in clinical settings who have been treated with substantially high doses of haloperidol or who have developed side effects on moderately low doses. For too many children, this experience has altered their lives significantly. They have become chronically depressed, have gained sufficient weight that they are considered obese, or have lost the ability to concentrate and learn in school. Although their tics are indeed less of a problem, the quality of their lives has not improved. Despite this, haloperidol, used carefully and cautiously, can be an important intervention.

PIMOZIDE. Pimozide (Orap), a diphenyl-butylpiperidine, is also a dopaminergic blocking agent with D_2 receptor selectivity. It has a similar response rate and side-effect profile to haloperidol. Approximately 70% to 80% of individuals with TS will respond to pimozide. Some studies indicate that side effects occur less frequently with pimozide than with haloperidol treatment (Chouinard & Steinberg, 1982; Moldofsky & Sandor, 1988). Others have reported no difference in side effects between pimozide or haloperidol (Shapiro et al., 1988). It may be true that some individuals tolerate and respond to one neuroleptic better than another. Early reports of EKG abnormalities, U waves and inverted T waves, raised concern about cardiotoxic properties of pimozide. Further clinical research studies have not supported these earlier findings (Moldofsky & Sandor, 1988). Nonetheless, in view of the concern raised by the earlier studies, it is recommended that EKG studies be done at baseline and yearly.

Treatment with pimozide usually begins at 1 mg daily, with gradual increments, every 5 to 7 days, up to 3 to 5 mg as a total daily dose. Some children with more severe symptoms require a higher dose, for example, up to 8 mg/day. Pimozide has a longer half-life than haloperidol and therefore allows a single dosing schedule.

Parents should be warned that TD is a possible development with long-term treatment or in rare cases, even after relatively short-term treatment. Because no one understands why some individuals develop TD and others do not, it is not possible to predict this when initiating neuroleptic treatment.

CLONIDINE. Clonidine (Catapres), an $alpha_2$-adrenergic receptor agonist, was developed as an antihypertensive agent and was first described by Cohen, Young, Nathanson, and Shaywitz (1979) as a treatment for TS 15 years ago. The effectiveness of clonidine in TS is thought to be related to the action of the $alpha_2$-adrenergic receptor agonist in reducing the release of norepinephrine from central noradrenergic neurons and thus serving as a modulating influence on the dopaminergic system. It is an alternative to the neuroleptics, and many clinicians use clonidine as a first choice because of its relative safety. Several well-controlled, double-blind studies have demonstrated varying results, some indicating efficacy, while others show no significant advantage of clonidine over placebo (Cohen et al.,

1979; Borison, Ang, Hamilton, Diamond, & David, 1983; Goetz et al., 1987; Leckman et al., 1991).

In the Goetz study (1987), subjects also were receiving neuroleptics, and the dose of clonidine was higher than the dose that has been found to be effective in other studies (7.5–15 μ/kg per day). This study did not find a significant difference between clonidine and placebo in the treatment of TS. In the most recent double-blind, placebo-controlled study, Leckman et al. (1991) demonstrated that using both clinical ratings and tic count ratings, clonidine was significantly superior to placebo in decreasing tics. The degree of improvement does not parallel that of the neuroleptic, but the side effects are much less.

The recommended starting dose for clonidine for children and adolescents is 0.05 mg (½ tablet) in the morning for approximately 3 to 5 days and increasing by 0.05 mg/day up to three times a day for younger children (below 12 years) and four times a day for adolescents, yielding a total daily dose of 0.15 to 0.2 mg. Gradual increases in the dose avoid some of the problems of sedation. Some children respond to smaller doses, such as 0.025 mg three times a day, while others respond to doses up to 0.35 mg/day. Greater efficacy is achieved if the dosing is divided by 3 to 4 hours during waking hours. For example, a child of 8 years might receive clonidine, 0.05 mg at 8:00 AM, 0.05 mg at noon, and 0.05 mg at 4:00 PM. The total dose and pattern of dosing are dependent on the response of the child. The recommended total daily dose is between 0.15 and 0.35 mg. The primary side effects are sedation, dry mouth, and dizziness.

Sedation and dry mouth usually subside after an adjustment to clonidine is made. Clonidine is used as an antihypertensive treatment and thus initially lowers the blood pressure. This might cause orthostatic hypotension or mild dizziness in some individuals. This can be remedied by lowering the dose slightly. Clonidine has been reported to be effective in reducing impulsivity and increasing the ability of the child to focus. Thus, with children who have both TS and attentional and impulsivity difficulties, clonidine may be effective in treating both types of symptoms.

DESIPRAMINE. Because approximately 50% of children who present with TS also have ADHD, pharmacotherapy needs either to address both symptoms or to target the most disabling symptoms. The most commonly used treatment for ADHD, the stimulant medications, also have been reported to exacerbate tics (Lowe, Cohen, Detlor, Kreminitzer, & Shaywitz, 1982). Because clonidine is effective for only about 40% to 45% of individuals who are treated, efforts have been made over the past few years to find alternative treatments for children with TS and ADHD. Desipramine (Norpramine), a tricyclic antidepressant, has been shown to be effective in treating ADHD, while not increasing tics (Hoge & Biederman, 1986; Riddle, Hardin, Cho, Woolston, & Leckman, 1988). Recent reports of the sudden death of four children who were taking desipramine have indicated concerns about the possible cardiotoxic effects of this specific tricyclic but not other tricyclics. This has led clinicians to proceed cautiously at the present time in the use of this agent until further clarification about safety is obtained.

FLUOXETINE. Fluoxetine (Prozac) is a specific inhibitor of neuronal serotonin reuptake and has been demonstrated as an effective and relatively safe treatment for OCD in children and adults (Riddle, Hardin, King, & Woolston, 1990: Jenike, Buttolph, Baer, Riccardi, Holland, 1989). Its effect on tic symptoms has been studied without evidence of significant results (Riddle et al., 1990). However, fluoxetine can be helpful for children with TS who experience obsessions and compulsions as their more troubling symptoms.

The major side effects of fluoxetine include behavioral activation, changes in sleep, and less frequently, abdominal discomfort. In a review of 24 children, ages 8 to 16 years, who were treated with fluoxetine ranging in doses from 20 to 40 mg/day, 50% demonstrated motor restlessness, sleep disturbance, social disinhibition, or a subjective sensation of excitation (Riddle et al., 1991). Lowering the dose or discontinuing the fluoxetine stopped these symptoms. Starting children on smaller doses of fluoxetine, such as 10 mg/day and gradually increasing to a therapeutic dose allows close monitoring of side effects, which appear to be dose related. Fluoxetine is currently available in liquid form, which allows for the administration of lower doses in children. Children and adolescents do not usually require a total daily dose in excess of 20 mg/day, and many may respond at lower doses.

Recently there has been public alarm concerning the possible association of suicidal ideation and fluoxetine. The causal relationship between fluoxetine and suicidal ideation remains unclear (King et al., 1991). Careful assessment of suicidal ideation before and during treatment with fluoxetine is recommended. As noted in published case reports, suicidal thought or behavior may not be preceded by symptoms of depression but rather, appear as a preoccupation with death and notions of inflicting self-harm (King et al., 1991).

CLOMIPRAMINE. Clomipramine (Anafranil), a tricyclic antidepressant, differs from other tricyclics because it not only affects norepinephrine levels, but also inhibits reuptake of serotonin. It is the most studied medication used to treat OCD in adults and children and has been shown to be superior to other tricyclic agents in reducing obsessive and compulsive symptoms in up to 50% of individuals studied (Thoren, Asberg, Cronholm, Jorenstedt, & Traskman, 1980; Flament, Rapoport, Murphy, Berg, & Lake, 1987; Leonard et al., 1989; Mavissakalian, Jones, Olson, & Pered, 1990). To date, clomipramine has not been systematically studied as a treatment for obsessive–compulsive symptoms in patients with TS, though clinical experience indicates that it may be as effective as fluoxetine. Some patients have been reported to experience an exacerbation of their tics on clomipramine, but the majority of TS patients respond to its antiobsessional action without a worsening of their tics (Caine, Polinsky, Ebert, Rapaport, & Mikkelsen, 1979; Yaryura-Tobias, 1975; Ratzoni, Hermesh, Brandt, Lauffer, & Munitz, 1990).

The usual starting dose of clomipramine is 25 mg/day, with increases in 25- to 50-mg increments every 5 days to symptom improvement or as tolerated. Children and adolescents generally respond to a dosage between 150 and 200 mg/day or 3 mg/kg per day for children, given in two to three divided doses (Leonard et al., 1989). The side effects of clomipramine, such as dry mouth, constipation, sweating, sedation, and orthostatic hypotension, are similar to those seen in other tricyclic antidepressants. In addition, side effects common to other serotonin reuptake inhibitors are seen, including nausea, tremor, and anorgasmia. Seizures have been reported rarely in individuals who have received doses up to 300 mg/day (Anafranil package insert). As with other tricyclic antidepressants, such as desipramine, there is the potential for development of prolongation of PR and QT intervals (Elliot & Popper, 1991). Children may be more vulnerable to the cardiotoxic side effects than adults (Ryan, 1990). With any child who receives clomipramine at any dose, EKGs should be obtained at baseline, during the upward adjustment, and periodically during long-term use.

SERTRALINE. Sertraline (Zoloft), a naphthalenamine, is structurally unique and chemically unrelated to other antidepressants (Doogan & Caillard, 1988). It exhibits greater selectivity for inhibition of serotonin uptake relative to norepinephrine uptake than either fluoxetine or the tricyclic antidepressants. Sertraline has been available and approved to treat adults with depression since March 1992. There are no published data in children or adolescents, though there is currently a multicentered study of the efficacy of sertraline in treating adolescents with major depression. Another industry-sponsored multicentered study also is looking at the efficacy of sertraline in treating children and adolescents with OCD. Preliminary studies (Jenike et al., 1990) in adults with OCD have been inconclusive.

The common side effects include gastrointestinal complaints, including nausea, diarrhea, and dyspepsia; tremor; dizziness; insomnia and somnolence; dry mouth and male ejaculatory delay. Compared with the tricyclic antidepressants, including clomipramine, sertraline is associated with a significantly lower incidence of the above side effects (Cohn, Shrivastava, & Mendels, 1990; Doogan & Caillard, 1988). Sertraline has an average plasma elimination half-life of 26 hours, with steady-state plasma levels achieved within 1 week. The usual starting dose for adolescents is 25 mg twice daily, increasing to 50 mg twice daily.

Summary

This chapter has presented an overview of the tic disorders in children and adolescents, concentrating on TS, with relevant confirmation for clinical nurse specialists and all nurses working with children in school, mental health, pediatric, or family practice settings.

This overview has reviewed the definition of tics and tic disorders, the prevalence in children of the major tic disorder, clinical description, natural history, associated features, etiology, differential diagnosis, assessment, and treatment. Case vignettes have been used to illustrate clinical examples.

TS encompasses a vast array of biologic, social, emotional, developmental, psychiatric, and neuropsychologic aspects. Nurses are in an ideal position to contribute on many levels because of the unique training in the biologic, medical, and psychosocial–developmental dimensions of clinical care. In addition to clinical care, nurses also have the advantage of contributing unique research skills that can address such issues as nongenetic factors influencing expression of severity or the impact on a child's development of a chronic illness that involves socially unacceptable symptoms.

Beyond this, nurses also have backgrounds in case management and team collaboration, both important aspects in the clinical care of children and adolescents with TS.

REFERENCES

Achenbach, T. M., & Edelbrock, C. S. (1981). Behavioral problems and competencies reported by parents of normal and disturbed children aged four through sixteen. *Monographs of the Society for Research in Child Development, 46* (1).

American Psychiatric Association (1994). *Diagnostic and statistical manual of mental disorders* (4th ed.). Washington, DC: American Association Press.

Apter, A., Pauls, D. L., Bleich, A., Zohar, A. H., Kron, S., Ratzoni, G., Dycian, A., Kotler, M., Weizman, A., Gadot, N., & Cohen, D. J. (1993). An epidemiological study of Gilles de la Tourette's syndrome in Israel. *Archives of General Psychiatry, 50* (9), 734–738.

Berg, C., Rapoport, J. L., & Flament, M. (1986). The Leyton Obsessional Inventory-Child Version. *Journal of the American Academy of Child and Adolescent Psychiatry, 25*(1), 84–91.

Borison, R. L., Ang, L., Hamilton, W. J., Diamond, B. I., & David, J. M. (1983). Treatment approaches in Gilles de la Tourette Syndrome. *Brain Research Bulletin, 11*(2), 205–208.

Bornstein, R. A., Carroll, A., & King, G. (1985). Relationship of age to neuropsychological deficit in Tourette's syndrome. *Developmental Behavioral Pediatrics, 6*, 285–286.

Burd, L., Kerbeshian, J., Wilkenheiser, M., & Fisher, W. (1986a). Prevalence of Gilles de la Tourette's syndrome in North Dakota adults. *American Journal of Psychiatry, 143*, 787–788.

Burd, L., Kerbeshian, J., Wilkenheiser, M., & Fisher, W. (1986b). Prevalence of Gilles de la Tourette's syndrome in North Dakota school-age children. *Journal of the American Academy of Child Psychiatry, 25*, 552–553.

Bruun, R. D. (1988). The natural history of Tourette's syndrome. In D. J. Cohen, R. D. Bruun, & J. F. Leckman (Eds.), *Tourette's Syndrome and Tic Disorders* (pp. 21–39). New York: John Wiley & Sons.

Caine, E. D., McBride, M. C., Chiverton, P., Bamford, K. A., Rediess, S., & Shiao, S. (1988) Tourette's syndrome in Monroe County school children. *Neurology, 38*(3), 472–475.

Caine, E. D., Polinsky, R. J., Ebert, M. H., Rapaport, H. L., & Mikkelsen, E. J. (1979). Trial of chlorimipramine and desipramine for Gilles de la Tourette syndrome. *Annals of Neurology, 6*, 305–306.

Chappell, P. B., Leckman, J. F., Riddle, M. A., Anderson, G. A., Listwack, S. J., Ort, S. I., Hardin, M. T., Scahill, L., & Cohen, D. J. (1990). Biological and genetic studies of Tourette's syndrome: Implications for treatment and future research. In S. I. Deutch, A. Weizman, & R. Weigman (Eds.), *Application of Basic Neuroscience for Child Psychiatry* (pp. 241–260). New York: Plenum Press.

Chouinard, G., & Steinberg, S. (1982). Type I tardive dyskinesia induced by anticholinergic drugs, dopamine agonists and neuroleptics. *Progress in Neuropsychopharmacology and Biological Psychiatry, 6*, 571–578.

Cohen, D. J., Young, J. G., Nathanson, J. A., & Shaywitz, B. A. (1979). Clonidine in Tourette's syndrome. *Lancet, ii*, 551–553.

Cohen, D. J., Riddle, M. A., & Leckman, J. F. (1991). Pharmacotherapy of Tourette's syndrome and associated disorders. In D. Shaffer (Ed.), *The Psychiatric Clinics of North America* (pp. 109–130). Philadelphia: W.B. Saunders.

Cohn, C. K., Shrivastava, R., Mendels, J. (1990). Double-blind multicenter comparison of sertraline and amitriptyline in elderly depressed patients. *Journal of Clinical Psychiatry, 51*(Suppl. B), 18–27.

Comings, D. E., & Comings, B. G. (1984). Tourette syndrome and attention deficit disorder with hyperactivity: Are they genetically related? *Journal of the American Academy of Child Psychiatry, 23*, 138–146.

Cooper, J. (1970). The Leyton Obsessional Inventory. *Psychological Medicine, I*, 48–64.

Doogan, D. P., & Caillard, V. (1988). Sertraline, a new antidepressant. *Journal of Clinical Psychiatry, 49*, 46–51.

Elliott, G. R., & Popper, C. W. (1991). Editorial: Tricyclic antidepressants: The QT interval and other cardiovascular parameters. *Journal of Child Adolescent Psychopharmacology, I*, 187–191.

Endicott, J., Spitzer, R. L., & Fleiss, J. L. (1976). The Clinical Global Scale: A procedure for measuring overall severity of psychiatric disturbance. *Archives of General Psychiatry, 33*, 776–771.

Erenberg, G., Cruse, R. P., & Rothner, A. D. (1986). Tourette syndrome: An analysis of 200 pediatric and adolescent cases. *Cleveland Clinic Quarterly, 53*, 127–131.

Fahn, S., & Erenberg, G. (1988). Differential diagnosis of the phenomena; a neurologic perspective. In D. J. Cohen, R. D. Bruun, & J. F. Leckman (Eds.), *Tourette's syndrome and Tic Disorder* (pp. 41–54). New York: John Wiley & Sons.

Ferrari, M., Mathews, W. S., & Barbas, G. (1984). Children with Tourette syndrome: Results of psychological tests given prior to drug treatment. *Developmental Behavioral Pediatrics, 5*, 116–119.

Flament, M., Rapoport, J., Murphy, D., Berg, C. J., & Lake, R. (1987). Biochemical changes during clomipramine treatment in childhood obsessive compulsive disorder. *Archives of General Psychiatry, 44*, 219–225.

Goetz, C. G., & Klawans, H. L. (1982). Gilles de la Tourette on Tourette Syndrome. In A. J. Freidhoff & T. N. Chase (Eds.), *Gilles de la Tourette Syndrome* (pp. 1–16). New York: Raven.

Goetz, C. G., Tanner, C. M., Wilson, R. S., Carroll, V. S., Como, P. G., & Shannon, K. M. (1987). Clonidine and Gilles de la Tourette syndrome: Double-blind study using objective rating methods. *Annals of Neurology, 21*, 307–310.

Goyette, C. H., Connors, C. K., & Ulrich, R. F. (1978). Normative data on Revised Connors Parent and Teacher Rating Scales. *Journal of Abnormal Child Psychology, 6*, 221–236.

Hoge, S. K., & Biederman, J. (1986). A case of Tourette's syndrome with symptoms of attention deficit disorder treated with desipramine. *Journal of Clinical Psychiatry, 47*, 478–479.

Jagger, J., Prusoff, B. A., Cohen, D. J., Kidd, K. K., Carbonari, C. M., & John, K. (1982). The epidemiology of Tourette's syndrome: A pilot study. *Schizophrenia Bulletin, 8*, 267–278.

Jenike, M. A., Buttolph, L., Baer, L., Riccardi, J., & Holland, A. (1989). Open trial of fluoxetine in obsessive-compulsive disorder. *American Journal of Psychiatry, 146*, 909–911.

Jenike, M. A., Baer, L., Summergrad, P., Minichiello, W. E., Holland, A., Seymour, R. (1990). Sertraline in Obsessive-Compulsive Disorder: A double blind comparison with placebo. *American Journal of Psychiatry, 147*(7), 923–928.

King, R. A., Riddle, M. A., Chappell, P. B., Hardin, M. T., Anderson, G. M., Lombroso, P., & Scahill, L. (1991). Emergence of self-destructive phenomena in children and adolescents during fluoxetine treatment. *Journal of American Academy of Child an Adolescent Psychiatry, 30*, 179–186.

Leckman, J. F., & Cohen, D. J. (1988). Descriptive and diagnostic classification of Tic Disorders. In D. J. Cohen, R. D. Bruun, & J. F. Leckman (Eds.), *Tourette's Syndrome and Tic Disorders* (pp. 3–20). New York: John Wiley & Sons.

Leckman, J. F., Riddle, M. A., & Cohen, D. J. (1988). Pathobiology of Tourette's syndrome. In D. J. Cohen, R. D. Bruun, & J. F. Leckman (Eds.), *Tourette's Syndrome and Tic Disorders* (pp. 103–118). New York: John Wiley & Sons.

Leckman, J. F., Towbin, K. E., Ort, S. I., & Cohen, D. J. (1988). Clinical assessment of Tic Disorder severity. In D. J. Cohen, R. D. Bruun, & J. F. Leckman (Eds.), *Tourette's Syndrome and Tic Disorders* (pp. 55–78). New York: John Wiley & Sons.

Leckman, J. F., Walkup, J. T., & Cohen, D. J. (1988). Clonidine treatment of Tourette's syndrome. In D. J. Cohen, R. D. Bruun, & J. F. Leckman (Eds.), *Tourette's Syndrome and Tic Disorders* (pp. 291–302). New York: John Wiley & Sons.

Leckman, J. F., Pauls, D. L., Peterson, B. S., Riddle, M. A., Anderson, G. A., & Cohen, D. J. (1992). Pathogenesis of Tourette's syndrome: Clues from clinical phenotype. In T. N. Chase, A. J. Friedhoff, & D.J. Cohen (Eds.), *Advances in Neurology* (pp. 15–24). New York: Raven Press.

Leckman, J. F., Hardin, M. T., Riddle, M. A., Ort, S. I., Stevenson, J., & Cohen, D. J. (1991). Clonidine treatment of Tourette's syndrome. *Archives of General Psychiatry, 48*, 324–328.

Leckman, J. F., Riddle, M. A., Hardin, M. T., Ort, S. I., Swartz, K. L., Stevenson, J., & Cohen, D. J. (1989). The Yale Global Tic Severity Scale: Initial testing of a clinician-rated scale of tic severity. *Journal of the American Academy of Child and Adolescent Psychiatry, 28*(4), 566–573.

Leckman, J. F., & Cohen, D. J. (1991). Tic Disorders. In M. Lewis (Ed.), *Child and Adolescent Psychiatry* (pp. 613–621). Baltimore: Williams & Wilkins.

Leonard, H. L., Swedo, S. E., Rapoport, J. L., Kolby, E. V., Lenane, M. C., Cheslow, D. L., & Hamburger, S. D. (1989). Treatment of obsessive-compulsive disorder with clomipramine and desipramine in children and adolescents: A double-blind crossover comparison. *Archives of General Psychiatry, 46*, 1088–1092.

Lowe, T. L., Cohen, D. J., Detlor, J., Kreminitzer, M. W., & Shaywitz, B. A. (1982). Stimulant medications precipitate Tourette's Syndrome. *Journal of the American Medical Association, 247*, 1729–1731.

Lucas, A. R., Beard, C. M., Rajput, A. H., & Kurland, L. T. (1982). Tourette's Syndrome in Rochester, Minnesota, 1968-1979. *Advances in Neurology, 35*, 267–269.

Mavissakalian, M., Jones, B., Olson, S., & Pered, J. M. (1990). The relationship of plasma clomipramine and N-desmethylclomipramine response in obsessive-compulsive disorder. *Psychopharmacology Bulletin, 26*, 119–122.

Moldofsky, H., & Sandor, P. (1988). Pimozide treatment of Tourette's syndrome. In D. J. Cohen, R. D. Bruun, & J. F. Leckman (Ed.), *Tourette's Syndrome and Tic Disorders* (pp. 281–289). New York: John Wiley & Sons.

Pauls, D. L., Kruger, S. D., Leckman, J. F., Cohen, D. J., & Kidd, K. K. (1984). The risk of Tourette's syndrome and chronic multiple tics among relatives of Tourette's syndrome patients obtained by direct interview. *Journal of the American Academy of Child Psychiatry, 23*, 134–137.

Pauls, D. L., & Leckman, J. F. (1986). The inheritance of Gilles de la Tourette's syndrome and associated behaviors: Evidence for autosomal dominant transmission. *New England Journal of Medicine, 315*, 993–997.

Pauls, D. L., Raymond, C., Stevenson, J., & Leckman, J. F. (1991). A family study of Gilles de la Tourette. *American Journal of Human Genetics 48* (1), 154–163.

Price, R. A., Kidd, K. K., Cohen, D. J., Pauls, D. L., & Leckman, J. F. (1986). A twin study of Gilles de la Tourette's syndrome. *Archives of General Psychiatry, 42*, 815–820.

Ratzoni, G., Hermesh, H., Brandt, N., Lauffer, M., & Munitz, H. (1990). Clomipramine efficacy for tics, obsessions and compulsions in Tourette's syndrome and obsessive compulsive disorder: A case study. *Biological Psychiatry, 27*, 95–98.

Regeur, L., Pakkenberg, B., Fog, R., & Pakkenberg, H. (1986). Clinical features and long term treatment with pimozide in 65 patients with Gilles de la Tourette's syndrome. *Journal of Neurology, Neurosurgery, and Psychiatry, 49*, 791–795.

Riddle, M. A., Hardin, M. T., Cho, S. C., Woolston, J. L., & Leckman, J. F. (1988). Desipramine treatment of boys with attention-deficit hyperactivity disorder and tics: preliminary clinical experience. *Journal of American Academy of Child Adolescent Psychiatry, 27*, 811–814.

Riddle, M. A., Hardin, M. T., King, R. A., & Woolston, J. L. (1990). Fluoxetine treatment of children and adolescents with Tourette's and obsessive compulsive disorders: Preliminary clinical experience. *Journal of American Academy of Child Adolescent Psychiatry, 29*, 45–48.

Riddle, M. A., King, R. A., Hardin, M. T., Scahill, L., Ort, S. I., & Leckman, J. F. (1990). Behavioral side effects of fluoxetine in children and adolescents. *Journal Child Adolescent Psychopharmacology, 1*, 193–198.

Riddle, M. A., Nelson, J. C., Kleinman, C. S., Rasmusson, A. M., Leckman, J. F., King, R. A., & Cohen, D. J. (1991). Sudden death in children receiving Norpramin: A review of three reported cases and commentary. *Journal of American Academy Child Adolescent Psychiatry, 30*, 104–108.

Ryan, N. D. (1990). Heterocyclic antidepressants in children an adolescents. *Journal of Child Adolescent Psychopharmacology, 1*, 21–31.

Scahill, L., Ort, S. I., & Hardin, M. T. (1991). Genetic epidemiology in child psychiatric nursing: Tourette's syndrome as a model. *Journal of Child and Adolescent Psychiatric Nursing, 4*, 154–161.

Scahill, L., Ort, S. I., & Hardin, M. T. (1993). Tourette's Syndrome, Part I: Definition and Diagnosis. *Archives of Psychiatric Nursing, 7*(4), 203–208.

Shapiro, A. K., Shapiro, E. S., & Young, J. G. (1988). *Gilles de la Tourette Syndrome* (2nd ed.). New York: Raven Press.

Shapiro, A. K., & Shapiro, E. S. (1988). Treatment of tic disorders with haloperidol. In D. J. Cohen, R. D. Bruun, & J. F. Leckman (Eds.), *Tourette's Syndrome and Tic Disorders* (pp. 267–280). New York: John Wiley & Sons.

Singer, H. S., & Walkup, J. T. (1991). Tourette Syndrome and other tic disorders: Diagnosis, pathophysiology, and treatment. *Medicine, 70*, 15–32.

Thoren, P., Asberg, M., Cronholm, B., Jorenstedt, L., & Traskman, L. (1980). Clomipramine treatment of obsessive compulsive disorder: I. A controlled clinical trial. *Archives of General Psychiatry, 37*, 1281–1285.

Towbin, K. E., Riddle, M. A., Leckman, J. F., Bruun, R. D., & Cohen, D. J. (1988). The clinical care of individuals with Tourette's syndrome. In D. J. Cohen, R. D. Bruun, & J. F. Leckman (Eds.), *Tourette's Syndrome and Tic Disorders* (pp. 329–352). New York: John Wiley & Sons.

Yarura-Tobias, J. A. (1975). Clomipramine in Gilles de la Tourette disease. *American Journal of Psychiatry, 132*, 1221.

Zahner, G. E. P., Clubb, M. M., Leckman, J. F., Pauls, D. L. (1988). The epidemiology of Tourette's syndrome. In D. J. Cohen, R. D. Bruun, J. F. Leckman (Eds.), *Tourette's Syndrome and Tic Disorders* (pp. 79–90). New York: John Wiley & Sons.

CHAPTER

21

Eating Disorders

Nicki Warren Potts

With the media's and society's emphasis on thinness, it is little wonder that body weight is a concern for many adolescent and young women.* Women who express dissatisfaction with their body shape and weight probably represent the mainstream of women. Because these concerns are present to some degree in most women in Western society, it is reasonable to question whether eating disorders represent the extreme point on a weight continuum or distinct diagnostic entities. Some authorities view eating disorders as a continuum ranging from unconcern with weight and normal eating to discontent with weight and benign dieting to the more serious eating pathology and psychosocial impairment of anorexia nervosa and bulimia nervosa (Garner & Garfinkel, 1980; Striegel-Moore, Silberstein, & Rodin, 1986). Other writers view eating disorders as distinct diagnostic entities and argue that there are fundamental differences in psychopathology between classic eating disorder syndromes and the milder expression of symptoms (Bruch, 1973; Crisp, 1970; Garfinkel & Garner, 1982; Selvini-Palazzoli, 1978).

Anorexia nervosa is a clinical syndrome characterized by voluntary refusal to eat and weight loss leading to body weight 15% below that expected for age and height. The term anorexia nervosa is a misnomer because the individual does not experience true loss of appetite until late in the illness. Appetite and hunger usually are increased but strongly resisted. Bulimia nervosa, commonly referred to as bulimia, is a clinical syndrome characterized by episodes of binge eating followed by purging techniques to prevent weight gain. Purging may take the form of fasting, self-induced vomiting, laxative abuse, or compulsive exercise.

Statistics indicate that one out of every 200 American girls will develop anorexia nervosa to some extent (National Institute of Child Health and Human Development, 1983). These statistics reflect a dramatic increase in prevalence in the last 2 decades. However, eating disorders have emerged only recently as clinical entities. Bulimia nervosa was first identified by the American Psychiatric Association (APA) in the *Diagnostic and Statistical Manual of Mental Disorders*, 3rd ed. (DSM III) in 1980.

Anorexia and bulimia are seen in a heterogeneous population. The individual who acquires these illnesses may come from intact families or divorced families. They may be academically outstanding or have learning disabilities. Thus, it is important to discard stereotypes when working with these patients.

Disorders of eating encompass a broad range of

*In an effort to avoid grammatical awkwardness, the author has used feminine pronouns throughout this chapter to refer to anorectic and bulimic individuals. This also reflects the fact that Anorexia and Bulimia are disorders that primarily affect women. This is not meant to imply that men cannot also suffer from Anorexia Nervosa and Bulimia Nervosa.

nursing, medical, psychologic, nutritional, and social problems. Eating disordered clients present a fascinating and often intimidating task for the nurse. This chapter provides an overview of the biologic, psychodynamic, familial, and sociocultural factors associated with eating disorders and a discussion of treatment modalities and nursing management.

Anorexia Nervosa

DEFINING CHARACTERISTICS

More than 95% of people with anorexia nervosa are female (Carino & Chmelko, 1983). Essentially, the same disorder occurs in males although approximately one tenth as often. Although most anorectics have been from white, middle- and upper-class families, more recent observations indicate that this social class and race distribution may have eroded in the 1970s (Garfinkel & Garner, 1982).

Anorexia typically begins in adolescent girls who are, or perceive themsevles to be, overweight. The age of onset is bimodal, with one peak at ages 12 and 13 and another at age 17. The weight loss usually is associated with a major change, such as the onset of menstruation, a family move, or going to college. Many clients can recall a remark made to them concerning their weight as the precipitant. The weight loss diet may begin sensibly but continues out of control. Weight loss is achieved by severe caloric restriction and exclusion of carbohydrates and fats. Additionally, weight gain is often avoided by use of purging techniques, such as fasting, self-induced vomiting, laxatives, or diuretics. Approximately 30% to 50% of the anorectic population engages in binge eating and vomiting (Casper, Elke, & Halmi, 1980).

Eating behavior becomes disorganized, and ritualistic habits surrounding food preparation and consumption can emerge. The individual becomes frantically preoccupied and obsessed with food. She often takes hours to finish even the smallest meal, cutting everything into miniscule size. Many females with anorexia are gourmet cooks and prepare lavish meals for family members. This preoccupation with food is consistent with events that occur during the process of starvation. Studies demonstrating the consequences of starvation (to simulate prisoner-of-war conditions) were conducted during World War II with healthy servicemen. As weight loss progressed, the men became more preoccupied with food and engaged in unusual eating behaviors, such as cutting up food to make meals last for hours. There was no diminution in the desire for food, and food became the dominant topic of all conversation and thinking (Keys, Brozed, Henschel, Mickelsen, & Taylor, 1950).

Anorectics are high achievers and strive for perfection in all aspects of their life. They tend to believe themselves a failure if they are not always successful. Parents typically characterize their daughter as devoted, compliant, and "perfect." Interpersonal relationships are invariably disturbed. The anorectic is frequently isolated and maintains interpersonal distance from family and peers. As a result, she fails to achieve the preadolescent confidence and competence and healthy ego strength.

Early in their illness, anorectics often feel euphoric about their weight loss. This feeling is thought to be mediated by endorphin and is comparable to a "runner's high." Depression follows the euphoria and may arise from starvation rather than the underlying psychiatric status. Suicide has occurred in chronic anorectic patients, and an overall mortality rate of 5% at 5 years after diagnosis has been reported (Swift, 1982).

PSYCHOLOGIC FEATURES

Disturbances in psychologic functioning are numerous and include the following:

- Relentless pursuit of thinness with body image disturbances of delusional proportions
- Faulty perception of inner sensations, including visceral sensations and affective states
- Pervasive sense of personal ineffectiveness
- Cognitive distortions

Dominating the psychologic features is a relentless pursuit of thinness with body image disturbances of delusional proportions. This drive for thinness goes far beyond normal dieting and may involve techniques such as purging to avoid weight gain. Losing weight or maintaining low weight to achieve a certain look are closely related to the struggle for self-control and an improvement in self-esteem. The disturbance in body image is evidenced by the individual's lack of recognition of the degree of her weight loss and by her preoccupation that a particular part of her body is still too fat. Emaciated in appearance, she believes she looks "normal" and strives to maintain that thinness (Bruch, 1978).

Faulty perception of inner sensations includes visceral sensations and affective states. She is unable to identify internal sensations of hunger and satiety. Hunger is denied, yet there are constant thoughts of food. She feels full after only a few bites. In the background of some of these individuals is a deficit in the parents' confirmation and response to child-initiated cues. This lack of response to the child's needs deprives her of the groundwork for body identity and leads to faulty perception of internal, visceral sensations. She is perplexed about differentiating between physiologic disturbances and emotional experiences. This faulty perception also extends to affective states. Patients describe a lack of awareness of feelings beyond primitive, helpless rage and anger (Bruch, 1973).

The third area of psychologic maladaptation is a pervasive sense of personal ineffectiveness. The individual feels helpless and ineffective in conducting her own life. The severe discipline over her body represents a desperate effort to overcome the panic about being powerless. She believes that throughout her life she has been on a path shaped by others. Who she is has been ignored and dismissed. She has not had a chance to develop herself. She has acted only in response to others' demands instead of doing what she wanted to do. Unable to live this way, she turns her body into the arena for struggle. Dieting becomes one area in which she seeks to gain control of her life and counteract her feelings of ineffectiveness and low self-esteem. Treating her body as an enemy, she tries to conquer and control it by denying her need for food and rest. Paradoxically, in this struggle with her body, she perpetuates the very denial of self that she is fighting against. The anorectic's defiance is not an expression of strength and independence but a defense against feeling she has no core personality and of being powerless and ineffective (Orbach, 1986).

The main cognitive distortion is a dichotomous or all-or-nothing, black-or-white form of reasoning (Garner & Bemis, 1982). The self and the world are viewed in terms of extremes; one is all good or all bad, with no middle ground. If one is not perfect, then the only other alternative is being a total failure.

PHYSICAL MANIFESTATIONS

The classic signs of anorexia nervosa are the direct effects of starvation. Usually the effects of starvation cause the individual to seek medical care. Below a critical weight, defined as 90% of ideal body weight, signs of physiologic compromise emerge as the body tries to mitigate the results of weight loss.

The most common physiologic changes involve fluid and electrolyte disturbances, cardiac irregularities, and gastrointestinal problems. Hypokalemia (<3.5 mEq/L) is one of the most serious manifestations of anorexia nervosa (Brotman, Rigotti, & Herzog, 1985) because of the important role potassium plays in cell function and neuromuscular transmission. Several mechanisms cause hypokalemia. A person who restricts food and fluids will have decreased circulating plasma volume and may have hypokalemia. Individuals who use laxatives or diuretics can develop hypokalemia because 80% of the body's potassium is excreted in urine and 20% through the feces (Dardis & Hofland, 1990). Vomiting also can cause hypokalemia. The signs and symptoms of hypokalemia include muscle weakness (lower extremities are affected first), abdominal distress, and constipation from impaired motility of intestinal smooth muscle.

Cardiac irregularities are caused by the decreased potassium levels and have been reported in up to 60% of clients (Garfinkel & Garner, 1982). These include sinus bradycardia, low amplitude, T-wave inversion, and atrioventricular block. Sudden death in anorectics has been linked to prolonged QT intervals (Brotman et al., 1985). Typically the individual restricts food and water or purges to eliminate calories, and hypovolemia or a decrease in the circulating fluid occurs. As a result of fluid depletion, the systemic arterial and venous blood pressure decrease. Bradycardia usually develops and reflects a decrease in metabolism.

Gastrointestinal problems are common and may limit weight gain. Gastric motility abnormalities include a feeling of early satiety after consuming a small amount of food, bloating, abdominal distention, and constipation.

The basic metabolic rate decreases during starvation as an energy-conserving mechanism and results in the individual feeling cold even in warm weather. The skin is commonly dry and cracking, with a yellowish discoloration thought to be due to increased carotene deposition. Often a fine downy hair, or lanugo, may cover the extremities, face, and trunk. The majority of female anorectics have amenorrhea and estrogen deficiency. When amenorrhea occurs, weight loss usually precedes it. However, in up to 25% of cases, amenorrhea occurs before weight loss (Herzog & Copeland, 1985).

DIAGNOSTIC CRITERIA

The DSM IV (APA, 1994) lists the following criteria for the diagnosis of anorexia nervosa:

- Refusal to maintain body weight over a minimal normal weight for age and height (e.g., weight loss leading to maintenance of body

CLINICAL EXAMPLE: MARY

Mary is a 5-ft, 3-in, 17-year-old high school senior admitted with a diagnosis of anorexia nervosa. Both parents are professionals; her father is a lawyer and her mother, a psychologist. Mary initially described her family as "very close and supportive—no problems at all." In actuality, her parents had divorced when she was 11. She lived with her brothers and sister with her father and stepmother. She appeared to cope fairly well with the domestic disruption, formed a good relationship with her stepmother, and excelled in school. In high school she made all "As," applied to and was accepted at several Ivy League universities, and received a National Merit Scholarship. After receiving this impressive array of accomplishments, Mary began to lose weight and refused to eat "fattening" foods. Her weight decreased 25 lb in 6 months. Her stepmother reported that she was preoccupied with meal planning and preparation at home yet ate very little food. She exercised excessively and would jump up and down even while studying. When her weight reached 75 lb, she was admitted to the hospital. Mary perceived herself as not emaciated and described her thighs as too heavy. She said the food she ate just sat in her stomach and caused it to "bloat."

In therapy, Mary revealed that the breakup of her parents' marriage had indeed caused her a great deal of distress. She firmly believed that it was up to her to make the "new, reconstructed family" work and that her "bad" feelings about the divorce would only upset her father and stepmother. She had never been able to make demands on other people and resolved to make the best of this situation. Additionally, Mary realized that she had no autonomous motivation for working hard and doing well in school. She had excelled because of her father's expectations. However, her feelings of self-worth increased considerably when she began to lose weight. During the course of therapy, Mary eventually understood that, prior to the anorexic episode, she had succeeded in dealing with life, but at the expense of developing any positive sense of who she was. She saw herself as being shaped by others' needs, rather than by anything she was or wanted for herself.

weight less than 85% of that expected) or failure to make expected weight gain during period of growth, leading to body weight less than 85% of that expected

- Intense fear of gaining weight or becoming fat, even though underweight
- Disturbance in the way in which one's body weight, size, or shape is experienced (e.g., the person claims to "feel fat" even when emaciated, believes that one area of the body is "too fat" even when obviously underweight)
- In postmenarcheal females, absence of at least three consecutive menstrual cycles when otherwise expected to occur (primary or secondary amenorrhea) (see Clinical Example: Mary)

ETIOLOGY

Most experts agree that there is inadequate evidence that a single pathway leads to anorexia nervosa. The current view is of a multidimensional, interactional model involving risk factors within the individual, family, and culture. Therefore, a description of the development of anorexia must address the biologic, psychodynamic, familial, and sociocultural perspectives.

BIOLOGIC THEORY. Although several neurochemical abnormalities have been noted in anorexia nervosa, it is difficult to distinguish those attributable to starvation from those that may be specific for the disease itself. In anorexia nervosa, the state of starvation produces extensive changes in hypothalmic and metabolic functioning.

However, some hormonal alterations cannot be attributed to starvation. For 70% of females, loss of menses, or amenorrhea, occurs shortly after the onset of the weight loss. In a significant proportion (estimates vary between 7% and 24%), amenorrhea appears to precede the weight loss (Herzog & Copeland, 1985). Cortisol production, which is decreased in starvation associated with other diseases, is increased in anorexia nervosa and returns to normal with weight recovery (Casper, Chatterton, & Davis, 1979; Hurd et al., 1977). Based on these neurochemical abnormalities, it has been proposed that there is an increased activity of the hypothalmic–pituitary–adrenal system that is out of proportion to the emaciation.

Additional support for a biologic theory is provided by investigators who have reported disturbances in levels of neurotransmitters in the brain. Specifically, norepinephrine and its metabolites are low in untreated anorectics, but with weight restoration, they increase to normal levels (Gross, Lake, Ebert, Ziegler, & Kopin, 1979). However, decreased levels of cerebral spinal fluid norepinephrine may persist even with long-term weight restoration, indicating abnormalities in norepinephrine metabolism (Kaye, Ebert, Raleigh, & Lake, 1984). This disturbance may indicate an underlying neurochemical abnormality in clients with anorexia nervosa.

PSYCHODYNAMIC THEORY. This theoretical viewpoint proposes that a major predisposition to anorexia nervosa relates to deficits in ego development during the first years of life that impair the individual's ability to function separately from the family. With little or no encouragement of independence during the individuation–separation phase, the child is deprived of autonomy and decision-making abilities. Therefore, she tends to be obedient and conform readily to others' expectations. The flaw in the child's development seems to lie in the interaction in the parent–child relationship. Materially, everything is provided for the child, but care is given according to the parents' decisions and convictions, with little attention to the child's needs or wants (Bruch, 1982).

Another similar viewpoint emphasizes developmental problems based on faulty interaction with the early primary caregiver, typically the mother. This has been further developed as a disturbance in the sense of self beginning at the level of the mirroring phase in which the mother is unable to see the child as herself (Rizzutto, Peterson, & Reed, 1981).

Regarding premorbid personality characteristics that predispose to anorexia nervosa, there is and has been considerable diversity of opinion. It is difficult to separate the psychopathologic characteristics that are possible precursors of the disorder from those that are byproducts of a serious illness or are secondary to starvation. However, several personality characteristics are unduly prominent. These include a reliance on approval from others, conformity, compliance, perfectionism, and a lack of responsiveness to inner needs. These qualities suggest an individual with extremely high personal expectations and a need to please others and conform to maintain a sense of self-worth. These passive characteristics make the individual extremely vulnerable to familial, peer, and cultural influences (Garfinkel & Garner, 1982).

FAMILY SYSTEMS THEORY. The exact role of the family in the development of anorexia nervosa is not clearly understood. However, it is suggested that certain family relationships are closely related to the development and maintenance of anorexia and that the illness plays an important role in maintaining the family homeostasis. Family relationships are characterized by poorly delineated boundaries between individual members and between the parent and child subsystems.

The child's psychologic and bodily functioning become the subject of undue family interest. Because parental control is maintained in a context of apparent concern, it becomes very difficult for the child to protest. Family members are taught to make their wishes known indirectly and in the spirit of self-sacrifice, thus making disagreement an act of betrayal.

Finally, the child's involvement in parental conflict is considered a key factor. Parental conflict is handled in maladaptive ways in which covert coalitions are formed. The child is openly encouraged to side with one parent against the other and may switch from one parent to another depending on the situation. The parents also may submerge their conflicts by blaming or protecting their sick child who is defined by them as the only family problem. The anorectic child thus becomes accustomed to diverting parental conflict onto herself (Minuchin, Rosman, & Baker, 1978).

SOCIOCULTURAL THEORY. The recent trend that idealizes the thin female body and the woman's changing role in society has been implicated in the increased incidence of anorexia nervosa. New and often contradictory roles and expectations for women, although a desirable transition, may pose adjustment problems for some. Women must maintain traditional standards of attractiveness while striving for the heightened demands of professional performance and success. (See the section on sociocultural etiology of bulimia nervosa for additional information.)

However, not all individuals exposed to these cultural pressures to be slim and perfect develop anorexia nervosa. Thus, the majority of evidence suggests that the disorder is multidetermined. In addition to these sociocultural factors, predispositions within the individual and certain familial characteristics are important in the expression of the disorder.

THERAPEUTIC AND NURSING MANAGEMENT

Effective treatment of anorexia nervosa involves nutritional rehabilitation to reverse the severe malnutrition, individual psychotherapy to correct the deficits and distortions in psychologic functioning, and family therapy to resolve disturbed patterns of interactions.

NUTRITIONAL REHABILITATION. The signs and symptoms of starvation usually require medical management in a hospital when weight loss reaches more than 25% of original weight. Bruch (1982) believes there is a critical weight, usually below 90 or 100 pounds, at which malnutrition maintains an abnormal mental state and creates psychologic problems that are biologically, not psychodynamically, determined. Inpatient treatment for a significantly underweight anorectic (under 75% of ideal weight) generally requires a stay of at least 3 months. In facilities with experienced personnel and comprehensive eating disorder programs, nasogastric tube feeding and hyperalimentation are virtually never required.

The client is expected to eat regular, balanced meals planned by a dietitian. Initially, choosing foods creates anxiety and aggravates fears about food, eating, and weight. Most clients tolerate a gradual increase in calories and amounts of food, beginning with 1200 to 1500 calories per day and adding 100 to 200 calories per day. A maximum of 3500 to 5000 calories per day is necessary to achieve the desired weight gain of approximately 2 pounds per week. A target weight is established by the entire health care team based on the weight at which the client functioned well prior to the illness and which is appropriate for age, height, and sex. Initially, the anorectic resists the target weight as "too heavy," but without a target she feels out of control and believes the staff want her to gain weight indefinitely. It is important to reassure the client that she will not be allowed to get fat (Akridge, 1989). The nursing staff must stress that the primary concern for her is regaining health through better nutrition. She should be informed early in treatment that initial weight gain results from fluid retention as the extracellular compartments expand but will become less extreme if the diet continues to be followed.

Symptom-oriented approaches, such as behavioral techniques, can pave the way for more insight-oriented therapy after nutritional restitution. However, opinions are divided about the role of these strategies in the refeeding process. Some experts consider them potentially dangerous because although they produce weight gain, they can result in external compliance without internal change in attitude. The client can literally eat her way out of the hospital.

Behavioral programs involve contracting with specific goals and rewards. Weight gain may lead to telephone, mail, visitor, or ground privileges. A clearly defined behavioral plan is communicated to the client and maintained through a unified team approach. The weight management program must be nonnegotiable. While the majority of clients strongly protest abdication of this control, most admit later that being relieved of the responsibility actually facilitated therapeutic progress.

PSYCHOTHERAPY. Individual psychotherapy is based on the premise that behavior is influenced by unconscious psychologic processes derived from early experiences. Disordered eating patterns are viewed as symptoms of unconscious conflicts and will resolve with insight (Geary, 1988). Psychotherapy is begun only after the anorectic has gained enough weight to concentrate and think clearly. Therapy is a lengthy and arduous process that begins during the hospitalization and continues on an outpatient basis. The goals of psychotherapy assist the client to do the following:

- Develop an initial sense of self and an understanding of the underlying conflicts.
- Develop a realistic perception of one's body.
- Develop more adaptive coping mechanisms to deal directly with painful inner conflicts, rather than indirectly through food and eating.
- Demonstrate and verbalize an enhanced self-worth and self-esteem.

In helping the client develop her genuine self, the nurse needs to maintain a balance between recognizing the strength that is manifested in the anorexia and relating to the person behind the anorexia. The anorectic brings two distinct selves into therapy. The easiest to meet is the anorectic defense or that part of her that reveals no needs. The other self is underdeveloped and unrecognized by the anorectic. The client has no sense of her own strength and needs the nurse's help in integrating these two selves (Orbach, 1986).

The nurse provides what Winnicott (1965) calls a "holding" environment in which the needy and hungry person can safely emerge. Building such an alliance has been called an art. The anorectic has developed intricate routines, such as wiping off her eating utensils between each bite, to build a barrier between her inner self and the world and to reinforce the idea that she is strong and impenetrable. She wants to relinquish her routines in this relationship; however, she feels caught in a dilemma, having no sense of self that exists outside of her anorexia. She wants and needs to be nurtured but has difficulty accepting it (Orbach, 1986).

Another aspect of the "holding" environment is provision of a carefully structured environment that ensures physical and emotional safety. The supportive structure during and after meals and snacks is necessary to interrupt the impulse to vomit or increase physical activity. In addition to interrupting these behaviors, the nurse helps the client to process feelings that trigger these reactions and teaches her to deal directly with these uncomfortable feelings.

FAMILY THERAPY. In a younger client population, 18 years or younger and living at home, the treatment of choice is family therapy using a systems approach (Minuchin et al., 1978; Selvini-Palazzoli, 1978). Work with the family begins during hospitalization but continues as part of ongoing treatment following discharge. In older clients, family therapy may be an integral part of treatment involving marital therapy and therapy with the family of origin.

According to Minuchin's approach, symptoms of an eating disorder develop in one family member, usually a child, but the child is only one part of a complicated system in need of help. The child's illness draws attention away from other family difficulties, especially parental conflicts, and stabilizes the equilibrium of the system. Resolution of family conflicts through therapy may remove the need to maintain the child's illness. The parents or siblings, like the client, may resist dealing with their own problems and prefer to focus exclusively on the anorectic child.

Most nurses focus on several dysfunctional interaction patterns within the family: enmeshment, overprotectiveness, and lack of conflict resolution (Minuchin et al., 1978). Enmeshment refers to an extreme form of proximity and intensity in family interactions. Boundaries defining the individual are so weak that functioning in an individually differentiated way is precluded. Family members intrude on each other's thoughts and feelings and speak for each other. During therapy sessions, the nurse can insist that all members speak for themselves. Two family members are not allowed to discuss a third member without that person's participation.

Overprotectiveness refers to the family members' high degree of concern for each other's well-being. The parents' overprotectiveness prohibits the children from developing autonomously or completely outside the family. It is important for the nurse to challenge overprotective operations and at the same time to support coping behavior in the anorectic child.

Lack of conflict resolution is seen in avoidance of conflicts and problems left unresolved. Usually a strong moral or religious code is used as the rationale for such avoidance. The lack of conflict is maintained as the parents use the child to stabilize their own relationship. The conflict avoidance transaction is among the most resistant dysfunctional characteristic of the family. In general, the nurse challenges conflict avoidance by creating boundaries that help the members to discuss and resolve their disagreements. When two members express a difference of opinion, the nurse may ask them to sit close to each other, using space to signal a boundary, and insist that they discuss the matter. He or she then blocks the attempts of other family members to help or intervene (Minuchin et al., 1978).

NURSES' REACTIONS TO THE ANORECTIC

Working with the anorectic can evoke a variety of feelings in the nurse. Generally, she experiences herself trying to connect with someone who has never truly related. The client attempts to protect the nurse and herself from her inner despair and hopelessness. When she does expose these feelings, she anticipates rejection and may retreat from the nurse's acceptance. The nurse may feel as though the client is attempting to control and manipulate the relationship just as she controls her food. It is important to take the feeling of being manipulated further and ask, "What is the client missing, and what can't she ask for directly?" Developing a therapeutic relationship with the anorectic is difficult, demanding, and challenging. Her self-contempt often arouses in the nurse strong feelings of compassion. It is common to want to nurture and protect her, yet this must be avoided (Box 21-1 and the Nursing Care Plan for Anorexia Nervosa).

Bulimia Nervosa

DEFINING CHARACTERISTICS

Bulimia nervosa is a psychiatric disorder characterized by binge eating, followed by purging techniques to compensate for the excessive food intake. Typically the binge behavior consists of uncontrolled, secretive consumption of large amounts of high-calorie or "forbidden" foods in a short period of time. For an episode of eating to be considered bulimic, it must fulfill the following two conditions: The person should regard the quantity of food as excessive, and it should be experienced as outside of voluntary control. What is of primary importance is how the episode is experienced by the individual, not the quantity of food eaten (Fairburn & Cooper, 1984). The binge is counteracted by a variety of purging methods to prevent weight gain, including self-induced vomiting, fasting, obsessive exercise, and laxative or diuretic abuse. The majority of bulimics purge by vomiting. This binge–purge cycle may be repeated from several times per week to several times per day.

Bulimia, like anorexia nervosa, is predominantly a female disorder; more than 90% of bulimic individuals are women. Bulimia nervosa is increasing

BOX 21–1 • ASSESSMENT PARAMETERS FOR ANOREXIA NERVOSA

ASK THE CLIENT

1. Are you very afraid of becoming fat?
2. Have other people told you that you look emaciated? Do you still feel fat?
3. Do you feel anxious before you eat? Do you feel guilty after you eat?
4. How do you feel about the way your body is proportioned?
5. How often do you weigh yourself or measure your body size?
6. Do you know what your medically recommended body weight is?
7. Do you want to become thinner than you are now?

DETERMINE

1. If the client has lost at least 15% of her minimal body weight as projected for her age and height
2. If the client weighs or measures herself once per day or more often
3. If the client menstruates at all, and if so, how regularly
4. If the client follows a rigid exercise regimen
5. If the client sometimes vomits or takes laxatives or diuretics after eating

in incidence, especially in college-age women. Estimates range from 5% to 20%. The typical bulimic is between the ages of 15 and 30, single, upwardly mobile, college-educated, and from an intact family of more than one child. There appears to be greater heterogeneity of socioeconomic status in bulimia than is usually cited for individuals with anorexia nervosa. The bulimic individual has always been within 10% of her ideal weight, although approximately one third to one half have a history of being slightly overweight. Approximately 10% to 30% have a probable previous history of anorexia nervosa (Johnson & Connors, 1987).

Another feature of bulimics is the intensity and prominence of their concerns with shape and weight. A morbid fear of fatness and sensitivity to weight gain are present. Because of their poor control of eating, they feel in constant danger of gaining weight and getting fat.

Individuals with bulimia also report significant impairment in all areas of their lives. As the disorder progresses, social isolation and life adjustment problems occur. Social withdrawal occurs as they become more involved with food.

Cognitive distortions in the bulimic are similar to those of the anorectic. Examples of these distorted thoughts include the following (Johnson & Connors, 1987):

- Dichotomous, all-or-none, or black-and-white thinking. The self and the world are viewed in extremes, such as "I'm a complete failure because I ate a bad food today."
- Control fallacy or faulty attribution involves viewing the self as externally controlled and helpless; for example, "When I get the urge to binge, I'm just helplessly overwhelmed, and I just do it."
- Magnification is the tendency to exaggerate the meaning or significance of a particular event; for example, "Being thin is the key to all success and happiness," or "Nothing else in life counts for anything unless you're thin."

PHYSICAL MANIFESTATIONS

Many of the physical problems and complications experienced by bulimics are side effects from the disordered eating or purging behavior. The rapid consumption of large amounts of food may cause acute gastric dilation with pain, nausea and vomiting, gastric rupture, and even death (Mitchell, Pyle, & Miner, 1982). Nutritional deficiencies and malnutrition can be associated with hair loss, brittle nails, fatigue, insomnia, weakness, and mood changes. Dental cavities, erosion of tooth enamel, and tooth discoloration are associated with frequent ingestion of highly sugared foods and the regurgitation of gastric acid. A painless enlargement of the parotid glands secondary to frequent stimulation from binge eating and vomiting results in a swollen appearance of the cheeks (Levin, Falks, & Dixon, 1980). The back of the hand may be calloused or scarred from repeated abrasion of the skin against the maxillary incisors during self-induced vomiting. The dental problems are subtle physical changes that may go unnoticed by an unsuspecting physician but are usually picked up by a dentist.

Vomiting results in electrolyte imbalances from loss of potassium, sodium, and chloride; muscle weakness; fatigue; constipation; and depression. Esophagitis and ulceration of the esophagus also may result from frequent exposure to acidic stomach contents (Goode, 1985). Menstrual irregularities occur in more than 40% of bulimics.

DIAGNOSTIC CRITERIA

Prior to the 1940s, bulimic behavior was reported as occurring in the context of anorexia nervosa. During the 1950s, binge eating was described among

NURSING CARE PLAN: Anorexia Nervosa

Nursing Diagnosis	Expected Outcome	Interventions
Alteration in Nutrition: Less than Body Requirements related to self-starvation	Regains weight within normal range for height and age	Implement diet management program.
		Weigh daily at the same time in a hospital gown.
	Demonstrates nutritionally adequate eating pattern	Supervise meals using firm, empathic approach.
		Avoid discussing food or somatic complaints.
		Monitor client for 2 hours after eating to prevent vomiting.
		Provide positive reinforcement for weight gain rather than for amount of food eaten.
Disturbance in Self-Concept: Body Image, related to inaccurate perception of body size	Demonstrates realistic attitudes and perception of body size	Point out misperceptions of body image.
	Displays evidence of developing self-esteem	Work with client to identify strengths.
	Demonstrates increased self-assurance	Teach assertion skills through modeling.
		Help client discriminate family's ideas and feelings as distinct from her own.
	Demonstrates less need to conform to rules and expectations of others	Encourage identification and expression of feelings.
		Avoid making evaluative statements about progress.
		Verbally recognize and reinforce genuine communication of feelings.
Ineffective Individual Coping related to inability to make decisions	Exhibits appropriate coping mechanisms	Encourage independent decision making.
		Offer positive reinforcement for independent problem-solving and appropriate decisions.
		Encourage client to reach own conclusions.
Alteration in Family Processes related to enmeshment of family members	Demonstrates more effective communication patterns	Observe family interactions.
		Explore source of guilt feelings and responsibility toward parents when expressed by client.
		Assist parents in working through guilt feelings.
		Teach parents how to show their caring appropriately.
		Teach parents how to reinforce appropriate behavior in child.
		Assist family to understand psychodynamics of anorexia nervosa and therapeutic treatment plan.
		Discuss community resources and support groups.

obese populations. It was not until the last decade that the occurrence of bulimic behavior among individuals without significant histories of weight disorder became apparent.

The diagnosis of bulimia nervosa may first be suspected from the presence of physical complications, such as fluid and electrolyte disturbances due to gastrointestinal losses, erosion of tooth enamel, abdominal complaints, and throat complaints. The diagnosis is established on the basis of criteria established in the DSM IV (APA, 1994):

- Recurrent episodes of binge eating (rapid consumption of a large amount of food in a discrete period of time)
- A feeling of lack of control over eating behavior during the eating binges
- Regular self-induced vomiting, use of laxatives or diuretics, strict dieting or fasting, or vigorous exercise to prevent weight gain
- A minimum average of two binge eating episodes and compensatory behavior to prevent weight gain per week for 3 months
- Self-evaluation unduly influenced by body shape and weight

ETIOLOGY

BIOLOGIC FACTORS. Examining biologic influences is crucial to understanding bulimia. An increasing body of literature has suggested that affective instability may be a genetic risk factor for bulimia (Hawkins & Clement, 1980; Johnson, Lewis, & Hagman, 1984). Bulimics experience substantial and frequent affective instability, including rapidly fluctuating moods with irritability, anxiety, fatigue, restlessness, despair, and agitation. The typical bulimic has a long-standing affective problem that predates the onset of the eating disorder (Johnson & Connors, 1987). However, no conclusions regarding the genetic transmission of bulimia through an affective disorder link can be made (Striegel-Moore et al., 1986).

Another biologic factor is the genetic predisposition for women to have higher body fat composition than men, a sex difference that appears to hold across all races and cultures. At the same time, the "ideal" female body is much thinner that the natural female figure. Furthermore, it appears that the body most women naturally have is incongruent with society's ideal female figure.

INTRAPSYCHIC FACTORS. Although there is too little research regarding the personality characteristics of bulimics, some consistent trends have emerged. Overall, bulimics appear to have significant problems identifying and articulating their internal states. It is likely that this difficulty contributes to feelings of being helpless in controlling internal states (self-regulation). They appear to have highly variable moods that fluctuate from persistent fatigue and depression to a feeling of agitation accompanied by impulse control difficulties, such as stealing or shoplifting, substance abuse, and suicidal behavior. Alcohol and drug abuse occur in 20% to 25% of bulimics, and a substantial percentage of bulimic clients are children of alcoholics. Consequently, they have long histories of feeling somewhat out of control and perhaps helpless in relation to their bodily experience. Unlike many anorectics who seem proud of their symptoms, most bulimics feel guilty, ashamed of their binge eating and purging, depressed, and out of control.

Another prominent personality trait is low self-esteem or profound feelings of ineffectiveness. Bulimic individuals' experience of themselves appears to be one of self-doubt and uncertainty. They have high self-expectations and are very harsh, critical, and punitive in evaluating themselves. They are self-conscious around others and highly sensitive to signs of rejection or disapproval. In spite of this sensitivity, however, they generally seek interpersonal relationships (Potts, 1984).

FAMILY FACTORS. The family environment of the bulimic is characterized as disengaged, chaotic, highly conflicted, and neglectful. Family members use indirect and contradictory patterns of communication and are deficient in problem-solving skills, nonsupportive of independent behavior, and less intellectually and recreationally oriented than nonbulimic families despite their high achievement orientation (Johnson & Connors, 1987). Children from this type of family generally feel disorganized, disconnected, and insecure.

SOCIOCULTURAL FACTORS. Obviously biologic and familial factors alone cannot explain why the incidence of bulimia nervosa has increased among a rather homogeneous group (15- to 25-year-old, middle to upper class, white, college-educated women in westernized countries). The broader sociocultural context and current cultural norms and stereotypes must be considered.

The current cultural emphasis on thinness plays a major role in the development of bulimia nervosa, as it does in anorexia. The movement toward a thinner ideal standard of feminine beauty is compounded by the fact that the population averages for weight have trended higher, largely as a result of better nutrition (Garner, Garfinkel, Schwartz, & Thompson, 1980). This creates a growing disparity between the real and ideal norms for body shape.

Societal changes accompanying the women's

movement, particularly the female sex role stereotype, in the 1960s and 1970s is another important cultural factor. It has been proposed that being concerned with one's appearance and making efforts to enhance and preserve one's beauty are central features of the female sex role stereotype. The pursuit of attractiveness, chiefly thinness, and beauty has been considered a feminine responsibility. Women at greatest risk for bulimia appear to have most deeply endorsed the traditional female sex role, valuing thinness and attractiveness. Bulimic women typically show stereotypically "feminine" behaviors, such as being dependent, eager to please, unassertive, and concerned with social approval (Boskind-White & White, 1983; Hawkins & Clement, 1980; Johnson et al., 1984). Cultural stereotypes for female behavior and roles are changing. However, many women who have achieved occupational success and financial independence continue to be unduly concerned about their weight and pursue thinness.

THERAPEUTIC AND NURSING MANAGEMENT

INPATIENT VERSUS OUTPATIENT TREATMENT. Due to the multidetermined nature of bulimia, effective treatment programs include a variety of modalities, such as individual, group, family, and marital psychotherapy; nutritional counseling; drug therapy; and support groups. Treatment usually is on an outpatient basis because most normal-weight bulimics do not require hospitalization. When bulimics are placed in a highly structured and supportive inpatient environment, they improve immediately. Unfortunately, many quickly relapse when discharged to their regular living situation. Therefore, discharge planning should begin early in their hospitalization.

Any approach to the client's problems should include an evaluation of the biologic, familial, psychologic, and sociocultural factors that have predisposed the individual toward ineffective behaviors and relationships. The goals of inpatient treatment include interrupting the binge–purge cycle, normalizing food intake by establishing healthy eating patterns, and restructuring cognitive distortions. By virtue of nursing's emphasis on the whole person within the family and cultural context, nurses are pivotal in the evaluation and treatment of eating disordered clients (Potts, 1984).

INDIVIDUAL PSYCHOTHERAPY. Several important perspectives can guide the nurse therapist in understanding the bulimic individual. The nurse must successfully create an interpersonal therapeutic relationship in which the bulimic can learn a variety of adaptive tools to manage her life. The nurse's initial task is to respond in a way that communicates that he or she is invested in learning how the bulimic client experiences the world and what can be done to improve her life. Forming a therapeutic alliance with her can only occur if the nurse truly empathizes with her experience, particularly her preoccupation with food, weight, and her body. The careful and persistent awareness and processing of the bulimic's reactions to the nurse's actions facilitate this alliance.

Directive interventions include behavioral strategies to interrupt the bulimic behaviors of binge eating and purging and to normalize eating. These may involve meal planning, goal setting, self-monitoring, and the exploration of alternative self-regulatory activities. Purge-delaying or purge-avoiding tactics may be valuable, such as phoning a friend, taking a bath, or walking. Cognitive approaches enable the client to examine the dysfunctional thoughts and to substitute more constructive ones. A typical cognitive distortion, such as "I ate a piece of cake. I've lost control, so I might as well eat all of it," can be replaced with "It's OK once in a while to eat a moderate amount of my favorite dessert. I do not need to eat the entire cake but will get back on my eating program immediately." Relapse-prevention techniques prepare the bulimic for occasional slips: A dysfunctional feeling, such as "This binge wipes out a month of abstinence; I'm back where I started," can be replaced by a planned response, "Nothing can take away what I accomplished this last month; I won't let one slip become a major setback" (Wooley & Wooley, 1985).

GROUP AND FAMILY THERAPY. Group treatment is extremely useful with bulimic clients. Regardless of whether the bulimic's family is actually involved in therapy, it is important to assume that they are "in the room" affecting the client's behavior and motivations. The therapeutic team often needs to function as "parents" to the family system as a whole (Johnson & Connors, 1987).

DRUG THERAPY. Drug therapy with antidepressants has shown promising results in the treatment of bulimics. In almost all of the short-term studies of antidepressants, a favorable response to medication has been obtained (Mitchell & Groat, 1984; Pope, Hudson, & Jonas, 1983; Walsh et al., 1982). A favorable response to medication is defined as diminution of binge eating and purging behaviors and a decrease in depressive, obsessive, and anxiety symptoms. Antidepressant medication is the only treatment that has been demonstrated in a controlled study to be highly effective for both bulimia and its associated symptoms, such as depression and food preoccupation. Pharmacotherapy is recommended for bulimics with concomitant major depressive disorder, substantial depressive or anxiety symptomatology, or a resistance to the usual psychotherapeutic interventions.

However, on an outpatient basis, antidepressants should not be given to individuals who are unreliable, acutely suicidal, abusing drugs and unwilling to stop, psychotic, or who have severe character pathology when a poor therapeutic relationship exists. While the evidence for antidepressant treatment of bulimia is still in its early stages, it is already stronger than the evidence for any other kind of treatment (Pope & Hudson, 1984).

SPECIAL TREATMENT ISSUES

Common countertransference issues may arise in working with eating disordered clients. Countertransference refers to feelings and reactions evoked in the therapist by the therapeutic interaction with a client. These issues may affect male and female staff.

SHARING SOCIETY'S OBSESSION WITH THINNESS. No one can be completely immune to society's obsession with thinness. Supporting the client's dissatisfaction with her body and agreeing with plans for severe dietary restriction are counterproductive.

REVULSION AT THE BINGE–PURGE BEHAVIOR. Binge eating can connote various negative messages for the nurse, such as being out of control, greedy, and self-indulgent. It is not uncommon for nurses and other members of the team to feel a sense of superiority at their own "self-control" because they do not binge eat. Self-induced vomiting can be particularly disgusting; however, the nurse must work through this attitude to discuss vomiting behavior matter-of-factly, rather than judgmentally.

ENVY OF THE CLIENT. Given the constant barrage of the cultural ideal for women, it is likely that most women in our society, including nurses, have a certain measure of body dissatisfaction. Some eating disordered clients are "attractive" according to societal standards and have glamorous professions, such as modeling or acting. Thus, female nurses may have to deal with feelings of envy about the client's attractiveness and thinness. The female nurse must come to terms with her own appearance, just as clients must.

THE NURSE WITH EATING OR WEIGHT PROBLEMS. Nurses must be prepared to face intense scrutiny about their own weight and to discuss personal weight-related issues nondefensively when necessary. Being aware of one's own weight-related issues and dealing with them through supervision or therapy are necessary when working with eating disordered clients. Nurses who are overweight must be prepared to discuss this explicitly. They need to be nondefensive about their weight and ask the client how she might feel about having an overweight nurse. This gives the client permission to discuss her feelings.

A slender nurse may have to deal with the client's envy and hostility that the nurse has something that the client desperately wants. Clients tend to make incorrect assumptions about the nurse being slender through willpower. The nurse must present reality by focusing on eating normally and still maintaining weight when one is at a natural body weight.

Clients will often ask about how the nurse became interested in eating disorders or if the nurse has ever had an eating disorder. If this is the case and if the client inquires, it can be helpful to tell the truth in brief, with an emphasis on the recovery period. For the nurse who has never had an eating disorder and is questioned about it, a reply about having experienced societal pressures regarding attractiveness is effective. It is important to ask if the nurses's lack of personal experience makes the client feel she cannot be understood. Presenting oneself as someone who has specific knowledge about eating disorders, combined with a readiness to discuss the client's feelings, will usu-

BOX 21–2 • ASSESSMENT PARAMETERS FOR BULIMIA NERVOSA

ASK THE CLIENT

1. Do you consume large amounts of food in brief periods of time (binge)?
2. Do you feel that once you begin eating this way, you can't stop?
3. Do you try to hide it when you eat this way?
4. Do you make yourself vomit or use laxatives or diuretics after a binge?
5. Do you feel anxious before a binge? Do you feel depressed and guilty after a binge?

DETERMINE

1. If the client's weight fluctuates 10 lb or more
2. If the client's parotid glands are enlarged from frequent vomiting (chipmunk facies)
3. The presence of dental caries and loss of enamel on the client's teeth
4. If the client has repeatedly tried to lose weight by dieting, fasting, or vomiting, or by taking laxatives, diuretics, or emetics

NURSING CARE PLAN: Bulimia Nervosa

Nursing Diagnosis	Expected Outcome	Interventions
Alteration of Fluid Volume: Deficit related to self-induced vomiting, laxative, or diuretic abuse	Fluid and electrolytes stabilize within normal limits	Monitor electrolyte levels daily. Record intake and output daily. Weigh daily on same scale before breakfast. Monitor vital signs, especially assessing for cardiac arrhythmias.
Alteration in Nutrition: Less than Body Requirements related to binging or purging	Normalization of eating behavior Nutritional status stabilizes without evidence of binging or purging	Obtain a detailed record of daily food intake. Consult with dietitian to develop weight-normalization plan. Provide structured environment for client to learn to control eating. Assure client that you will not allow "runaway" weight gain to occur. Assist client in exploring overvaluation of thinness. Assist client to express feelings about losing control of eating, rapid weight gain, and urge to vomit.
Disturbance in Self-Concept related to disturbed perceptions of body size and shape	Regains a realistic body image Develops realistic attitudes about body size and shape	Assist client to express feelings and concerns about body image. Consistently point out misperceptions about body image. Provide support for accurate perceptions. Assist client to verbalize positive affirmations about own body (e.g., "I am healthy and energetic at my ideal weight").
Ineffective Individual Coping related to inability to control eating habits	Demonstrates effective individual coping, free from uncontrolled binge or purge behavior	Explore patterns of behaviors that occur before binge or purge episodes. Assist client to find adaptive ways of coping with feelings, anxiety, and stressors. Assist client to identify times of neediness, loneliness, dissatisfaction with life, and so forth and to develop alternative ways to nurture self at these times.

ally alleviate these concerns (Johnson & Connors, 1987) (Box 21-2 and Nursing Care Plan for Bulimia).

Summary

This chapter discusses the incidence and clinical syndromes of anorexia and bulemia. Etiologic theories of eating disorders include biologic, psychodynamic, family systems, and sociocultural factors. Therapeutic management of eating disorders involves nutritional rehabilitation, psychotherapy, family therapy, group therapy, and pharmacological therapy. Concerns of nurses also are addressed in the chapter.

REFERENCES

Akridge, K. (1989). Principles and practice: Anorexia nervosa. *Journal of Obstetric, Gynecologic, and Neonatal Nursing, 18,* 25–30.

American Psychiatric Association. (1980). *Diagnostic and statistical manual of mental disorders* (3rd ed.). Washington DC: Author.

American Psychiatric Association. (1994). *Diagnostic and sta-*

tistical manual of mental disorders (4th ed.). Washington DC: Author.

Boskind-White, M., & White, W. (1983). *Bulimarexia: The binge-purge cycle.* New York: W. W. Norton.

Brotman, A. W., Rigotti, N., & Herzog, D. B. (1985). Medical complications of eating disorders: Outpatient evaluation and management. *Comprehensive Psychiatry, 26,* 258–272.

Bruch, H. (1973). *Eating disorders: Obesity, anorexia nervosa, and the person within.* New York: Basic Books.

Bruch, H. (1978). *The golden cage: The enigma of anorexia nervosa.* Cambridge: Harvard University Press.

Bruch H. (1982). Anorexia nervosa: Therapy and theory. *American Journal of Psychiatry, 139,* 1531–1538.

Carino, C. M., & Chmelko, P. (1983). Disorders of eating in adolescence: Anorexia nervosa and bulimia. *Nursing Clinics of North America, 18,* 343–352.

Casper, R. C., Chatterton, R. T., & Davis, J. M. (1979). Alteration in serum cortisol and its binding characteristics in anorexia nervosa. *Journal of Clinical Endocrinology Metabolism, 49,* 406–411.

Casper, R. C., Elke, E. D., & Halmi, K. A. (1980). Bulimia: Its incidence and clinical importance in patients with anorexia nervosa. *Archives of General Psychiatry, 37,* 1030–1040.

Crisp, A. H. (1970). Anorexia nervosa: "Feeding disorder," "nervous malnutrition," or "weight phobia?" *Review of Nutrition and Dietetics, 12,* 452–504.

Dardis, P. O., & Hofland, S. L. (1990). Anorexia nervosa: Fluid-electrolyte and acid-base manifestation. *Journal of Child Psychological Nursing, 3,* 85–90.

Fairburn, C. G., & Cooper, P. J. (1984). The clinical features of bulimia nervosa. *British Journal of Psychiatry, 144,* 238–246.

Garfinkel, P. E., & Garner, D. M. (1982). *Anorexia nervosa: A multidimensional perspective.* New York: Brunner/Mazel.

Garner, D. M., & Bemis, K. M. (1982). A cognitive-behavioral approach to anorexia nervosa. *Cognitive Therapy and Research, 6,* 123–150.

Garner, D. M., & Garfinkel. P. E. (1980). Socio-cultural factors in the development of anorexia nervosa. *Psychological Medicine, 10,* 647–656.

Garner, D. M., Garfinkel, P. E., Schwartz, D., & Thompson, M. (1980). Cultural expectations of thinness in women. *Psychological Medicine, 47,* 483–491.

Geary, M. C. (1988). A review of treatment models for eating disorders: Toward a holistic nursing model. *Holistic Nursing Practice, 3,* 39–45.

Goode, E. T. (1985). Medical aspects of the bulimic syndrome and bulimarexia. *Transactional Analysis Journal, 15,* 4–11.

Gross, H. A., Lake, C. R., Ebert, M. H., Ziegler, M. G., & Kopin, E. J. (1979). Catecholamine metabolism in primary anorexia nervosa. *Journal of Clinical Endocrinology Metabolism, 49,* 805–809.

Hawkins, R. C, & Clement, P. F. (1980). Development and construct validation of a self-report measure of binge eating tendencies. *Addictive Behaviors, 5,* 219–226.

Herzog, D. B., & Copeland, P. M. (1985). Eating disorders. *New England Journal of Medicine, 133,* 295–303.

Johnson, C., & Connors, M. E. (1987). *The etiology and treatment of bulimia nervosa: A biopsychological perspective.* New York: Basic Books.

Johnson, C., Lewis, C., & Hagman, J. (1984). The syndrome of bulimia. *Psychiatric Clinics of North America, 7,* 247–274.

Kaye, W. H., Ebert, M. H., Raleigh, M., & Lake, C. R. (1984). Abnormalities in CNS monoamine metabolism in anorexia nervosa. *Archives of General Psychiatry, 41,* 350–355.

Keys, A., Brozed, J., Henschel, A., Mickelson, O., & Taylor, H.L. (1950). *The biology of human starvation* (Vol. 1). Minneapolis, MN: University of Michigan Press.

Levin, P. A., Falks, J. M., & Dixon, K. (1980). Benign parotid enlargement in bulimia. *Annals of Internal Medicine, 93,* 827–829.

Minuchin, S., Rosman, B. L., & Baker, L. (1978). *Psychosomatic families: Anorexia nervosa in context.* Cambridge, MA: Harvard University Press.

Mitchell, J. E., & Groat, R. (1984). A placebo-controlled double-blind trial of amitriptyline in bulimia. *Journal of Clinical Psychopharmacology, 4,* 186–193.

Mitchell, J. E., Pyle, R. L., & Miner, R. A. (1982). Gastric dilatation as a complication of bulimia. *Psychosomatics, 23,* 96–99.

National Institute of Child Health and Human Development. (1983). *Facts about anorexia nervosa.* Bethesda, MD: U.S. Government Printing Office.

Orbach, S. (1986). *Hunger strike: The anorectic's struggle as a metaphor of our age.* New York: W.W. Norton.

Pope, H. G., & Hudson, J. I. (1984) *New hope for binge eaters.* New York: Harper & Row.

Pope, H. G., Hudson, J. I., & Jonas, J. M. (1983). Antidepressant treatment of bulimia: Preliminary experience and practical recommendations. *Journal of Clinical Psychopharmacology, 3,* 274–281.

Potts, N. L. (1984). Eating disorders: The secret pattern of binge/purge. *American Journal of Nursing, 84,* 32–35.

Rizzuto, A. M., Peterson, R. K., & Reed, M. (1981). The pathological sense of self in anorexia nervosa. *Pediatric Clinics of North America, 4,* 471–487.

Selvini-Palazzoli, M. P. (1978). *Self-starvation: From individuation to family therapy in the treatment of anorexia nervosa.* New York: Jason Aronson.

Striegel-Moore, R. H., Silberstein, L. R., & Rodin, J. (1986). Toward an understanding of risk factors for bulimia. *American Psychologist, 41,* 246–263.

Swift, W. J. (1982). The long-term outcome of early onset anorexia nervosa: A critical review. *Journal of American Academy of Child Psychiatry, 21,* 38–46.

Walsh, B. T., Stewart, J. W., Wright, L., Harrison, W., Roose, S. P., & Glassman, A. H. (1982). Treatment of bulimia with monoamine oxidase inhibitors. *American Journal of Psychiatry, 139*(12), 1629–1630.

Winnicott, D. W. (1965). *The maturational process and the facilitating environment.* London: Hogarth Press.

Wooley, S. C., & Wooley, O. W. (1985). Intensive outpatient and residential treatment for bulimia. In D. M. Garner & P. E. Garfinkel (Eds.), *Handbook of psychotherapy for anorexia nervosa and bulimia* (pp. 391–430). New York: The Guilford Press.

CHAPTER

22

Chemical Dependency

Valerie A. Woodard

Trends

Use of alcohol and illicit drugs by high school students has generally declined since peaks in the late 1970s and early 1980s. The percentage of high school seniors who had used any illicit drug was 64.4% in 1982 (Johnston, O'Malley, & Bachman, 1991) but dropped to 40.7% in 1992, (Johnston, O'Malley, & Bachman, 1993). However, according to 1992 survey results, while seniors showed improvement, eighth graders significantly increased their use of marijuana, cocaine, D-lysergic acid diethylamide (LSD), other hallucinogens, and, to a lesser degree, inhalants (Johnston et al., 1993). Surveyors suggest that less public attention to the problems of drug use in recent years may have contributed to increased use of some drugs by younger children.

DRUG DEPENDENCE

Physical dependence (neuroadaptation) describes physiologic changes in response to long-term psychoactive drug use so that cessation or reduced dosage results in aversive withdrawal symptoms. Negative reinforcement occurs when drugs are taken to alleviate these symptoms.

Symptoms of withdrawal represent a rebound phenomenon. Symptoms are generally the opposite of intoxicating drug effects. Marked physiologic symptoms can accompany withdrawal from CNS depressants and opioids; subjective, rather than physical, symptoms may accompany withdrawal from amphetamines, cocaine, and cannabis. Withdrawal from hallucinogens, phencyclidine (PCP), and inhalants is not significant (APA, 1994).

Tolerance occurs when the same amount of drug produces less effect so that more must be taken to achieve the desired result. Tolerance may develop to some drug effects more than to others. Drugs within the same class are often cross tolerant and can be used to relieve withdrawal symptoms. Reverse tolerance, or "kindling," refers to what appears to be increased receptor sensitivity after repeated drug use. This may increase the risk of seizures.

Psychological dependence refers to loss of control over drug use and the sometimes compulsive need to repeat its subjective effects despite negative consequences.

Mechanism of Psychoactive Drug Actions

All psychoactive substances affect the brain by enhancing or inhibiting neurotransmitters. These are chemical messengers that affect mood and behavior by passing information from neuron to neuron.

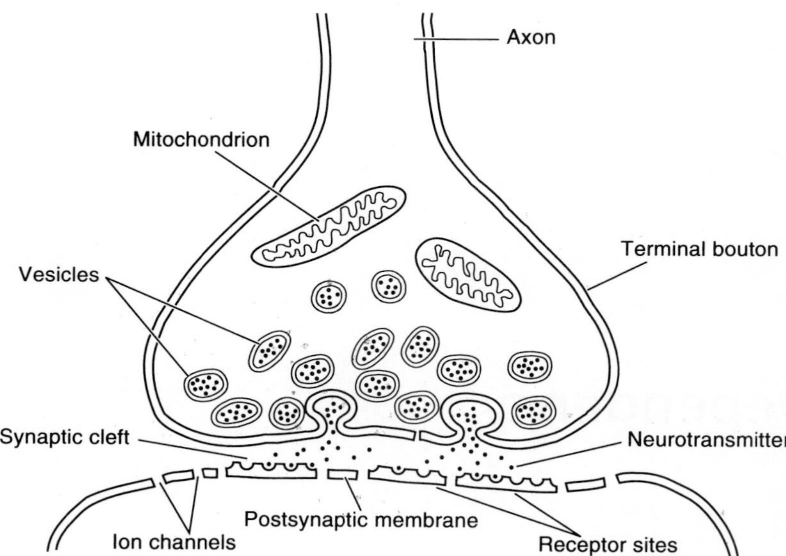

FIGURE 22–1 • Close-up of a synapse. Molecules of neurotransmitter are enclosed in vesicles in the terminal bouton of the axon. Two vesicles are shown fused to the presynaptic membrane, releasing neurotransmitter into the synaptic cleft. The neurotransmitter initiates activity in the postsynaptic neuron by binding to receptor sites in the postsynaptic membrane. (From Martin, M. B., Owen, C. M., & Morihisa, J. M. [1987]. An overview of neurotransmitters and neuroreceptors. In R. E. Hales and S. C. Yudofsky [Eds.], *The American Psychiatric Press textbook of neurosychiatry*. Washington, DC: American Psychiatric Press. Copyright 1987 by the American Psychiatric Press, Inc. Reprinted by permission.)

Once released, the neurotransmitter crosses the synaptic space between neurons and binds to a postsynaptic receptor. There, its effects may be excitatory, promoting passage of the chemical message, or inhibitory, stopping or retarding it (Fig. 22-1). Neurotransmitters that are usually inhibitory include dopamine (DA), γ-aminobutyric acid (GABA), and serotonin (5-hydroxytryptamine—5-HT). Those neurotransmitters that are usually excitatory include acetylcholine (ACH), glutamate, and norepinephrine (NE). When neurotransmitters finish their work, they are either enzymatically destroyed, or they return to the presynaptic neuron in a process called reuptake.

The reward and pleasure centers of the brain have been identified along the mesocorticolimbic circuits of DA (Jaffee, 1990) (Fig. 22-2). Stimulation of these areas with food, electricity, or a variety of drugs results in increased DA (Jaffee, 1990), suggesting a strong role for this neurotransmitter in the mechanism of reinforcement. Common involvement of 5-HT systems is also suggested (Gold, 1993). Withdrawal from a variety of drugs may be caused by rebound hyperactivity of the NE-containing, brain stem nucleus, called the locus coeruleus (Gold, 1993).

Central Nervous System Depressants (Barbiturates, Ethanol)

EFFECTS

Barbiturates and ethanol, the alcohol in beverages, produce CNS depression with initial calming effects that can progress to sleep, coma, and fatal cardiorespiratory depression at higher doses. Cross-tolerance develops between CNS depressants, so when taken separately, the effect of each is decreased. However, taken in combination, these drugs compete for the same metabolic liver enzymes and circulate longer, potentiating the effects of each. The result can be a fatal overdose.

WITHDRAWAL

Physical dependence on barbiturates and ethanol can produce potential life-threatening physiologic symptoms of withdrawal when the drug is removed. Symptoms of autonomic nervous system hyperactivity and possible seizures are the opposite of intoxicating effects. In heavy, chronic users, withdrawal can progress to delirium, hyperthermia, and cardiovascular collapse. Severe withdrawal symptoms may be treated with tapered doses of the same or a cross-tolerant sedative or benzodiazepine (BZ). Nurses can monitor the need for medication using severity assessment scales that numerically quantify withdrawal symptoms (Foy, March, & Drinkwater, 1988; Kinney & Severinghaus, 1991). The goal is to manage symptoms and decrease the risk of seizures without oversedating. Most adolescents do not progress beyond minor withdrawal symptoms that respond to reassurance and do not need medication.

The extent to which child or adolescent alcohol abuse impairs development is not known. However, alcohol does interfere with nutritional metabolism. It disrupts endocrine systems necessary for bone, muscle, and sexual develoment; it causes neurologic and neuropsychologic deficits in areas such as memory and cognition, and liver damage has been found in alcohol-abusing adolescents (Arria, Tarter, & VanThiel, 1990)

MECHANISMS OF ACTION

The action of barbiturates and ethanol in CNS depression is in part related to their enhancement of the inhibitory neurotransmitter GABA (Rall, 1990) at its large receptor sites embedded in brain cell membranes. A single dose of ethanol increases DA production, possibly contributing to its positive reinforcement (Tabakoff, Hoffman, & Petersen, 1990). Barbiturates (Rall, 1990) and ethanol (Weight, 1989) also inhibit the excitatory neurotransmitter glutamate. A compensatory increase in glutamate receptors (up-regulation) may contribute to hyperexcitability and seizures during ethanol withdrawal (Tabakoff et al., 1990). Repeated ethanol withdrawals are progressively severe, possibly due to kindling (Goodwin, 1988).

Opioids

MECHANISM OF ACTION

The opioids are a group of drugs that bind to various opioid receptors where they act as morphine agonists (mimic morphine), antagonists (initiate no action), or agonist–antagonists and partial agonists (mixed actions). The three major opioid receptors, mu (μ) for morphine, kappa (κ), and delta (δ) appear to inhibit synaptic transmission, in part by decreasing the release of excitatory neurotransmitters (Jaffee & Martin, 1990).

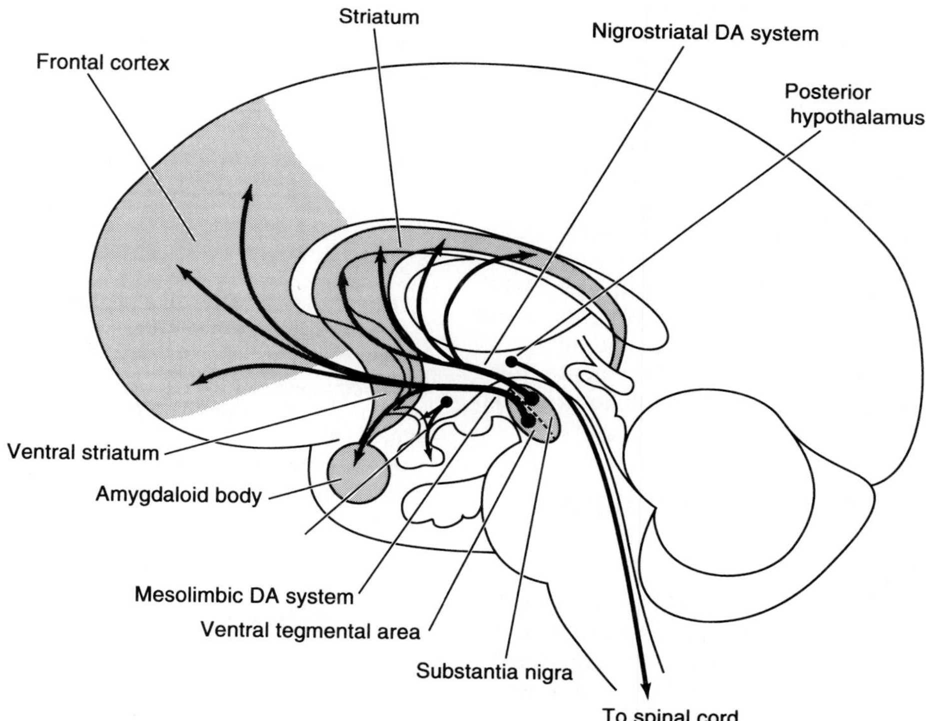

FIGURE 22–2 • Dopaminergic pathways. The nigrostriatal DA system originates in the substantia nigra and terminates in the main dorsal part of the striatum. The ventral tegmental area gives rise to the mesocorticolimbic DA system, which terminates in the ventral striatum, amygdaloid body, frontal cortex, and some other basal forebrain areas. The tuberoinfundibular DA system innervates the median eminence as well as the posterior and intermediate lobes of the pituitary, and dopamine neurons in the posterior hypothalamus project to the spinal cord. (From Heimer, L. [1983]. *The human brain and spinal cord: Functional neuroanatomy and dissection guide* [p. 234]. New York: Springer-Verlag. Copyright 1983 by Springer-Verlag. Reprinted by permission of the author.)

The reinforcing effects of μ opioids appear to be associated with activation of DA circuits, although findings are unclear (Jaffee & Martin, 1990). Most opioids that cause abuse and dependence are μ agonists (Jaffee, 1989). Morphine and its agonists act primarily at μ receptors with features including euphoria, analgesia, drowsiness, decreased gastrointestinal motility, respiratory depression, and miosis. Antagonists, such as naloxone and nalorphine, can reverse the effects of opioids by displacing them at receptors.

TOXICITY AND WITHDRAWAL

Opioid overdose is a medical emergency. Pupils may be pinpoint or dilated if there is anoxia. Coma, cardiac arrhythmia, and convulsions may develop. Death may follow respiratory depression in combination with pulmonary or cerebral edema (Schuckit, 1989). Treatment may include administration of an opioid antagonist that reverses symptoms within minutes and can precipitate withdrawal.

Withdrawal symptoms include tremor, craving, flu-like lacrimation and rhinorrhea, abdominal pain, and muscle spasm. Some symptoms may reflect increased NE activity (Jaffee, 1989). Withdrawal does not usually constitute a medical emergency. Tapered doses of methadone are used in detoxification of adult opioid addicts, but this is rare in adolescent management. Methadone is a μ agonist with analgesic effects but without the "high" of heroin.

Adolescent opioid use is associated with delinquency, which precedes it (Kraus, 1981). Rage and aggression also are common in heroin addicts, suggesting opioids may function to self-medicate these powerful affects (Khantzian, 1985). Opioids are taken through all routes of administration.

Central Nervous System Stimulants

EFFECTS AND PATTERNS

The behavioral and subjective effects of amphetamines and cocaine are similar. Psychostimulant use is energizing and associated with grandiosity. Khantzian (1985) suggests stimulant users select these drugs to self-medicate depression or feelings of inadequacy.

Cocaine free base (crack) smoking and intravenous stimulant use can lead to abuse within weeks or months compared to the slower addictive liability of intranasal or oral routes. This is due to almost immediate euphoric effects followed by a dysphoric "crash," leading to repeated dosing in cycles of "binges" or "runs." Abuse may develop more rapidly in adolescents than in adults. A sample of teens who called the "800-COCAINE" helpline progressed from first use to dysfunction in 1.5 years compared with more than 4 years for adults (Washton & Gold, 1987). Callers also revealed a profile of the cocaine-addicted adolescent (Table 22-1).

EUPHORIA

Cocaine and smokeable street forms of methamphetamine ("Ice" or "Glass") have been clinically described as the most powerfully reinforcing drugs available. Their euphoric effects are thought to result primarily from enhancement of DA by blocking its reuptake, and amphetamine also stimulates its release (Jaffee, 1989; 1990). New understanding of cocaine addiction comes from cloning the gene for the DA transporter protein that removes DA from the synapse (reuptake) (Mathias, 1992) This is the action cocaine blocks, producing its "high." The intensity of cocaine reinforcement is illustrated by monkeys who self-administer the drug until death (Deneau, Yanagita, & Seevers, 1969) dramatizing its supremacy over other drives. A survey of 500 callers to 800-COCAINE showed more than half preferred cocaine to food, sex, and social relationships (Washton & Gold, 1987).

TABLE 22–1 Profile of Cocaine-Addicted Adolescents

A random sample of 100 teenage callers to the "800-COCAINE" helpline revealed a profile of the cocaine-addicted adolescent:

Missed days at school	75%
Significant drop in grades	69%
Drug-related disciplinary problems	48%
Expelled	31%
Sold drugs	44%
Stealing from family, friends, employer	31%
Cocaine-induced seizures and loss of consciousness	19%
Automobile accidents	13%
Suicide attempts	14%
Violent behavior	27%

From Washton, A. M., & Gold, M. S. (1987). "Recent trends in cocaine abuse: A view from the national hotline, '800-COCAINE.'" In B. Stimmel (Ed.), *Cocaine: Pharmacology, addiction, and therapy* (pp. 42–43). New York: The Haworth Press, 1987.

TOXICITY

Cocaine and amphetamines are potent sympathomimetics. They block reuptake of the sympathetic nervous system neurotransmitter NE (Jaffee, 1990). Toxicity is characterized by sympathetic nervous system hyperactivity evidenced by elevated vital signs that can progress to extreme elevations in blood pressure and temperature, convulsions and cardiovascular shock (Schuckit, 1989). Repeated subthreshold doses of cocaine may lead to seizures, as an apparent result of kindling. Vasoconstriction, a hallmark of cocaine toxicity, is associated with ischemia of myocardial and skeletal muscle and of the intestines. The latter may follow body packing (rupture of condoms packed with cocaine and ingested) (Cregler, 1989). Other medical emergencies include respiratory failure and subarachnoid hemorrhage (Gold, 1993). Mixtures of cocaine with alcohol or heroin (speedballs), increase the risk of acute overdose reactions. Cardiac arrhythmia, tachycardia, mycarditis, infarct, and sudden death may follow recreational cocaine use, not just massive doses (Isner et al., 1986). Death from amphetamine toxicity, although uncommon, is related to hyperpyrexia, seizures, and shock (Mirin & Weiss, 1983). CNS stimulants also can precipitate a psychosis with paranoid delusions, hallucinations, or formication.

WITHDRAWAL: DYSPHORIA, CRAVING, ANHEDONIA

Stimulant withdrawal is experienced as dysphoric, but it does not have the physiologic symptoms of withdrawal from CNS depressants. Craving and withdrawal may be due to DA depletion in brain reward areas, when the return of synaptic DA to the presynaptic neuron is blocked, and DA is lost through metabolism (Dackis & Gold, 1988). Chronic cocaine use may similarly deplete NE after acutely stimulating it, thus possibly accounting for dysphoric withdrawal symptoms such as depression and anhedonia (Dackis & Gold, 1988).

Gawin and Kleber have described three phases of cocaine withdrawal starting with a depressive "crash" followed by symptoms that include anxiety, anhedonia, and craving, and ending with an indefinite period of craving triggered by environmental cues (Gawin & Kleber, 1986).

A program of "extinction," repeated exposure to unreinforced cues, has been developed by O'Brien et al. (1988). There is no definitive pharmacologic treatment for cocaine toxicity or withdrawal, but research includes drugs that are DA agonists (Gold, 1993) and development of an enzyme that would act like a vaccine to reduce cocaine's addictive qualities (Morrell, 1993).

Hallucinogens

GENERAL ATTRIBUTES

Hallucinogens are a family of drugs that may be synthetic (LSD), or derived from plants or fungi (Schuckit, 1989). They have in common the ability to alter perceptions, thoughts, and feelings. Many resemble amphetamines and are structurally similar to neurotransmitters, especially serotonin, but it it not known exactly how they affect the brain (Schuckit, 1989). Hallucinogens are usually taken episodically. They are not strong reinforcers, and there is no significant withdrawal. Sensory stimuli are intensified and may be mixed. Synesthesias, hearing colors and seeing sounds, may occur, as well as distortions of body image. There may be a loss of boundaries with fear of self-fragmentation or a sense of union with the universe (Jaffee, 1989). Perceptual effects may be accompanied by anxiety, depression, or paranoia (APA, 1994).

INTOXICATION AND TOXICITY

Frank hallucinations, perceptions of people or things that are not there, may occur with dosage.

Hallucinogens may precipitate panic, flashbacks, or psychosis with paranoid delusions or hallucinations (Schuckit, 1989). Nursing can provide a supporting milieu structure and reassurance that hallucinations are drug-induced and will subside. Maintaining verbal contact provides reality orientation.

Hallucinogens also cause adrenergic-like symptoms such as tachycardia, dilated pupils, and tremor. Convulsions, cardiovascular collapse, and extreme temperature elevations are particular risks with an overdose of methylene dioxyamphetamine (MDA) and methylene dioxymethamphetamine (MDMA), known as "ectasy" (Schuckit, 1989).

LSD

LSD, perhaps the most commonly abused hallucinogen, is an extremely potent drug that may produce frank hallucinations at low doses (Schuckit, 1989). It is 100 times more potent than psilocin and psilocybin, the active ingredient in psychoactive mushrooms, and 4000 times more potent than the peyote cactus product, mescaline (Jaffee, 1990; Schuckit, 1989). Fatal accidents, suicide (Jaffee, 1990), and homicide (Hollister, 1984) have occurred during LSD intoxication. It can be smoked, ingested, and injected and is often dissolved on sugar cubes, blotter paper, or gelatin squares.

PCP

PCP (angel dust) has CNS depressant, CNS stimulant, hallucinogenic (Jaffee, 1989), sympathomimetic, cholinergic (Schuckit, 1989), and anesthetic effects that may be attributable to general enhancement and disruption of neurotransmitters. It has been shown to block reuptake of DA, NE, and 5-HT (Jaffee, 1989) and increase acetylcholine (Schuckit, 1989). Its behaviorial effects may also relate to inhibition of the excitatory neurotranmitter glutamate (U.S. Department of Health and Human Services, 1991)

PCP is taken for its euphoric effects but it also can produce panic, belligerence, assaultiveness, and bizarre, self-injurious behavior without apparent perception of pain. Restraints should be avoided to prevent muscle damage, but therapeutic holding may be indicated. Toxicity also may include psychosis, coma, convulsions, high temperature and blood pressure, and cardiac or respiratory failure (Schuckit, 1989). Nursing measures include providing safety, reducing stimuli, and monitoring vital functions. "Talking down" is not effective. Collaborative measures may include reducing fever with cool soaks or a hypothermic blanket, and possible anticonvulsant or antihypertensive medication.

Cannabinoids

The main psychoactive ingredient of the marijuana plant (cannabis) is delta-9-tetrahydrocannabinol (THC). Today's THC has four times the potency of the THC of the 1970s (Schwartz, Hoffman, & Jones, 1987). The sinsimilla (seedless) plant variety, in great demand by adolescents, has six times the THC concentration of most earlier THC (Schwartz et al., 1987).

EFFECTS

THC may be smoked or ingested. It has both stimulant and sedative properties (Mirin & Weiss, 1983). Perceptual distortions occur as vivid, visual images and sensory intensification. Users experience feelings of unreality and a distorted sense of time. Larger doses may precipitate frank hallucinations (Schuckit, 1989). Other complications include panic, paranoia, persecutory delusions, and flashbacks. Cardiovascular effects include dose-related tachycardia and injected conjunctiva. Withdrawal symptoms have been described (Jaffee, 1990), but a syndrome has not been established. Supportive care and reassurance usually are sufficient.

MECHANISM OF ACTION

A receptor responsive to psychoactive cannabinoids has been identified (Herkenham et al., 1990; Marx, 1990), and several possible natural brain molecules that bind to it are under study (Barinaga, 1992). High levels of the receptor are in the movement control centers of the cerebellum, cognitive and memory areas of the cerebral cortex, and hippocampus (Marx, 1990) and more diffusely in the hypothalamus and amygdala (Herkenham et al., 1990). These limbic structures are along DA reward circuits. It is proposed that the effects of THC result from enhancement of DA along these circuits by blocking reuptake and by modulating opioid receptors (Gardner & Lowinson, 1991). THC is fat soluble and is readily stored in lipid-rich tissues of the brain, testes, lungs, and ovaries, where it may remain approximately 45 days with slow release back into the blood stream (Macdonald, 1989).

ADVERSE PHYSICAL EFFECTS

THC use is associated with short-term memory impairment and decreased ability to store information, impaired driving skills (Murray, 1986), reproductive dysfunctions (Maykut, 1984), and a possible amotivational syndrome (APA, 1994). Smoking three to four THC cigarettes daily can produce chronic bronchitis and epithelial change equal to that of 20 tobacco cigarettes (Wu, Tashkin, Djahed, & Rose, 1988). Compared with smoking cigarettes, approximately three times more tar is inhaled, and one third more is retained after smoking THC (Wu et al., 1988). Tar condensate is carcinogenic. THC use can exacerbate preexisting schizophrenia (Jaffee, 1990), seizures in epileptics (Schuckit, 1989), and angina in patients with coronary artery disease (Jaffee, 1989). Escalating dysfunction is described in the lives of 35 teenagers before and after heavy marijuana use (at least four times weekly for at least 4 months) (Table 22-2).

Inhalants

Inhalant use has resisted the dramatic downward trend of some other drug groups. Young children are at particular risk. Among eighth graders. 17.4% of those surveyed in 1992 had used inhalants, making them the only class of drugs used at a substantially higher rate in grade 8 than in grades 10 or 12

TABLE 22–2 Adolescents' Self-Assessment of Problems Before and After Frequent Marijuana Use

	Before Marijuana		After Marijuana	
	No.	*%*	*No.*	*%*
Poor school grades	11	31	31	89
Vandalism	6	17	14	40
Conflicts with parents	16	46	32	92
Depression	6	17	21	60
Explosive temper	6	17	20	57
Feeling of worthlessness	6	17	20	54
Suicide attempt	0	0	7	27
Visit to psychiatrist or other mental health professional	11	31	24	60

From Schwartz, R. H., Hoffman, N. G., & Jones, R. (1987). Behavioral, psychosocial, and academic correlates of marijuana usage in adolescence. *Clinical Pediatrics, 26*(5), 268. Copyright 1987 by The International Publishing Group. Reprinted with permission.

(Johnston et al., 1993). Inhalants include volatile solvents, aerosols, anesthetics, and volatile nitrites. They may be sniffed or huffed (inhaled by mouth) directly or from soaked cloth. Aerosol spray, glue, or solvent-soaked fabric may be placed in a paper bag that is then placed over the user's head. Effects occur within minutes and last up to 45 minutes (Schuckit, 1989). Nitrous oxide, used as a propellant for whipped cream, also is abused for its euphoric and hallucinogenic effects. Amyl nitrite, used to treat angina, and butyl nitrite, an ingredient of room odorizers, are abused as aphrodisiacs.

MECHANISMS OF ACTION

The effect of inhalants on consciousness is similar to that of CNS depressants. Initial intoxicating effects, reached by most inhalants, are excitatory and euphoric, followed by CNS depression, disorientation, and behavioral disinhibition (McHugh, 1987). In the final stages, ataxia, stupor, seizures, and cardiorespiratory arrest may occur (McHugh, 1987). Solvents may act by disordering neuronal membranes and generally disrupting neurotransmitter systems (Schuckit, 1989).

TOXICITY

Volatile solvents and aerosols contain mixtures of toxic chemicals, including acetone, benzene, toluene, dichlorofluoromethanes and trichlorofluoromethanes, ketones, and petroleum products (U. S. Department of Health & Human Services, 1987). Impairments associated with various chemicals include anemias, neuropathies, hepatitis, possible liver or kidney failure (Schuckit, 1989), and encephalopathy in children (King, Day, Oliver, Lush, & Watson, 1991). Potentially fatal cardiac arrythmia and respiratory depression are particular risks with solvent or aerosol use (Schuckit, 1989). Sudden sniffing death has been reported in children who inhale the contents of paper bags containing aerosol spray (Bass, 1970). There is no apparent withdrawal syndrome, but the relapse rate is high. Nursing measures for inhalant intoxication include close monitoring of vital signs and level of consciousness and support of vital functions (see Tables 22–3 and 22–4).

Origins of Substance Abuse

Current consensus supports a multifactorial etiology of substance abuse, with psychosocial, genetic, and environmental influences converging to increase or protect against a child's vulnerability to chemical dependency.

GENETIC INFLUENCES

Substantial research, especially adoption studies that separate genetic and environmental influences, supports a genetic predisposition for compulsive use of at least a subtype of alcoholism (Bohman, Sigvardsson, & Cloninger, 1981; Goodwin, 1979) and possibly for other psychoactive drugs (Cadoret, Troughton, O'Gorman, & Haywood, 1986). Possible biological vulnerability also is supported by identification of a genetic variant for the DA D_2 receptor that may be associated with severe alcoholism (Blum et al., 1990), but findings are inconsistent (Turner et al., 1992). New research also suggests a variant of this receptor may play a role in polysubstance abuse vulnerability (Smith et al., 1992).

Other biological markers for alcoholism have also been identified (Whelan, 1992), including those associated with children of alcoholics (COAs), indicating their possible genetic loading. COAs, for example, were found to have a less intense reaction to alcohol than those persons with a negative family history (Schuckit, 1989). Children of two alcoholic parents also are more likely than children of one parent or no alcoholic parents to proceed more rapidly from first intoxication to treatment for alcoholism (McKenna & Pickens, 1981), and more adolescent sons of alcoholics than sons of nonalcoholics were found to have neuropsychological

TABLE 22–3 Actions of Six Psychoactive Drug Groups

Psychoactive Substances	Street Name	Intoxication	Toxicity/Overdose	Withdrawal
Barbiturates Ethanol		Sense of well-being followed by disinhibition, impaired judgement, slurred speech, incoordination, unsteady gait	Marked central nervous system (CNS) depression (especially respiratory function), stupor, coma, psychosis	Autonomic hyperactivity, nausea or vomiting, tremor, seizures, insomnia, delirium, hyperthermia, cardiovascular collapse
Opioid agonists Morphine Heroin Fentanyl Methadone	 Horse, H, Harry China white	Euphoria followed by dysphoria; drowsiness, analgesia, pupil constriction, impaired attention/memory, decreased respiratory rate	Pinpoint pupils (or dilation with anoxia), coma, shock, pulmonary or cerebral edema, respiratory failure	Lacrimation, rhinorrhea, perspiration, yawning, dilated pupils, piloerection (goose flesh), chills, diarrhea, aching, tremor, nausea, vomiting, abdominal pain
CNS stimulants Amphetamines Methamphetamines Cocaine	 Bennies, dexies ice, glass, crank snow, crack	Euphoria, increased energy and sexual interest, decreased appetite, tremor, dilated pupils, nausea, vomiting, chills, tachycardia, increased blood pressure	Arrhythmias, high blood pressure, hyperthermia, convulsions, cardiovascular shock, panic, paranoid delusions, formication, hallucinations, delirium	Depression; insomnia, then hypersomnia; decreased appetite, then hyperphagia; agitation, then fatigue; anhedonia, persistent craving
PCP	Angel dust	Euphoria, belligerence, assaultiveness, sweating, increased blood pressure or heart rate, nystagmus, numbness, muscle rigidity, seizures	Panic, violence, catatonia, psychosis, flashbacks, increased temperature and blood pressure, convulsions, coma, cardiorespiratory failure	—
Hallucinogens LSD Psilocybin and psilocin DMT, DET Mescaline (Peyote) DOM, STP MDA MDMA	 Acid, sugar Shrooms Businessman's trip (DMT) Bad seed Peace Love Bug Ecstasy	Hallucinations, euphoria, depersonalization, derealization, synesthesia, pupil dilation, increased vital signs, incoordination, tremor	Panic, flashbacks, depression, anxiety, paranoia, delusions, hallucinations, confusion; high temperature, convulsions, cardiovascular collapse (particular risk with MDA & MDMA)	—
Cannabinoids Marijuana Hashish Hashish oil	 Reefer Hash	Euphoria, paranoia, inability to gauge time, social withdrawal, memory impairment, incoordination, injected conjunctiva, increased appetite, tachycardia	Panic, flashbacks, paranoia, delusions, hallucinations	Possible irritability, restlessness, decreased appetite, insomnia, tremor, chills

(continued)

TABLE 22–3 Actions of Six Psychoactive Drug Groups *(Continued)*

Psychoactive Substances	Street Name	Intoxication	Toxicity/Overdose	Withdrawal
Inhalants		Euphoria, belligerence, dizziness, nystagmus, incoordination, slurred speech, nausea and vomiting, tremor, stupor, coma	Panic, disorientation, emotional lability; cardiac arrythmia, CNS depression (solvents)	—
Volatile solvents				
Aerosols				
Anesthetics				
Nitrous oxide	Laughing gas			
Volatile nitrites	Snappers			
Amyl, Butyl	Poppers			

Sources: American Psychiatric Association. (1994). *Diagnostic and statistical manual of mental disorders* (4th ed.). Washington, D.C.: Author.
Schuckit, M. A. (1989). *Drug and alcohol abuse: A clinical guide to diagnosis and treatment* (3rd ed.). New York: Plenum.
Wilford, B. B. (1981). *Drug abuse: A guide for primary care physicians.* Chicago: American Medical Association.
Jaffee, J. H. (1990). Drug addiction and drug abuse. In A. G. Gilman, T. W. Rall, A. S. Nies, & P. Taylor (Eds.), *Goodman and Gilman's the pharmacological basis of therapeutics* (8th ed.) (pp. 522–573). New York: Pergamon Press.

deficits in areas such as memory, language processing, and attention (Tarter, Hegedus, Goldstein, Shelly, & Alterman, 1984).

PSYCHOSOCIAL RISK FACTORS

Social science research in the last decade has identified a plethora of psychosocial risk factors that predict later substance use or abuse. But some findings are inconsistent. Researchers suggest this reflects different paths to substance abuse, with combinations of risk factors unique to each adolescent. Newcomb, Maddihean, and Bentler (1986) found that out of 10 risk factors, the total number, not a particular set, predicted substance use or abuse.

AGE AT FIRST USE

Substantial research supports early drug use as a strong predictor of later, more serious drug involvement (Kandel, 1982). Robins and Przybeck (1985) found that when drug use began prior to age 15, close to one half of the men and two fifths of the women studied later met Diagnostic and Statistical Manual, 3rd ed., (DSM III) criteria for a drug disorder.

ACHIEVEMENT-RELATED FACTORS

Poor school performance (Kandel, 1978; Zucker & Gomberg, 1986), truancy (Zucker & Gomberg, 1986), and low academic aspirations and motivation (Jessor & Jessor, 1977; Kandel, 1978) have been found to precede initiation or later abuse of alcohol or illicit drugs.

INDEPENDENCE

Value placed on independence has consistently distinguished future users and nonusers of marijuana (Kandel, 1978). This is described by Jessor and Jessor (1977) as freedom from adult control, expressed in behaviors considered age inappropriate.

LOCUS OF CONTROL

Some evidence suggests early adolescent COAs are more likely than others to believe events in their lives are beyond their control (Windle, 1990). However, findings are inconsistent with respect to an external rather than internal locus of control as antecedent to adolescent substance use or abuse (Windle, 1990).

SELF-ESTEEM

The self-esteem and self-derogation theory of substance abuse (Kaplan, 1980) postulates that substance use or abuse is one deviant alternative used to boost self-esteem in response to negative self-attitudes that follow rejection by one's normative membership group. In a 3-year study of 3148 seventh graders, Kaplan (1977) found an increase in self-rejecting attitudes preceded deviant behaviors,

TABLE 22–4 Nursing Interventions for Acute Intoxication and Withdrawal

Acute Intoxication and Withdrawal	Basis
For All Psychoactive Drugs	
1. Identify drug(s) and amount taken. Obtain a drug history, specimens for toxicology (blood, urine, emesis), and blood chemistries. (C)*	Drug identification enables an estimate of recovery time, drug-specific treatment. Blood chemistries and evaluate liver, kidney, and respiratory function.
2. Maintain constant observation.	Prevent self-injury. Observation enables early identification of change in physical, mental state.
CNS Depression (occurs with CNS depressant, opioid, and inhalant intoxication)	
1. Monitor vital signs, pupil response, level of consciousness, cardiac, respiratory status ISO. Support vital functions: airway, respiration (oxygen therapy, resuscitation), circulation (open IV line). (C)*	Depression of cerebrocortical, cardiac, and respiratory centers can precipitate respiratory depression, cardiac arrhythmia, coma. Pupils are pinpoint in opioid toxicity and dilate in hypoxia.
2. Use gastric lavage, activated charcoal, castor oil, diuresis, hemodialysis as ordered. (C)*	Prevent further absorption; promote rapid excretion of CNS depressants.
3. Administer an opioid antagonist (usually naloxone) as ordered. (C)* Monitor for withdrawal symptoms.	If symptoms are due to opioid toxicity, they will reverse within minutes and may precipitate withdrawal.
4. Administer IV glucose as ordered. (C)*	Glucose will reverse symptoms due to hypoglycemia.
5. Provide adequate nutrition. Administer thiamine, vitamin, and mineral preparations as ordered. (C)* Provide a well-balanced diet.	Wernicke's encephalopathy (seen in chronic adult alcoholics) is associated with thiamine deficiency. Alcohol interferes with metabolism of most vitamins and nutrients.
CNS Stimulation (occurs in CNS stimulant, hallucinogen, and PCP intoxication and in CNS depressant withdrawal)	
1. Monitor and support vital functions.	CNS hyperactivity can precipitate convulsions, extreme elevations in BP and temperature, shock.
2. Use gastric lavage, ammonium chloride, cranberry juice, diuresis as ordered. (C)*	Promote excretion in PCP and CNS stimulant toxicity.
3. Use a severity assessment scale to evaluate CNS depressant withdrawal (Foy et al., 1988; Kinney & Severinghaus, 1991).	Scales quantify symptoms as a guide to possible treatment with a cross-tolerant drug.
4. Administer a pentobarbital challenge as ordered in sedative–hypnotic withdrawal. (C)*	Determine the degree of tolerance as a guide to treating withdrawal with tapered doses of a cross-tolerant drug.
5. Apply cool soaks and hypothermic blanket as ordered. (C)*	Hyperthermia may result from sympathetic nervous system overactivity.
6. Monitor for seizures. Maintain seizure precautions. Protect from aspiration and administer anticonvulsant medication as ordered (usually diazepam). (C)*	CNS hyperactivity can cause seizures. Diazepam increases the seizure threshold by enhancing GABA.
7. Provide adequate nutrition, including a nutritional consultation as indicated.	CNS stimulants decrease appetite and cause weight loss.
Hallucinations may be associated with hallucinogen, PCP, stimulant, inhalant, THC use and CNS depressant.	
1. Provide structure, support, and reassurance that hallucinations are drug induced and will subside.	Hallucinogens can produce panic, especially in naïve users.
2. Provide reality orientation through verbal contact.	Loss of reality contact may accompany hallucinations.
3. Protect from injury to self or others. Remove sharps. Provide a quiet, stimulus-free environment.	Panic and hallucinations can precipitate injurious behavior. Bizarre or violent behavior may accompany drug toxicity. "Talking down" is not effective in PCP toxicity.

(continued)

TABLE 22–4 Nursing Interventions for Acute Intoxication and Withdrawal *(Continued)*

Acute Intoxication and Withdrawal	Basis
4. Avoid physical restraint. A therapeutic hold is preferable. If restraint is necessary, use soft restraint.	Restraint can exacerbate panic. Muscle contractions during restraint are associated with hyperthermia, rhabdomyolysis, and myoglobinuric renal failure in PCP toxicity.

*(C) indicates collaborative functions.

Sources: Doenges, M. E., Townsend, M. C., & Moorhouse, M. F. (1989). *Psychiatric care plans: Guidelines for client care.* Philadelphia: F.A. Davis.

Foy, A., March, S., & Drinkwater, V. (1988). Use of an objective clinical scale in the assessment and management of alcohol withdrawal in a large hospital. *Alcoholism: Clinical and Experimental Research, 12*(3), 360–364.

Kinney, J., & Severinghaus, J. (1991). Overview of medical management. In J. Kinney (Ed.), *Clinical manual of substance abuse* (pp. 91–112). St. Louis: Mosby-Year Book.

Kulberg, A. (1986). Substance abuse: Clinical identification and management. *Pediatric Clinics of North America, 33*(2), 325–361.

Schuckit, M. A. (1989). *Drug and alcohol abuse: A clinical guide to diagnosis and treatment* (3rd ed.). New York: Plenum.

including drug use. However, research findings are inconsistent with respect to self-esteem as a risk factor for substance abuse (Windle, 1990).

ATTITUDES

Kandel (1978) describes a process of anticipatory socialization in which adolescents develop attitudes favorable to drug use prior to actually use. This includes the belief that THC, hard liquor, and other illicit drugs are not harmful and that THC should be legalized (Kandel, 1978). Negative attitudes toward drugs may be a protective factor. Use of THC and cocaine declined among 1990 high school seniors, as perceived risk of harm increased (Johnston et al., 1991).

SENSATION SEEKING

Sensation seeking is a strong predictor of substance use (Andrucci, Archer, Pancoast, & Gordon, 1989). Sensation seekers are defined as those willing to take risks to obtain stimulation and arousal (Zuckerman, Ball, & Black, 1990).

SOCIABILITY

Drug experimenters, primarily with THC, were the psychologically healthiest group compared with frequent users and abstainers, in a study that followed children from preschool to age 18 (Shedler & Block, 1990). Frequent users showed relative maladjustment prior to initiation of drug use. These researchers suggest that rather than reflecting deviance, experimentation by otherwise well-adjusted adolescents may be an age-appropriate expression of differentiation and limit testing, whereas drugs may have a different psychologic meaning for maladjusted youngsters (Shedler & Block, 1990).

SEXUAL AND PHYSICAL ABUSE

A study by the Chemical Abuse/Addiction Treatment Outcome Registry (CATOR) found 37% of 625 adolescent girls and 5% of 1146 boys reported sexual abuse; the figures for physical abuse were 32% and 29%, respectively (Harrison & Hoffman, 1989). In general, sexual abuse victims initiate substance use earlier than nonvictims and are more likely to identify escape from family problems as a motivating factor (Harrison, Hoffman, & Edwall, 1989).

PEER INFLUENCE

The peer group is consistently found to be one of the most powerful influences on adolescent drug behavior (Kandel, 1982). It is a particularly strong influence on initiation to use of THC (Kandel, 1982). Peer influence occurs through the nearly equal effects of socialization, when one friend influences another, and selection, where adolescents with similar values seek each other (Kandel, 1982).

FAMILY INFLUENCE

The child's initition into drug use is influenced by parental use of alcohol or psychoactive drugs, by parental attitudes about drugs, and by the parent–child relationship (Kandel, 1982). The influence of each factor varies with the stage of drug use. Parental influence has been found to be especially strong on adolescent involvement with illicit drugs other than THC, but peer influence supercedes that of parents in initiation to the THC use (Kandel, 1978).

DUAL DIAGNOSIS

A dual diagnosis, particularly depression, attention-deficit/hyperactivity disorder (AD/HD), or conduct disorder, is commonly associated with adolescent substance abuse. A concurrent psychologic disorder has important prognostic implications. The presence of neurologic risk factors and more pathologic personality test scores was associated with less favorable treatment outcome in a study of 94 chemically dependent adolescents (Knapp, Templer, Cannon, & Dobson, 1991).

DEPRESSION AND SUICIDALITY. An estimated 60% to 80% of adolescent substance abusers are depressed on admission for treatment (Kaminer, 1991). Depression that accompanies or follows substance abuse, as part of withdrawal, will likely subside within 2 weeks of abstinence. However, prior depression can be expected to persist and may require antidepressant medication. Psychoactive substances seem to be a risk factor for adolescent suicide, but it is unclear if they are causative or secondary to depression.

CONDUCT DISORDER AND AGGRESSION. Delinquent (Kandel, 1978), deviant-prone (Jessor & Jessor, 1977), and antisocial, aggressive behavior (Zucker & Gomberg, 1986) have consistently been found to precede substance use.

However, severe polydrug use may help maintain delinquent behavior. The CATOR report showed that 1 year after completing treatment for substance abuse, arrest rates were 45% for relapsed youth compared with only 16% for those who remained abstinent (Harrison & Hoffman, 1989).

HYPERACTIVITY. Childhood hyperactivity has been linked to adolescent substance abuse as a risk factor (Gittleman, Mannuzza, Shenker, & Bonagura, 1985). However, hyperactivity may be only a risk factor when it occurs with conduct disorder (Gittleman et al., 1985) or aggression (Loney, 1988).

Adolescent Development and Substance Abuse

COGNITIVE AND MORAL DEVELOPMENT

Cognition and moral values develop in parallel stages (Liebert, Poulos, & Marmor, 1977). Substance abusing adolescents may become arrested in this development when drug abuse begins. Many are stuck at the level of concrete operational thinking, where behavior is guided by consequences and external authority, rather than by a desire to conform to convention, the next higher developmental stage. Transition to this stage can be promoted in treatment by encouraging adolescents to adopt milieu and group norms (Nowinski, 1990). Drug use avoids the cognitive turmoil that accompanies transition to higher cognitive and moral levels, where one's own principles and principles of social order are the final reference for decision making. Drug use promotes dependence by forcing adults to step in and set limits. Promoting cognitive and moral growth is an important part of treatment that cannot occur through reliance on behavior modification and external control (Nowinski, 1990). Approaches that promote internalization of values and control include a milieu environment that models prosocial norms and exercises in values clarification, problem solving, and role playing issues of moral conflict.

EGO IDENTITY

The task of adolescence is establishment of an ego identity, according to psychoanalyst Erik Erikson (Liebert et al., 1977). This is sought through role experimentation, which may include drug use, and is achieved with definition of a social role. Failure to find and commit to a role by the end of adolescence results in role confusion and identity diffusion. The highest rate of drug experimentation has been found in youths with identity diffusion (Jones & Hartmann, 1988).

SEPARATION–INDIVIDUATION

Child psychologist Peter Blos (1979) describes a second separation–individuation stage of development in which adolescents move toward autonomy by disengaging from emotional dependence on internalized, infantile parental ties. In rejecting dependence on internalized parental objects, it is theorized that the adolescent must regress to rework earlier conflict (Blos, 1979). Characteristics of this process include a return to "action language" (Blos, 1979, p. 155), the search for new love objects outside the family, and mourning the loss of parental ties (Davis, 1985). As a separate identity is reconstructed, some parental values are retained, and others discarded in what Blos calls "selective overhaul" (Blos 1979, p. 180). Alternate life-styles, including drugs, may be used to demonstrate separateness. Drugs also may be used to act out the conflict between emancipation from parental control and a desire to remain attached by rejecting parental standards while creating dependency.

In the first separation at 18 to 36 months of age, the child learns to tolerate physical separateness from the mother by internalizing her image and self-soothing functions. Failure of this developmental task, leaves children depressed, angry, and deficient in internalized ego functions such as frustration, tolerance, impulse control, and affect regulation (Masterson, 1988). Adolescents with ego weakness experience the second separation–individuation as intensely anxiety-producing.

Khantzian (1977) suggests that drugs are used to cope with painful affects in the absence of internalized defenses. Grandiosity (brashness, exhibitionism, entitlement) also may serve this defensive purpose, a dynamic recognized by the nursing diagnosis Defensive Coping. Treatment goals for these adolescents include the following:

- Promoting internalization of ego functions to support separation
- Promoting insight into the role of alcohol and drugs as interfering with this process

Limit setting and consistency provide an external source of control. A supportive, empathetic milieu environment helps the adolescent internalize control. Recognizing feeling states (or alexithymia) and making the connection between feelings and drug use is difficult for those who are chemically dependent (Gabbard, 1990). Helping them identify and tolerate unpleasant feelings enables substituting verbalization for acting out (Gabbard, 1990).

Progression of Drug Use

THE GATEWAY DRUGS

Studies have consistently shown that progression of adolescent drug use follows sequential stages (Kandel, 1975). Alcohol and cigarettes act as "gateways" to use of drugs farther along in the sequence. However, progression through the stages is not inevitable. Many adolescents discontinue use at a particular stage (Kandel, 1975). The sequence starts with use of beer or wine (stage I), followed by tobacco or hard liquor (stage II). Marijuana (stage III) is a crucial step between legal and other illegal drug use (stage IV), greatly increasing the risk of progression (Kandel, 1975). The probability is very small that an adolescent will use drugs, such as LSD or heroin, without first using marijuana (Kandell, 1975).

Nursing Process

ASSESSMENT

Goals of substance abuse assessment include the following:

- Identifying the level of substance abuse involvement
- Motivating the child or adolescent toward treatment
- Matching the child's or adolescent's needs to appropriate treatment levels and modalities

Assessment also provides a basis for the initial nursing diagnosis. The assessment interview can motivate the desire for treatment by promoting insight and presenting options. Choice of treatment level includes outpatient counseling, school- or community-based programs, or residential treatment. Treatment modalities include adjunctive psychotherapy, family therapy, medical evaluation or treatment, personal and social skills training, and special academic or vocational services. Areas of evaluation include the following:

1. The level of substance use involvement
   The stage of progression in drug use
   The stage of progression from experimentation to dependence
2. Physical assessment
   Signs of intoxication, withdrawal, adverse physical effects
3. Psychological assessment
   Reality orientation
   Defenses, ego deficits, and strengths
   Level of moral and cognitive development, ego identity, issues of separation–individuation or enmeshment
   Potential for violence
   Concurrent problems (depression, conduct problems, hyperactivity, eating disorders, learning problems)
4. Biologic risk factors
   Family history of substance abuse
   Family history of associated disorders (antisocial behavior, AD/HD, depression)
5. Psychosocial risk factors
   Personal, peer, and family risk factors, codependency issues, physical or sexual abuse
6. Contributing or precipitating stressors
   Losses
   Legal problems
7. Protective factors
   Personal strengths and support systems

Treatment

OUTCOME

There is not a great deal of information about treatment outcome for adolescent substance abuse, but favorable outcome has been found in association with being female, having few legal problems and few neurologic risk factors, and having assets such as a higher verbal IQ and more emotional health than adolescents with a less positive treatment result (Knapp et al., 1991). The CATOR study of adolescent substance abuse treatment completers showed post-treatment abstinence was associated with regular aftercare and self-help group attendance, parental Alanon attendance, (Hoffman, Streed, & Harrison, 1990;1991), and treatment completion (Harrison & Hoffman, 1987)(Fig.22-3).

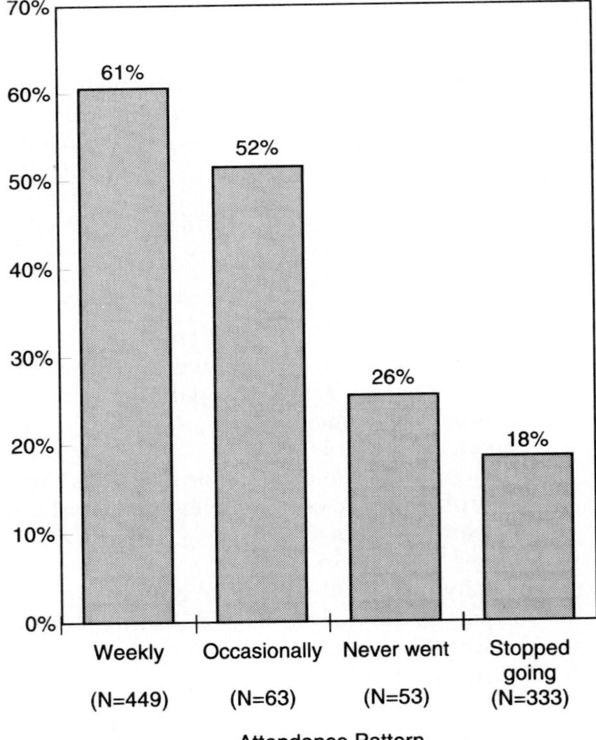

FIGURE 22–3 • One-year abstinence rates for support group attenders. (From Harrison, P. A., & Hoffman, N. G. [1989]. *CATOR report: Adolescent treatment completers one year later* [p. 51]. St. Paul, MN: The Ramsey Clinic. Reprinted by permission.)

TREATMENT PHASES

EARLY TREATMENT. Denial of substance abuse or that it is the cause of other problems in the adolescent's life is common in early treatment. One treatment goal is to enable honest evaluation of one's behavior by promoting recognition of those defenses, such as rationalization, projection, denial, and repression, that are in the way (Marlatt, 1985).

Assisting adolescents to associate substance abuse with resulting problems in their lives and challenging faulty logic promotes insight into defensive behavior. Group process is especially helpful in confronting denial.

SOCIAL SKILLS TRAINING. After the adolescent has identified substance abuse as a problem, he or she can begin to work on other maladaptive interpersonal patterns that contribute to vulnerability. Social skills training considers substance abuse a learned behavior that functions to achieve goals, such as popularity or stress reduction, that the adolescent is otherwise unable to achieve due to poor personal and social competence (Botvin & Wills, 1985). Skills deficits can lead to social rejection, which increases susceptibility to substance use. Mastery of social skills furthers the goal of internalizing control. Within the milieu, nurses can help children or adolescents apply new skills, including the following:

- Assertiveness
- Relaxation
- Problem solving
- Specific Refusal Skills
- Anger management
- Self-esteem building
- Stress management
- Values clarification

RELAPSE. Researchers have just begun to examine adolescent relapse. Fifty-seven percent of 924 adolescents in the CATOR study relapsed within 1 year after treatment, although 23% of those were brief relapses (Harrison & Hoffman, 1989). Factors predicting relapse included a history of multiple arrests, nonacceptance of the diagnosis of chemical dependency, and friends' use of drugs after treatment (Streed et al., 1990/1991). Peer influence on relapse is very strong. In one study, 60% of adolescent relapses involved direct social pressure, approximately one third of the relapses were triggered by attempts to cope with negative feelings, and close to 27% identified interpersonal conflict as a precursor (Brown, Vik, & Creamer, 1989).

Relapse begins with warning signs, including return of addictive thinking used to justify relapse, re-

CLINICAL EXAMPLE: JOE

Sixteen-year-old Joe was brought to the hospital by his parents for evaluation. They were concerned about his recent failing grades and escalating noncompliance at home. They said Joe had been well behaved until 8 months ago. Joe's mother was upset that he no longer spent time with his regular friends but instead hung out with a new group of 17- and 18-year-olds, some of whom had dropped out of school. Joe had been truant 21 days out of the last grading period. Assessment revealed that Joe had started drinking at age 14, shortly after a major family move. He had progressed from beer to hard liquor, which he had consumed daily for close to 1 year, usually drinking to intoxication. Joe reported two blackouts and two failed attempts to "cut down." He also had smoked marijuana three to five times weekly for the last 6 months. This began just after a breakup with his girlfriend. Joe acknowledged things sometimes got "out of hand," but maintained he could "handle it" if his parents would "just get off [his] back."

NURSING CARE PLAN

Nursing Diagnosis: Ineffective Denial related to fear of loss of substance use, evidenced by denial of negative consequences

Short-Term Goal: The adolescent will verbalize an understanding of the association between substance use and problems in his life, including impaired family relationships, failing grades, and truancy by ______ (date).

Long-Term Goal: The adolescent will identify defensive coping mechanisms and verbalize an understanding of how they function to enable substance use by discharge.

Discharge Criteria: The adolescent will verbalize an understanding of the defenses he uses to enable substance use and identify substance use as a problem.

Nursing Interventions: The nurse will:

1. Encourage the adolescent to explore the problems in his life and how they relate to substance use by writing a drug use autobiography and presenting it to his group by ______ (date).
2. Provide nonjudgmental feedback when forms of denial are demonstrated.
3. Provide education about defensive behavior, and give positive feedback when the adolescent demonstrates awareness of defensive avoidance.
4. Assist the adolescent to complete step one of AA in a program workbook.

Nursing Diagnosis: Powerlessness related to polysubstance abuse or dependence, evidenced by failed attempts at control

Short-Term Goal: The adolescent will verbalize feelings of powerlessness over ability to control substance use by ______ (date).

Long-Term Goal: The adolescent will verbalize acceptance of the need for treatment.

Discharge Criteria: The adolescent will verbalize responsibility for a plan to maintain abstinence.

Nursing Interventions: The nurse will:

1. Encourage the adolescent to explore feelings associated with loss of control and to ask for feedback from his group.
2. Assist the adolescent to complete steps one through three in a 12-step workbook, with presentations to his group starting ______ (date).
3. Assist the adolescent to explore options and develop a plan to increase his personal power (setting realistic goals, developing sobriety-based interests) by ______ (date).
4. Assist the adolescent to attend a youthful AA or NA group and obtain a sponsor by ______ (date).

Nursing Diagnosis: Ineffective Individual Coping related to inadequate coping skills, evidenced by psychoactive substance use following episodes of stress

Short-Term Goal: The adolescent will verbalize feelings associated with the family move and breakup with his girlfriend and understanding of how feelings relate to substance use by ______ (date).

Long-Term Goal: The adolescent will learn and demonstrate positive coping skills to replace substance use by discharge.

Discharge Criteria: The adolescent will verbalize acceptance of responsibility for a plan to maintain new ways to cope.

Nursing Interventions: The nurse will:

1. Assist the adolescent to express and label feelings of loss and stress and how they relate to substance use.
2. Assist the adolescent to use opportunities in the milieu to apply positive coping skills to deal with stress and loss and to develop a plan for ongoing maintenance (commitment to regular aftercare, daily moral inventory, directory of sources of support).

(continued)

CLINICAL EXAMPLE: JOE (*Continued*)

Nursing Diagnosis: Knowledge Deficit related to misconception and denial of information about the effects of drugs on mood, behavior, and physiology, evidenced by continued use despite negative consequences.

Short-Term Goals: The adolescent will verbalize understanding of the effects of drugs on the body and life process by ______ (date).

Long-Term Goals: The adolescent will develop a plan for life-style change by discharge. The adolescent will demonstrate knowledge of how drugs affect the body and commit to a plan for life-style change.

Nursing Interventions: The nurse will:

1. Provide the adolescent with factual information about the emotional, behavioral, and physiologic effects of drugs on the body in drug education classes three times weekly.
2. Provide the adolescent with information about the process of addiction and recovery in group sessions two times weekly.

Doenges, M. E., Townsend, M. C., & Moorhouse, M. F. (1989). *Psychiatric care plans: Guidelines for client care.* Philadelphia: F. A. Davis.

Townsend, M. C. (1991). *Nursing diagnosis in psychiatric nursing: A pocket guide for care plan construction* (2nd ed.). Philadelphia: F. A. Davis.

surgence of unmanageable feelings, and self-defeating behaviors (Gorski, 1990). In relapse prevention, adolescents identify their individual relapse warning signs and practice new coping responses.

Attending self-help groups, such as Alcoholics Anonymous (AA) or Narcotics Anonymous, helps maintain treatment gains. Adolescents should be introduced to these groups during treatment and begin working the 12 steps of AA, which provide a value system and framework for life-style change (see Clinical Example: Joe).

REFERENCES

American Psychiatric Association. (1994). *Diagnostic and statistical manual of mental disorders* (4th ed.). Washington, DC: Author.

Andrucci, G. L., Archer, R. P., Pancoast, D. L., & Gordon, R. A. (1989). The relationship of MMPI and sensation seeking scales to adolescent drug use. *Journal of Personality Assessment, 53*(2), 253–266.

Arria, A.M., Tarter, R.E., & VanThiel, D.H. (1991). The effects of alcohol abuse on the health of adolescents. *Alcohol Health and Research World, 15*(1), 52–57.

Barinaga, M. (1992). Pot, heroin unlock new areas of neuroscience. *Science, 258,* 1882–1884.

Bass, M. (1970). Sudden sniffing death. *Journal of the American Medical Association, 212*(12), 2075–2079.

Blos, P. (1979). *The adolescent passage: Development issues.* New York: International Universities Press.

Blum, K., Noble, E. P., Sheridan, P. J., Montgomery, A., Ritchie, T., Jagadeeswaran, P., Nogami, H., Briggs, A. H., & Cohn, J. B. (1990). Allelic association of human dopamine D_2 receptor gene in alcoholism. *Journal of the American Medical Association, 263*(15), 2055–2060.

Bohman, M., Sigvardsson, S., & Cloninger, C. R. (1981). Maternal inheritance of alcohol abuse. *Archives of General Psychiatry, 38,* 965–969.

Botvin, G. J., & Wills, T. A. (1985). Personal and social skills training: Cognitive-behavioral approaches to substance abuse prevention. In C. S. Bell & R. Battjes (Eds.), *Prevention research: Deterring drug abuse among children and adolescents* (pp. 8–49). Rockville, MD: National Institute on Drug Abuse Research Monograph 63.

Brown, S. A., Vik, P. W., & Creamer, V. A. (1989). Characteristics of relapse following adolescent substance abuse treatment. *Addictive Behaviors, 14,* 291–200.

Cadoret, R. J., Troughton, E., O'Gorman, T. W., & Haywood, E. (1986). An adoption study of genetic and environmental factors in drug abuse. *Archives of General Psychiatry, 43,* 1131–1136.

Cregler, L. L. (1989). Adverse health consequences of cocaine abuse. *Journal of the National Medical Association, 81*(1), 27–35.

Dackis, C. A., & Gold, M. S. (1988). Psychopharmacology of cocaine. *Psychiatric Annals, 18*(9), 528–530.

Davis, I. P. (1985). *Adolescents: Theoretical and helping perspectives.* Boston: Kluwer-Nljhoff Publishing.

Deneau, G., Yanagita, T., & Seevers, M. H. (1969). Self-administration of psychoactive substances by the monkey. *Psychopharmacologia* (Berl), *16,* 30–48.

Foy, A., March, S., & Drinkwater, V. (1988). Use of an objective clinical scale in the assessment and management of alcohol withdrawal in a large hospital. *Alcoholism: Clinical and Experimental Research, 12*(3), 360–364.

Gabbard, G. O. (1990). *Psychodynamic psychiatry in clinical practice.* Washington, DC: American Psychiatric Press.

Gardner, E. L., Lowinson, J. H. (1991). Marijuana's interaction with brain reward systems: Update 1991. *Pharmacology Biochemistry and Behavior, 40,* 571–580.

Gawin, F. H., Kleber, H. D. (1986). Abstinence symptomology and psychiatric diagnosis in cocaine abusers. *Archives of General Psychiatry, 43,* 107–113.

Gittleman, R., Mannuzza, S., Shenker, R., & Bonagura, N. (1985). Hyperactive boys almost grown up: I: Psychiatric status. *Archives of General Psychiatry, 42,* 937–947.

Gold, M.S. (1993). *Cocaine.* New York: Plenum Publishing Corp.

Goodwin, D. W. (1979). Alcoholism and heredity. *Archives of General Psychiatry, 36,* 57–61.

Goodwin, F. K. (1988). Alcoholism research: Delivery on the promise. *Public Health Reports, 103*(6), 569–574.

Gorski, T. T. (1990). The Cenaps model of relapse prevention: Basic principles and procedures. *Journal of Psychoactive Drugs, 22*(2), 125–133.

Harrison, P. A., & Hoffman, N. G. (1987). *CATOR 1987 report. Adolescent residential treatment: Intake and follow-up findings.* St. Paul, MN: Ramsey Clinic.

Harrison, P. A., & Hoffman, N. G. (1989). *CATOR report. Adolescent treatment completers one year later.* St. Paul, MN: Ramsey Clinic.

Harrison, P. A., Hoffman, N. G., & Edwall, G. E. (1989). Differential drug use patterns among sexually abused adolescent girls in treatment for chemical dependency. *International Journal of Addictions, 24*(6), 499–514.

Herkenham, M., Lynn, A. B., Little, M. D., Johnson, M. R., Melvin, L. S., de Costa, B. R., & Rice, K. C. (1990). Cannabinoid receptor localization in brain. *Proceedings of the National Academy of Sciences of the United States of America, 87*(5), 1932–1936.

Hoffman, N. G., Streed, S. G., & Harrison, P. A. (1990/1991). Adolescent treatment: Success rates soar when key elements are present. *Adolescent Counselor,* 19–21.

Hollister, L. E. (1984). Effects of hallucinogens in humans. In B. L. Jacobs (Ed.), *Hallucinogens: Neurochemical, behavioral, and clinical perspectives* (pp. 19–33)). New York: Raven Press.

Isner, J. M., Estes, III, N. A. M., Thompson, P. D., Costanzo-Nordin, M. R., Subramanian, R., Miller, G., Katsas, G., Sweeney, K., & Sturner, W. Q. (1986). Acute cardiac events temporally related to cocaine abuse. *The New England Journal of Medicine, 315*(23), 1438–1443.

Jaffee, J. H. (1989). Psychoactive substance use disorders: Drug dependence: Opioids, nonnarcotics, nicotine (tobacco), and caffeine. In H. I. Kaplan & B. J. Sadock (Eds.), *Comprehensive textbook of psychiatry* (Vol. 1) (5th ed.) (pp. 642–685). Baltimore: Williams & Wilkins.

Jaffee, J. H. (1990). Drug addiction and drug abuse. In A. G. Gilman, T. W. Rall, A. S. Nies, & P. Taylor (Eds.), *Goodman and Gilman's the pharmacological basis of therapeutics* (8th ed.) (pp. 522–573). New York: Pergamon Press.

Jaffee, J. H., & Martin, W. R. (1990). Opioid analgesics and antagonists. In A. G. Gilman, T. W. Rall, A. S. Nies, & P. Taylor (Eds.), *Goodman and Gilman's the pharmacological basis of therapeutics* (8th ed.) (pp. 485–522). New York: Pergamon Press.

Jessor, R., Chase, J. A., & Donovan, J. E. (1980). Psychosocial correlates of marijuana use and problem drinking in a national sample of adolescents. *American Journal of Public Health, 70*(6), 604–613.

Jessor, R., & Jessor, S. L. (1977). *Problem behavior and psychosocial development: A longitudinal study of youth.* New York: Academic Press.

Johnston, L. D., O'Malley, P. M., & Bachman, J. G. (1991). *Drug use among American high school seniors, college students, and young adults, 1975–1990, 1.* (DHHS Publication No. ADM 91-1813). Washington, DC: U.S. Government Printing Office.

Johnston, L. D., O'Malley, P. M., & Bachman , J. G. (1993). *National survey on drug use from the monitoring the future study, 1975-1992* (Vol.1). (NIH Publication No. ADM 93-3597) Washington, D.C.: U.S. Government Printing Office.

Jones, R. M., & Hartmann, B. R. (1988). Ego identity: Developmental differences and experimental substance use among adolescents. *Journal of Adolescence, 11,* 347–360.

Kaminer, Y. (1991). Adolescent substance abuse. In R. J. Frances & S. I. Miller (Eds.), *Clinical textbook of addictive disorders* (pp. 320–347). New York: The Guilford Press.

Kandel, D. (1975). Stages of adolescent involvement in drug use. *Science, 190*(Nov. 28), 912–914.

Kandel, D. B. (1978). Convergences in prospective longitudinal surveys of drug use in normal populations. In D. B. Kandel (Ed.), *Longitudinal research on drug use* (pp. 3–38). Washington, DC: Hemisphere-Wiley.

Kandel, D. B. (1982). Epidemiological and psychosocial perspectives on adolescent drug use. *Journal of the American Academy of Child Psychiatry, 21*(4), 328–347.

Kaplan, H. B. (1977). Increase in self-rejection and continuing/discontinued deviant response. *Journal of Youth and Adolescence, 6*(1), 77–87.

Kaplan, H. B. (1980). Self-esteem and self-derogation theory of drug abuse. In D. J. Lettieri, M. Sayers, & H. W. Pearson (Eds.), *Theories on drug abuse: Selected contemporary perspectives* (pp. 128–131). Rockville, MD: National Institute on Drug Abuse Research Monograph 30.

Khantzian, E. J. (1977). The ego, the self, and opiate addiction: Theoretical and treatment considerations. In J. D. Blaine & D. A. Julius (Eds.), *Psychodynamics of drug dependence* (pp. 101–117). Rockville, MD: National Institute on Drug Abuse Research Monograph 12.

Khantzian, E. J. (1985). The self medication hypothesis of addictive disorders: Focus on heroin and cocaine dependence. *American Journal of Psychiatry, 142*(11), 1259–1264.

King, M. D., Day, R. E., Oliver, J. S., Lush, M., & Watson, J. M. (1981). Solvent encephalopathy. *British Medical Journal, 283,* 663–664.

Kinney, J., & Severinghaus, J. (1991). Overview of medical management. In J. Kinney (Ed.), *Clinical manual of substance abuse* (pp. 91–112). St. Louis: Mosby-Year Book.

Knapp, J. E., Templer, D. I., Cannon, W. G., & Dobson, S. (1991). Variables associated with success in an adolescent drug treatment program. *Adolescence, 26*(102), 305–317.

Kraus, J. (1981). Juvenile drug abuse and delinquency: Some differential associations. *British Journal of Psychiatry, 139,* 422–429.

Liebert, R. M., Poulos, R. W., & Marmor, G. S. (1977). *Developmental psychology* (2nd ed.). Englewood Cliffs, NJ: Prentice-Hall.

Loney, J. (1988). Substance abuse in adolescents: Diagnostic issues derived from studies of attention deficit disorder with hyperactivity. In E. R. Rahdert & J. Grabowski (Eds.), *Adolescent drug abuse: Analysis of treatment research* (pp. 19–26). Rockville, MD: National Institute on Drug Abuse Research Monograph 77.

Macdonald, D. I. (1989). *Drugs, drinking, and adolescents* (2nd ed.). Chicago: Year Book Medical Publishers.

Marlatt, G. A. (1985). Cognitive assessment and intervention procedures for relapse prevention. In G. A. Marlatt & J. R. Gordon (Eds.), *Relapse prevention* (pp. 201–279). New York: The Guilford Press.

Marx, J. (1990). Marijuana receptor gene cloned. *Science, 249*(Aug. 10), 624–649.

Masterson, J. F. (1988). *Search for the real self.* New York: The Free Press.

Mathias, R. (1992). Scientists clone gene essential to understanding cocaine addiction. *NIDA Notes, 7*(2), 2–4.

Maykut, M. O. (1984). *Health consequences of acute and chronic marijuana use.* New York: Pergamon Press.

McHugh, M. J. (1987). The abuse of volatile substances. *Pediatric Clinics of North America, 34*(2), 333–340.

McKenna, T., & Pickens, R. (1981). Alcoholic children of alcoholics. *Journal of Studies on Alcohol, 42*(11), 1021–1029.

Mirin, S. M., & Weiss, R. D. (1983). Substance abuse. In E. L. Bassuk, S. C. Schoonover, & A. J. Gelenberg (Eds.), *The practitioner's guide to psychoactive drugs* (2nd ed.) (pp. 221–291). New York: Plenum.

Morrell, V. (1993). Enzyme may blunt cocaine's action. *Science, 259,* 1828.

Murray, J. B. (1986). Marijuana's effects on human cognitive functions, psychomotor functions, and personality. *The Journal of General Psychology, 113*(1), 23–55.

Newcomb, M. D., Maddahian, E., & Bentler, P. M. (1986). Risk factors for drug use among adolescents: Concurrent and longitudinal analysis. *American Journal of Public Health, 76*(5), 525–531.

Nowinski, J. (1990). *Substance abuse in adolescents and young adults.* New York: W.W. Norton.

O'Brien, C. P., Childress, A. R., Arndt, I. O., McLellan, A. T., Woody, G. E., & Maany, I. (1988). Pharmacological and behavioral treatments of cocaine dependence: Controlled studies. *Journal of Clinical Psychiatry, 49*(2, Suppl.), 17–22.

Perry, T. A. (1989/1990). Glass and ice. *Adolescent Counselor, 18.*

Rall, T. W. (1990). Hypnotics and sedatives; ethanol. In A. G. Gilman, T. W. Rall, A. S. Nies, & P. Taylor (Eds.), *Goodman and Gilman's the pharmacological basis of therapeutics* (8th ed.) (pp. 345–382). New York: Pergamon Press.

Robins, L. N., & Przybeck, T. R. (1985). Age of onset of drug use as a factor in drug and other disorders. In C. L. Jones & R. J. Battjes (Eds.), *Etiology of drug abuse: Implications for prevention* (pp. 178–192). Rockville, MD: National Institute on Drug Abuse Research Monograph 56.

Schuckit, M. A. (1989). *Drug and alcohol abuse: A clinical guide to diagnosis and treatment* (3rd ed.). New York: Plenum.

Schwartz, R. H., Hoffman, N. G., & Jones, R. (1987). Behavioral, psychosocial, and academic correlates of marijuana usage in adolescence. *Clinical Pediatrics, 26*(5), 264–270.

Shedler, J., & Block, J. (1990). Adolescent drug use and psychological health. *American Psychologist, 45*(5), 612–628.

Smith, S. S., O'Hara, B. F., Persico, A. M., Gorelick, D. A., Newlin, D. B., Vlahvo, D., Solomon, L., Pickins, R., & Uhl, G. R. (1992). Genetic vulnerability to drug abuse. *Archives of General Psychology, 49*, 723–727.

Streed, S. G., Harrison, P. A., & Hoffman, N. G. (1990/1991). The bottom line: Medical care costs, arrests drop sharply after treatment. *Adolescent Counselor*, 22–25.

Tabakoff, B., Hoffman, P. L., & Petersen, R. C. (1990). Advances in neurochemistry: A leading edge of alcohol research. *Alcohol Health & Research World, 14*(2), 138–143.

Tarter, R. E., Hegedus, A. M., Goldstein, G., Shelly, C., & Alterman, A. I. (1984). Adolescent sons of alcoholics: Neuropsychological and personality characteristics. *Alcoholism: Clinical and Experimental Research, 8*, 216–222.

Turner, E., Ewing, J., Shilling, P., Smith, T. L., Irwin, M., Schuckit, M., & Kelsoe, J.R. (1992). Lack of association between an RFLP near the D_2 dopamine receptor gene and severe alcoholism. *Biological Psychiatry, 31*, 285–290.

U.S. Department of Health and Human Services. (1987). *The second triennial report to Congress: Drug abuse and drug abuse research* (DHHS Publication No. ADM 87-1486). Washington, DC: U.S. Government Printing Office.

U.S. Department of Health and Human Services (1991). *Drug abuse and drug abuse research: The third triennial report to Congress.* (DHHS Publication No. ADM 91-1704). Washington, DC: U.S. Govenment Printing Office.

Washton, A. M., & Gold, M. S. (1987). Recent trends in cocaine abuse: A view from the national hotline, "800-COCAINE." In B. Stimmel (Ed.), *Cocaine: Pharmacology, addiction, and therapy* (pp. 31–49). New York: The Haworth Press.

Weight, F. F. (1989). Inhibition by ethanol of NMDA-activated ion channels. *Alcohol Health & Research World, 13*(4), 352–354.

Whelan, G. (1992). Biological markers of alcoholism. *Australian and New Zealand Journal of Medicine, 22*, 209–213.

Windle, M. (1990). Temperament and personality attributes of children of alcoholics. In M. Windle & J. S. Searles (Eds.), *Children of alcoholics: Critical perspectives* (pp. 129–167). New York: The Guilford Press.

Wu, T. C., Tashkin, D. P., Djahed, B., & Rose, J. E. (1988). Pulmonary hazards of smoking marijuana as compared with tobacco. *The New England Journal of Medicine, 318*(6), 347–351.

Zucker, R. A., & Gomberg, E. (1986). Etiology of alcoholism reconsidered. *American Psychologist, 41*(7), 783–793.

Zuckerman, M., Ball, S., & Black, J. (1990). Influences of sensation seeking, gender, risk appraisal and situational motivation on smoking. *Addictive Behaviors, 15*, 209–220.

UNIT

V

Treatment Modalities

CHAPTER

23

Play Therapy

Deane L. Critchley

Therapists in the 1920s treating disturbed young children recognized that the child's method of communication and exploration of the world was through play. Thus, therapy became an effort at understanding the meaning of play as an expression of the child's troubles and problems. Psychoanalysts who pioneered play therapy tried to understand the unconscious meaning of play. In the early 1920s, Hug-Helmuth (1921) first used play as a therapeutic tool. During the same decade, Klein (1932) and Freud (1928) elaborated on the symbolic meanings and uses of play in a therapeutic relationship with a child.

Play is a medium for expressing feelings, exploring relationships, and attempting new solutions to ongoing problems. Play primarily offers a unique opportunity for developing a therapeutic relationship between therapist and child (Kanner, 1948). As the alliance with the therapist develops, the child is able to be less guarded about expressing feelings and is more free and open to new relationships and behaviors. Therapeutic play provides opportunities for the child to develop self-understanding, self-acceptance, and self-mastery (Oremland, 1988). Hidden and threatening content is spontaneously presented in the nonthreatening interpersonal atmosphere of the session.

Play therapy is used for diagnosis and treatment of childhood emotional and behavioral disorders. In this chapter, play is discussed in terms of its therapeutic purposes and goals unrelated to the practice setting. Play therapy methods and techniques are discussed with clinical illustrations. The stages in the therapeutic play relationship are discussed broadly, as are selected issues inherent in the work with parents. Finally, research on treatment outcome is highlighted.

History of Play Therapy

The focus of play therapy has broadened from the traditional psychoanalytic focus on the child's unconscious to include the child's conscious cognitions, observable behaviors, recent experiences, family interactions, and peer and social interactions. Play techniques for use with families were also developed (Critchley, 1982a; Scharff, 1989), in schools (Nickerson, 1973), in preschools (Brody, 1978), and in other community settings. Play therapists have used a variety of play materials, including board games, puppets (Irwin, 1985), art materials, music (Moreno, 1985), food (Raynor & Manderino, 1989), and computers (Johnson, 1984). They also have begun to use paraprofessionals and parents as direct agents of therapeutic change (Berlin & Critchley, 1982; Ginsberg, 1976).

Play therapists need to understand how play normally develops in children and how play behavior changes as the child develops. This chapter is based on certain assumptions. The first is that the reader will have some theoretical background in

Barbara Schoen Johnson: CHILD, ADOLESCENT AND FAMILY PSYCHIATRIC NURSING, © 1994 J.B. Lippincott Company

child development, psychodynamics, and psychopathology. There are extensive and excellent writings in these areas that cannot be covered here. Second, the author assumes that most clinicians beginning their work with children have had some experience with adult psychotherapy. Thus, general principles of psychotherapeutic techniques are not presented except as they relate specifically to the treatment of children. The appreciation of diverse cultural and socioeconomic factors and their important implications for effective clinical work cannot be overstated, and such knowledge by the reader is assumed.

Finally and most importantly, it is assumed that readers interested in psychotherapeutic work with children will receive ongoing education and clinical training in their work with child patients and their families to assist in learning the details and refinements of psychotherapeutic technique. Such supervised training is essential in the mastery of clinical work. No chapter or book can replace supervised experience; it can only complement it (Critchley, 1987).

This chapter introduces the novice child therapist to the world of children. Some of the major ideas the beginning worker needs to keep in mind are reviewed and there are suggestions about how to proceed in the phases of clinical work with children and families. The suggestions are supported whenever possible by principles and rationale so that the reader has some basis for judging their usefulness and applicability.

What Is Meant by Play?

No single, comprehensive definition of play exists. The most widely used definition is given by Erikson (1950). He describes play as an ego function that expresses the child's bodily and social processes as mediated through the self. Play is generally thought to be the antithesis of work: It is fun!

In the literature, certain elements are generally considered to typify play behavior. Play is pleasurable (Plant, 1979; Weisler & McCall, 1976). Play is inherently complete. It does not depend on external rewards or other people early in its development (Plant, 1979). Play behavior does not occur in novel or frightening situations (Piaget, 1962; Switsky, Haywood, & Isett, 1974).

Play may use fantasy during certain developmental stages. Both play and fantasy allow an emotional release that would not be permitted within the framework of existing reality and that modify reality and make it less threatening. Games with rules do not generally fit within the standard definition of play. In games there is some sense of an implied task or goal. Games are sometimes viewed as an intermediate phase between the spontaneous play of young children and the often overregulated play behavior of adults.

Berlin (1986) points out that the increased use of games in therapeutic work with children to some extent reflects a change in the types of children being seen in treatment. Increasingly, therapists are seeing children with serious psychopathology resulting from severe neglect or physical or sexual abuse. These children use little verbal communication. It is common to find that such children come from homes where talking with parents or among adults is unusual. The behavioral problems these young children experience are part of an orientation that emphasizes action rather than speech. Consequently, play therapy that uses games has become an increasingly important method of establishing therapeutic communication.

Play can serve many functions: It can help in learning basic skills and social skills, in exploring the environment, and in acquiring and imitating desired adult roles. Play can help the child relax, release excess energy, and master situations or conflicts and anxiety (Berlin & Critchley, 1989; Critchley, 1982b; Jack, 1987). The function of play is always secondary to its being fun and is something of which the child is usually unaware.

Purpose and Goals of Play Therapy

Goals and interventions used in play therapy need to be individualized according to the child's specific needs, conflict areas, and problem behaviors. There are, however, certain purposes for and goals of treatment that apply broadly to play therapy.

The overall purpose of play therapy is to help free the child of conflicts and resulting problem behaviors. Another purpose identified in recent years is to reduce the effects of early traumatic experiences, thus providing the child with an opportunity for more optimal growth and development. Specifically, conflict reduction and amelioration of serious childhood trauma, such as physical abuse, enhances the child's adaptability and flexibility in responding to life experiences.

Treatment goals include new learning about the self and the environment; helping the child and family develop new expectations, roles, and relationships; and helping the child develop more adaptive coping skills. Achieving these goals in play therapy requires intervention in multiple areas, depending on the child's strengths and areas of need. These areas include changes in the child's pathology, especially ego functioning; alterations in social adaptation and school functioning; and changes in the family's interaction patterns.

Stages of Play Therapy

Dividing play therapy into stages is arbitrary and rigid but necessary for didactic purposes.

INITIAL STAGE

In early play therapy sessions, the therapist often continues the assessment of the child's difficulties. Additional contact with parents, interactions with the child, and observations of the child's play help the therapist gather additional data about areas of strength and conflict and the specific factors that contribute to the child's difficulties (Critchley, 1979; 1992). The therapist uses all information obtained in determining treatment goals and the necessary direction that therapy should take to meet those goals.

In addition, the therapeutic relationship with the child and parents begins in this initial stage. Successful treatment depends on a good working relationship with the child in which he or she feels comfortable in talking and interacting with the therapist. Developing a collaborative relationship with the child and parents is seen as necessary by most therapists regardless of theoretical orientation.

Another important feature of this early treatment period is structuring the therapeutic process. The child becomes familiar with the setting and the length and frequency of sessions and learns about the limits that may be imposed on his or her behavior within the playroom.

Children are generally told that they can play with any of the materials and talk about anything they wish; they are encouraged to express themselves freely. Most therapists accept a wide range of behaviors from the child. However, certain behaviors are generally considered to be unacceptable and require intervention from the therapist. Most therapists agree that limits need to be set against hitting or other physically aggressive behavior toward the therapist or the child. Most therapists would not permit the child deliberately to destroy materials in the playroom. Other situations that might require limit setting could include the child insisting on multiple trips to the bathroom during sessions in the absence of a physical need or inappropriate demonstrations of physical affection. Setting limits may range from simple statements that certain behaviors are unacceptable to physical restraint in extreme cases, such as when a child attempts to physically harm himself or herself or the therapist.

Generally, few limits are needed and are invoked only as the situation requires. The therapist does not present a list of rules to the child at the beginning of therapy. Rather, as necessary, the therapist sets limits in such a way as to convey continued acceptance of the child while clarifying the unacceptability of certain behaviors.

Limit setting can be therapeutic by providing the child with a lesson in self-control, giving the child a sense of security, and reassuring the child that anxiety-provoking fantasies cannot be acted out (Ginott, 1964; Reisman, 1973). Limit setting is one example of why dividing therapy into stages is generally artificial. Although providing guidelines for acceptable behavior in therapy often occurs during the initial phase, it may be necessary and appropriate to set limits at any time during treatment.

MIDDLE STAGE

Resolving conflict and bringing about healthy personality change occurs throughout therapy but is most evident during the middle stage of treatment. Using the information obtained during assessment and the developing child–therapist relationship, the therapist works to effect positive changes. The treatment methods used depend on the orientation of the therapist and the nature of the child's problems. An analytically oriented therapist may interpret the child's play behaviors or verbalizations in an attempt to bring the child's unconscious conflicts into awareness to deal with them in an emotionally constructive way. On the other hand, a client-centered therapist may use a technique such as reflection of feelings to clarify the nature of the child's feelings, to emphasize that they can be understood, and thus help promote personal growth. The use of these and other techniques depends on the nature of the child–therapist interactions in any session and the therapist's view about what needs to be done to move the child toward specific treatment goals.

TERMINATION STAGE

During this period, several issues need to be considered. First, although the initial problems for which the child has entered therapy may have been resolved, other issues may have developed during the course of treatment that may require further treatment. The criteria used to judge the appropriateness for termination are primarily deciding whether the child's development has been facilitated and whether any serious developmental delays continue. Once the decision to terminate has been made, the therapist needs to explore how it can best be accomplished; for example, how many more sessions will be required to deal with the remaining issues? These issues include working through the child's and parents' feelings of separation and rejection.

After the therapist, parents, and child decide to terminate therapy, they also reach an agreement on the number of sessions before ending treatment. During this time separation issues are raised, future plans are made, and loose ends are resolved. This period permits the child to lessen his or her dependency on the therapist and to function more independently (West, 1987). It is often useful to schedule sessions at longer intervals to help decrease the child's reliance on the therapist and to make a final assessment about the need for further work and the appropriateness of termination. A significant part of termination is to make the child and parents aware that the therapist is available if unexpected problems arise later.

Some therapists will make an appointment for a specific follow-up visit to assess how the child and parents are doing some time after the end of treatment. Follow-up often is important for at least two reasons. First, it provides an opportunity for the child to discuss any problems that may have developed subsequent to treatment, so these can be explored. Second, follow-up information provides the therapist with data regarding the effectiveness of the child's treatment. Although information from the child and parents is subjective, it can provide useful clinical data.

The Process of Play Therapy

The actual process of therapy can be learned only through practice. Each therapy situation is a unique experience as the therapist and child live through each hour together. Process refers to those interpersonal interactions that occur during the course of the play therapy experience. The focus is on the movement within the relationship as a result of the interaction between therapist and child and the effort to understand the various aspects of interaction as they evolve. Change in a child as a result any specific hour may or may not occur. The changes that do occur may reflect developmental progression or regression and are a part of the process.

STAGES OF PROCESS

Some writers see the therapeutic process as moving through predictable stages. Moustakas (1955) stresses a parallel between normal emotional development in the early years of life within the family and the emotional growth seen in a therapeutic relationship. He identifies the following levels of the therapeutic process. Initially, he sees the child expressing generalized negative feelings throughout play. The child then moves to expressing ambivalent or hostile feelings and then to expressing direct negative feelings about parents, siblings, and others. At the next level, the child is able to express positive and negative feelings, although ambivalently, directed toward parents, siblings, and others. Finally, the child is able to express clear, distinct, and generally realistic feelings, both positive and negative, with positive feelings predominating in the play. Moustakas believes that the therapeutic relationship provided in play therapy gives the child opportunities to develop emotional maturity and to grow through the expression and exploration of the various levels of the emotional process.

Axline (1947) sees children undergoing a process similar to that described by Moustakas. She believes that when play therapy is successfully concluded, the child assumes responsibility for his or her own feelings and for expressing these feelings honestly and openly because these attitudes have been facilitated by a nonintrusive therapist.

Berlin (1986) describes the play therapy process with physically abused children as slowly developing some trust in the therapist; testing out the trust through play, such as building and destroying block houses; playing out anger and hate toward doll figures; and finally involving the therapist as a partner in war games and later in constructive play activities.

MANIFESTATIONS OF PROCESS

Anyone who has engaged in psychotherapeutic work with clients is undoubtedly familiar with the processes of resistance, transference, and countertransference. This chapter points out their unique aspects in work with children.

Resistance usually is thought of as an unconscious inhibition about expressing to others one's feelings and thoughts. These interferences with communication usually are the result of adults' repressive attitudes in the child's past life inhibiting free communication. Abused children lack a trust of adults, which is a conscious resistance to be overcome (Bow, 1988).

Resistance usually becomes apparent in the initial sessions. Children in general are more frightened and resistive to therapy than adults. There are a number of possible reasons for this. Children are less powerful than adults. The differences in size, strength, power, and knowledge stem from actual repeated experiences and provide the impetus to exaggerate the differences the child imagines. Children are to some degree afraid of their parents and other adults. Children's concepts of punishment and of parents and other adults in authority tend to be somewhat primitive, exaggerated, and frightening.

Children may be "magical" in their thinking. Chronologically the child is closer to or actually uses primary process thinking or prelogical reasoning. One needs to remember the lack of sophistication of the child. A child is brought up essentially with only one conceptual frame of reference, that of the parents. The child unquestionably believes that this is not only the true frame of reference (reality), but the only one.

Harter (1983) argues persuasively that the child's cognitive level has important implications for therapeutic work. Harter believes that interpretation is not useful with young children. She asserts that the preoperational child's cognitive style is one of association because the boundary between realism and fantasy is ambiguous for the child at this cognitive level. Inhelder and Piaget (1954) have described that preoperational children have not yet mastered the complexities of language and thus create their own system of symbols and signifiers, those found in make-believe play. Consequently, direct interpretations made by the therapist are not likely to be understood. The therapist's behavior and the developing relationship are thus more important than interpretation.

TRANSFERENCE AND COUNTERTRANSFERENCE ISSUES

Children are known to project on the therapist overtly and covertly the feelings, attitudes, and expectations they have experienced in their interactions with their parents (Brody, 1961; Markowitz, 1964). Transference reactions in children are in part altered because of the significance of the child's parents in their present life. However, conflicts experienced by the child are expressed in the transference. Children have no other way of feeling about and interacting with other adults than in the ways they have learned to feel and behave toward their parents.

Discussions of countertransference (i.e., the therapist's feelings and attitudes toward the child) are uncommon outside the area of child psychoanalysis. Factors that have been identified as contributing to countertransference in work with children include the child's unpredictable, narcissistic expressions of impulse; the tendency to act out unconscious material in treatment; and cultural factors (Critchley, 1991). Such behaviors sometimes result in the therapist experiencing anxiety that their own unresolved childhood feelings will emerge. Kabcenell (1974) postulates that the "naughty" child threatens the analyst's sense of competence and the ability to structure the analytic situation. Papers describing sexual countertransference feelings and thoughts in work with children are rare (Christ, 1973; Yandell, 1973).

The phenomena of fear and hate are rarely mentioned in the literature on countertransference in work with adults or children. Winnicott's (1949) classic paper on "Hate in the Countertransference" describes the hateful feelings that work with psychotic or antisocial patients can arouse and how the therapist needs to recognize the feelings provoked by the patient and use them constructively in the treatment process. Berlin (1987) describes how adults who work with sexually abused children must deal effectively and honestly with the children's ability to elicit hate in adults before they can benefit from any positive relationships.

Empathy is a powerful therapeutic tool in working with children. Ornstein (1976) describes how interpretations that reflect the therapist's empathy for the child (i.e., an emotional awareness of the child's frightening feelings, such as hate or violence) tends to reduce resistance and negative transference while encouraging positive transference. Empathy facilitates the child's more open involvement in play and verbal behaviors.

In addition to the specific transference–countertransference feelings identified previously, the therapist often has positive feelings, such as "rescue fantasies," that can be a major stumbling block in treatment (Critchley, 1991). Such feelings seem to be much more intense and frequent in work with children. These feelings and their intensity are natural in work with children and can be put to therapeutic use. If not understood, such feelings may seriously interfere with treatment (Berlin, Critchley, & Rossman, 1984).

Models of Play Therapy

All therapy models for children, other than the nondirective, use therapist behavior, selected play materials, or both to guide the child's expression of feelings or behavior. A number of therapy models have been designed specifically for dealing with particular problems. For example, Kuhli (1983) has developed a technique using two houses. The child is encouraged to express feelings to help him or her deal with the separation difficulties experienced during parental divorce or changes in placement. In general, directive therapies emphasize content or the relationship. That is, a focus on content uses play and play materials as a means of eliciting fantasies and the child's unconscious wishes. Here the content and the release of feeling are critical. A focus on the therapeutic relationship uses play, play materials, and structure to provide the child with familiar tools with which to relate to the therapist. Here, the actual content of the play assumes less importance than its use by the child in relating to the therapist as a nonthreatening, interested adult and promotes the child's psychological growth (Allen, 1934).

Clearly, all therapists introduce play materials that will stimulate productive content. Also, the therapist's reactions influence the child's use of the materials. However, for the sake of greater organization and clarity, the play therapy approaches described are discussed under the headings of content and relationship focus. The methods presented are only a few of the many available. The ones presented tend to be used widely or are significant examples of the category they represent (Schaefer, 1985).

CONTENT-FOCUSED PLAY THERAPY APPROACHES

PSYCHOANALYTIC. The most well-known and influential of the content-focused child treatment approaches are the psychoanalytic. The basic approach remains much the same as developed by Freud and Klein. Format and style have changed, but the approach changes the procedures not the basic principles or assumptions. The assumptions are that a nonintrusive adult or adults, will facilitate play that reflects unconscious conflicts that can then through the therapist's comments, interpretations, or behaviors become conscious. This is the essence of conflict reduction.

STRUCTURED PLAY THERAPY. This approach is based on Levy's release therapy (1939). The therapist selects materials believed to be relevant to the child's problems. Structured play therapy as developed by Hambridge (1955) sets up the specifics of the play situation to recreate the stressful events or anxiety-inducing situation and therefore reduces the child's stressful feelings.

THE MUTUAL STORY TELLING TECHNIQUE. Gardner (1971) developed a technique based on the traditional therapeutic practice of eliciting stories from children about their drawings, dolls, and other productions. The child is asked to make up a story with the therapist's help. The therapist may describe the characters or settings and ask the child to make up a story. The therapist begins the story, and the child continues creating plots and narrative. The therapist retells the story with alternative outcomes to present the child with healthier adaptations and outcomes. Kestenbaum (1985) discusses children's use of fantasy and imaginative play through story telling as a therapeutic technique in psychoanalytic-oriented play therapy.

RELATIONSHIP-FOCUSED PLAY THERAPY APPROACHES

NONDIRECTIVE PLAY THERAPY. This approach developed by Axline (1947) is based on the client-centered approach Rogers (1951). In nondirective play therapy, the therapist leaves the responsibility and direction of movement to the child. Nondirective or client-centered play therapists hold that the strengths for self-development are best activated by the child at his or her own pace and direction. The goal of nondirective therapy is the child's acceptance of himself or herself, which is considered a necessary ingredient for a feeling of self-worth. The therapist demonstrates acceptance of the child through responses showing empathic understanding. The therapist's role is to help the child feel free to express feelings and thoughts and to experience pleasure in that process, which facilitates a sense of responsibility for her or his own feelings and behaviors and eventually the ability to evaluate them for himself or herself.

THERAPLAY. Jernberg (1979) developed Theraplay based on the assumption that a deficiency in emotionally positive infantile sensory stimulation experiences can lead to later emotional problems. Such deficits could include parental failure to provide tactile or verbal and auditory stimulation for the child or the child's inability to process such stimulation. Without this early stimulation, the child fails to develop self-confidence and trust in others.

The techniques of Theraplay are designed to remediate the child's stimulation deficit; the therapist uses tickling, stroking, other physical contact, and prolonged eye contact. Jernberg (1979) has begun including the parents as therapists to strengthen the parent–child relationship through the stimulation activities.

BEHAVIORAL APPROACHES. These approaches are aimed primarily at specific problem behaviors, especially noncompliance (Forehand & King, 1977) and hyperactivity (Patterson, Jones, Whittier, & Wright, 1965). Reward and contingency methods are used to modify unacceptable behaviors. Parents may be brought into the playroom. Because the focus is on producing appropriate interpersonal responses, such as self-control, the goal of improving relationships is clear. When parents or therapists participate in the playroom with the child, they strive to model desirable behaviors for the child or to respond to the child in ways that interrupt inappropriate behavior patterns and reinforce positive responses (See Clinical Example: Jerry).

Child Group Play Therapy Approaches

As with many new approaches, group therapy with children developed out of the perceived limitations of other treatment approaches (Helmer & Laliberte, 1987). Individual psychotherapy did not provide children with peer experiences or prepare them to function more appropriately in groups. Initially, efforts were made to provide adjuncts to individual treatment that met these needs, such as activity clubs, scouting, and other activities. Such groups were not successful for children with problems in relating to their peers.

In 1943, Slavson first outlined the theory and clinical techniques of a treatment approach he called activity group therapy (AGT). The primary goal of AGT is to provide socialization experiences that were not possible in individual therapy and usually did not occur in traditional social experiences. Slavson's conceptual orientation is psychoanalytic. He believes that the therapeutic group environment needs to be permissive and noncontrolling because this affords children the opportunity to express their thoughts and feelings through play and action. Similar AGT structures were developed by Redl (1944), Axline (1947), and Ginott (1961). All AGT approaches stress ego development, but all have slightly different emphases. Schiffer (1969) modified the basic AGT approach for use with preschool and early school-age children.

Slavson (1943) noted that many children were too disturbed to function in the nondirective AGT model and believed they might better respond to a more structured and interpretation-focused group. This belief led to the development of activity–interview group psychotherapy (AIGP). This format is characterized by individual patient–therapist interpretative interactions and by group discussions and interpretation intended to facilitate resolution of the members' problems. Schiffer (1984) provides an excellent description of AGT and AIGP models.

Behavioral models of group psychotherapy developed in the 1960s as an alternative to psychodynamic and client-centered therapies (Rose, 1967). Behavioral proponents stressed the need to define and operationalize specific, measurable therapeutic goals. In the early 1970s, two major texts on behavioral group treatment appeared (Graziano, 1972; Rose, 1972). Behavioral group models have dealt with cognitive–developmental age differences (Weisselberger, 1977), the relationship between specific approaches and type of psychopathology (Plenk, 1978), the role of parents (Gaines, 1981), and length of treatment (Rhodes, 1973).

GROUP VERSUS INDIVIDUAL CHILD TREATMENT

Individual and group treatment cannot always be differentiated on the basis of goals. While each seeks to help the child resolve basic adjustment problems, group treatment has a primary socialization purpose in addition to other goals. The two approaches cannot be differentiated on the basis of theoretical framework because both types have been conceptualized using psychoanalytic, client-centered, and behavioral models. There is considerable overlap in the patient populations treated with group or individual psychotherapy. The therapist's role can be similar depending on theoretical orientation in terms of developing the therapeutic alliance, outlining goals, attending to the process, and dealing with termination issues.

Groups provide opportunities to develop a number of relationships; child–therapist, child–child, and the entire group–therapist in contrast to only the child–therapist relationship in individual therapy. Advocates of group psychotherapy believe these additional relationships have therapeutic value. Be-

CLINICAL EXAMPLE: JERRY

Jerry, age 5½ years, was brought in by his parents for a diagnostic evaluation because he had been a "terror" for the last 6 months. He repeatedly tried to hit his 11-month-old sister. His physical attacks on his mother and fighting with peers in kindergarten had intensified. He was expelled from kindergarten and, much of the day, was locked in his room to prevent attacks on his sister and mother. Jerry's father, an engineer, was often away from home. He could control Jerry, but their wrestling and rough horseplay, which both had enjoyed until a year ago, was not now possible because Jerry tried to bite and scratch his father, despite the spankings he received for such behavior.

Jerry's history indicated a normal pregnancy and birth. During the first 4½ years of life, Jerry was advanced in reaching physical and psychologic milestones. He was an affectionate, playful child who got along well with children in preschool. He loved for his mother to read to him at bedtime and recognized many words in his books. Because of his father's absences, he clung more to his mother.

He began at age 3½ to demand that he sleep in his parents' bed when his father was away, which he was not permitted to do. Jerry continued to seek to wrestle with his father and enjoyed their "hikes" in the woods. Jerry's mother had been quite concerned when, at age 3½ or 4, he began to show his penis to girls in preschool, but she had been reassured by the teacher that this was normal behavior. Jerry's assaultive behavior began a few months after the birth of his sister during a prolonged absence of his father from home.

In the playroom with his male therapist, Jerry looked with disdain at all the toys on the shelves and demanded to know why he was here. The therapist said he understood Jerry was very angry; he hit and hurt people so people didn't like him, and that probably meant he must be feeling pretty bad inside. Jerry snorted and aimed a kick at a large wooden truck. He was then told he could play with all the toys, but he could not break them or hurt himself or the therapist. With that statement, Jerry made a dash for the door saying, "I'm leaving." When the therapist held the door closed, Jerry stared intently at the therapist who guessed out loud that "Jerry might like to kick the therapist, but he'd better not try because he would be held so he could not move." After glaring at the therapist and calling him an "S.O.B.," Jerry walked away from the door and sat in the middle of the floor looking defiant. The therapist sat on the floor, put a couple of flexible dolls in a toy truck, and pushed it toward Jerry. Jerry looked indifferently at the truck. When one of the dolls fell out, the therapist exclaimed, "Boy, that one really fell on his head, I wonder if he got broken?" though Jerry did not reply, there was a slight smile on his lips. At the end of the hour, he quietly returned to his parents.

In the next hour, the doll family was available, leaning against the doll house. Jerry glanced at them and went to the dart game (the darts had no points but had rubber suction cups). While they played a game, the therapist commented that he would stand about 3 ft farther away from the target to make it a more equal game. Jerry accepted this and showed unusual dexterity with the darts and won three games quickly. The therapist cheered each good throw and moaned at his own bad shots, and Jerry began to smile and then chuckle. After five games, Jerry turned to a ring toss game. He and the therapist were evenly matched. The therapist continued his praise of good shots, which elicited pleased smiles from Jerry. At the end of the hour, he boasted to his mother that he beat the therapist at darts.

The therapist met with both parents and explained to them that Jerry was faced with the need to work out severe oedipal problems and acute sibling rivalry aggravated by his father's absences and his parents' failure to deal with his hostile behavior in a clear and consistent way. A 3- to 4-month period of once-a-week play therapy was suggested with parent sessions two times a month, to which the parents agreed.

Jerry, like other neurotic children, seemed to know why he was in the playroom. He came eagerly to the playroom. In the third session, after a brief game of darts, he turned to exploring the box containing toy soldiers, space men, and space monsters. He lined up the soldiers against the space monsters and, making appropriate noises, fought a fierce battle in which the soldiers were demolished. "No one can beat these space monsters. Nobody," he shrieked. "That space monster scares me," the therapist yelled back. The therapist then assembled a set of space soldiers, and both made battle noises as their armies fought. Jerry decided the space monsters won. For the next 3 weeks, battles were fought with Jerry and his space monsters killing the therapist's armies. In the fourth week, he appeared to respond to the therapist's previous repeated comments about how angry and ferocious those monsters were and how they must hate everybody and how nobody could like them. By finding a laser jet gun for the spacemen to use to destroy the monsters, he then took charge of the spacemen and had the therapist control the army of space monsters that Jerry's spacemen demolished.

(continued)

CLINICAL EXAMPLE: JERRY (*Continued*)

Gradually Jerry moved from the space creatures to the family in the house. Various family members were hurt or killed by a space monster. Jerry would not identify the family members. Once when the monster had hurled a female figure over the roof of the house, the therapist offered the ambulance to Jerry as a way of getting the woman to the hospital. At first Jerry refused it, but later would place whichever doll had been mauled by the monster into the ambulance. The ambulance always crashed into several cars and trucks driven by the therapist and barely made it to the hospital in time to save the doll. This play lasted 5 weeks.

The parents reported in their sessions that Jerry was much easier to live with and much less angry and hostile at home. They had in the meantime established a clear set of contingencies and rewards based on Jerry's behaviors. After a week of testing to see if his parents would be consistent, Jerry began to settle down. Jerry's mother and father had worked through the impact of the father's absences on her. The father worked out a temporary arrangement to be home for 3 months and then to fly in from his jobs each weekend.

In the next phase of therapy lasting 4 weeks, Jerry ran over the daddy doll and the baby doll repeatedly. The therapist helped verbalize Jerry's apparent gleeful feelings. The therapist would say, "You are bad. You deserve being run over." Jerry would smile. He made sure that each doll made its hazardous trip to the hospital to be saved. When he finally ran over the mommy doll, the therapist invited Jerry to become his assistant surgeon in the hospital to make her well. In the next 2 weeks, Jerry made himself the chief surgeon who took care of the mommy doll and made her well. The therapist's comments about how great a doctor Jerry had become pleased him. For several seeks, all the members of the doll family had accidents, including for the first time, the boy doll. Jerry as the surgeon always made them well, with much praise for his skill from the therapist.

Jerry lost interest in the doll family, found the puppets, and with the therapist enacting the parts of the mother and the giant, Jerry enacted the roll of Jack in *Jack and the Bean Stalk.* Jerry as Jack always brought the gold back to mother and eluded the giant with great shouts of glee. When asked where Jack's father was, he would say, "Oh, he's off somewhere." This play lasted 3 weeks.

During the last 2 weeks of therapy, Jerry would snuggle up to the therapist, wanting to be read to from Grimm's fairy tales. He also liked a book about dragons and their families. Sometimes he would draw a character from a story, especially the wolf in *Little Red Riding Hood* and how scared the wolf was when the hunter jumped out.

Jerry was seen for follow-up 6 weeks after treatment ended. He was doing well behaviorally both in kindergarten and at home. This example is a much condensed description of 6 months of treatment.

DISCUSSION

This case illustrates the complication of oedipal conflicts by acute sibling rivalry. These problems were compounded by the father's absences, which made him unavailable to help with discipline and to reduce Jerry's fantasies and fears about his father's death while he was away on trips.

The work with the parents centered around resolving the mother's anger at her husband for being away so much and not sharing her burdens. Some resolution occurred. The need for a behavioral program to help control Jerry's behavior at home was clear, and the parents were able to develop clear rules, rewards, and contingencies that gradually became effective.

In play therapy in the first hour, the therapist's firmness seemed to present an adult attitude Jerry was looking for, especially when coupled with statements that lessened his angry, hostile feelings. Being allowed to express aggression through the dart game and winning without retaliation by the therapist was reassuring. It led to playing out his anger and hatred about his family through the war games. He was then able to transfer his expressions of hostility to the doll family when the generalized violence and the destruction of the therapist's armies were permitted and answered with understanding of these feelings. Rescuing the family figures who were hurt was a necessary way of providing restitution for the hostile feelings Jerry now centered on family members. The hidden anger toward his mother was finally expressed and resolved. His fear that he would lose her love and that the baby would take his place was reduced as the therapist helped him to be the powerful surgeon who could cure (i.e., "make up" for) his hateful feelings. Secure in the relationship with the therapist, he could enact aggressive, oedipal stories like *Jack and the Bean Stalk* with great enjoyment.

cause optimal personality development requires successful integration into groups outside the immediate family, group therapy provides the child with a therapeutic social environment that functions as a preliminary to more traditional social experiences. It also helps resolve crippling rivalries.

Advocates of individual therapy assume that the child's problems need to be handled through individual treatment before adequate progress can be made toward group functioning or that the process of individual treatment occurs simultaneously with changes in the broader social milieu. Group advocates believe that group experiences have a profound effect on each individual's specific problems and that these problems begin to resolve within the context of the group, and the whole group begins to function more adaptively. Finally, a sense of social responsibility develops through cooperation and mutual respect. Group treatment often is more appealing to the child than individual treatment because there are many activities and experiences, and for some children, it is less emotionally threatening than individual therapy.

Determining Treatment Progress

Haworth (1964) and Swanson (1970) discuss criteria for identifying change during therapy, always taking into account the child's cognitive–developmental level. The three general areas suggested for assessment of change are related to changes in play activity and content, relationship to the therapist, and self-image and self-esteem.

Changes in play activity and content are noted in shifts from accidental, impersonal, and aggressive behaviors with dolls and toys to more purposeful and less aggressive play in which the child assumes responsibility for his or her actions. That is, a child is more likely to say, "I pushed the doll down," rather than "The doll fell down." Regressive play also is decreased. More constructive play occurs with less fantasy play. Attribution of good and bad qualities toward play figures occurs initially, then this same capacity is seen with family members. Verbal communication becomes more mature and frequent.

Changes in relationship to the therapist are seen with diminished resistance to or need for limit setting and with an increased ability to accept the end of the hour and to participate in putting things away. The child has less concern about other children seen by the therapist. In general, there is a more open relationship and a greater tendency to accept and enjoy the therapist's accepting and empathic comments.

Changes in the child's self-image are revealed by a greater interest in and acceptance of his or her sexual identity and a greater capacity for insight and self-evaluation. The child is able to compare earlier feelings or behaviors with current ones. The child demonstrates a more positive self-image and sense of self-worth.

One cannot be certain how much change is the result of the psychotherapy and how much is the result of the developmental process. The changes enumerated provide good clinical data about the child's progress and are generally useful in evaluating progress in treatment.

Working with Parents

An area that is discussed relatively little in the child psychotherapy literature is working with the child's parents. Children in treatment need the support of their parents to enhance their progress in treatment. Parental support permits the child to use the therapy experience most effectively.

Current social and cultural changes within American society have led to varied and significant changes in family life. Parenthood, which was previously taken for granted as a family responsibility, has changed greatly in today's society. Changing values and sex roles; high divorce rates; increasing number of single-parent, mostly female-headed, families; high family mobility; and fewer economic resources are contributing to massive and pervasive changes in family life. Guidelines for parents, once available through one's own heritage, extended family, friends, neighborhood, and community, are no longer as relevant or accessible in today's rapidly changing world.

It is a particularly difficult decision for parents to seek help for their child. Often they delay seeking help in the hope that the child's symptoms and suffering will simply disappear. Occasionally this happens, but frequently it does not, and the stigma of seeking treatment contributes to parental delay. Almost every parent makes the decision to seek help for their child with struggle and pain. Whether immediately apparent or not, such suffering will be present in almost every parent. It is important that the therapist not lose sight of the parents' pain and deal with their suffering with respect and tact.

The most common and the initial approach to working with parents falls under the rubric of parent guidance. This process assumes that the parents have relatively good ego functioning and identify with the goals of treatment. Parent guidance is basically supportive.

The literature on parent work describes a wide spectrum of issues as parent guidance. Sandler, Kennedy, and Tyson (1980) discuss general goals. They see parent guidance as a means of providing ongoing emotional and practical support to the parents that enhances their self-esteem and supports the child's treatment. Additionally, parent guidance needs to provide information about growth and development and help in child management. Discussions in the literature agree that parent guidance does not make use of interpretation and that the therapist deals with conscious and preconscious material.

Swanson (1970) identifies three major objectives in working with parents of children in treatment. These include maintaining an alliance with the family so that they will continue to support the child's treatment; obtaining information from parents about events in the life of the child and family; and working together with the parents to create or alter characteristics of the child's environment that contribute to the child's difficulties or hinder the child's emotional growth and development.

Chethik (1989) identifies similar objectives and identifies several other areas requiring work with the parents: general difficulties in either parent's life that interfere with the ability to effectively parent; differences in childrearing beliefs and techniques; and the stress of having a child in treatment (e.g., feelings of guilt, a sense of failure, rivalry or competition with the therapist).

In some situations, the work with the parents needs to go beyond guidance. When unconscious conflicts of the parents or between parent and child are major issues in the child's need for treatment or the parent displays major individual psychopathology, then the parent(s) requires treatment. Such treatment is best provided by a therapist other than the one treating the child.

Authors have described a need to deal with some of the unconscious aspects of the parent–child relationship. Writers who have discussed this type of work with parents include Fraiberg (1954), Levy (1937), Slavson (1952), and Szurek (1952). Chethik (1989) describes this level of work with parents as a process of ego-clarification and limited insight therapy. While the work focuses on treatment of the parent–child relationship, the work often results in change in other areas of the parent's life beyond the capacities for parenting. Current concerns about work with parents often center on abusive, neglecting parents who had little nurturance in their own childhood. Work with these parents must focus on helping them to feel cared about and supported. They can then, in time, give more to their child (See Clinical Example: Freddy).

Individual Child Therapy—Outcome Research

There are limited outcome studies on psychoanalytic and client-centered individual treatment of children, and these are of poor quality. A review of child psychotherapy research by Barrett, Hampe, and Miller (1978) reported only two psychoanalytic research studies (Heinieke, 1969; Heinieke & Strassman, 1975) and six client-centered studies; one examines process (Moustakas & Schlalock, 1955) and the rest, outcome (Bills, 1950a; 1950b; Cox, 1953; Dorfman, 1958; Seeman, Barry, & Ellinwood, 1964) during the last 30 years.

In general, the outcome studies have indicated small gains in the treatment groups over comparison groups. The methodology used in all of these studies had many flaws. There is clearly insufficient evidence provided by this small number of studies to support or reject the effectiveness of individual child psychotherapy. The continued use of these approaches indicates their practical value, and many case illustrations document their worth. There continues to be a need to provide greater empiric documentation of their value.

More research has evaluated the effectiveness of behavioral approaches to individual child treatment. Problem areas successfully treated with behavioral approaches include academic and school difficulties (Hallahan, Lloyd, Kauffman, & Loper, 1983; Lahey & Drabman, 1981), hyperactivity and attentional disorders (Barkley, 1983), conduct disorders and juvenile delinquency (Kazdin & Frame, 1983), social skills deficits (Bornstein, Bellack, & Herson, 1980; Siegel & Ridley-Johnson, 1985), problem behaviors of autistic and retarded children (Schreibman, Koegel, Charlop, & Egel, 1982), and somatic disorders (Siegel, 1983).

The amount and quality of research on the various behavioral approaches vary greatly. Some research has been through well-controlled experimental designs, while others have been single-case studies. Notably lacking are long-term follow-up studies of the behavioral treatment of childhood disorders.

A few comparative outcome studies have investigated the efficacy of behavioral and other approaches in the treatment of childhood disorders

CLINICAL EXAMPLE: FREDDY

At age 6, Freddy was an impulsively aggressive child who had had problems with peer relationships since beginning school. Other children and his teacher were overwhelmed at the intensity of his rages.

Freddy's parents had divorced when he was 3 years old. The divorce had been difficult for everyone. Freddy and his mother had an overly close relationship, and he felt responsible for "driving" his father away. Because the parents had joint custody, both in terms of physical custody and decision making, Freddy spent equal time with each parent. The therapist saw the parents separately as their mutual antagonism made joint meetings unproductive.

Much of the early work with the parents focused on the difficulties both parents were having disciplining Freddy. He often simply would not follow directions or comply with expectations. He would climb on the furniture, refuse to go to bed, and come for meals when he was ready. Both parents felt a need to give in to Freddy's wishes. His mother wondered if he were a "fragile" child, while his father tended to ignore Freddy's disruptive behavior. In examining the reasons for their reluctance to set limits with Freddy, both parents realized they felt extremely guilty at how the divorce had affected Freddy. They each felt they had caused Freddy a great deal of pain and anguish. Once they achieved this understanding, they became aware that the discipline problems at home were creating problems for Freddy at school. Both parents were then able to develop more effective discipline techniques. They were able not only to expect compliance from Freddy, but also to set up appropriate expectations for him, such as helping to fold his clothes and put them away, picking up his toys, and cleaning his room.

As each parent discussed the divorce, they revealed some of their mutual rage and bitterness that followed. The father disclosed how he hated to answer the telephone because his ex-wife frequently called to confront him with his failings and to make yet another demand. The mother expressed how the divorce and her ex-husband had treated her unjustly. She had supported her husband through graduate school, and they had an understanding that he would support her through her graduate work. Now, because of the divorce, this was not happening. In addition, she felt the burden of being a single parent fell more heavily on her because of her greater financial constraints. As the parents individually were able to express their bitterness and frustration with each other and felt that they were heard, they were then able to work together around issues involving Freddy.

During the first phase of the parental work, it was necessary to help the parents understand how Freddy's attachment to his parents had been affected by the divorce. A child of Freddy's age and developmental level would be experiencing increased affection for his mother and a need for closeness, while at the same time an intensified sense of competition and rivalry with his father.

When this information was shared with the parents, Freddy's mother raised a problem she had previously avoided. She described Freddy as seeking to kiss her on the lips and of "accidentally" touching her breasts. The therapist discussed all children's needs for physical affection and physical closeness and that this need can be expressed in sexualized behaviors if there is no close male figure to prohibit such behavior. The mother was able to use this information in formulating more appropriate expectations and limits about physical contact and self-care behaviors. For example, she let Freddy take his own bath because a boy his age needed the "privacy."

When Freddy's mother broke up with a boyfriend who had been living with them for approximately 1 year, Freddy was very upset for several weeks. The therapist explained to Freddy's mother that having the boyfriend in the home had helped Freddy control some of his wishes for excessive closeness with her. When his mother talked with Freddy about his reaction to her boyfriend's leaving, Freddy told her that it seemed as if he drives everyone away, his Daddy too. His mother was very direct in telling Freddy that the separations were from the adults' decisions, not Freddy's behavior.

Another issue that surfaced in the parental work was the identification of underlying issues when Freddy's aggressive behaviors intensified. After a period of relative calm, Freddy suddenly began repeatedly attacking several boys in his class. Freddy complained that the other boys started it; one of them cut his arm, and another "almost tore my arm off." When the therapist explored this behavior with the parents, it was revealed that Freddy's paternal grandfather had recently had emergency surgery for an embolism in his leg. Freddy became very anxious. With encouragement, Freddy's father talked with him about his grandfather. Freddy expressed anxiety about the possibility of his grandfather dying or having his leg cut off. Once Freddy's concerns were discussed realistically by his father, Freddy

(continued)

CLINICAL EXAMPLE: FREDDY *(Continued)*

visibly relaxed. It was as if Freddy feared that the violence inside him might affect his grandfather. He slept peacefully for the first time in a week, and his fighting in school disappeared.

DISCUSSION

This example illustrates a number of the characteristics in working with parents. One aspect is that of dealing with the problems of the parents as individuals that interfere with their effectiveness as parents. Freddy's parents were both relatively well-integrated people who were supportive of Freddy's treatment and who generally functioned well in other aspects of their lives. Their divorce, however, had left many residual scars that at times interfered with their parenting abilities. Both parents felt guilty about the impact of the divorce on Freddy and tried to make it up to him by minimizing his frustration and avoiding limit setting. Freddy's mother at times dealt with her own loneliness by intensifying her attachment to her son. When these patterns of behavior were brought to their attention, the parents responded effectively. Also, the opportunity for the parents to vent their feelings individually about their failed relationship permitted them to put the past in better perspective and to work together more effectively to meet Freddy's needs.

Another component of parent guidance is the need for the therapist to help the parents better understand the developmental process in relation to their child. A major issue with these parents was to help them understand how underlying oedipal dynamics were affected by the divorce. Understanding these dynamics helped both parents modify their physical interactions with Freddy in more age-appropriate ways.

The therapist also helped the parents understand some of the specific psychodynamics underlying Freddy's behavior. This is another aspect of parent work. Freddy was a counterphobic child in that when he became frightened, he often projected fears and "identified with the aggressor." This dynamic explained much of his aggressive behavior. There were many opportunities to help the parents understand that when Freddy became overly aggressive, he was often frightened. The therapist and parents could clearly trace Freddy's aggressiveness and worries about his arm to his grandfather's surgery. The parents' increasing ability in the course of Freddy's treatment to help him understand the "scary" roots of his aggressiveness enhanced the overall therapeutic process.

(De Leon & Mandell, 1966; Young & Turner, 1965). Comparative studies of pharmacotherapy and behavioral techniques in treating hyperactive children have shown behavioral approaches to be equally effective or superior in dealing with such problems as disruptive behavior and excessive activity levels (Christensen & Sprague, 1973)

Children's Group Therapy—Outcome Research

In the last 20 years, there have been numerous studies on group treatment with children. They range from comparisons of a single approach (Kelly & Matthews, 1971), to comparisons of multiple approaches (Randolph & Hardage, 1973), and behavioral models (Berry, Turone, & Hardt, 1980). Patient populations have ranged in age from 6 to 12 years, and the degree of psychopathology has varied from psychosis to mild adjustment problems. Most studies have dealt with mildly disturbed children and emphasized measuring the child's social and academic adjustment within the school setting (Berry et al., 1980).

The behavioral group models tend to have the more favorable outcome results (Abramowitz, 1976). This result may or may not be due to better study design. It does not imply that other group models are not effective because many of the nonbehavioral group studies were less methodologically sound.

Although there are many more outcome studies on group than on individual child therapy approaches, both areas reveal similar problems. The research is generally flawed in design or methodology and limited in scope. As a result, no definitive conclusions can be drawn about the effectiveness of either individual or group treatment with children. More controlled clinical research is necessary in both areas.

Summary

This chapter presents an overview of individual and group play therapy with children, the ways in which psychotherapy with children differs from that with adults, and the general and specific factors contributing to psychotherapeutic change.

The purpose and goals of play therapy are discussed, as are the stages and process of treatment. Play therapy models are described in terms of whether their focus was content or relationship and examples given. A clinical illustration of individual therapeutic treatment with a child is presented. Clinically important treatment issues, such as goal setting, limits, resistance, transference and countertransference, are described. The rationale for work with parents is presented, and a clinical illustration of such work is discussed. Studies on the effectiveness of individual and group play therapy with children are reviewed.

REFERENCES

Abramowitz, C. V. (1976). The effectiveness of group psychotherapy with children. *Archives of General Psychiatry, 33* 320–326.

Allen, F. (1934). Therapeutic work with children. *American Journal of Orthopsychiatry, 4*, 193–202.

Axline, V. (1947). *Play therapy: The inner dynamics of childhood.* Boston: Houghton Mifflin.

Barkley, R. A. (1983). Hyperactivity. In R. J. Morris & T. R. Kratochwill (Eds.), *The practice of child therapy.* New York: Pergamon.

Barrett, C. L., Hampe, E. I., & Miller, L. C. (1978). Research on child psychotherapy. In S. L. Garfield & A. E. Bergin (Eds.), *Handbook of psychotherapy and behavior change* (2nd ed.). New York: John Wiley & Sons.

Berlin, I. N. (1986). The use of competitive games in play therapy. In C. Schaefer & S. Reid (Eds.), *Home play: Therapeutic uses of childhood games.* New York: John Wiley & Sons.

Berlin, I. N. (1987). Some transference and countertransference issues in the playroom. *American Academy of Child and Adolescent Psychiatry, 26*, 101–107.

Berlin, I. N., & Critchley, D. L. (1982). The work of play for parents of schizophrenic children. *Child Psychiatry and Human Development, 13*, 111–119.

Berlin, I. N., & Critchley, D. L. (1989). The therapeutic use of play for mentally ill children and their parents. In C. Schaefer & J. Briesmeister (Eds.), *Handbook of parent training.* New York: John Wiley & Sons.

Berlin, I. N., Critchley, D. L., & Rossman, P. G. (1984). Current concepts in milieu treatment of seriously disturbed children and adolescents. In M. Shore & F. Mannino (Eds.), *Psychotherapy of children: Vol. I: Psychotherapy: Theory, research and practice* (pp. 118–131). Washington, D.C.: American Psychiatric Association.

Berry, K. K., Turone, R. J., & Hardt, P. (1980). Comparison of group therapy and behavioral modification with children. *Psychological Reports, 46*, 975–978.

Bills, R. E. (1950a). Nondirective play therapy with retarded readers. *Journal of Consulting Psychology, 14*, 140–149.

Bills, R. E. (1950b). Play therapy with well adjusted retarded readers. *Journal of Consulting Psychology, 14*, 246–249.

Bornstein, M. R., Bellack, A. S., & Hersen, M. (1980). Social skills training for highly aggressive children. *Behavior Modification, 4*, 173–186.

Bow, J. N. (1988). Treating resistant children. *Child and Adolescent Social Work Journal, 5*, 3–15.

Chethik, M. (1989). *Techniques of child therapy.* New York: The Guilford Press.

Christ, A. E. (1973). Sexual countertransference problems with a psychotic child. In S. A. Szurek & I. N. Berlin (Eds.), *Clinical studies in childhood psychoses.* New York: Brunner/Mazel.

Christensen, D. E., & Sprague, R. L. (1973). Reduction of hyperactive behavior by conditioning procedures alone and combined with methylphenidate (Ritalin). *Behavior Research and Therapy, 11*, 331–334.

Cox, P. N. (1953). Sociometric status and individual adjustment before and after play therapy. *Journal of Abnormal and Social Psychology, 48*, 354–356.

Critchley, D. L. (1979). Mental status examinations with children and adolescents: A developmental approach. *Nursing Clinics of North America, 14*, 429–441.

Critchley, D. L. (1982a). A developmental perspective for the treatment of families with young children. In I. Clements & D. Buchanan (Eds.), *Family therapy: A nursing perspective.* New York: John Wiley & Sons.

Critchley, D. L. (1982b). Therapeutic group work with abused preschool children. *Perspectives in Psychiatric Care, 20*, 79–85.

Critchley, D. L. (1987). Clinical supervision as a learning tool for the therapist in milieu settings. *Journal of Psychosocial Nursing and Mental Health Services, 25*, 18–22.

Critchley, D. L. (1991). Multicultural aspects of countertransference with children and adolescents in milieu settings. In R. L. Hendron & I. N. Berlin (Eds.), *Psychiatric inpatient care of children and adolescents* (pp. 207–220). New York: John Wiley & Sons.

Critchley, D. L. (1991). Nursing's contributions to a psychiatric inpatient treatment milieu for children and adolescents. In R. L. Hendron & I. N. Berlin (Eds.), *Psychiatric inpatient care of children and adolescents* (pp. 250–263). New York: John Wiley & Sons.

Critchley, D. L. (1992). Role of developmental theory in child and adolescent mental health assessment. In P. West & C. Evans (Eds.), *Psychiatric and mental health nursing care of children and adolescents.* Frederick, MD: Aspen.

De Leon, G., & Mandell, W. A. (1966). A comparison of conditioning and psychotherapy in the treatment of functional enuresis. *Journal of Clinical Psychology, 22*, 326–330.

Dorfman, E. (1958). Personality outcomes of client-centered child therapy. *Psychology Monographs, 73*, 3 Whole No. 456.

Erikson, E. (1950). *Childhood and society.* New York: W.W. Norton.

Forehand, R., & King, H. E. (1977). Noncompliant children: Effects of parent training on behavior and attitude change. *Behavior Modification, 1*, 93–108.

Fraiberg, S. (1954). Counseling for the parents of the very young child. *Social Casework, 35*, 47–57.

Freud, A. (1928). *Introduction to the technique of child analysis.* New York: Nervous and Mental Disease Publishing.

Gaines, T. (1981). Structured activity discussion group psychotherapy for latency-age children. *Psychotherapy: Theory, Research and Practice, 18*, 537–541.

Gardner, R. (1971). *Therapeutic communication with children: The mutual storytelling technique.* New York: Science House.

Ginott, H. G. (1961). *Group psychotherapies with children.* New York: McGraw-Hill.

Ginott, H. G. (1964). The theory and practice of "therapeutic intervention" in child treatment. In M. Haworth (Ed.), *Child psychotherapy.* New York: Basic Books.

Ginsberg, B. G. (1976). Parents as therapeutic agents: The usefulness of Filial therapy in a community mental health center. *American Journal of Community Psychology, 4*, 47–54.

Graziano, A. M. (1972). *Group behavior modification for children.* New York: Pergamon.

Hallahan, D. P., Lloyd, J. W., Kauffman, J. M., & Loper, A. B. (1983). Academic problems. In R. J. Morris & T. R. Kratochwill (Eds.), *The practice of child therapy.* New York: Pergamon.

Hambridge, G. (1955). Structured play therapy. *American Journal of Orthopsychiatry, 25*, 601–617.

Harter, S. (1983). Cognitive-developmental considerations in the conduct of play therapy. In C. E. Schaefer & K. J. O'Connor (Eds.), *Handbook of play therapy.* New York: John Wiley and Sons.

Haworth, M. (1964). *Child psychotherapy.* New York: Basic Books.

Heinieke, C. M. (1969). Frequency of psychotherapeutic sessions as a factor affecting outcome: Analysis of clinical ratings and test results. *Journal of Abnormal Psychology, 74*, 533–560.

Heinieke, C. M., & Strassman, L. H. (1975). Toward more effective research on child psychotherapy. *Journal of the American Academy of Child Psychiatry, 14*, 561–588.

Helmer, L. S., & Laliberte, M. (1987). Assessment groups for preschool children: A preventive program. *Archives of Psychiatric Nursing, 1*, 334–340.

Hug-Helmuth, H. (1921). On the technique of child analysis. *International Journal of Psychoanalysis, 2*, 287–305.

Inhelder, B., & Piaget, J. (1954). *The growth of logical thinking from childhood to adolescence.* New York: Basic Books.

Irwin, E. (1985). Puppets in therapy: An assessment procedure. *American Journal of Psychotherapy, 39*, 389–400.

Jack, L. W. (1987). Using play in psychiatric rehabilitation. *Journal of Psychosocial Nursing and Mental Health Services, 25*, 17–20.

Jernberg, A. M. (1979). *Theraplay.* San Francisco: Jossey-Bass.

Johnson, R. (1984). High tech play therapy. *Techniques, 1*, 128–133.

Kabcenell, R. (1974). On countertransference. *The Psychoanalytic Study of the Child, 29*, 22–33.

Kanner, L. (1948). *Child psychiatry.* Springfield, IL; Charles C. Thomas.

Kazdin, A. E., & Frame, C. (1983). Aggressive Behavior and conduct disorder. In R. J. Morris & T. R. Kratochwill (Eds.), *The practice of child therapy.* New York: Pergamon.

Kelly, E. W., & Matthews, D. B. (1971). Group counseling with discipline problem children at the elementary school level. *School Counseling, 18*, 273–278.

Kestenbaum, C. (1985). The creative process in child psychotherapy. *American Journal of Psychotherapy, 39*, 479–489.

Klein, M. (1932). *The psychoanalysis of children.* London: Hogarth Press.

Kuhli, L. (1983). The use of two houses in play therapy. In C. E. Schaefer & K. J. O'Connor (Eds.), *Handbook of play therapy.* New York: John Wiley & Sons.

Lahey, B. B., & Drabman, R. S. (1981). Behavior modification in the classroom. In W. E. Craighead, A. E. Kazdin, & M. J. Mahoney (Eds.), *Behavior modification: Principles and applications.* Boston: Houghton Mifflin.

Levy, D. M. (1937). Attitude therapy. *American Journal of Orthopsychiatry, 7*, 103–113.

Levy, D. M. (1939). Release therapy. *American Journal of Orthopsychiatry, 9*, 713–736.

Markowitz, J. (1964). The nature of the child's initial resistances to psychotherapy. In M. Haworth (Ed.), *Child psychotherapy.* New York: Basic Books.

Moreno, J. (1985). Music play therapy: An integrated approach. *Arts in Psychotherapy, 12*, 17–23.

Moustakas, C. (1955a). The frequency and intensity of negative attitudes expressed in play therapy. *Journal of Genetic Psychology, 86*, 301–325.

Moustakas, C., & Schlalock, H. B. (1955). An analysis of therapist-child interaction in play therapy. *Child Development, 26*, 143–157.

Nickerson, E. (1973). The application of play therapy to a school setting. *Psychology in the Schools, 10*, 362–365.

Oremland, E. K. (1988). Mastering developmental and critical experiences through play and other expressive behaviors in childhood. [Special issue] Play in health care settings. *Children's Health Care, 16*, 150–156.

Ornstein, A. (1976). Making contact with the inner world of the child: Toward a theory of psychoanalytic psychotherapy with children. *Comprehensive Psychiatry, 17*, 3–36.

Patterson, G., Jones, R., Whittier, J., & Wright, M. (1965). A behavior modification technique for the hyperactive child. *Behavioral Research and Therapy, 2*, 217–226.

Piaget, J. (1962). *Play, dreams and imitation in childhood.* New York: Norton.

Plant, E. (1979). Play and adaptation. *The Psychoanalytic Study of the Child, 34*, 217–232.

Plenk, A. M. (1978). Activity group therapy for emotionally disturbed preschool children. *Behavioral Disorders, 3*, 210–218.

Randolph, D. L., & Hardage, N. C. (1973). Behavioral consultation and group counseling with potential dropouts. *Elementary School Guidance Counseling, 7*, 204–209.

Rayner, C. M., & Manderino, M. A. (1989). "Color your life": An assessment and treatment strategy for children. *Journal of Child and Adolescent Psychiatric Mental Health Nursing, 2*, 48–51.

Redl, F. (1944). Diagnostic group work. *American Journal of Orthopsychiatry, 14*, 53–67.

Reisman, J. (1973). *Principles of psychotherapy with children.* New York: John Wiley & Sons.

Rhodes, S. L. (1973). Short-term groups of latency-age children in a school setting. *International Journal of group Psychotherapy, 23*, 204–216.

Rogers, C. E. (1951). *Client-centered therapy.* Boston: Houghton Mifflin.

Rose, S. D. (1967). A behavioral approach to group treatment of children. In E. J. Thomas (Ed.), *The sociobehavioral approach and applications to social work.* New York: Council on Social Work Education.

Rose, S. D. (1972). *Treating children in groups: A behavioral approach.* San Francisco: Jossey-Bass.

Sandler, J., Kennedy, H., & Tyson, R. (1980). *The technique of child psychoanalysis.* Cambridge, MA: Harvard University Press.

Schaefer, C. E. (1985). Play therapy. [Special issue] Children's play. *Early Child Development and Care, 19*, 95–108.

Scharff, J. S. (1989). Play with young children in family therapy: An extension of the therapist's holding capacity. [Special issue] Children in family therapy: Treatment and training. *Journal of Psychotherapy and the Family, 5*, 159–172.

Schiffer, M. (1969). *The therapeutic play group.* New York: Grune & Stratton.

Schiffer, M. (1984). *Children's group therapy: Methods and case histories.* New York: Free Press.

Schreibman, L., Koegel, R. L., Charlop, M. H., & Egel, A.

(1982). Autism and childhood schizophrenia. In A. B. Bellack, M. Hersen, & A. E. Kazdin (Eds.), *International handbook of behavior modification and therapy.* New York: Plenum.

Seeman, J., Barry, E., & Ellinwood, C. (1964). Interpersonal assessment of play therapy outcome. *Psychotherapy: Theory, Research and Practice, 1*, 64–66.

Siegel, L. J. (1983). Psychosomatic and psychophysiological disorders. In R. J. Morris & T. R. Kratochwill (Eds.), *The practice of child therapy.* New York: Pergamon.

Siegel, L. J., & Ridley-Johnson, R. (1985). Anxiety disorders of childhood and adolescence. In P. H. Bornstein & A. E. Kazdin (Eds.), *Handbook of clinical behavior therapy with children.* Homewood, IL: Dorsey.

Slavson, S. R. (1943). *An introduction to group therapy.* New York: The Commonwealth Fund.

Slavson, S. R. (1952). *Child psychotherapy.* New York: Columbia University Press.

Swanson, F. L. (1970). *Psychotherapists and children.* New York: Pitman Publishing.

Switsky, H., Haywood, H., & Isett, R. (1974). Exploration, curiosity and play in young children: Effects of stimulus complexity. *Developmental Psychology, 10*, 321–329.

Szurek, S. A. (1952). Some lessons from the efforts at psychotherapy with parents. *American Journal of Psychiatry, 109*, 296–302.

Weisler, A., & McCall, R. (1976). Exploration and play: Resume and redirection. *American Psychologist, 31*, 492–508.

Weisselberger, D. (1977). Developmental phases in activity-interview group psychotherapy with children. *Journal of Group Dynamics and Psychotherapy, 8*, 20–26.

West, J. (1987). Ending or beginning: A discussion of the theory and practice of termination procedures in play therapy. *Journal of Social Work Practice, 1*, 49–65.

Winnicott, D. (1949). Hate in the countertransference. *International Journal of Psychoanalysis, 30*, 69–77.

Yandell, W. (1973). Therapeutic problems related to the expression of sexual drives in children. In S. A. Szurek & I. N. Berlin (Eds.), *Clinical studies in childhood psychoses.* New York: Brunner/Mazel.

Young, G. C., & Turner, R. (1965). CNS stimulant drugs and conditioning treatment of nocturnal enuresis. *Behavior Research and Therapy, 3*, 93–101.

CHAPTER

24

Individual Therapy

Susan Mace Weeks

Child psychiatric and mental health nursing is a developing area of nursing specialization. It offers a broad practice domain with a multiplicity of theories providing vast opportunities for making a positive impact on clients. Nurses' challenge is to develop a societal view of our authority to practice within specialized areas. Individual therapy with children and adolescents provides nurses with the opportunity to establish an arena of practice within the domain of nursing (McBride, 1988).

Child and adolescent individual therapy is a therapeutic modality through which psychiatric and mental health nurses can use their skills and knowledge to produce positive changes within society. Such changes will be the proving ground for nurses to earn societal recognition of nursing's potential as a profession. Child and adolescent psychiatric and mental health nurses are being underused (Pothier, Norbeck, & Laliberte, 1985), particularly in the realm of individual therapy. It is, therefore, a challenge to increase our expertise and visibility in this role.

This chapter provides a historic overview and understanding of child and adolescent individual therapy, as well as knowledge in the application of the nursing process in the individual therapy setting. Specialized techniques, various client populations, and therapist qualities also are examined. Finally, recommendations for areas of future investigation and involvement are offered.

Historic Perspective

Individual therapy as a therapeutic modality evolved from 19th century techniques developed by Josef Breuer, Jean-Martin Charcot, and Sigmund Freud (Ford & Urban, 1963). The theories and techniques developed by these physicians were expanded and refined by numerous theorists, including Alfred Adler, J. L. Dollard, Karen Horney, Carl Jung, Neal Miller, Otto Rank, and Carl Rogers (Levin, 1978).

Because of the variety of viewpoints, it has been difficult to develop a systematic and controlled definition of individual therapy. However, therapists basically agree on the general characteristics of individual therapy. Individual therapy involves two people interacting in a confidential manner that assists the client to develop interpersonal intimacy with the therapist based on mutual trust and respect. When individual therapy is used with children and adolescents, the goals and techniques are modified to facilitate positive client outcomes. These modifications are discussed throughout this chapter.

Individual therapy within the realm of child and adolescent psychiatric and mental health nursing is structured around the nursing process. This structure provides a systematic and consistent method of moving the client toward desired goals. It also provides an objective manner of understanding an often subjective therapeutic modality.

Assessment

The initial stage of individual therapy is focused on obtaining a thorough and accurate assessment of the client's difficulties and desired outcomes. Using a structured assessment approach provides an essential foundation on which to construct a therapeutic interview relevant to the client's progress (Cline, 1979). The primary components of the assessment are the nursing history, interview, and interaction.

An accurate history directs future therapeutic interactions and functions as a helpful indicator of prognosis. The history, which is often obtained from the client's parent or guardian, should include demographic, medical, and psychosocial information. A review of developmental milestones provides essential clues to the etiology of the present difficulty. A behavioral questionnaire and educational and family information are necessary to complete the therapist's mental picture of the client's history (Cline, 1979). If the history is obtained in written form, it should be reviewed with the parent or guardian in a verbal interview.

The nurse may obtain further written data from the client (depending on age) through the use of incomplete sentences, structured questionnaires, and self-rating behavioral checklists. The client interview continues the data collection process. It is important to obtain the following information: growth and development; physical status; emotional status; cultural and socioeconomic background; activities of daily living; coping mechanisms; patterns of interaction; the client's perception of, and satisfaction with, his or her health status; the client's goals; and human and material resources (Stuart & Sundeen, 1979).

Family, school, and peer assessments are additional useful tools. The mental status examination for a child, such as the example developed by Sanchez (Johnson, 1989), provides a helpful and easy-to-use structure for assessing a child. During the assessment phase, the nurse therapist's focus should be problem identification, which will lead to the development of nursing diagnoses.

Nursing Diagnosis

A thorough assessment of the child or adolescent may yield areas of concern, which can be translated into nursing diagnoses. The statement of an accurate nursing diagnosis is fundamental to appropriate and successful intervention and is the determinant of future action.

The nursing assessment highlights areas of concern. Typical concerns obtained from a nursing assessment of a child include difficulty with attachment bonds, object relatedness, and separation–individuation. Concerns frequently elicited from a nursing assessment of an adolescent include difficulties with self-esteem, body image, identity formation, independence, sexuality, and social roles (Stuart & Sundeen, 1979). These areas of concern are then transposed into nursing diagnostic statements. Common nursing diagnoses may be found in Box 24-1.

Planning

After identifying nursing diagnoses, the nurse sets goals with the client and plans future intervention. Client involvement in the planning process helps to prevent noncompliance or sabotage and strengthens family support. When identifying goals and objectives, the nurse must address the affective realm and behavioral measures of progress. The planning stage also includes priority setting and outlining discharge criteria.

Intervention

Individual therapy with children and adolescents may seek to work through current difficulties, prevent problems, or rehabilitate following disorder or trauma. The desired focus of individual therapy derives from the nursing diagnoses.

The primary components of an effective therapeutic relationship are trust and motivation. The nurse therapist must demonstrate a consistent and reliable presence to the client. In addition, the nurse therapist determines whether the goal of the individual therapy is supportive, educational, or directed toward the integration of newly learned adaptive patterns.

Broad outcomes of therapeutic relationships include improved self-understanding, symptom reduction, development of a consistent sense of self, ability to use foresight and have fun, desire to be with others but able to be alone, and ability to make choices (Johnson, 1989). The nurse may pursue these outcomes by discussing the topics identified in the nursing assessment and by encouraging the client to address areas of concern not verbalized.

Nursing interventions strive to help the client

BOX 24–1 • NURSING DIAGNOSIS STATEMENTS

Nursing Diagnoses				Related Factors
Self-Care Deficit	→	Related to	→	Disturbed self-concept
Altered Thought Processes	→	Related to	→	Sensory-perceptual alterations
Altered Nutrition	→	Related to	→	Maturational crisis
Sleep Pattern Disturbance	→	Related to	→	Situational crisis
Impaired Verbal Communication	→	Related to	→	Social isolation
High risk for Violence	→	Related to	→	Fear
Impaired Impulse Control	→	Related to	→	Anxiety
Ineffective Individual or Family Coping	→	Related to	→	Inadequate support systems
Impaired Social Interaction	→	Related to	→	Withdrawal
Altered Growth and Development	→	Related to	→	Powerlessness
Knowledge Deficit	→	Related to	→	Neurlogic deficit

make important connections between behaviors and feelings, such as self-criticism and low self-esteem. Individual therapy seeks to help the child or adolescent differentiate between thoughts, feelings, and behaviors. The client is encouraged to express genuine emotions, and the nurse therapist unconditionally accepts the client and his or her feelings.

Transference and countertransference issues are inevitable in the course of individual therapy. Therefore, the nurse therapist must maintain a relationship with a clinical supervisor to ensure that the client is provided with optimal treatment.

Evaluation

It is difficult to define success in therapeutic relationships. The number of variables impacting the therapy are considerable, including the client, family, therapist, setting, and length of treatment. Few studies have attempted to define successful individual therapy with children and adolescents; those that have addressed this issue have focused on narrow characteristics (Oliver, Searight, & Lightfoot, 1988).

The nurse evaluates the effectiveness of individual therapy by comparing the client's current status to the previously identified affective and behavioral goals and discharge criteria. When the discharge criteria have been met, termination is appropriate. At times the nurse may reassess the client, set new goals, or alter existing goals.

The nurse therapist involves the client and family in the evaluation stage. Termination should be handled in a bridging manner, which allows the client and therapist to let go of the therapeutic relationship without eroding the therapeutic outcome (West, 1984).

Specialized Techniques Used in Individual Therapy

Individual therapy in its classic, historic form occurred in an outpatient setting and consisted primarily of verbal interaction. Today, however, nurse therapists have adapted individual therapy techniques to a variety of settings and populations to meet the needs of a wider range of clients. This section examines specialized techniques and adaptations of individual therapy used in various clinical settings and with various client populations.

Individual therapy with children and adolescents often is used in conjunction with inpatient hospitalization. As the most restrictive of treatment options, inpatient hospitalization is limited to client situations that are unresponsive to other forms of treatment. Mental health clients should always receive the least restrictive appropriate treatment option (Dalton, Muller, & Forman, 1989).

Today's health care environment is trying to find innovative methods to make inpatient and other

TABLE 24–1 Techniques Used in Individual Therapy with Children

Technique	Description	Reference
1. Analogy	Use of cartoon characters and animals for story creation	Baird, 1984
2. Elective brief therapy	For children and adolescents who have suffered loss	Turecki, 1982
3. "Color your life"	To help children progress from action to verbal expression	Raynor & Manderino, 1989
4. Psychoanalytic psychotherapy	Emphasis on the meaning of behavior in resolving internal conflicts	Sholevar, Burland, Frank, Etczaty, & Goldstein, 1989
5. Metaphor	For adolescents between the stages appropriate for play therapy and direct verbalization	Saari, 1986
6. Innovative technique for resistant children	Ventriloquist figures, family word association, magic tricks, balloon animal therapy	Bow, 1988
7. Story telling	To increase fantasy and imaginative play	Kestenbaum, 1985
8. Mutual story telling	Therapist offers a return story to introduce healthier options	Stirtzinger, 1983
9. Puppets	For use with hospitalized children	Alger, Linn, Beardslee, 1985
Puppetry	To increase reflection and verbalization; to distinguish fantasy from reality	Irwin, 1985
10. Symbolic communication	Music, art, and body movement to resolve grief issues	Segal, 1984
11. Movement therapy	To examine the relationship between physical manifestations and psychic representations	Weber, 1984
12. Bibliotherapy	To express feelings and gain insight	Cohen, 1987

Alger, I., Linn, S., & Beardslee, W. R. (1985). Puppetry as a therapeutic tool for hospitalized children. *Hospital and Community Psychiatry, 36*(2), 129–130.

Baird, F. (1984). The use of analogy in individual psychotherapy with young and pre-adolescents: "Superman, Bimbo and the big, grey wolf." *Journal of Adolescence, 7*(3), 285–293.

Bow, J. N. (1988). Treating resistant children. *Child and Adolescent Social Work Journal, 5*(1), 3–15.

Cohen, L. J. (1987). Bibliotherapy: Using literature to help children deal with difficult problems. *Journal of Psychosocial Nursing, 25*(10), 20–24.

Irwin, E. C. (1985). Puppets in therapy: An assessment procedure. *American Journal of Psychotherapy, 39*(3), 389–400.

Kestenbaum, C. J. (1985). The creative process in child psychotherapy. *American Journal of Psychotherapy, 39*(4), 479–489.

Raynor, C. M., & Manderino, M. A. (1989). "Color Your Life." An assessment and treatment strategy for children. *Journal of Child and Adolescent Psychiatric and Mental Health Nursing, 2*(2), 48–51.

Saari, C. (1986). The use of metaphor in therapeutic communication with young adolescents. *Child and Adolescent Social Work Journal, 3*(1), 15–25.

Segal, R. M. (1984). Helping children express grief through symbolic communication. *Social Casework, 65*(10), 590–599.

Sholevar, G. P., Burland, J. A., Frank, J. L., Etczaty, M., & Goldstein, J. (1989). Psychoanalytic treatment of children and adolescents. *Journal of the American Academy of Child and Adolescent Psychiatry, 28*(5), 685–690.

Stirtzinger, R. M. (1983). Story telling: A creative therapeutic technique. *Canadian Journal of Psychiatry, 28*(7), 561–565.

Turecki, S. (1982). Elective brief psychotherapy with children. *American Journal of Psychotherapy, 36*(4), 479–488.

Weber, I. (1984). Body boundaries and the developing self in movement therapy. *Pratt Institute of Creative Arts Therapy Review, 5,* 41–48.

TABLE 24–2 Target Issues for Specific Client Populations

Population	Therapeutic Targets	Reference
1. Children of divorce	Faulty interaction patterns	Oppawsky, 1988–1989
2. Head injured children	Behavioral changes	Hartman, 1987
3. Language and speech disordered children	Social interaction	Kotsopoulos & Boodoosingh, 1987
4. Suicidal children	Decreasing environmental stressors	Frances & Pfeffer, 1987
5. Sexually abused children	Separation or abandonment, denial and repression, regression, psychologic defenses	McDonough & Love, 1987; Damon, Todd, & MacFarland, 1987; Shapiro & Dominiak, 1990
6. Psychosomatic children	Sick role and family systems	Stark & Blum, 1986
7. Depressed children	Relationships versus withdrawal, anger, social support, introjection	Cytryn & McKnew, 1985; O'Connor, 1986
8. Adopted children	Attachment issues	Lyle, Coyle, & Mooney, 1983
9. Conduct disordered children	Modeling, behavioral therapy	Webster-Stratton, 1984
10. High-risk infants and toddlers	Attachment, separation, aggression	Phillips, 1982
11. Abused preschool children	Trust, object relations, separation or individuation	Critchley, 1982
12. Aphasic children	Depression, anxiety, communication	Pachalska, 1982
13. Autistic children	Object relations, separation or individuation	Tustin, 1988
14. Learning disabled children	Self-esteem, relationships	Golden, 1985
15. Eating disordered children	Depression, gender identity	Oehler & Burns, 1987

Critchley, F. L. (1982). Therapeutic group work with abused preschool children. *Perspectives in Psychiatric Care, 20*(2), 79–85.
Cytryn, L., & McKnew, D. H. (1985). Treatment issues in childhood depression. *Psychiatric Annals, 15*(6), 401–403.
Damon, L., Todd, J., & MacFarland, K. (1987). Treatment issues with sexually abused young children. *Child Welfare, 66*(2), 125–137.
Frances, A., & Pfeffer, C. R. (1987). Reducing environmental stress for a suicidal ten-year-old. *Hospital and Community Psychiatry, 38*(1), 22–24.
Golden, L. B. (1985). A critical case study of play therapy. *Journal of Child and Adolescent Psychotherapy, 2*(4), 286–290.
Hartman, S. (1987). Patterns of change in families following severe head injuries in children. *Australian and New Zealand Journal of Family Therapy, 8*(3), 125–130.
Kotsopoulos, A., & Boodoosingh, L. (1987). Language and speech disorders in children attending a day psychiatric programme. *British Journal of Disorders of Communication, 22*(3), 227–236.
Lyle, I., Coyle, N., & Mooney, S. (1983). Psychotherapy with children to be adopted: Two cases. *Residential Group Care and Treatment, 2*(1–2), 73–100.
McDonough, H., & Love, A. J. (1987). The challenge of sexual abuse: Protection and therapy in a child welfare setting. *Child Welfare, 66*(3), 225–235.
O'Connor, K. (1986). The interaction of hostile and depressive behaviors: A case study of a depressed boy. *Journal of Child and Adolescent Psychotherapy, 3*(2), 105–108.
Oehler, J. M., & Burns, M. J. (1987). Anorexia, bulemia, and sexuality: Case study of an adolescent inpatient group. *Archives of Psychiatric Nursing, 1*(3), 163–171.
Oppawsky, J. (1988–89). Family dysfunctional patterns during divorce: From the view of the children. *Journal of Divorce, 12*(2–3), 139–152.
Pachalska, M. K. (1982). Prevention of the state of social dependence of patients afflicted with aphasia. *American Journal of Social Psychiatry, 2*(3), 51–53.
Phillips, N. K. (1982). Intervention with high-risk infants and toddlers. *Social Casework, 63*(10), 586–592.
Shapiro, S., & Dominiak, G. (1990). Common psychological defenses seen in the treatment of sexually abused adolescents. *American Journal of Psychotherapy, 44*(1), 68–74.
Stark, T., & Blum, R. (1986). Psychosomatic illness in childhood and adolescence: Clinical considerations. *Clinical Pediatrics, 25*(11), 549–554.
Tustin, F. (1988). Psychotherapy with children who cannot play. *International Review of Psychoanalysis, 15*(1), 93–106.
Webster-Stratton, C. (1984). Randomized trial of two parent-training programs for families with conduct-disordered children. *Journal of Consulting and Clinical Psychology, 52*(4), 666–678.

treatments as effective as possible, such as focusing on short-term inpatient stays (Dalton, Bolding, Woods, & Daruna, 1987). One research study identified individual therapy as the most effective treatment modality used in an inpatient hospitalization (Loff, Trigg, & Cassels, 1987).

Parents and family may be involved in treating children and adolescents in individual therapy through parent counseling, therapy, and supportive and educational groups. Numerous studies support the use of family therapy in conjunction with individual therapy (Braverman, Hoffman, & Szkrumelak, 1984; Salin, 1985; Sider & Clements, 1982; Steinhauer & Tisdall, 1984).

Group, biologic, behavioral, and social therapeutic modalities are other effective therapies for the individual and family (Bromfield & Pfeifer, 1988; Fine, 1982). Some innovative inpatient units are encouraging the hospitalization of an entire family on the same multigenerational unit and have shown positive treatment results (Combrinck, Gursky, & Brendler, 1982).

Many innovative techniques have been researched and used in individual therapy with children and adolescents (Table 24-1).

Client Populations

Individual therapy is a broad technique that is effective with a variety of client populations. Regardless of the client's specialized characteristics or needs, the nursing process serves as the format through which the nurse therapist conducts individual therapy. However, the focus issues, interventions, and goals vary with different client populations. Table 24-2 highlights target therapeutic issues for various client populations.

Therapist Qualities

Numerous theorists have described desirable therapist qualities. Carl Rogers' ideas are applicable to the nurse therapist role in individual therapy with children and adolescents. In 1951 Rogers outlined the primary conditions necessary for a therapeutic relationship: empathy, respect, warmth, genuineness, self-disclosure, concreteness, confrontation, and immediacy of the relationship.

Other studies have concurred with Rogers' theory. For example, Mace (1986) demonstrated that empathy is a positive correlate to a nurse's commitment to his or her profession. Kahn (1987) found that appropriate therapeutic self-disclosure assists in decreasing client anxiety, providing support, modeling effective communication and responsibility, and confronting distortions of reality. The effective and appropriate use of a therapeutic self is vital in attaining positive outcomes in individual therapy with children and adolescents.

Future Perspectives

A number of recent studies have examined future action necessary to strengthen the role of psychiatric and mental health nursing in the care of children and adolescents. Areas requiring professional attention include federal policy, funding, research, classification, and recruitment (McBride, 1988; Murphy & Hoeffer, 1987; Pothier, 1988a; 1988b). Pursuit of these areas will enhance nursing's role and effectiveness in individual therapy with children and adolescents.

REFERENCES

Braverman, S., Hoffman, L., & Szkrumelak, N. (1984). Concomitant use of strategic and individual therapy in treating a family. *American Journal of Family Therapy, 12*(4), 29–38.

Bromfield, R., & Pfeifer, G. (1988). Combining group and individual psychotherapy: Impact on the individual treatment experience. *Journal of the American Academy of Child and Adolescent Psychiatry, 27*(2), 220–225.

Cline, F. W. (1979). *Understanding and treating the difficult child.* Evergreen, CO: Evergreen Consultants.

Combrinck, G. L., Gursky, E. J., & Brendler, J. (1982). Hospitalization of single-parent families of disturbed children. *Family Process, 21*(2), 141–152.

Dalton, R., Bolding, D. D., Woods, J., & Daruna, J. H. (1987). Short-term psychiatric hospitalization of children. *Hospital and Community Psychiatry, 38*(9), 973–976.

Dalton, R., Muller, B., & Forman, M. A. (1989). The psychiatric hospitalization of children: An overview. *Child Psychiatry and Human Development, 19*(4), 231–244.

Fine, P. (1982). Play and family therapy as care skills for child psychiatry: Some implications of Piaget's theory for integrations in training and practice. *Child Psychiatry and Human Development, 13*(2), 79–96.

Ford, D. H., & Urban, H. B. (1963). Systems of psychotherapy: A comparative study. New York: John Wiley & Sons.

Johnson, B. S., Ed. (1989). *Psychiatric mental health nursing: Adaptation and growth.* Philadelphia: J.B. Lippincott.

Kahn, E. E. (1987). The choice of therapist self-disclosure in psychotherapy groups: Contextual considerations. *Archives of Psychiatric Nursing, 1*(1), 62–67.

Levin, M. T. (1978). *Psychology: A biographical approach.* New York: McGraw-Hill.

Loff, C. D., Trigg, L. J., & Cassels, C. (1987). An evaluation of consumer satisfaction in a child psychiatric service: Viewpoints of patients and parents. *American Journal of Orthopsychiatry, 57*(1), 132–134.

Mace, S. L. (1986). *Empathy and commitment to nursing of*

baccalaureate nursing students. Unpublished Master's Thesis. Denton: Texas Woman's University.
McBride, A. B. (1988). Coming of age: Child psychiatric nursing. *Archives of Psychiatric Nursing, 2*(2), 57–64.
Murphy, S. A., & Hoeffer, B. (1987). The evolution of subspecialties in psychiatric and mental health nursing. *Archives of Psychiatric Nursing, 1*(3), 145–154.
Oliver, J. M., Searight, H. R., & Lightfoot, S. (1988). Client characteristics as determinants of intervention modality and therapy progress. *American Journal of Orthopsychiatry, 58*(4), 543–551.
Pothier, P. C. (1988a). Child mental health problems and policy. *Archives of Psychiatric Nursing, 2*(3), 165–169.
Pothier, P. C. (1988b). Graduate preparation in child and adolescent psychiatric and mental health nursing. *Archives of Psychiatric Nursing, 2*(3), 170–172.
Pothier, P. C., Norbeck, J. S., & Laliberte, M. (1985). Child psychiatric nursing: The gap between need and utilization. *Journal of Psychosocial Nursing and Mental Health Services, 32*(7), 18–23.
Salin, L. (1985). We're o.k., they're o.k. *Family Therapy Networker, 9*(4), 31–37.
Sider, R. C., & Clements, C. D. (1982). Family or individual therapy: The ethics of modality choice. *American Journal of Psychiatry, 139*(11), 1455–1459.
Steinhauer, P. D., & Tisdall, G. W. (1984). The integrated use of individual and family psychotherapy. *Canadian Journal of Psychiatry, 29*(2), 89–97.
Stuart, G. W., & Sundeen, S. J. (1979). *Principles and practice of psychiatric nursing.* St Louis: C.V. Mosby.
West, J. (1984). Ending or beginning? A discussion of the theory and practice of termination procedures in play therapy. *Journal of Social Work Practice, 1*(2), 49–65.

CHAPTER

25

Family Therapy

Doris S. Greiner and Alice S. Demi

Family therapy is more than a mode of treatment; it is a way of thinking. Philosophically, it differs greatly from an individual approach or a group approach. The aim of family therapy is to see the family from a comprehensive perspective. Because family therapy conceptualizes emotional and behavioral problems broadly, multiple ways of intervening are appropriate. Although not all emotional and behavioral problems require family therapy, many problems are best treated by family therapy. Even when family therapy is not specifically indicated, the approaches often are useful in augmenting other therapeutic modes.

Family therapy is an especially important treatment mode for families with children or adolescents. When family members' needs are not met, emotional and behavioral problems often develop. Any member of the family may exhibit these problems; however, it is most often the child or adolescent who signals the family distress through emotional or behavioral symptoms. Thus, the child's or adolescent's symptoms often provide the incentive for the family to seek therapy and subsequently to recognize and deal with the multiple aspects of the problem.

Furthermore, the family progresses through several developmental stages during the childrearing years. During these stages of family development, individual developmental needs and tasks often conflict with family developmental needs and tasks. The multiple changes and conflicting needs and tasks produce stress and result in family disequilibrium. Fortunately, this disequilibrium brings with it the potential for change and growth. During these periods of disequilibrium, family therapy is more likely to produce therapeutic changes in a shorter time than when the family is in a state of relative calm and equilibrium.

In this chapter a brief overview of the various family therapy approaches is presented. Bowen's family systems approach (Bowen 1976; 1978; Kerr & Bowen 1988) is described in detail and its application demonstrated. Differences between family-focused nursing practice and family therapy as practiced by nurses are discussed. Finally, some contemporary critiques of family therapy approaches are addressed.

OVERVIEW OF FAMILY THERAPY APPROACHES

Theoretical approaches to family therapy are diverse and often conflicting. Family therapists share many common assumptions about family structure and function; however, they also hold significantly different views on the nature and origin of family dysfunction and on treatment approaches. Many attempts have been made to sort the various therapies into specific categories, but none of these attempts provides discrete, mutually exclusive categories. Jones (1980) divided family therapy approaches into integrative, psychoanalytic, multigenerational, structural, interactional, social network, and behavioral. Gurman and Knisern (1981) divided the approaches into psychoanalytic, intergenerational, systems, and behavioral approaches. Goldenberg and Goldenberg (1985) divided the approaches into psychodynamic, experiential–humanistic, Bowenian, structural, communication, and behavioral.

The approach used by Goldenberg and Goldenberg (1985) provides a conceptually clear method of classifying the various theories based on seven variables: time frame (past or present), role of the unconscious, emphasis on insight or action, role of the therapist, unit of analysis, theoretical underpinnings, and the goal of therapy. Because of its clarity, this classification approach is used to present an overview of the major theoretical perspectives (Table 25-1).

Psychodynamic Approach

The major theoretical foundation for psychodynamic family therapy is psychoanalysis. Major interest is placed on the individual, with emphasis on how the family members feel about each other and how they deal with each other. The therapist functions in a neutral role and makes interpretations of individual and family behaviors. The goals of treatment are insight, increased ego functioning, more satisfactory object relations, increased psychologic maturity, and reduced interlocking pathologies. The focus in therapy is on the past, and interventions are designed to explore early experiences. Unconscious processes are of major interest, because it is assumed that repressed material results in unresolved conflicts in the present. Increased insight results in greater understanding, resolution or reduction of conflict, intrapsychic change, and increased interpersonal competency. Some of the theorists and clinicians using this approach are Ackerman, Bell, Boszormenyi-Nagy, Framo, and Skynner.

Experiential–Humanistic Approach

The theoretical foundations for experiential–humanistic family therapy are existentialism, humanistic psychology, and phenomenology. The target of interest is the dyad and the problems that occur between the members of the dyad. The therapist assumes an active role and functions as facilitator of growth. The goals of treatment are growth, more satisfactory interaction patterns, clearer communication, and greater self-actualization. The focus in therapy is on the present; data are obtained from observation of the family members in the therapy sessions. Unconscious motivation is considered unimportant, whereas free choice and self-determination are of primary importance. Increased self-awareness leads to free choice, responsibility, and change. Theorists and clinicians using this approach include Kempler, Satir, and Whitaker.

Structural Approach

The theoretical bases for structural family therapy are structural family theory and systems theory. The target of therapy is the family's current organization and alignments; thus, coalitions, boundaries, and power are analyzed. The goal of treatment is to change family organization and structure by changing relationships. The role of the therapist is to manipulate family structure and thus change dysfunctional interactional patterns.

Family and systems theories propose that earlier transactional patterns are carried over into current family structure; therefore, treatment focuses on present and past. Therapy is based on the assumptions that action precedes understanding and that change in interaction patterns is more important than insight. Learned habits and roles are more significant causes of family problems than unconscious processes. Minuchin is the major theorist using this approach.

Communication Approach

The theoretical bases for family communication therapy are communication theory, systems theory, and behaviorism. The targets of therapy are dyads and triads. Faulty interpersonal communication between two or more family members is hypothesized as the cause of family problems and symptoms.

The therapist takes a very active role in therapy, is problem-focused, prescriptive, manipulative, and often uses paradoxic interventions. The goal of treatment is to change dysfunctional behaviors between family members and consequently, to reduce or eliminate the problems and symptoms. The focus of therapy is on the present, because the assumption is that the problems or symptoms

(text continues on page 362)

TABLE 25–1 A Comparison of Six Theoretical Viewpoints in Family Therapy

Dimension	Psychodynamic	Experiential/ Humanistic	Bowenian	Structural	Communication/ Strategic	Behavioral
Major time frame	Past; history of early experiences needs to be uncovered.	Present; here-and-now data from immediate experience observed.	Primarily the present, although attention is also paid to one's family of origin.	Present and past; family's current structure is carried over from earlier transactional patterns.	Present; current problems or symptoms are maintained by ongoing, repetitive sequences between people.	Present; focus on interpersonal environments that maintain and perpetuate current behavior patterns.
Role of unconscious processes	Unresolved conflicts from the past, largely out of the person's awareness, continue to attach themselves to current objects and situations.	Free choice and conscious self-determination are more important than unconscious motivation.	Earlier concepts suggested unconscious conflicts, although now recast in interactive terms.	Unconscious motivation is less important than repetition of learned habits and role assignments by which the family carries out its tasks.	Family rules, homeostatic balance, and feedback loops determine behavior, not unconscious processes.	Problematic behavior is learned and maintained by its consequences; unconscious processes are rejected as too inferential and unquantifiable.
Insight versus action	Insight leads to understanding, conflict reduction, and ultimately intrapsychic and interpersonal change.	Self-awareness of one's immediate existence leads to choice, responsibility, and change.	Rational processes are used to gain self-awareness into current relationships, as well as intergenerational experiences.	Action precedes understanding; change in transactional patterns are more important than insight in producing new behaviors.	Action-oriented; behavior change and symptom reduction are brought about through directives rather than interpretations.	Actions prescribed to modify specific behavior patterns.
Role of therapist	Neutral; makes interpretations of individual and family behavior patterns.	Active facilitator of potential for growth; provides family with new experiences.	Direct but nonconfrontational; detriangulated from family fusion.	Stage director; manipulates family structure to change dysfunctional sets.	Active; manipulative; problem-focused; prescriptive, paradoxic.	Directive; teacher, trainer, or model of desired behavior; contract negotiator.

Unit of study	Focus on individual; emphasis on how family members feel about one another and deal with each other.	Dyad; problems arise from interaction between two members (for example, husband and wife).	Entire family over several generations; may work with one dyad (or one partner) for a period of time.	Triads; coalitions, subsystems, boundaries, power.	Dyads and triads; problems and symptoms viewed as interpersonal communications between two or more family members.	Dyads; effect of one person's behavior on another; linear view of causality.
Major theoretical underpinnings	Psychoanalysis.	Existentialism; humanistic psychology; phenomenology.	Family systems theory.	Structural family theory; systems.	Communication theory; systems, behaviorism.	Behaviorism; social learning theory.
Goals of treatment	Insight, psycho-sexual maturity, strengthening of ego functioning; reduction in interlocking pathologies; more satisfying object relations.	Growth, more fulfilling interaction patterns; clearer communication; expanded awareness; authenticity.	Maximization of self-differentiation for each family member.	Change in relationship context to restructure family organization and change dysfunctional transactional patterns.	Change dysfunctional, redundant behavioral sequences ("games") between family members to eliminate presenting problem or symptom.	Change in behavioral consequences between people to eliminate maladaptive or problematic behavior.
Major theorists or practitioners	Ackerman, Framo, Boszormenyi-Nagy, Stierlin, Skynner, Bell	Whitaker, Kempler, Satir	Bowen	Minuchin	Jackson, Erickson, Haley, Madanes, Selvini-Palazzoli, Watzlawick	Patterson, Stuart, Liberman, Jacobson, Margolin

From Goldenberg, I., & Goldenberg, H. (1991). Family therapy: An overview (3rd ed.). Pacific Grove, CA: Brooks/Cole.

are the result of ongoing interactions of family members. Unconscious processes are unimportant; rather, family rules, homeostatic mechanisms, and feedback are important factors influencing family functioning. Insight also is unimportant; rather, changes in family functioning are brought about through prescription, not interpretation. Some of the clinicians and theorists associated with this approach are Erickson, Haley, Madanes, Jackson, and Selvini-Palazzoli.

Behavioral Approach

The theoretical bases for behavioral family therapy are behaviorism and social learning theory. The targets of therapy are dyads; one person's behavior is hypothesized to have a direct effect on another's behavior. The therapist assumes a very directive role, serving as a teacher of, and a role model for, desired behavior. Emphasis is placed on mutual contracting. The therapist strives for precision in identifying the problem, measuring change quantitatively, and conducting research to validate effectiveness of the treatment modality. The goal of therapy is to change the behavior of the dyads and thus eliminate the problem or symptom. The focus of behavioral family therapy is on the present interpersonal environment that elicits or maintains the behavioral patterns. Insight has no relevance in this approach. Action is prescribed to achieve goals. A major assumption of the theory is that problem behaviors and symptoms are learned and maintained through behavioral reinforcement. Major theorists and clinicians using this approach are Lieberman, Margolin, Patterson, and Stuart.

Bowenian Approach

The theoretical basis for Bowen's family therapy is family systems theory. The target of therapy is the entire family over several generations; however, the therapist may work with one dyad or one individual before, or while working with, the larger family system. The therapist assumes a direct but nonconfrontational role and works to remain detriangulated from the family system. The goal of therapy is to maximize self-differentiation of each family member. The focus of therapy is primarily the present, but attention also is paid to patterns of behavior in the family of origin.

In Bowen's earlier work, he emphasized unconscious processes, but more recently he has emphasized the role of interaction in the etiology of family problems. Bowen proposes that, through rational processes, family members can gain self-awareness into current relationships and into intergenerational processes. Bowenian therapy is widely practiced by therapists in various disciplines, including nursing.

BOWEN FAMILY SYSTEMS THEORY

The clinical examples presented in this chapter are conceptualized from a Bowen family systems framework. This framework offers the clinician a broad yet sufficiently specific perspective from which to view anxiety, relationships, treatment, and the interactive process present in all aspects of clinical work. Various clinical techniques can be incorporated within this conceptualization while maintaining theoretical consistency.

Assessment of anxiety is an initial and continuing process in any clinical work. Within the Bowen conceptualization, anxiety, acute and chronic, is a central variable. Anxiety is fundamental to human relationships. Patterns of handling anxiety are experienced most vividly in nuclear and extended family relationships. The triangle is the concept that describes the direct or immediate experience of anxiety; when tension arises between two individuals, a third will be involved by the two to relieve the immediate tension. This is observable in squabbles between children when one "tells" on the other. The third person is being triangled into the problem situation. Likewise, when parents experience an increase in tension in their relationship and begin to focus on what one of the children is or is not doing, that child becomes the third point in an emotional triangle. This is an automatic process that usually happens outside of awareness. With time, patterns develop within systems for handling chronic anxiety. Family members who are interested and able to think about emotional issues can recognize patterns of handling anxiety. Clinicians can certainly observe these patterns and use them as a basis for planning short- and long-term intervention.

In making an initial assessment of a clinical problem, the therapist assumes that the tension of anxiety has increased and that the therapist is vulnerable to becoming a third point in an anxious triangle in the family system. Bowen asserts that even one contact with a family therapist, who is experienced by the family system as a calm presence, can have a positive effect. The therapist's objective is to be involved with the individual(s) without entering into and replicating the automatic emotional triangling patterns that the family system uses to handle anxiety.

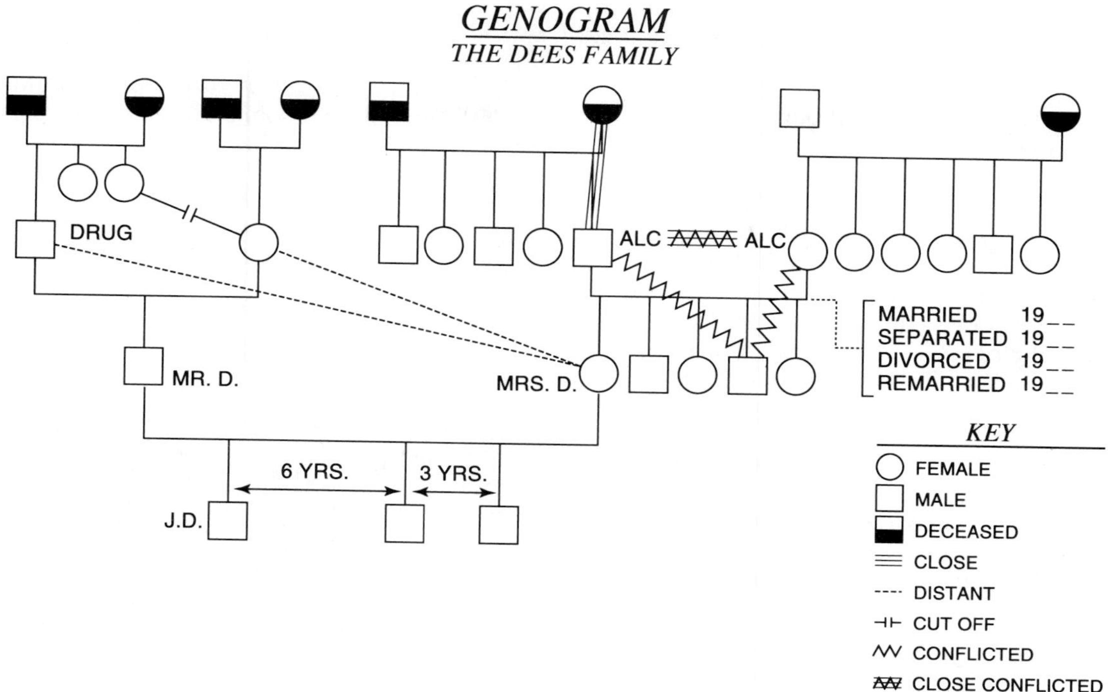

FIGURE 25–1 • Genogram for the Dees family. The genogram is used as a graphic representation of family information. Sibling position, a concept within Bowen theory, is immediately apparent. First born children are on the left of the line between their parents. Each sibling follows in order of birth. A child born six years before the next sibling, Jim's position, is functionally in the position of an only child. The nuclear family concept that hypothesizes patterns of handling emotionality in a family is illustrated here. Mrs. Dees' parents are both experiencing dysfunction related to heavy alcohol use, and they both continue active conflictual relationships with their second son. This relationship is also conceptualized as an ongoing emotional triangle. Information is added to a genogram as work proceeds, providing a dynamic reference point for planning family intervention.

To assess the problem, the therapist hears a description of the problem from as many points of view as possible or appropriate. During the description of the problem, the therapist elicits information about anxiety and how is it experienced. Factual information about the family system also emerges. The therapist organizes this information into a genogram (Fig. 25-1), which is explained to family members. The explanation is brief or lengthy, depending on their interest and degree of emotionality related to what they are experiencing or describing. The intent of the therapist is to assist family members to think about the emotional processes in which they are caught.

A second concept of the Bowen systems theory is that of differentiation of self. Thinking and emotion are to some extent fused in all individuals. The more differentiated these functions are within an individual, the more that person will be free to proceed with life plans and experience life's possibilities. When these functions are highly fused, the individual is vulnerable to the emotionality of others and becomes active in endless triangles. In an individual with limited self-differentiation, behavior is comfort seeking and automatic.

The third concept of Bowen's theory is that of the nuclear family. An initial assessment always includes information about the nuclear family. A relatively stable amount of emotionality is brought to a new family unit by the partners creating the unit, whether in a marriage or in another type of stable relationship. The couple develops ways of handling closeness and distance. The addition of children to the family system leads to new patterns for handling emotionality. Parents include their children to varying degrees in these new patterns. Nuclear families typically handle emotionality by four patterns—distance, conflict, dysfunction in a spouse, and projection to one or more children. When symptoms of emotional dysfunction appear in a child, a nuclear family process of projection to a child is a starting point for planning intervention.

Application to a Family with an Adolescent Achievement Issue

Mrs. Dees originally came to treatment when her own anxiety increased to an unmanageable level after learning of an incest issue in her family of origin. She had thought that the alcoholism of both of her parents was her primary issue and developed ways for handling the related stress. Mrs. Dees was very shaken when she learned from her maternal aunt that the maternal grandfather had sexually abused both the aunt and Mrs. Dees' mother as little girls and that Mrs. Dees' mother, the oldest daughter, had taken responsibility for the safety and security of the four younger siblings, with only partial success (see the genogram in Fig. 25-1).

After initial work with these family of origin issues, Mrs. Dees wanted to involve her husband in her therapy work. Mrs. Dees hoped to address the discomfort in relationships with her husband's family. The potential for triangling by including the husband in therapy was assessed and discussed before and after he joined the ongoing therapy.

Mrs. Dees, Mr. Dees, and the therapist examined nuclear family processes. The situation of their oldest child, Jim, emerged as that of a triangled, or projected, child. At age 15, Jim was into a second year of school failure. His parents were aware that he had experimented with alcohol and marijuana. When the father became anxious, he immediately focused on the son. The father was certain that heavy drug involvement was inevitable. Exploring the question of drug use in the father's family revealed the presence of a mystery. Mr. Dees' father had been jailed at some point in his own youth, presumably for a drug-related incident. Mr. Dees was not willing to discuss this with his father (a first-choice intervention) but was willing to consider the ways in which his own anxiety about drugs might influence his behavior with his son.

Both parents came from families in which boundaries were unclear. In Mrs. Dees' family, emotional issues were potentially explosive. Abandonment of responsibility and alcohol abuse were continuing problems in her family. According to Mr. Dees, his mother assumed responsibility for everything in his family. The message that both Mr. and Mrs. Dees had learned in their families of origin was that men are not to be trusted and that women have to watch men very carefully. They both watched their son carefully. Jim did not take responsibility for his own behavior. This became increasingly clear as Jim's parents responded to questions about responsibility and attempted to think through their responsibilities *to* him, as separate from their responsibility *for* him. (This is not a clear distinction, which discourages many families from persisting in the process.)

These parents did persist in addressing the responsibility issue and were able to explore options for relating to their son that were previously unimaginable to them. A vivid example of such an option was that of acknowledging that school might not be the best place for Jim to be spending his time, because he clearly was not using school for its intended purpose. At age 17, before the end of 11th grade, Jim chose to leave school. Anxiety accompanied this decision for all involved. Continual effort was made on the part of both parents to problem solve with their son without taking responsibility for his decision making.

During the following months, Jim became involved in intermittent drug- and alcohol-related situations in ways that could not go unnoticed by his parents, because they received telephone calls during the night from the police. With each episode, the parents attempted to think about the situation and their own reactions to it. Decisions had to be made about actions to be taken. In each of these situations, they made decisions and then used regularly scheduled therapy sessions (every other week) to examine their feelings and actions. Some decisions were affirmed by the parents as positive, and some were modified considerably after careful thought. Differences in the views of each parent were clarified and examined. They monitored varying degrees of conflict, distance, and potential for dysfunction.

Jim has now passed a high school equivalency examination and completed one term in college. He is working toward a self-determined goal of attending college in another state. His parents continue to observe and accept his decision-making process and attempt to clarify the decisions they want and need to make in relation to their son.

Several other concepts of Bowen's theory were evident in the Dees family. The concepts of family projection process and multigenerational transmission process describe the emotional projection that occurs in repeated patterns over generations. The extended families of both parents demonstrated patterns of over-responsibility and irresponsibility. The contract for therapy with this couple was to examine family emotional patterns and plan for change. Change occurs in an emotional system when individuals clarify their own part in negative processes and take positions of responsibility for their own behavior. Change is never something someone else should or should not do. While examining responsibility in their relationship with their son, both parents were clarifying their relationship to each of their parents and to other extended family members. Mrs. Dees was more verbal and therefore this process was more explicit. Her parents continue to use alcohol. Distance and confusing bids for closeness, sometimes of a sexual nature, are among the ongoing issues she continues to define.

The potential for cutoff is great in this family, and at an earlier point in the marriage, Mrs. Dees had cut off from her husband's parents. The concept of emotional cutoff demonstrates the potential for handling emotionality by permanent distancing. Rather than addressing emotional issues in the relationships in which they originate and in a way that allows for growth, individuals stop active participation in the relationships. The emotionality continues and expresses itself in other relationships. If Mrs. Dees cut herself off from her own parents, whose behavior is at times extremely anxiety producing, it is doubtful that she would have been as free to think responsibly about her relationship with her own son. Thus, she would be more likely to behave in controlling ways that would increase the chances of her son behaving irresponsibly. The pattern for triangling alcohol into relationships already exists in this family system. The son's experimentation with alcohol could easily have become a way of handling the distress of age-appropriate decision-making.

Sibling position is the last Bowenian concept to be discussed here. Based originally on the work of Toman (1961), it provides an initial set of hypotheses about personality characteristics and usual functioning based on order of birth and number, sex, and spacing of siblings. Mrs. Dees was an oldest sister, Mr. Dees an only child. Oldest sisters are prone to have learned a great deal about leadership and caretaking in the small social group composed of siblings. This was true of both Mrs. Dees and her mother. Mr. Dees was an only child. Toman hypothesizes that only sons have not had the kinds of group relationship experiences that siblings have had, nor have they observed parental interaction with other children in the family. At a less than conscious level, only sons are prone to think that their way is the only way and that what they wish to happen will happen. Openly discussing with a couple how much their experiences match the descriptions of usual sibling functional positions can be a way of exchanging a great deal of information rapidly. Mrs. Dees identified that her own "oldest daughter" tendencies were very strong, as had her own mother's been. However, when Mrs. Dees was a teenager, her family had become chaotic with parental drinking, separations, divorces, and remarriages. The timing of Mrs. Dees' first request for therapy, when her own son was a teenager, was theoretically predictable.

In summary, the concepts of Bowen family systems theory directed the assessment of the problem, the planning, and the intervention. The aspect of therapy with this couple that involved their adolescent son has been highlighted, illustrating application of the concepts of Bowen's theory. The son was seen only once by the therapist and once by a school counselor for evaluation. The plan for intervening in the son's failure to achieve and alcohol and drug experimentation was to work with the parents to clarify responsibility issues in all of their relationships, specifically those in their families of origin.

Concurrently, therapy helped the parents think about anxious issues that involved their son and clarify their responsibility *to* him and *for* him. These were ongoing concerns, and they learned to pose questions to themselves. The answers the parents formulated changed as their son matured. They also learned to identify issues or behaviors to which they were almost certain to react anxiously and to catch themselves before responding reactively. In an early session, the father said, "I feel the need for a big post to grab onto. My anger comes over me like a great wind, and if I had something to hold on to, I might be able to stop myself from being blown away by it and saying and doing things that don't do a bit of good anyway." Mr. Dees was able to use an imaginary post during that period to stop his destructive emotional processes.

Evaluation of the direction and continuing usefulness of this work is made explicit at periodic intervals. One approach to evaluation with the Dees was to review with them the case material written for this chapter. They both confirmed the accuracy, validating that what was written reflected their understanding. However, Mrs. Dees observed that so much of the richness of the experience is not captured in a clinical description. Mr. Dees simply went on with the work, using this opportunity to initiate discussion of an issue he had raised earlier but had not pursued.

CLINICAL EXAMPLE: SCOTT FAMILY

Mr. Scott and his wife brought his 9-year-old daughter, Suzie, to a public mental health center because they were concerned about the child's destructive behavior. As in many families, regardless of the therapy setting, they saw the child as the only problem and asked the therapist to fix the child's problem. Suzie was the only child of either parent, her natural mother having died in childbirth.

In the assessment phase of work with this family, Mr. Scott revealed that he and Suzie had lived with his mother prior to marrying his present wife. Although both grandmothers had an investment in the child, each for complex reasons, the stepmother was minimally invested in the child. The therapist used the concept of triangles to identify processes that were repeating themselves, without getting caught in the reasons for the triangling. Separate sessions with the child and with the parents focused on what was happening and who had what part in the process and finding a safe emotional space and a safe physical space in which the child could grow.

Suzie eventually described abusive behavior on the part of the stepmother. She said, "I know I should not have hit my mother, but when she picked up the knife and came toward me, I got scared." Because public protective agencies were already investigating this family, the therapist did not need to make any further report. Within a few weeks of the discussion of abuse, the father decided that it would be best for Suzie to go back to live with her maternal grandmother. The therapist did not know what had prompted this shift in Mr. Scott's position. Previously he had not taken a stand that would be contrary to the wishes of anyone. His decision though, was counter to the paternal grandmother's wishes, supported by the stepmother, and a cause for rejoicing on the part of the maternal grandmother. In three monthly follow-up sessions, the family's anxiety level appeared to be markedly decreased, and no behavior problems were reported by the maternal grandmother, teachers, or the child.

COMPARISON OF FAMILY-FOCUSED NURSING WITH FAMILY THERAPY

Family-focused nursing practice has many elements in common with family therapy. Both conceptualize the family as a system and focus interventions on the system rather than on individuals. Both have similar goals, but they differ in their emphasis on specific goals. Goals common to both approaches are to reduce anxiety, facilitate problem solving, mobilize support, stimulate motivation, provide education, effect behavioral changes and role changes, facilitate normative and non-normative transitions, and change interpersonal processes. Family-focused nursing practice is more likely to focus on the goals related to problem solving, support, motivation, education, and normative transitions, whereas family therapy is more likely to focus on the goals related to interpersonal processes, non-normative transitions, behavioral changes, and role changes. Clearly, there is much overlap between the two groups regarding goals.

The emphasis on specific goals may be heavily influenced by the setting in which the nurse is employed and by the types of clients generally seen in that setting. Families that present in public clinics often pose different challenges than families in private settings. Differences often include the kinds of problems that the families bring, the time and energy that the families have to address their problems, and general family resources. Therefore, in the public clinic setting, therapy is often short-term, intense, and crisis oriented, as the Clinical Example for the Scott family illustrates.

Nurses' Preparation for Practice

The preparation of nurses for practice in family-focused nursing and family therapy differs markedly. Ideally the preparation for family-focused nursing practice should be at the graduate level. In practice, however, much family-focused care is provided by nurses who do not have a master's degree. Most baccalaureate-prepared nurses have some preparation for family-focused care, and they provide this care in a number of settings, such as community health, home health, and parent–child nursing. In contrast, the nurse family therapist always has at least a master's level education, which includes theory and supervised practice of family therapy; ideally, the preparation includes post-master's course work, extensive clinical supervision, and specialist certification.

Nurses practicing family-focused care and family nurse therapists must have the knowledge and skills necessary to complete a thorough assess-

CLINICAL EXAMPLE: NOONAN FAMILY

Mrs. Noonan contacted her pediatrician during the first week of school. She reported that her first-born daughter, Jane, had started school that week and that she had been extremely upset each morning about going to school, cried, and clung to her mother when arriving at school. She calmed down in school only when the mother was present. She was sure that Jane would settle down, but the problem seemed to be getting worse rather than better. The pediatrician referred Mrs. Noonan to a private child psychiatric clinic where she was seen by a nurse therapist. In the initial interview, the nurse intervened in the mother's anxiety and learned that the mother had had similar distress when entering school for the first time. The nurse also learned that during the month prior to beginning school, the mother experienced a major loss, the death of her father, whom she continues to mourn.

The nurse therapist assigned specific behavioral tasks to modify the interaction of mother and child. The mother was invited to continue to work with the therapist for three sessions to evaluate and refine the behavioral assignments and to explore continuing personal loss issues. If a family-focused nurse in the pediatrician's office had seen Mrs. Noonan initially, the nurse may have been able to intervene in her anxiety and make the behavioral prescriptions and thus may have dealt as effectively with the presenting problem as did the nurse therapist. The brief therapy provided by the nurse therapist was useful but, in this case, not essential.

ment of families undergoing transitions and develop a plan of care. The family-focused nurse practitioner is likely to deal with families facing normative and non-normative transitions, whereas the family nurse therapist is more likely to deal with families facing non-normative transitions. Furthermore, the family nurse therapist is more likely to deal with families with more complex or severe dysfunction. The Clinical Example for the Noonan family demonstrates the potential for greater application of family-focused care.

The major area of difference between the two types of nurse practitioners is the type and range of treatment interventions. The family-focused nurse tends to use direct, straightforward interventions, such as teaching or role modeling; the family nurse therapist may use these interventions but also more diverse, subtle, or complex interventions, such as paradoxic intention and intergenerationally focused, brief interventions.

CRITIQUE OF CONTEMPORARY FAMILY THERAPY APPROACHES

Family therapy is undergoing a revolution incited by feminists who have criticized some of the basic premises of family therapy (Conn, 1990; Gelman, 1990; McGoldrick, Anderson, & Walsh, 1989). Specific abuses of traditional family therapy approaches include sexual stereotyping; blaming the family, particularly the mother, for problems (such as schizophrenia) that do not have a psychodynamic etiology; and considering the family ahistorically.

Feminists recognize and deplore the power imbalance between men and women that exists in society today. They assert that family structure and function are expected to be male dominated and that women are expected to assume the primary responsibility for parenting and domestic work. Most family therapy theorists have been male, and their writings have dominated theoretical developments in the field. These writings have perpetuated the imbalance of power and devaluing of women in the family therapy setting, thus exacerbating the problems related to the emancipation of women. While most family nurse therapists are female, these women often work with male cotherapists or are supervised by male therapists. Thus, the influence of the dominant male view that perpetuates the oppression of women within the family is constant. Some family nurse therapists are unaware of these forces, while others are well attuned to these issues. For nurse therapists who identify with the feminist perspective, there is the danger of crossing over the line between therapy and advocacy.

Goldner (1985), Carter and McGoldrick (1988), and Walters, Carter, Papp, and Siverstein (1988) have been leaders in sensitizing the family therapy profession to the feminist critique. They assert that common family therapy techniques are to "hit the mother and coddle the father," the rationalization being that because the mother is the most involved and motivated, she can take the heat, while the father cannot. He is likely to drop out of therapy if not coddled. Another problem is the belief that "mothers can and fathers can't"; thus, the person who needs to change is the mother. Some women are refusing to play the roles they have traditionally played in society; this leads to changes in family structure and function that may be stressful. Unfortunately, the tendency is to blame the woman for precipitating these stressors, rather than to recognize the equal rights of the woman. This promother attitude must be balanced with the recognition that the potential exists to create the reverse problem, father blaming.

Leslie and Cosick (1989) summarized some of the challenges feminist therapy offers traditional family therapy:

1. Individual choice or responsibility needs to be considered instead of looking only at mutually created patterns of interaction.
2. Power inequalities need to be recognized instead of simply assuming inequality.
3. Individual family members should be identified as clients, instead of identifying the entire family as the client.
4. The therapist should choose a therapy approach that incorporates a more equal relationship with clients.
5. Therapists should recognize that symptoms in a family may be naturally occurring manifestations of oppression in society, instead of simple manifestations of systems difficulties in a family unit.
6. Families need to be able to talk about gender issues, such as money and power, in therapy.
7. Therapists need to help families develop ways of functioning based on competence, instead of on gender.
8. The assumption that therapy is "value free" needs to be discarded.

Feminist therapy and most of the traditional systems-based family therapy are incompatible. The Bowen-based family therapy described in this chapter is congruent with seven of the eight challenges to family therapy as proposed by Leslie and Cosick (1989). For example, working toward increased differentiation is highly compatible with the first feminist challenge that emphasizes individual choice and responsibility. The two approaches differ on the perspective of who is the client. In challenge number three, Leslie and Cosick propose that individual family members, not the entire family, should be identified as the client. In the Bowen perspective, the entire family is perceived as the client, with recognition that individuals are inseparable from their families; although the family is the client, the major goal of therapy is to increase the functioning effectiveness of individuals within the family. Clearly, much work is needed to integrate feminist philosophy into family therapy approaches, while recognizing the constantly changing sociocultural milieu that affects our attitudes and behaviors.

Summary

When working with children and adolescents, family issues are a major consideration. This chapter presents an overview of the theories and approaches that inform the practice of family therapy. In addition, examples are presented of family therapy using a Bowenian approach. Nurses who practice family therapy are in a position to affect significant and life-changing interventions. A feminist perspective challenges everyone who works with families to integrate these concepts into their practice.

REFERENCES

Bowen, M. (1976). Theory in the practice of psychotherapy. In P. J. Guerin (Ed.), *Family therapy*. New York: Gardner Press.

Bowen, M. (1978). *Family therapy in clinical practice* (pp. 42–90). New York: Jason Aronson.

Carter, B., & McGoldrick, M. (Eds.) (1988). *The changing family life cycle: A framework for family therapy* (2nd ed.). New York: Gardner Press.

Conn, V., & Hirschmann, M. (1990). The case for and against family systems theory. *Journal of Child and Adolescent Psychiatric/Mental Health Nursing, 3*, 29–33.

Gelman, D. (1990). Fixing the between. *Newsweek*, 42–43.

Goldenberg, I., & Goldenberg, H. (1985). *Family therapy: An overview* (2nd ed). Monterey, CA: Brooks/Cole.

Goldner, V. (1985). Feminism and family therapy. *Family Process, 24*(1), 31–48.

Gurman, A., & Knisern, D. (Eds.). (1981). *Handbook of family therapy.* New York: Brunner/Mazel.

Jones, S. (1980). *Family therapy: A comparison of approaches.* Bowie, MD: Brady.

Kerr, M., & Bowen, M. (1988). *Family evaluation: An approach based on Bowen theory.* New York: Norton.

Leslie, L., & Cosick, M. (1989, November). Teaching feminist family therapy: A faculty and student perspective. Paper presented at annual meeting of The National Council of Family Relations, New Orleans, LA.

McGoldrick, M., Anderson, C., & Walsh, F. (Eds.) (1989). *Women in families: A framework for family therapy.* New York: Norton.

Toman, W. (1961). *Family constellation.* New York: Springer Publishing.

Walters, M., Carter, B., Papp, P., & Silverstein, O. (1988). *The invisible web: Gender patterns in family relationships.* New York: The Guilford Press.

CHAPTER

26

Group Therapy

Charlotte Gilbert

Groups are naturally occurring phenomena for children and adolescents. According to Crockett (1984), peer interactions may provide opportunities for children's psychologic development, such as the formation of close relationships with other people, the development of social skills that promote positive social interactions, and understanding self and others. Because modern western culture does not recognize adult status until many years past childhood, another benefit of peer groups is that they help bridge the void between the worlds of child and adult (Vorrath & Brendtro, 1974). Overall, the peer group provides important opportunities for youth to meet as equals within their own generation, communicate, understand others' points of view, get along with others, compare self with others, define one's social role, and perfect one's social skills (Cole & Cole, 1989; Grunebaum & Solomon, 1980; 1982; Redston-Iselin, 1987; Sahler & McAnarey, 1981).

Group Interventions

Peer affiliations in the form of group activity are much the norm during preadolescence and adolescence. Therefore, group interventions may be more akin to the norm and less threatening than other forms of therapy, such as individual therapy, and group reinforcement is often more powerful for many children than individual reinforcement (Rose & Edleson, 1987). Rose and Edleson propose that additional benefits of group interventions with children and adolescents experiencing emotional or behavioral problems include feedback about behaviors that are annoying or pleasing to others, knowledge of cognitions that are self-defeating or self-enhancing, toleration of others, and opportunities to practice new behaviors, such as learning the skills involved in giving and receiving critical feedback and advice.

Overall, group interventions provide a mechanism for peers to fulfill needs related to socialization, identity, and competence in a context other than family. The process of group therapy provides members with support, identification with others in similar circumstances, and the ego strength to work through problematic issues (Loomis, 1979; 1991; Siepker, Lewis, & Kandaras, 1985; Yalom, 1985), thus reducing member isolation and loneliness.

The approach, membership, length, and content of group interventions with children, adolescents, and families vary. Often group therapy models must be adapted given the reality of issues in a therapy setting, such as leadership changes, inclusion of sibling pairs, and parental resistance (Moss, 1984). Moss proposes that behavioral change can be facilitated in a group under less than ideal circumstances when basic parameters are held fast, such as guidelines for each specific group, maintainance of structure, and learning from the experiences of others.

Group interventions provide the child and adolescent psychiatric-mental health clinical nurse specialist with a unique opportunity to treat the responses of children, adolescents, and families to actual or potential health problems in a context more reflective of the real world, the social context. Therefore, this chapter describes group interventions often used with children, adolescents, and families. Issues related to child development, research, and implications for nursing practice and research are discussed.

Developmental Considerations

Children and adolescents mature with time, and the influence of development is seen in peer relationships and cognitive ability (Grunebaum & Solomon, 1980; 1982; Shirk, 1988). Because group therapists are concerned with peer interaction, client insight, and the use of interpretation, they must be knowledgeable of the influence of development on peer relationships and cognition.

DEVELOPMENTAL STAGES OF PEER RELATIONSHIPS

According to Grunebaum and Solomon (1982) peer groups have distinct developmental stages that include toddlerhood, preschool, middle childhood, and adolescence. The toddler (1 to 3 years) has limited language skills, and play is parallel rather than cooperative. The skills of the preschool child (3 to 6 years) reflect further development. The child is verbal; engages in cooperative play; shares; pretend plays with another; reacts to the emotions of others; engages in sociodramatic play; joins in simple cooperative games, such as building a house with blocks; and experiences positive exchanges with others so that aggression becomes modulated and decreased. During middle childhood (6 to 9 years), children begin to perceive the other's perspective, empathize, and learn that their emotions and those of others may be calculated, controlled, disguised, or feigned (Grunebaum & Solomon, 1982). Cognitive maturity allows the child to plan and carry out long sequences of purposive activities, exercise self-control, and submit voluntarily to rules of games. Friendships are usually with people of the same gender. During adolescence (12 to 16 years), the youth is able discern differing social perspectives, achieve psychologic independence from family, and form attachments to peers.

COGNITIVE DEVELOPMENT

Child psychotherapy has traditionally assigned a major role to self-understanding as a means for promoting emotional and behavioral change. Therefore, the second developmental issue of importance to the child and adolescent group therapist is cognitive development.

Traditional therapy approaches emphasize the importance of careful timing of interpretations and focus on the emotional readiness of the child or the quality of the therapeutic relationship. For example, therapeutic communication may arouse within the child unacceptable or intolerable feelings like guilt or sadness, and the child may avoid further discussion of the topic. One of the reasons usually given for the lack of response to a therapeutic intervention has been resistance on the part of the child (Schaffer & Pollak, 1987; Shirk, 1988). Resistance is defined as any individual or group level behavior that is used defensively in place of the stated task of talking about personal and interpersonal issues, feelings, and concerns and is characterized by silences, talking about irrelevant subjects, or acting out (Scheidlinger, 1985). The cognitive–developmental perspective suggests that many resistances may be a result of interpretations that are composed of psychologic constructs that might or might not be in the cogitive repertoire of the child (Shirk, 1988).

Children's understanding of the causes of behavior becomes more psychologic with increasing age (Shirk, 1988). Preschoolers, young children, and school-age children understand behavioral events in terms of external situational causes, and when confronted with therapeutic efforts to consider internal determinants, children may appear resistant and focus on solutions in the external environment. Older school-age children and adolescents are more likely to consider behavioral events in terms of internal causes; this is a behavior dependent on cognitive development and the ability to understand psychologic concepts and processes. Therefore, it is important to consider that a child's externalization of his or her difficulties might not be the result of defensive motivation, but rather an expression of a cognitive component of a particular developmental period (Shirk, 1988).

Group Intervention Models

HISTORIC DEVELOPMENT

In a review of the literature related to child and adolescent group psychotherapy, Rachman and Raubolt (1984) report that Moreno, Aichhorn, Redl, Slavson, Gabriel, and Wollan were pioneers in the development of group work with adolescents during the early to mid-20th century. They disregarded adolescence as a separate developmental stage in the life cycle, and early groups included children who were between the ages of 8 and 15 years. The groups were created in response to societal needs and because of a paucity of therapists with didactic and clinical experience working with delinquent children and adolescents, clients of child guidance clinics, or the schools. Activity was the medium of early groups; educational activities, crafts, and play were emphasized in an atmosphere that fostered social awareness, development of potentialities, and respect for democratic principles.

Group interventions used with children and adolescents include a variety of models, such as play group therapy, relationship-oriented group psychotherapy, peer therapy, activity group therapy, behavior group therapy, psychoeducational group interventions, and adolescent group psychotherapy. In general, interventions with young children tend to be more play and activity oriented, and verbalization is more likely to be used in interventions with older children and adolescents who have greater cognitive and verbal abilities. Group interventions have focused on a variety of problems experienced by children and adolescents, such as abused, preschool children (Critchley, 1982); children with chronic illness (Nathan & Goetz, 1984); children with parents who abuse substances (Owen, Rosenberg, & Barkley, 1985); children in women's shelters (Gilbert, 1988a); bereaved preschool and school-age children (Masterman & Reams, 1988); and girls who were sexually abused (Gilbert, 1988b).

Common Characteristics of Group Interventions

The purpose of group therapy is closely related to the purpose of nursing care: to diagnose and treat human responses to actual or potential health problems (Loomis, 1979; 1991). Within the group, members have the opportunity to maintain existing healthy behaviors, alter some existing behaviors, and learn new behaviors. Loomis suggests that the primary advantage of group therapy rests with the variety of people with similar problems or objectives who work on them together. In the process, they find that they are less alone and isolated, because sharing human problems is one of the benefits of group therapy.

CURATIVE FACTORS

All groups are hypothesized to possess mechanisms, curative factors that promote behavioral change (Yalom, 1985). Curative factors include the following:

- Instillation of hope—others have endured or changed, and so can I
- Universality—the event or feeling experienced is similar to that of others
- Imparting of information—health care teaching and sharing in which a cognitive component usually preceeds behavioral change
- Altruism—sharing a part of self with others, support and assistance of others
- Corrective recapitulation of the family group—group members and therapist represent a symbolic family
- Group cohesiveness—all factors that act on all members to remain in group
- Interpersonal learning—insight
- Imitative behavior—group members model behavior on that of other members
- Development of socialization techniques—social skills
- Catharsis—expression of feelings
- Existential factors—recognition that life may be unfair and that each person bears responsibility for their behavior (Loomis, 1991; Yalom, 1985)

In a study of adolescent group members, adolescents reported that the most helpful curative factors were catharsis, interpersonal learning, existential factors, group cohesiveness, and relationship formation (Corder, Whiteside, & Haizlip, 1981).

Group Psychotherapy for Children

ACTIVITY THERAPY GROUPS

Group psychotherapy for children and adolescents began with Slavson, the originator of activity groups (Slavson, 1943; Slavson & Schiffler, 1975). Activity therapy groups were developed for prepubertal children between age 9 through puberty. The purpose of the activity group was to facilitate the expression of conflicted feelings through a sustained relationship with a permissive therapist and peers for 3 to 4 years. Interpretations of behavior were avoided, and resistance and other defense mechanisms were not explored.

Slavson and Schiffler (1975) consider knowledge of child development and specific issues common to particular developmental periods important in group work with children and adolescents. Groups for preschoolers, age 4 to 5 years, include male and female children who engage in parallel play and symbolic sibling rivalry. During the latency period, age 6 to 12 years, children experience a transition to an expanded environment of new adults and peers. Whereas latency-age groups may include members of both genders who engage in play games with rules, Slavson and Schiffler (1975) suggest that early adolescent groups need therapist consistency and limits. Middle adolescent groups may include members of both genders, between the ages of 15 and 16 years, and are similar to adult groups because verbalization and discussion are the primary modes of communication.

According to Slavson and Schiffler (1975), the structure of the group demands consideration of variables, such as number of sessions, length of each session, and mix of members. In activity group therapy, an additional important consideration is that of space and equipment, which have the potential to facilitate the child's expression of conflicted feelings, such as pounding tools, clay, checkers, cards, and so forth. The size of the group and the length of sessions vary in activity groups. Groups for older children may have as many as six to eight children; five children may be the maximum for preschool and nursery groups. The number of members also may be influenced by the diagnosis and presenting problem of each child; the productivity of the group depends on a blend of aggressive and passive children and those who fall within this continuum. The length of each session may range from 90 minutes to 2 hours. Younger children's groups may be 75 minutes, and older children and adolescent groups may be as long as 2 hours.

The role of the activity therapist is permissive and facilitative of the expression of member conflict through appropriate activity and discussion. Important qualities of the therapist include the ability to attend to multiple children and the ability to tolerate children's activities and negative behaviors. Therapists, especially beginning therapists, need supervision to work through feelings associated with multiple behaviors exhibited by members in group and to determine appropriate equipment to facilitate each member's expression of conflicted feelings. For example, the therapist must not react personally to the behavior of the child. The therapist must convey the sense that he or she is not only in control of his or her own feelings, but is in control of the group and will not allow any child to be physically or emotionally hurt in the group (Slavson & Schiffler, 1975).

Phases of group described by Slavson and Schiffler (1975) include initial, middle, and termination. During the initial phase of group, children begin to know each other, form subgroups for play, and develop autonomy through games and imagination. The middle phase of therapy finds members engaging in symbolic play, which reflects individual and group conflicts and is interspersed with verbalization by the children. Separation and termination occur as the children's problems are resolved.

GROUP PLAY THERAPY

Ginott (1958; 1961; 1975) was an early proponent of group play therapy for children. According to this psychoanalytic model, emotional problems originate from faulty experiences in child–parent–sibling relationships. Therefore, group play therapy is the treatment of choice for many children between the ages of 3 and 9 years. This is because the group provides a corrective experience in which members modify behavior in exchange for acceptance as a result of corrective relationships with an adult as substitute parent and with peers as substitute siblings. The focus of treatment in play group therapy is the individual child; no group goals are set, and no group cohesion is sought.

In group play therapy, the dynamics are the same as those in psychotherapy and include relationship, catharsis, insight or ego strengthening, reality testing, and sublimation (Slavson, 1976). Slavson states that catharsis is an essential factor in all psychotherapy, and through play and language, repressed feelings are unfolded. Therefore, play under specially set conditions and in the presence of a permissive, understanding adult is a form of communication and catharsis. Slavson considers play as the most suitable means for children to communicate the content of the unconscious and the distress that the pressures of their environment create. Play also facilitates sublimation; for example, anger and aggression are subliminated and displaced through the use of play equipment, such as a hammer.

Several factors are important to the structure of group play therapy. Open membership, or the admission of new children, is permitted to replace children who terminate or drop out of treatment (Ginott, 1958; 1961; 1975). To maximize the effectiveness of the group model, Ginott also suggests that the group should consist of children with dissimilar syndromes so that each child is exposed to people and behavior different from and complementary to their own. Ginott recommends a small balanced group consisting of only a few quiet children and no more than two aggressive children. Age and gender of group members also are important components; groupmates should not differ in age by more than 12 months, and groups for school-age children should be the same gender. Ginott proposes that limits be addressed only when needed because they may challenge aggressive children and inhibit the submissive ones.

The role of the leader in group play therapy is one of a neutral but friendly substitute parent (Ginott, 1958; 1961; 1975) who responds to the acts and verbalizations of group members to help them acquire insight. According to Ginott, the medium of group provides the therapist with the opportunity to plan insight-provoking incidents so that disturbed youngsters will express repressed feelings toward family members and authority figures.

Group play therapy provides two media for catharsis, play and talk, so that each child can use their preferred symbolic language. This model presents members with opportunities to obtain insight nonverbally about self and relationships with parents and peers, without interpretations and explanations and often the result rather than the cause of improvement (Ginott, 1958; 1961; 1975). For example, Slavson (1976) believes that children's insight is more perceptive when it is brought about by hearing uncanny remarks about situations, themselves, or others. Through the medium of play group therapy, children find that they are accepted by other children and the therapist; the children find that they are loved and worthy of love, so the children achieve a more wholesome self-image and perception of self-worth (Slavson, 1976).

RELATIONSHIP-ORIENTED GROUP PSYCHOTHERAPY

This model is based on a developmental, psychodynamic approach to group therapy with preschoolers, school-age children, and adolescents. The focus of this model is on individual dynamics and group dynamics (Siepker et al., 1985). The goal of relationship-oriented group therapy is to facilitate behavioral, personality, and emotional change in a group of children to increase their personal satisfaction and interactions with significant others. Group process has recognizable stages, and each stage has goals, tasks, and milestones that are observable and understandable and that can be used to accomplish individual and group treatment goals.

Siepker et al. (1985) state that the stages of group development in this model are preparation, exploration, cohesion, termination, and closure. During the preparation stage (de Neuhaus, 1985), initial contacts are made with group candidates and parents, and beginning relationships between child and therapist are established. The therapist plans the structure of the group and considers the age and stage of development of group members, group size, the length of each session, and the number of sessions. Optimal group size for children's groups is between five and seven children. Groups are usually closed unless there is a need to replace members. The length of each session depends on whether the structure will be verbal, activity oriented, or a combination of both. Discussion groups of 45 minutes are typical for latency-age and young adolescent groups, whereas 60- to 90-minute discussion groups are typical for older adolescents. Highly anxious groups may only be able to tolerate 10 minutes of discussion. Groups may be conducted for 6 months to 1 or 2 years. Short-term groups are usually conducted for 3 to 6 months, and diagnostic groups may be as short as four sessions.

Siepker et al. (1985) delineate other stages of group development. The exploration stage begins with the first session and continues until the group has achieved an identity. Anxiety occurs as children begin to value the group and realize that they must change to maintain group membership. This stage ends as the child commits self to the group and accepts controls. During the cohesion stage, members experience an intense psychologic closeness, and the work of group is best accomplished at this time. The termination stage occurs as the group recognizes that the end of the group is a reality and concludes with the final session. Siepker et al. (1985) also propose a stage of group development, closure, which is rarely considered by other therapists or theorists. The authors state that this stage extends from the final session of group to the implementation of recommendations for the future care of children and the resolution of the therapist's feelings for the children and the group.

Also, according to Siepker et al. (1985), the relationship-oriented therapist must have prior training, course work, or supervision in group work with children and adolescents. In this model, the therapist is active, involved, and sensitive to the psychosocial needs of the members and to the manifestations of member disturbance. Child and adolescent group therapists must like children, be able to give and take affection but not have a strong need to be liked by group members, be able to play and communicate verbally and nonverbally, and be able to tolerate frustration and children's expression of conflict through activity. The role of the therapist is to create a predictable atmosphere that motivates learning about self and others and provides security, acceptance, limits, and respect. The therapist uses therapeutic communication to focus on member relationships and uses simple interpretations that focus on the present, defenses, and behavior seen in group.

PEER THERAPY

Grunebaum and Solomon (1980; 1982) propose a group intervention method based on peer relationships. They suggest that the importance of peer relations for adjustment is unknown to most group therapists. The group treatment approach fosters friendship skills and assists the child to overcome early social deficits through the use of peer group techniques, such as role taking, empathy, conflict resolution, cooperative sharing, and dramatic play.

According to Grunebaum and Solomon (1980), the group leader in this model of therapy is that of participant–facilitator, and the role of the leader is to foster the cohesion of group members and facilitate their attachment to the group. Grunebaum and Solomon believe that the role of the leader in this model is more akin to the leader of the nursery-group, play, or latency-group leader than the classic psychoanalyst, because the peer group leader is knowledgable about peer relationship development and is motivated to foster peer relationships within the group as the medium of therapy.

Grunebaum and Solomon (1982) cite several implications for group therapists when using this model. They suggest that criteria for selection of group members should include an evaluation of peer developmental history to determine appropriateness for group; group members should not differ too drastically in levels of social development because group members will not tolerate major differences. Grunebaum and Solomon also suggest that group treatment should be less verbal, therapists should be less inclined to view doing and acting as resistances, and they should pay more attention to peer interactions. They propose the use of props, subgroups, games, food, music, and art for groups lacking the ability to relate as peers and techniques such as role taking, psychodramatic methods, activity therapy, and the rehearsal of important events to promote peer interaction.

Stages of group development are included in the peer interaction model of Grunebaum and Solomon (1980). Initially, group members are thought to be bound by a common meeting place and feelings about the leader; at this stage, peer relationships are relatively unimportant. In the next stage of development, members develop bonds with other group members, often on basis of superficial similarities, such as gender and age. Gradually, the group evolves toward mutual relationships as they learn to take into account their similarities and differences. During the later phase, group members increase their empathetic communication and achieve a more intense level of peer involvement and disclosure (Grunebaum & Solomon, 1982).

MULTIMETHOD GROUP THERAPY

Rose and Edleson (1987) espouse a multimethod approach to group therapy that is characterized by different methods of change, including behavior therapy, that are integrated or selectively used in the assessment, intervention, and generalization of change. Interaction is proposed as the basis of group process, and a peer-group approach is espoused as the most appropriate context for teaching and learning interpersonal skills. Targets of change include specific behaviors or cognitions a child may use in response to a given member's problems. The role of the group leader is active. For example, the leader can modify group norms, facilitate attainment of individual and group treatment goals by modifying the group's cohesiveness, and provide guidance and protection for group members.

Phases identified in this approach include planning, assessment, orientation, intervention, and termination. During the planning stage, the purpose of the group is established, potential members are assessed and recruited, and decisions are made as to group structure and physical environment (Rose & Edelson, 1987). Rose and Edleson propose that the assessment phase is paramount to an empiric approach; it determines the specific targets of intervention and identifies the client's personal resources for working toward achievement of goals. Data are collected during all phases of group: before treatment, immediately after treatment, and some time after treatment. A variety of assessment tools may be used: personality inventories and checklists, role play tests, sociometric tests, diaries, self-observation, direct observation of group members or individuals when not in the group, postsession questionnaires, and interviews. The orientation phase consists of imparting information to members, parents, and teachers as to the purposes of group, the methods to be used, and potential goals. Group contracts usually are in writing and signed by members, parents, and group leader; they delineate responsibilities of parents and children, the agency, and the group leader.

During the intervention phase, procedures are explained to members, and intervention strategies are applied (Rose & Edelson, 1987). Sociorecreational activities, especially games, are included in every session, usually at the end, as a means of keeping the attraction to the group high. At the end of every meeting, children are assigned homework for home, school, playground, or any other nongroup location. The children specify what, when, where, or with whom certain behaviors or cognitions are manifested within a given time. The goal of this phase is generalization of change; that is, the therapist is interested in the process of transferring what the child has learned in the group to the outside world and maintaining what he or she has learned beyond the end of treatment. The strategy is homework. The purpose of the latter is to create an opportunity for the children to try out in the real world what they learned in group and lessen dependence on the group leader.

Rose and Edelson (1987) state that clients are prepared for the termination of group by developing a plan to apply what they learned in group and after the group ends. The children design activities appropriate to practicing their newly learned skills. Within 2 to 3 months following group, there may be a booster session in which children have the opportunity to discuss their achievements and any new problems.

PSYCHOEDUCATIONAL GROUP INTERVENTIONS

A significant recent trend is the development of the time-limited or short-term group (Rose, 1985; Schneidlinger, 1984). The number of sessions are time-limited, and the group is homogeneous; that is, the group is bound by a common concern. Psychoeducational groups are a further development of the short-term group intervention. They are theme centered, short term, and include an educational component. Group dynamics are directed toward the mastery of various symptoms, habits, developmental milestones, organizational problems, normative crises, or traumatic life crises (Ettin, Heiman, & Kopel, 1988).

The active use of didactics and structured exercises to teach and work along the central focus differentiates psychoeducational from traditional process groups (Ettin et al., 1988). Each lesson or session addresses common concerns and helps members move from recognition through self-understanding to self-acceptance and the active assimilation of new perspectives. Exercises are specific to the needs of members, appropriate to overall goals of the group, and consistent with the phases of treatment process.

The group format provides a setting for the therapist to disseminate knowledge while working along the shared focus and simultaneously learning from the experiences of the members. The role of the leader is that of content expert and task organizer. The group leader is expert in subject matter. He or she develops a group protocol that allows materials to be ordered and structured according to group dynamic principles and that is consistent with members' evolving ability to take in the material. A knowledge of group dynamics and group process is critical: the choice, order, and method of presenting didactic material is matched with evolving group processes and linked to the developing receptivity of participants (Ettin et al., 1988).

The material in a psychoeducational group is presented in sequential order, and it is difficult to add members once a short-term group is underway (Ettin et al., 1988). Some dropout (15% to 35%) is considered normal. Therefore, it is practical to begin a group at the upper member limit and screen and select members who are most likely to attend the maximum number of group sessions. As with other group models, once individual appropriateness for the group is decided, the goal of the psychoeducational model is to match members similar enough to relate and work together and different enough to present a wide continuum of possible perspectives, feelings, and coping strategies around a common concern.

The number of sessions is preestablished and may range from six to 20, with a norm of eight to 12. Ettin et al. (1988) caution that the fewer the number of sessions, the more the group resembles crisis intervention in that the leader is placed in an authoritative role of expert or provider, and the members are in the dependent role of novice or receiver. The greater the number of sessions, the more the group resembles traditional open-ended therapy discussion group, and the leader's role shifts to teacher or facilitator or interactive participant or observer; members' complementary roles are learner or discussant or initiator or respondent. Ettin et al. (1988) caution that as the number of sessions increases, members' latent dynamics come to the fore, and affect-laden material is increasingly stimulated. It then becomes more difficult to stay within the chosen focus and to adhere to a directed task-focused approach.

The psychoeducational model recognizes group phases: pregroup, orientation, working, and termination. During the pregroup phase, appropriate members are selected and prepared for group by imparting information about the goals, rules, procedures, and common focus of the group. Throughout the orientation phase, the common focus (problem) of the group is portrayed, members are taught basic terminology and concepts, and members are encouraged to share and compare experiences. The working or production phase is characterized by dissemination of didactic material, structured skills training, and discussion. Members become more reliant on each other and less on the leader. During the termination or graduation phase, there is less emphasis on new material and skill acquisition and more attention to cognitive and emotional closure. Members review the experience of group, including meaningful components of the program; say goodbye; and discuss plans for the future.

ADOLESCENT GROUP PSYCHOTHERAPY

Group can be a substitute family for the adolescent, a transitional object encountered before going into the world; however, according to Scheidlinger (1985), outpatient adolescent group psychotherapy is not widely practiced and is underrepresented in the literature. Scheidlinger believes that outpatient group psychotherapy is a treatment of choice for adolescents for the following reasons: within the group, there can be sufficient anonymity to promote sharing thoughts and feelings, and group may be more acceptable to the adolescent than a psychotherapist's office. Additional benefits of group are opportunities for vicarious absorption of benign experiences of other members and insights. Also, the inclusion of members of both genders provides opportunities for discussion of sexual concerns and the practice of social skills.

The role of the therapist in this model is to help group members verbalize negative feelings, especially those toward adults (Scheidlinger, 1985). The therapist must possess knowledge of issues related to adolescence and group, in addition to skill and stamina to understand and deal with provocative testing and group level resistances that are often seen in adolescent groups, usually in the early phases. Scheidlinger cautions that the therapist must be alert to being cast in the role of real parent or other hated adults or behaving like one of the gang. Techniques used to facilitate group process include discussion, role play, family sculpting, and refreshments.

Scheidlinger (1985) identifies specific themes that characterize the initial, middle, and termination of group therapy. Prior to group, it is suggested that potential members have the opportunity to be prepared and establish a minimal working alliance with the therapist. Some potential members engage in individual therapy for several months prior to group therapy. During the initial phase of group, the struggle within the group is one of trust between the adult and group members; themes suggestive of this phase include hostility and contempt for parents and complaints about school authorities. The middle phase of adolescent group psychotherapy is characterized by belief in the confidentiality of group and consolidation of the therapeutic alliance. Therefore, the therapist can pose questions for individual and group discussion, confront group members with their defensive maneuvers, and offer relevant interpretations (Scheidlinger, 1985). Themes related to this phase of group include life situations, such as separation–individuation issues at home and in the group. During the termination phase, the group is concerned with working through themes of mourning and loss and relapses into problem behavior.

Although there are a variety of approaches to group interventions for children and adolescents, most interventions include some eclectic components. For example, Gilbert (1988a) was faced with the need to provide mental health intervention for children in a women's shelter. A time-limited, structured group approach was determined to be an appropriate modality because more children could be treated in group than in other therapies by a scarce resource, a therapist, skilled in group and child development; issues common to children who have experienced family violence could be worked through by more children in a group context; and the isolation and secretiveness of family violence could be reduced for more children in group. Due to the differing developmental needs of the children, the issues of family violence, and the behavioral problems manifested by the children, an eclectic theoretical approach was used and included relationship-oriented group therapy (Siepker et al., 1985), behavioral components of multimethod group therapy (Rose & Edleson, 1987), and Yalom's (1985) curative factors of universality, catharsis, and altruism. Art was used to help the children communicate issues important to them, and provide opportunities for member interaction. Group members, mothers, and the shelter director evaluated the group experience positively.

There are numerous models of group interventions for children and adolescents. Regardless of the approach, all models value the ability of group interventions to assist members to work through problems in a social context, identify group development phases, and require therapists or leaders to be expert in child growth and development and group principles.

Group Interventions with Families

Most families constitute the best means of fostering the long-term development of children and adolescents, and groups, whether psychodynamic, educational, process, or support, have been adapted to address problems faced by families (Kennedy & Keeney, 1987). Group interventions with families address a myriad of problems, such as mothers who are mentally retarded (Wayne & Fine, 1986); mothers with the diagnosis of borderline disorder and their children (Holman, 1985); grandparents who raise emotionally disturbed grandchildren (Kennedy & Keeney, 1987); and parents with children who have attention deficit disorder (Pond & Gilbert, 1987). The latter groups are discussed in more depth.

Kennedy and Keeney (1987) note that grandparents raising emotionally disturbed grandchildren constantly face the reality of full-time responsibility for emotionally disturbed grandchildren and the shattered dream of the "golden retirement years." Kennedy and Keeney designed a psychotherapy group to meet the needs of grandparents raising emotionally disturbed grandchildren. The major therapeutic task of the grandparent group was the resolution of conflictual feelings about the biologic parent. Other issues addressed in group included child management issues, emotional demands of the parental role, and individual needs. An additional benefit of group was the reduction of isolation; grandparents soon realized that others were experiencing similar problems (Kennedy & Keeney, 1987).

Parents who have children with attention-deficit hyperactivity disorder are subject to internal and external criticism regarding the management of their children (Pond & Gilbert, 1987). Pond, a nurse educator and parent of a child with this disorder, and Gilbert, a child psychiatric clinical nurse specialist, offered a short-term, educational support group for parents of children with this disorder. The purpose of the group was to offer guidance and assistance to parents of hyperactive children. Didactic material was presented in a supportive atmosphere and included education about the disorder, management approaches at home and at school, and stress management. Group members provided positive evaluations of their group experience: Participants enhanced their parenting skills, increased knowledge of the disorder and its management, and received support from members.

Group interventions, especially those based on psychoeducational models, hold promise for work with families. Group interventions provide families with opportunities to work through common issues in a nonjudgmental atmosphere. Members also may benefit from decreased isolation and loneliness and the chance to help others with similar problems.

Research Related to Group Interventions

There is a paucity of research-based information related to group interventions with children and adolescents (Siepker et al., 1985; Scheidlinger, 1985; Slavson & Schiffler, 1975). Several examples of research that has focused on group interventions are discussed here. Bornstein, Bornstein, and Walters (1988) conducted an empiric study of a short-term, 6-week, group treatment program for children of divorce. The 31 children between the ages of 7 to 14 years were randomly assigned to either a treatment group or a control group conducted by a male and female cotherapist. Each week specific issues experienced by children of divorce were discussed, such as information needs, communication skills, clarification of feelings, problem solving, anger management, and support. Premeasures and postmeasures were administered to the children, their parents, and teachers. No significant differences were found between the treatment and control groups, except that the experimental group reported increased conflict between parents and self over time, but the parents did not confirm this increase. The researchers suggest that the discrepancy may have resulted from the child's perceptual set; that is, prior to initiation of the program all children were informed that the group experience would help them to work through divorce-related problems, and the child may have expected that the discussions would generate increased conflict between themselves and their parents (Bornstein et al., 1988). Implications for therapists who conduct group interventions with children and adolescents include knowledge of cognitive development and feedback about communication.

Another study sought to determine adolescents' perception of the usefulness of Yalom's (1985) curative factors (Corder et al., 1981). Adolescents reported that the most helpful curative factors were catharsis, interpersonal learning, existential factors, group cohesiveness, and the importance of relationships. The adolescents did not identify insight as beneficial. The researchers suggest that the results of the study provide some implications for group interventions for adolescents and therapists, namely, the increased use of techniques that structure and the opportunities for peer feedback about behavior, such as role play and psychodrama. Other suggestions include pretherapy training sessions in which techniques are taught to group members to enhance the constructive expression of feelings and feedback about behavior and training programs for therapists that focus on techniques that facilitate the expression of emotions, such as anger.

Bernfield, Clark, and Parker (1984) state that a neglected area of research concerns group process. The researchers suggest that one approach to measuring the process material of a group would be to classify all members' acts within a group into three categories: 1) task roles that help the group accomplish its task; 2) group roles that assist the group to maintain itself as a group; and 3) individual roles that do not assist the group in any way. Task roles were defined as problem identification, information seeking, information giving, and feasibility testing. Group building and maintenance included coordinating, mediating, facilitating, supporting, and following. Individual roles were defined as blocking, withdrawing, digressing, and seeking recognition. The model proposed by Bernfield et al. values task and group building roles and discounts individual roles as nonfunctional with respect to group growth. The researchers studied 22 Canadian adolescent inpatients between the ages of 13 to 17 years who attended group therapy. The number of sessions ranged from five to 40, with a median of 15. One-hour group sessions were divided into three 10-minute observation periods.

Results of the study indicated that in the early stages of group development, there was a higher proportion of group and individual roles compared to midstage, and in the later stages of group, there was a higher proportion of group roles and a lower proportion of individual roles (Bernfield et al., 1984). Additional findings suggested that group behavior was positively related to treatment length. Patients in short-term treatment demonstrated reduced group behavior, and those who attended group for a longer time (more than 15 sessions) exhibited increased group behavior. Clinical observations in the residential milieu supported a parallel between changes in group behavior and improvement in the residential setting.

Treatment efficacy is another area that calls for research attention. Because much current information is based on findings from adult research, the need exists to determine components of group treatment that are effective specifically for children and adolescents. A study conducted by Fine, Forth, Gilbert, and Haley (1991) sought to to assess the long-term impact on depressive symptoms of two forms of short-term (12 weeks) group treatment for depressed adolescents. Adolescents were randomly assigned to either a therapeutic support group or a social skills group. Results of the study indicated that adolescents in the therapeutic support group had significantly reduced depressive symptoms and increased self-concept immediately following group treatment and at the 9-month follow-up. Adolescents in the social support group did not manifest significant results following group treatment but did demonstrate equivalent improvement at the 9-month follow-up. The researchers propose that individuals in the throes of mood disturbance may require a supportive atmosphere before they can approach a more cognitive task like social skills. Therefore, Fine et al. (1991) suggest that a combined approach be used in group treatment for depressed adolescents commencing with a therapeutic support component in early sessions and the introduction of a social skills approach in later sessions.

Gilbert (1990, unpublished dissertation) conducted a study of a structured short-term (8 weeks) group intervention for sexually abused girls based on a review of the literature and clinical experience (Gilbert, 1988b). Gilbert used the Roy adaptation model (Roy, 1984) to structure the research questions and the study. Forty-seven girls between the ages of 9 and 14 years participated in the study. Subjects who had been sexually abused were randomly assigned to a treatment group and received the structured group nursing intervention (SGNI) (n = 17) or a control group and received standard agency treatment (n = 13). Seventeen girls who had not been sexually abused volunteered for a comparison group and did not receive treatment. Although four modes are acknowledged in the Roy adaptation model, the modes studied were self-concept, role-function, and interdependence. Subjects were tested four times, pretest and three posttests at 2-month intervals. Although group members, caseworkers, parents, and therapist evaluated the SGNI positively, and scores were in the direction desired on variables studied (self-concept, loneli-

BOX 26–1 • CULTURAL IMPLICATIONS OF GROUPS WITH CHILDREN

An area of concern in child psychiatric nursing is the need to reflect national trends related to changing demographic, cultural, and ethnic populations. According to Costantino, Malgady, and Rogler (1988b), culturally sensitive programs include the following characteristics: accessibility of mental health programs for people who differ culturally; the selection of traditional therapy models that coincide with the perceived cultural characteristics of the identified population; and the incorporation of the cultural characteristics of a specific group into the standard treatment modality.

Costantino, Malgady, and Rogler (1988b) developed a group therapy model that was sensitive to the needs of adolescents of Puerto Rican heritage at risk for mental illness due to minority status and bilingual or bicultural conflicts. This population is noted to underuse and have little success with traditional therapies. Based on the results of previous research (Costantino, Malgady, & Rogler, 1985; Costantino, Malgady, & Rogler, 1988a), the researchers initiated a group intervention based on a folk heroine or hero model for adolescents who were Puerto Rican. Fourteen females and seven male Puerto Rican students, between the ages of 11 to 14 years, were divided into three groups of six, seven, and eight students each. Nine sessions were conducted by a therapist who was Puerto Rican and a cotherapist. Each group session lasted 2 hours. All materials were prepared in English and Spanish, and either language was used in group. Although invited to attend group, only one group had mothers in attendance. Mothers' participation in group consisted of reading the biographies of heroes or heroines in Spanish, sharing personal experiences, and role playing.

The researchers (Costantino, Malgady & Rogler, 1988b) found that adolescents reported the benefits of group as valuing the biographies of Puerto Rican heroes and heroines, increasing sense of pride in their cultural heritage, increasing knowledge of self and others, and clarifying adolescent vocational interest.

REFERENCES

Costantino, G., Malgady, R. G., & Rogler, L. H. (1986). Cuento therapy: A culturally sensitive modality for Puerto Rican children. *Journal of Consulting and Clinical Psychology, 54,* 639–654.

Costantino, G., Malgady, R. G., & Rogler, L. H. (1988a). *Cuento therapy: Folktales as a culturally sensitive psychotherapy for Puerto Rican children.* Maplewood, NJ: Waterfront Press.

Costantino, G., Malgady, R. G., & Rogler, L. H. (1988b). Folk hero modeling therapy for Puerto Rican adolescents. Special issues: Mental health research and service issues for minority youth. *Journal of Adolescence, 11,* 155–165.

ness, role function), all participants in the study demonstrated improved scores on all measures administered.

In addition to the call for research on group interventions, culturally sensitive issues also need to be addressed, as described in Box 26-1.

Implications for Nursing

Group interventions provide numerous opportunities to demonstrate nursing expertise in defined populations with specific problems. Nurses need to develop clinical models of group interventions that address the human responses of children, adolescents, and families to actual or potential health problems. In addition, group interventions must reflect cultural sensitivity to changing cultural, ethnic, and demographic patterns in the United States.

Nursing research must provide evidence of the effectiveness of nursing models of group interventions. This author believes that an empiric, or outcome, perspective, and a qualitative, or process, perspective are needed to determine which group intervention approach is most effective for a specific member problem and the effectiveness of each session toward meeting group goals. Triangulation methodology may be most appropriate because it has the ability to provide a quantitative and qualitative perspective (Duffy, 1987; Jick, 1979; Murphy, 1989).

Summary

Group interventions for children and adolescents are of recent origin. Early group interventions were activity oriented and combined children of differing developmental and chronologic ages. In general, group interventions with children and adolescents are underused and are less likely to be found in the clinical or research literature. Siblings in particular are a neglected population; a paucity of literature relates to group psychotherapeutic interventions for siblings. In addition to activity therapy groups, current group interventions include group play therapy, peer group therapy, relationship-oriented group therapy, psychodynamic group psychotherapy, behavior group therapy, and psychoeducation groups for children, adolescents, or families. These approaches reflect a multitude of perspectives on conducting group therapy with children and adolescents.

Groups for families vary in philosophic perspective and have undergone considerable adaptation to address the current needs of families, such as grandparents raising emotionally disturbed grandchildren. One group intervention, the psychoeducation model, has gained in popularity in recent years. Psychoeducational groups provide an educational approach to a common problem experienced by group members in a supportive environment.

Group interventions for children, adolescents, and families merit nursing attention, both clinical and research, for several reasons. Group interventions are akin to peer groups, which are developmentally appropriate for children and adolescents. They provide opportunities for the treatment of human responses to actual or potential health problems in a social context. Group interventions also allocate a scarce resource, nurse therapists skilled in child growth and development and group therapy, to a larger number of children.

Nurse clinicians, theorists, and researchers who value group interventions have the opportunity to contribute to the discipline and science of nursing. Group interventions designed and conducted by child and adolescent psychiatric-mental health nurses that incorporate principles of development, cultural sensitivity, and group therapy offer the potential for effective therapeutic interventions with children, adolescents, and families. These interventions can promote adaptive human responses to actual or potential health problems. Nurse clinician theorists have the opportunity to develop models of group interventions that use a nursing theoretical perspective, and nurse researchers have the opportunity to provide qualitative and empiric data about the effectiveness of nurse-developed or nurse-led group interventions. To paraphrase a statement made by Martha Rogers in regard to challenges that nursing must address now and in the future, Rogers said that nurses must "get with it." This clinician believes that "get with it" also applies to child and adolescent psychiatric and mental health nurses who value group interventions with children, adolescents, and families.

REFERENCES

Bernfield, G., Clark, L., & Parker, G. (1984). The process of adolescent group psychotherapy. *International Journal of Group Psychotherapy*, *34*(1), 111–126.

Bornstein, M. T., Bornstein, P. H., & Walters, H. A. (1988). Children of divorce: Empirical evaluation of a group-treatment program. *Journal of Clinical Child Psychology*, *17*(3), 248–254.

Cole, M., & Cole, S. R. (1989). *The development of children*. New York: Scientific American Books.

Corder, B. F., Whiteside, L., & Haizlip, T. M. (1981). A study of curative factors in group psychotherapy with adolescents. *International Journal of Group Psychotherapy*, *31*(3), 345–355.

Critchley, D. L. (1982). Therapeutic group work with abused preschool children. *Perspectives in Psychiatric Care*, *20*(2), 79–85.

Crockett, M. S. (1984). Exploring peer relationships. *Journal of Psychosocial Nursing and Mental Health Services*, *22*(10), 18–25.

de Neuhaus, M. S. (1985). Stage 1: Preparation. In B. B. Siepker & C. S. Kandaras (Eds.), *Group therapy with children and adolescents: A treatment manual* (pp. 54–85). New York: Human Sciences Press.

Duffy, M. E. (1987). Methodological triangulation: A vehicle for merging quantitative and qualitative research methods. *Image: The Journal of Nursing Scholarship*, *19*(3), 130–133.

Ettin, M. F., Heiman, M. L., & Kopel, S. A. (1988). Group building: Developing protocols for psychoeducational groups. *Group*, *12*(4), 205–225.

Fine, S., Forth, A., Gilbert, M., & Haley, G. (1991). Group therapy for adolescent depressive disorder: A comparison of social skills and therapeutic support. *Journal of American Academy of Child and Adolescent Psychiatry*, *30*(1), 79–85.

Holman, S. L. (1985). A group program for borderline mothers and their toddlers. *International Journal of Group Psychotherapy*, *35*(1), 79–93.

Gilbert, C. M. (1988a). Children in women's shelters: A group intervention using art. *Journal of Child and Adolescent Psychiatric and Mental Health Nursing*, *1*(1), 7–13.

Gilbert, C. M. (1988b). Sexual abuse and group therapy. *Journal of Psychosocial Nursing and Mental Health Services*, *26*(5), 19–23.

Ginott, H. G. (1958). Play-group therapy: A theoretical framework. *International Journal of Group Psychotherapy*, *8*, 410–418.

Ginott, H. G. (1961). *Group psychotherapy with children*. New York: McGraw-Hill.

Ginott, H. G. (1975). Group therapy with children. In G. M. Gazda (Ed.), *Basis approaches to group psychotherapy and group counseling* (2nd ed.) (pp. 272–294). Springfield, IL: Charles C. Thomas.

Gottschalk, L. A. (1990). The new psychotherapies in the context of new developments in the neurosciences and biological psychiatry. *American Journal of Psychotherapy, 44*(3), 321–339.

Grunebaum, H., & Solomon, L. (1980). Toward a peer theory of group psychotherapy: On the developmental significance of peers and play. *International Journal of Group Psychotherapy, 30*(1), 23–49.

Grunebaum, H., & Solomon, L. (1982). Toward a theory of peer relationships II: On the stages of social development and their relationship to group psychotherapy. *International Journal of Group Psychotherapy, 32*(3), 283–307.

Jick, T. D. (1979). Mixing qualitative and quantitative methods: Traingulation in action. *Administrative Sciences Quarterly, 24*, 602-601.

Johnson, M. L. (1988). Use of play therapy in promoting social skills. *Issues in Mental Health Nursing, 9*, 105–112.

Kennedy, J. F., & Keeney, V. T. (1987). Group psychotherapy with grandparents rearing their emotionally disturbed grandchildren. *Group, 11*(10), 15–25.

Loomis, M. E. (1979). *Group process for nurses.* St. Louis: C.V. Mosby.

Loomis, M. E. (1991). Group therapy. In G. K. McFarland & M. D. Thomas (Eds.), *Psychiatric mental health nursing: Application of the nursing process* (pp. 767–779). Philadelphia: J.B. Lippincott.

Lothstein, L. (1985). Group therapy for latency age Black males: Unplanned interventions, setting, and racial transferences as catalysts for change. *International Journal of Group Psychotherapy, 35*(4), 603–623.

Masterman, S. H., & Reams, R. (1988). Support groups for bereaved preschool and school-age children. *American Journal of Orthopsychiatry, 58*(4), 562–570.

Moss, N. G. (1984). Child therapy groups in the real world. *Journal of Psychosocial Nursing and Mental Health Services, 22*(3), 43–48.

Murphy, S. A. (1989). Multiple triangulation: Application in a program of nursing research. *Nursing Research, 38*(5), 294–297.

Nathan, S. W., & Goetz, P. (1984), Psychosocial aspects of chronic illness: Group interactions in diabetic girls. *Children's Health Care, 13*(1), 24–29.

Owen, S. M., Rosenberg, J., & Barkley, D. (1985). A group treatment approach for children of alcoholics. *Group, 9*(3), 31–42.

Pond, E. F., & Gilbert, C. M. (1987). A support group offers help for parents of hyperactive children. *Children Today, 16*(6), 23–26.

Rachman, A. W., & Raubolt, R. R. (1984). The pioneers of adolescent group psychotherapy. *International Journal of Group Psychotherapy, 34*(3), 387–413.

Redston-Iselin, A. (1987). Adolescent psychiatric nursing. In G. W. Stuart & S. J. Sundeen (Eds.), *Principles and practice of psychiatric nursing* (2nd ed.) (pp. 897–924). St. Louis: C.V. Mosby.

Rose, S. R. (1985). Time-limited treatment groups for children. *Social Work with Groups, 8*(2), 17–27.

Rose, S. D., & Edleson, J. L. (1987). *Working with children and adolescents in groups.* San Francisco: Jossey-Bass.

Roy, C. (1984). *Introduction to nursing: An adaptation model* (2nd ed.). Englewood Cliffs, NJ: Prentice-Hall.

Sahler, O. J., & McAnarney, E. R. (1981). *The child from three to eighteen.* St. Louis: C.V. Mosby.

Schaffer, S., & Pollack, J. (1987). Listening to the adolescent therapy group. *Group, 11*(3), 155–164.

Scheidlinger, S. (1985). Group treatment of adolescents: An overview. *American Journal of Orthopsychiatry, 55*(1), 102–111.

Scheidlinger, S. (1984). Short-term group psychotherapy for children: An overview. *International Journal of Group Psychotherapy, 34*(4), 573–585.

Shirk, S. R. (1988). Causal reasoning and children's comprehension of therapeutic interpretations. In S. R. Shirk (Ed.), *Cognitive development and child psychotherapy* (pp. 53–89). New York: Plenum Press.

Siepker, B. B., Lewis, L. H., & Kandaras, C. S. (1985). *Relationship-oriented group psychotherapy with children and adolescents.* New York: Human Sciences Press.

Slavson, S. R. (1976). Play group therapy. In C. Schaefer (Ed.), *The therapeutic use of child's play* (pp. 241–259). New York: Jason Aronson.

Slavson, S. R., & Schiffler, M. (1975). *Group psychotherapies for children: A textbook.* New York: International Universities Press.

Slavson, S. R., & Schiffler, M. (1943). *An introduction to group psychotherapy.* New York: International Universities Press.

Sturkie, K. (1983). Structured group treatment for sexually abused children. *Health and Social Work, 8*(4), 299–308.

Vorrath, H. H., & Brendtro, L. K. (1974). *Positive peer culture.* Chicago, IL: Aldine Publishing.

Wayne, J., & Fine, S. B. (1986). *Group work with retarded mothers. Social Casework, 67*(4), 195–202.

Yalom, I. (1985). *The theory and practice of group psychotherapy* (3rd ed.). New York: Basic Books.

CHAPTER

27

Information Processing Approaches

Anne DuVal Frost

This chapter explains the application of information processing approaches for individual therapy and psychosocial programs. These applications are based on the cognitive framework of information processing explained in Chapter 7. The benefits of this approach appear to be in the efficiency of a condensing mechanism to transform perceptions or increase learning by using culturally and developmentally appropriate themes or subjects.

Theoretical Review

A goal of individual therapy and psychosocial programs is to facilitate a reconstruction of nontherapeutic information stored in long-term memory (LTM). The process requires environmental stimuli (analogy, axiom, story) that activate a "computer search" in LTM. This search promotes not only identification and understanding of the stimulus, but also agreement or disagreement. There is always a tendency to try to fit new stimuli into the current structure of LTM. Therefore, novel stimuli (e.g., intellectual twist, humor, alarm) have the greater potential for a "no fit" conclusion from LTM and a need for mixing or reconstruction in short-term memory (STM). The limited space in STM is used most effectively by developing a context of prior knowledge to act as an organizing structure with which new information can be linked or associated. This context, or mnemonic, not only assists in the reconstruction of information and storage in LTM, but also acts as a triggering device for recall and continued rehearsal and integration of new ideas or information. The most efficient mnemonic is a "many to one," in which a single slogan, theme, or story framework can be used to store or trigger multiple associations.

Mnemonic strategies, such as slogans and themes in individual therapy and story contexts in psychosocial programs, can be developed by using the following formula:

C—chunking of new information in a context of
R—relevant
I—imagery-provoking
P—prior knowledge that increases
R—rehearsal with
N—novel associations for new storage

Individual Therapy

MARCIE

Three-year-old Marcie was referred by her mother, Kathy, for being an "extremely difficult child." She reportedly terrorized her parents and two older sisters, ages 5 and 4, with inconsistent demands and if unmet, waves of temper tantrums. Marcie's parents responded to the temper tantrums first with reason, then with screams or isolation in her room.

Barbara Schoen Johnson: CHILD, ADOLESCENT AND FAMILY PSYCHIATRIC NURSING, © 1994 J.B. Lippincott Company

During assessment, Marcie appeared to be very bright, perhaps gifted, and concerned with ghosts. She explained that the ghosts came into her room at night and scared her. When asked what helped when the ghosts came, Marcie stated that she "would run to Mommy and Daddy's room to spend the night." This scenario was validated by Kathy, who added that each incident precipitated parental anger because of disrupted sleep and lack of energy for the next day.

Marcie also demonstrated the need for control, an apparent stimulus for temper tantrums, with a voracious desire to win the games played in therapy. Her need for control and lack of ego strength was corroborated by a furrowed brow and adamant "no" when it was time to stop play and leave the session. However, distraction, such as who would be the leader out of the room, proved an effective incentive.

The fear of ghosts was a natural developmental response to the "eye for an eye, tooth for a tooth" sense of justice of a preoperational child. Marcie lived in expectation of even greater retaliation than that which she had received. To help her gain control over irrational fears and break the cycle of nightmares, she was given a small cardboard "magic wand," which she was to use with a rhyme reminiscent of the familiar, "Rain, rain, go away; come again another day." The new rhyme, "Ghost, ghost, go away; I don't want to play," provided a novel twist that stimulated Marcie's attention for rehearsal. She asked in a surprised tone if ghosts really played. Her LTM store was obviously comparing the fearful associations about ghosts with the new information. I encouraged this "mixing" in STM with a reminder about Casper, the friendly ghost. This was followed by a short film strip about Casper, which Marcie operated and controlled on the "toy" projector. The concrete imagery of a friendly Casper, also an analogy for a small child whose well-intended antics are often misunderstood, seemed to provide some relief, as evidenced by the repetitious request for the filmstrip.

Kathy reported "stunning" results with the "magic wand" with a single exception. One night, Marcie awoke, could not find her wand, and reinstituted the old scenario that had been eliminated for 2 weeks. The next day, Kathy and Marcie visited the toy store for a plastic wand that was too big to lose.

CRIPRN SUMMARY. "Ghost, ghost, go away; I don't want to play," provides a many-to-one chunking rhyme for associating new information for diminishing the violent image of ghosts. In addition the rhyme was relevant to Marcie's developmental thinking and her need for a greater sense of control. The concrete imagery of a friendly, misunderstood ghost based on prior knowledge of Casper and a popular nursery rhyme created interest in rehearsal. The rehearsal was enhanced by the novel intellectual twist regarding the characteristics of ghosts, as well as a previously unacknowledged form of magical control.

In conjunction with therapy for Marcie, several meetings were held with her parents. Rather than strategies for every incident, a philosophy of "distract and diffuse" was suggested. The limited size of the mnemonic and the alliteration support recall for many possible interventions. It was explained that Marcie's need for control might be influenced by being intellectually precocious and the youngest of three. The many ramifications could be summarized by her apparent inability to "walk her talk," (another short alliterative mnemonic). In other words, her verbal ability made her appear more capable and open to reason than her preoperational stage allowed. Both parents agreed that they often "lumped" Marcie with her sisters instead of treating her as the 3-year-old that she is. Using Marcie's developmental predisposition to "magical thinking" to distract and therefore diffuse potential power struggles, it was suggested that narratives featuring concrete images of mythical characters might replace previous, abstract pleadings to "be good, considerate, and thoughtful of others." The parents embraced the idea and reported successful results within days. For example, when Marcie characteristically began to struggle over which chair she would sit in for breakfast, Kathy announced, "The fairy godmother was here last night and tapped her magic wand on this chair" (pointing to one that was not the focus of the trouble and one usually occupied by a parent). Marcie quickly ran to that chair, and breakfast proceeded smoothly. When the daily struggle over what to wear began, Kathy explained, "On Tuesdays, the fairy princesses in the fairy godmother's court always wear pink" (or whatever the color of the outfit that Kathy thought Marcie might prefer for the day). Eventually Marcie would ask the color of choice for the princesses for that day.

Marcie's parents were highly enthusiastic about their newly developed parental effectiveness. Their understanding of a mnemonic framework was evidenced by their report that the DND (distract and diffuse) plan was better than the former TNT plan and that explosions had been cut to a new low.

CRIPRN SUMMARY. Distract and diffuse provides a many-to-one chunking slogan for associating new information about parental discipline strategies that are relevant to the developmental level of a preoperational child. The concrete axiom is not imagery provoking itself but is associated with the concrete images of fairy tale characters that are the basis for its implementation. The alliteration is part of prior knowledge and the meaning of the words. The interest in rehearsal was enhanced by the "civilized" approach to discipline through fantasy play. This provided a novel intellectual twist to a previous value of "Spare the rod, and spoil the child."

During parent consultations it became clear that Kathy had a stringent superego and was struggling with the need for perfection in the role demands of parent, wife, and professional. The need appeared related to Kathy's former care of her mother. Kathy's mother had died after a lengthy hospitalization while she was pregnant with Marcie. Kathy had been the daily caretaker and primary advocate for navigating a bureaucratic, and often unsympathetic, health care system. Kathy became so bonded with her mother that this child of the 60s relinquished her feminist, avant garde framework for the traditional tenants of the Catholic Church, presumably important to her mother. This included attending daily Mass on behalf of her mother. This surrogate return to the church haunted Kathy after her mother's death with guilt about her failure to be a "good Catholic girl." She felt that her mother could see all of the things that she had done that were alien to the Church's teachings. Kathy focused on her premarital sexual behavior. Although not promiscuous by most standards, her behavior, she felt, might be interpreted as such by the strict definition of Catholic teachings. Treatment progressed with a new DND mnemonic because of its positive association of success with Marcie. In this context, DND would represent "disobey and develop, giving Kathy permission to refresh her so-called disobedient stage for healthy repossession of self and future development.

A quote was introduced from Oscar Wilde, "Disobedience in the eyes of anyone who has read history is man's original virtue." With a shiver, Kathy stated, "How perfect for a Woodstock hippie . . . Oscar Wilde was my mother's favorite." Needless to say, the rest of the session was devoted to conjecture about this seemingly powerful coincidence. Transference could not have had a better facilitator.

The following axioms also were used to act as mnemonics for ongoing deliberation and transformation of LTM:

> There are few chaste women who are not tired of their trade (La Rochefoucauld, *Maxims*).
>
> Our vocabulary is defective: we give the same name to a woman's lack of temptation and a man's lack of opportunity (Ambrose Bierce, *The Devil's Dictionary*).
>
> Chastity—the most unnatural of the sexual perversions (Aldous Huxley, *Eyeless in Gaza XXVIII*).

Kathy continues in treatment at the time of this writing but recently stated "I have found my old self." She explained that this realization was based, in part, on a sudden dissatisfaction with her wardrobe. Most of the clothes had been bought before and shortly after her mother's death. Kathy now considered them dowdy and has decided to replace them with a "fresh, new, current look."

CRIPRN SUMMARY. "Disobey and develop" provides a many-to-one chunking slogan for associating new information about moral values that are relevant to the development of a less stringent superego. The concrete axiom is not imagery provoking itself but is associated with images of credible writers and poets respected for their insight and wisdom. The effectiveness of the previous "distract and diffuse" slogan had been stored as prior knowledge and the familiar alliteration. Rehearsal was enhanced by the novel permission to "act out." Permission to do the opposite of what Kathy thought she had been taught was both alarming and exciting.

LYNNE

Lynne, age 47, came for consultation about the possible effect of her stress on her 6-year-old daughter. She explained the immediate family constellation as her husband Tommy; a 28-year-old son, Bob, who had been a drug addict since high school; a 22-year-old daughter, Karen, who was "fine"; a daughter, Carol, who had died 4 years earlier at age 7; and her adopted 6-year-old, Claire.

Lynne explained that she was very worried about her son, who had been in several rehabilitation programs but had left the last one prematurely, a few months earlier. She stated that he was not doing well. Lynne said that she had been having such severe panic attacks and that she had recently sought emergency room care for a possible heart attack. The emergency room examination and a subsequent battery of tests by a private physician revealed no biophysical concerns.

Assessment of family dynamics revealed a codependency framework focused on Bob. Family interventions included financial bail outs and frequent phone calls across country to check on him. Further systems assessment revealed a number of recent deaths among friends and family, which included a niece, two nephews, and Bob's friend, all young adults. These deaths (some drug-related), the death of her daughter, and Bob's continued history of dugs and "street life" resulted in a supposition that Lynne could lose her son. When confronted with the possibility that her panic attacks related to a fear of Bob's death, Lynne looked shocked but responded immediately with, "I don't think I would survive." Further exploration revealed a fear that her husband and older daughter would not survive such a loss. Negating the presenting reason for consultation, Lynne felt 6-year-old Claire would do "OK."

It seemed obvious that therapy should focus on releasing Lynne from responsibility for Tommy and Karen's vulnerability and from her role in the family's pattern of codependency. This included validation of the potential loss of Bob and Bob's right to choices. The first issue was organized around the provocative mnemonic of "Sometimes it is easier to die than to live." While this was initially frightening, discussing the "uphill battle" of addiction and the analogy of a lifelong battle with cancer seemed helpful.

Next, the near-death experience and its reported characteristics were discussed. Comparing the associations of the pain of death with the novel ideas about the comfort of death, stimulated attention and rehearsal. Lynne worked on transforming death as an experience of suffering to an experience of gentle transition.

Then the issue of codependency was analyzed. At a moment of great frustration when Lynne was saying, "Why can't he just do what he should?" The therapeutic retort was, "It sounds as if Bob's addiction is as strong as yours." Again the novel and provocative concept stimulated rapt attention and an interest in rehearsal. Lynne's reply of "but I'm not addicted" was followed by "You may be addicted to Bob." Lynne was then asked to examine her inability to stop the bail outs and oversolicitous communications as an addictive pattern. Again, the shock that she and the family might be using problematic behavior as inflexible as Bob's increased Lynne's willingness to see the unproductive influence of codependency.

The next step of shedding responsibility for Bob's rehabilitation (other than being there for him with appropriate fiscal support for treatment) was to use an analogy of prearranged marriages reminiscent of the European heritage of this family and a likely LTM store. When asked if she would consider choosing a wife for Bob, Lynne laughed and said, "Of course not." "But aren't you trying to choose his life-style?" "Yes, but that's to protect him." Again the therapeutic retort, "but do you have any more right to protect him than to choose a wife for him?" Lynne's response, "but if we don't protect him, he will die," was met by, "but it may be easier to die" and "to die may be a choice."

These excerpts represent the major mnemonic themes. After 11 sessions, Lynne no longer experienced panic attacks and had discarded the tranquilizer prescribed by her internist. She also reported telling her husband to stop his addiction. They are no longer making daily phone calls or sending money. Lynne is sending humorous cards but as she stated, no advice.

CRIPRN SUMMARY. "Sometimes it is easier to die than to live," provides a many-to-one chunking slogan for associating new information about the potential choices and fate of Lynne's addicted son. It is relevant to acknowledge the repressed fear that was causing Lynne's panic attacks. The concrete slogan is not imagery provoking itself but was quickly associated with prior knowledge of images of battles (uphill battle) and the ravages of war. Rehearsal was enhanced by the novel suggestion that addiction is a chronic battle and the alarming intellectual "twist" that death might be preferable to life.

Characterizing Lynne's behavior as an addiction to Bob became a many-to-one chunking theme that clarified supportive versus codependent interventions that are relevant to ego-enhancing experiences for all members of the family. While the concrete slogan is not imagery provoking itself, it was associated with the "wasted" images of what Lynne called "druggies." Rehearsal was enhanced by the novelty of alarm when it was suggested that Lynne's behavior, like her son's, was harmful.

JULIA

Eighteen-year-old Julia frequently compromised the development of friendships with males and females. Shortly after the initiation of a relationship, she began self-criticism, conducting an inventory of all of the things "wrong" with her. She was consistently convinced that no one would like her when they found out what she was really like.

To facilitate her awareness of an overactive superego and the practice of a self-fulfilling prophecy, Julia was asked what she considered the greatest symbol for rules and authority. Her reply of the Supreme Court Justices provided a concrete, imagery-provoking analogy for a stringent superego.

It was suggested that every time Julia began a relationship, she seemed symbolically to telephone Washington to alert all nine justices to start frowning and shaking their fingers in disapproval. The therapist also acted out this provocative mock response as the "picture was painted." Julia, looking slightly alarmed, added, "So what you're saying is I should fire at least half?" She smiled at the humor of the therapist's suggestion to "fire all nine and substitute them with a fairy godmother."

CRIPRN SUMMARY. "Fire the Justices" became the organizing therapeutic theme and slogan for Julia when considering her psychodynamics and behavioral consequences. The many-to-one chunking slogan was a relevant analogic symbol for a stringent superego. The concrete imagery of black-robed judges being replaced by a kindly fairy godmother was an effective use of prior knowledge associated with these symbols. Julia eagerly tested the application through repeated rehearsal, admitting the effectiveness of the novelty by saying, "Every time I think of those funny judges shaking their fingers at me, I laugh and then say, get lost!"

Psychosocial Programs

Community-based psychosocial programs pose practice challenges that differ from individual therapy. The group constellation, prose format, and one-time presentation of most programs require that a responsive chord between nurse and clients be struck at the outset. Learning can be facilitated and a student–teacher relationship avoided by the use of a media mnemonic. A media mnemonic uses a media-promoted theme, character, or narrative that is socially and culturally familiar to the learner and provides relevant association with the health information. A media mnemonic incorporates the client's sociocultural tools, limiting the amount of effort necessary to understand new information by providing familiar associations. The media mnemonic also may evoke feelings of partial "ownership" of the curriculum and associations of entertainment and fun.

FAMILY VIOLENCE AND "THRILLER"

Michael Jackson's video "Thriller" was used for a group of three female adolescents who were referred by their high school guidance teacher for a variety of symptoms that included academic negligence, sexual acting out, and possible substance abuse. The guidance counselor suspected substance abuse and family violence in their homes. Two of the adolescents had previously tried and "given up" individual therapy.

At the contracting meeting, the adolescents demonstrated disdain, skepticism, and general resistance to further treatment. The therapist suggested an initial contract of three sessions of music video, telling the clients that a different video would be used for each session, the first being "Thriller." This occurred at the height of the video's popularity, and response to its novel use was reflected in interest and questions, such as "What's this all about?" and "You mean we're just going to watch videos?"

It was explained that while most videos were entertaining, they often dealt with meaningful issues. The clients were assured that the therapist would act as a resource and that the extent and direction of the discussion would be guided by them.

The dialogue of the first session began with an enthusiastic clamor about Michael Jackson. As the video story unfolded, a young man (Michael Jackson) was proposing under a moonlit sky to his girlfriend. This romantic scene abruptly changed to one of fear as the young man dramatically transformed into a werewolf. His girlfriend's ineffective screaming and lack of escape attempts stimulated reactions of disbelief from the clients and general concerns about female vulnerability to sexual assault.

The fearful scene of impending violence changed to one of relief when the two characters were shown as "players within a play." They were still in the role of boyfriend and girlfriend but as members of a movie audience watching the scene just described. This relief was followed by a postmovie walk home by the couple. Their route took them through a poorly lit cemetery suddenly populated by partially decayed residents rising from their graves. When the girlfriend turned for protection to her formerly solicitous date, she discovered that he too had become a ghoulish monster.

The predominant theme of boyfriend-turned-monster continued throughout the video. This plus the disarming music and extraordinary dancing seemed to lower resistances and stimulate discussion. The discussion focused on adults who "one minute sell you a bill of goods and the next minute are too drunk to fix dinner or are trying to slap you around."

This representative statement led to client sharing of similar family experiences with parents compromised by substance abuse. The painful life-style characterized by inconsistency, lack of trust, self-doubt, and general helplessness was acknowledged by all three clients. A clear outcome of the session was the realization of a shared experience so often denied in children of substance abusers.

"Thriller" initiated two successive three-part series of music videos followed by individual therapy for two of the clients. The guidance counselor reported a change in attitude by all three clients and "a greater openness to discussion."

CRIPRN SUMMARY. "Thriller" provided a many-to-one chunking context with a sequence of story events in a relevant analogy of caretaker to monster that represents the lived experience of children of substance abusers. The concrete characters and actions of the video provided stimuli for imagery representations. The familiarity of "Thriller" provided a context of prior knowledge usually associated with pleasure and entertainment. Rehearsal of new information was enhanced by the video's novel use and perhaps because it provided a context that "belongs" to the adolescent culture.

FUN WITH THE FLINTSTONES

Slides of Flintstone cartoons were used with latency-aged children to foster confidence in their cognitive and psychosocial competencies. The setting for the cartoons is a stone age civilization with contemporary values and life-style. The two featured families are the Flintstones and the Rubbles. The adult males, Fred and Barney, repeatedly used poor assessment skills and therefore ineffective interventions for daily crises. Although well-intended, their "pie in the sky" plans seldom resulted in successful outcomes.

Their wives, Wilma and Betty, represent the sound, reality-oriented decision making of wise parents. Fred and Barney are reminiscent of impulsive, error-prone children. Fortunately the wives' response to Fred and Barney is always one of tolerance, forgiveness, and support.

The children were seemingly delighted with the vulnerability of the adults. With ongoing discussion of the cartoons' events, they appeared more willing to view their own problem-solving skills with less defensiveness. An 8-year-old boy stated, "If Fred can mess up and try again, so can I." A classmate stated, "Fred never really gets upset with himself. Every day seems to be a new start."

CRIPRN SUMMARY. The Flintstones cartoons provided a many-to-one chunking context with a sequence of story events in a relevant analogy of "good guys" who try hard, fail, and try again. The concrete characters provided stimuli for imagery representations. The familiarity of the cartoon series provided a context of prior knowledge usually associated with entertainment and fun. Rehearsal of new information was enhanced by the novel use of the cartoons and the humorous dilemmas of Fred and Barney.

OVER THE RAINBOW

A case study of Dorothy Gale in the Land of Oz was presented to young adolescents as a context to stimulate discussion about the relationship between developmental needs and conflicts and their impact on family relationships, academic success, and evolving independence. The following case summary was distributed to each participant. It was used as a quick review before excerpts from a video of the original 1939 MGM movie were discussed.

Dorothy is a young adolescent living with her aunt and uncle on a Kansas farm. She has a small white dog named Toto whom she adores. As the story begins, Dorothy is frantically seeking help for a situational crisis involving Toto. Miss Gulch, a cruel spinster neighbor, arrives to take Toto to the sheriff where he will supposedly be destroyed for attempting to bite her. Dorothy's Auntie Em and Uncle Henry appear powerless to intervene. Toto is placed in Miss Gulch's bicycle basket but escapes a few minutes after the dark journey begins and returns to Dorothy.

At this point, a tornado suddenly strikes the farm and carries Dorothy, Toto, and the farmhouse swirling "over the rainbow" to the land of Oz. Oz at first appears beautiful, and Dorothy finds herself the heroine of the little people called the Munchkins, because the farmhouse landed on the Wicked Witch of the East and killed her. A celebration is in progress when yet another crisis begins. The Wicked Witch of the West appears and threatens revenge on Dorothy and Toto for killing her sister. Magical intervention comes in the form of Glinda, the good witch of the North.

When the Wicked Witch is gone, Dorothy tells Glinda that she wants to go home to Kansas. Glinda suggests that she enlist the aid of the Wizard of Oz and sets her off on the yellow brick road that will take her to the Emerald City, where the Wizard lives. Along the way, she and Toto acquire three traveling companions who decide that the Wizard might be able to help them attain the things they most want: a brain for the Scarecrow, a heart for the Tinman, and the courage for the Cowardly Lion. When they reach the Emerald City and are granted an audience with the seemingly powerful Wizard, they are given a task to complete before he will assist them: to return with the broomstick of the Wicked Witch of the West.

Fortified with group support, Dorothy and her companions face numerous trials requiring intelligence, mutual concern, and bravery. They successfully destroy the Wicked Witch by "melting" her with a bucket of water and return triumphantly to the Wizard, broomstick in hand. It is then that they discover that the Wizard has no extraordinary powers and is "but a mere man."

Once more Glinda appears to help Dorothy recognize her own ability to return to Kansas. Dorothy says goodbye to her three companions who are now fully aware of their inherent strengths and abilities. In fact, they will take over the responsibilities of running Oz in place of the now defunct Wizard.

Dorothy suddenly finds herself back in Kansas surrounded by her concerned and loving family and friends. Dorothy leaves us with her profound realization that "there's no place like home."

CRIPRN SUMMARY. "The Wizard of Oz" provided a many-to-one chunking context with a sequence of story events in a relevant analogy of the adolescent's strivings for independence and the concomitant ambivalence of leaving home. The concrete characters and events provided stimuli for imagery representations. The familiarity of "The Wizard of Oz" provided a context of prior knowledge usually associated with entertainment and fun. Rehearsal of new information was enhanced by the novel use of the movie and perhaps because the movie is a popular artifact of American culture.

SMURF

Four 6-year-olds vigorously compete in a relay race. The first one who reaches the finish line yells, "I'm the winner. Now I have three checks and a smurf prize." Another 6-year-old is successful in advancing past her peers in a game of "red smurf, green smurf" ("red light, green light"). At the completion, she announces, "See, I followed the directions. I'm a great Smurf!"

These children were part of a program called SMURF (Frost, 1984a). This is a mnemonic for social motivation using recreation and fantasy. The children were referred by their classroom teacher for consistently disruptive behavior. An average day found them sitting more in the school corridor than in their classroom.

In the SMURF program, these children were engaged in sensorimotor activities designed to give practice and recognition to their increasing ability to control their bodies from impulsive discharge. Fantasy was used through SMURF games and the symbolic role playing of the Smurf cartoon characters. Self-accountability was strengthened through each nursing intervention. One of the most successful strategies for practicing impulse control in the classroom was a rhyme the children were directed to use in a whisper to themselves: "Smurfs are great; Smurfs can wait."

CRIPRN SUMMARY. SMURF provided a many-to-one chunking context with the story "line" and characters of the popular Smurf television cartoons in a relevant analogy of responsible, yet error-prone, children and kind, but limit-setting, adults. The concrete characters and cartoon stories provided stimuli for imagery representations. The familiarity of the Smurfs provided a context of prior knowledge usually associated with entertainment and fun. Rehearsal was enhanced by the novel use of a Smurf context of play in a grade-school setting.

THE THREE LITTLE KITTENS

A parent education program, "the good side of bears, wolves, and witches," used slides of familiar nursery rhymes and fairy tales to associate early childhood principles of growth and development. The use of "Goldilocks and the Three Bears" is discussed with a summary of related research in Chapter 7; the curriculum script for "Goldilocks" from the research study is given in Box 27-1 to clarify the difference in presentation of information in a didactic format, story grammar, and media mnemonic.

The story of the "Three Little Kittens" was presented during the prototype program for the research study as a representation of the relationship between a mother and her children and the limit-setting strategies of one particular system.

As we recall from the familiar rhyme, the three kittens have lost their mittens. Their mother's response is, "What? Lost your mittens? You naughty Kittens. Then you shall have no pie." One of the first parental comments was, "I don't blame the mother cat for being angry. After all, do you know the cost of mittens today?" She continued by surmising that the mother cat most likely had "on record" numerous warnings for the kittens not to remove their mittens when playing outside. The group then considered the appropriateness of withdrawal of food as a punishment and explored the special significance of sweets.

As the story progresses, we learn that the kit-

(text continues on page 391)

BOX 27–1 • PROGRAM SCRIPT, "GOLDILOCKS AND THE THREE BEARS"

INSTRUCTIONS

The characters and events in "Goldilocks and the Three Bears" will be used as a teaching strategy to illustrate developmental reactions of an older sibling, Goldilocks, to the arrival of a younger sibling, Baby Bear.

Before explaining developmental principles, let's review the story of "Goldilocks and the Three Bears." It begins with Mama, Papa, and Baby Bear taking a walk in the woods. Goldilocks, lost and frightened, comes upon their house and goes in to seek comfort. She finds three bowls of porridge on the table. She tries Papa Bear's bowl but it is too hot; she tries Mama Bear's bowl but it is too cold; she tries Baby Bear's bowl, and "it is just right," so she "eats it all up." Goldilocks then seeks a comfortable chair. She rejects Papa and Mama Bear's chairs as being too hard and too soft but accepts Baby Bear's as being "just right." At that moment, to her horror, Baby Bear's chair breaks. Next, Goldilocks decides to take a nap but rejects Papa and Mama Bear's beds as being too hard and too soft but accepts Baby Bear's bed as being "just right." Goldilocks falls asleep, only to be awakened by the return of the three bears. Terrified, she leaps from the bed and runs out of the house to the astonishment and bewilderment of the bears.

"Goldilocks and the Three Bears," while an entertaining children's story, also contains a theme of sibling rivalry. Goldilocks, who represents the older sibling, once the "fair-haired" or favored child, feels rejected by parents who have become "bears." The alliance of the parents and new baby, as represented by the three bears, sets Goldilocks apart as different and alone. She fears retaliation from parents who have become wild animals. Being "lost in the woods" represents the helplessness and anxiety resulting from the change in once-familiar routines and relationships. This program explains how the intellectual and emotional stages of development of children 3 through 5 years of age cause children to think illogically and misinterpret their parents' good intentions. If parents understand the developmental thought processes of young children, which differ greatly from adult thought processes, they may be better able to prevent stress and future problems for the older sibling. In addition, this knowledge also may build parental confidence and decrease the stress of parenting.

Let's take a closer look at "Goldilocks and the Three Bears" for developmental explanations:

Goldilocks' fears and anxiety are due in part to her thinking process, which differs greatly from that of adults. The thinking of 3- through 5-year-old children is egocentric. This does not mean that they are selfish; they just have only one way to view a situation. They assume that their personal view is shared by everyone else. This prevents empathy with others and forces rejection of statements or behaviors that appear contradictory to their own. Likewise, children age 3 through 5 interpret the impact of all events according to how the events affect their own comfort and happiness. Therefore, when Goldilocks' parents explained that there would be a new baby, she was interested in how the event would affect her routine and the relationship with her parents. When the parents' time, energy, and affection had to be shared, Goldilocks may not have believed statements, such as, "We have enough love for two children" or "You'll learn to love the baby." Without concrete demonstrations of love and attention, such statements of adult logic would be rejected. Instead, such statements may foster anger or alienation.

The inability to accept such parental statements is complicated by an aspect of egocentrism called "magical" thinking. In magical thinking, Goldilocks assumes that all events are directly influenced by her thoughts or actions. In addition, the association between influence and event, or cause and effect, are often illogical. For example, the 3- through 5-year-old may associate stating the rhyme, "Rain, rain, go away. Come again another day," with the eventual cessation of the rain.

Likewise, Goldilocks may assume that her behavior influenced the arrival of the new baby. Because a child age 3 through 5 measures "good and bad" behavior according to the ability to follow parental rules and expectations, he or she may interpret the new baby as punishment for "bad" behavior. In other words, Goldilocks may think that if she had done more to please her parents and make them happy, they would not have needed another child. Identifying the behaviors that usually please parents, Goldilocks may further assume that had toys been put away more frequently or teeth brushed more effectively, there would have been less parental dissatisfaction and less need for another child.

There is little wonder that such primitive thinking may cause Goldilocks to feel angry and anxious. It is easy to understand how she could feel lost and view parents as strange and threatening. The fact that the bears went for a walk by themselves emphasizes how left out and alone the older sibling may feel.

The next three story events—eating Baby Bear's porridge, breaking Baby Bear's chair, and sleeping in Baby Bear's bed—all represent attempts by the older sibling to decrease feelings of anger and anxiety.

Tasting Papa Bear's and Mama Bear's porridge but finding that Baby Bear's was best represents Goldilocks' longing to gain her former family position of being the baby. Eating Baby Bear's porridge is an unconscious

(*continued*)

BOX 27–1 • PROGRAM SCRIPT, "GOLDILOCKS AND THE THREE BEARS" (*Continued*)

symbolic attempt to gain Baby Bear's power to influence the way Mama and Papa Bear focus their time and attention. Parents often report that the older sibling asks to taste the baby's food or to drink from the baby's bottle.

Testing Papa and Mama Bear's chairs but finding Baby Bear's chair "just right" again represents the older sibling's desire to regain the former family position of being the baby and foregoing the challenge of acting more "grown up." Breaking Baby Bear's chair just by sitting on it represents the inevitable and natural aggression that Goldilocks feels for Baby Bear. The baby's toys and possessions are a representative target of aggression when, in reality, Goldilocks would like to see Baby Bear "broken" and thrown away. While children may not act on their feelings and break the baby's possessions, parents should assume that feelings of aggression are usually present.

Testing Papa and Mama Bear's bed and finding that Baby Bear's bed was "just right" is the third confirmation of wanting to avoid growing up and instead to regain the position of baby and family life as it used to be. Parents often tell stories of the older sibling getting into the baby's crib or trying to reclaim some outgrown piece of equipment once theirs but now being used by the baby.

The next part of the story, the three bears returning home to find the empty bowl, broken chair, and Goldilocks sleeping in Baby Bear's bed, is very frightening. Being caught in misdeeds is frightening because the child age 3 through 5 thinks of justice as "an eye for an eye and a tooth for a tooth." This means that Goldilocks expects retaliation that duplicates her misbehavior. For example, for breaking the chair, she expects the bears to break something of hers, or if the chair is only symbolic of wanting to hurt the baby, then there is the fear that the bears will hurt her. Therefore, Goldilocks may exaggerate the bears' logical response and expect the harsh violent consequences of wild animals that far outweigh the misdeed.

This expectation of exaggerated retaliatory parental response is just as common for thoughts as for deeds. Children 3 through 5 years old believe that thoughts have the same power as deeds. Therefore, they believe that these thoughts can cause harm and therefore bring punishment.

In the story, when Goldilocks is discovered in Baby Bear's bed, she jumps up and runs out, "never to return to that house again." This represents an opportunity to be allowed to get away with angry thoughts and escape from harsh punishments. Punitive parental responses will result in excessive guilt. Logical explanations usually are lost in the illogical thinking of the child. Therefore, the type of response most supportive of the child's developmental stage should reflect a preestablished set of consistent age-appropriate limits, rules, and expectations. When a child does not fulfill an expectation, an opportunity is needed to "undo" or make up for the misbehavior. This may mean assisting in a repair or becoming a supervised helper in the care of the baby.

However, it is much harder to provide support for the older sibling when there are no behavioral clues to angry thoughts. While you may not be aware of the child's anger, the child believes that the parent is always aware of his or her thoughts. Again, egocentrism causes the child to think that his or her view is the only one. Angry thoughts may make the child as anxious as "misdeeds" because of the same expectation of retaliation. To provide developmental support, the child should be allowed to "get away" with angry thoughts. In other words, if parents assume that angry thoughts are a natural response to sibling rivalry, the child's day should be planned to include opportunities to turn negative thoughts and deeds into positive accomplishments. The more the child feels that his or her specific behaviors and tasks satisfy parental rules and expectations, the more the child can escape feelings of being naughty with the accompanying expectation of punitive punishment and feelings of guilt.

SUMMARY

Goldilocks represents the once favored fair-haired older child.

"Lost in the woods" represents replacement by the baby for failure to please the parents.

The bears represent the expectation of harsh punishments of "an eye for an eye and a tooth for a tooth" sense of justice.

Eating Baby Bear's porridge represents an attempt to gain the baby's power to influence parental time and attention.

Breaking Baby Bear's chair represents the typical aggressive thoughts and deeds toward the baby.

Sleeping in Baby Bear's bed represents an attempt to regain the former position in the family and the way things used to be.

Escape from the Bear's house represents running from the guilt of punitive punishments for either thoughts or deeds.

The years 3 through 5 are important as a foundation for later development. Accurate assessment of children's thinking and behavior is an important key to supportive responses.

tens respond to their mother's anger with sadness at having failed. With vigorous efforts, they search for the mittens in an attempt to "undo" the broken rule. When the mittens are found, the kittens immediately tell their mother of their success. Mother's response is, "What? Found your mittens? You good little kittens. Then you shall have some pie."

Again the topic of food was discussed, this time in regard to its appropriateness as a reward. There also was concern about the positive and negative aspects of what some parents considered a form of bribery.

Again returning to the story, in their eagerness to eat the pie, the kittens have not removed their mittens. Once more the kittens are in the shameful position of presenting what the reader assumes is another broken rule. Again mother's response is, "What? Soiled your mittens? You naughty kittens."

At this point, some mothers became outraged that the kittens were "set up" for failure. The rationale was that small children are impulsive in their efforts to enjoy treats. It was suggested that the mother cat should have given more supervision with gentle reminders that must be repeated to overcome a child's distractibility.

The group's discussion concluded that the mother recognized the kittens' despair and suggested an appropriate alternative to the dilemma because the kittens then proudly report to their mother that their mittens are washed. The mother's response is, "What? Washed your mittens? You darling kittens!"

The last two lines of the story gave special closure to the mother–child relationship. Mother cat says, "but I smell a rat close by! Hush, hush, hush!"

Several mothers concluded that the message strongly indicated that whether one's values determined the kitten's behavior as good or bad, such judgment would not affect the ultimate responsibility of the parent as one of acceptance, support, and protection from both physical and emotional harm.

CRIPRN SUMMARY. "The Three Little Kittens" provided a many-to-one chunking context with a sequence of story events in a relevant analogy of parenting with regard to discipline and nurture. The concrete characters and plot provided stimuli for imagery representations. The familiarity of "The Three Little Kittens" provided a context of prior knowledge usually associated with the parental pleasure of entertaining one's child. Rehearsal of new information was enhanced by the nursery rhyme's novel use and its disarming association with parental nurture in the American culture.

Summary

This chapter describes the application and usefulness of information processing in therapy with children, adolescents, and their families. Metaphors, analogies, anecdotes, and axioms are concrete cognitive mechanisms that can help the client make therapeutic gains. STM, LTM, and external memory are explained. Chunking, imagery, and mnemonic strategies are explored. The use of mnemonic strategies in psychiatric-mental health nursing is still new but offers promise for time- and cost-efficient interventions that yield effective results.

REFERENCES

Frost, A. D. (1984a). The use of smurfs for increased body control and self accountability. *Journal of Holistic Nursing, 2*(a), 38–42.

Frost, A. D. (1984b). The use of rock music to assist adolescent sexual identity. *Imprint, 13*(4), 36–42.

CHAPTER

28

Behavior Management

N. Margaret Brunett and Sue Cutbirth

Behavior management is a term that is widely used in child and adolescent psychiatric nursing practice. The effectiveness of patient outcome, that is, adaptive behavior change, depends on the practitioner's knowledge, skill, and ability in applying behavior management principles in the practice setting or milieu. The psychiatric nurse applies behavior management principles in everyday practice in inpatient and outpatient settings. The child and adolescent psychiatric nurse must have a clear conceptual picture of behavior management and its principles to influence adaptive behavior changes.

This chapter offers a conceptual definition of behavior management and its theoretical framework. Behavior management principles are identified and operationally defined (Box 28-1). Child and adolescent Clinical Examples illustrate the application of the nursing process and behavior management nursing interventions.

Historic Review

Behavior therapy with children originated around the turn of the 20th century. Lightner Witmer, the founder of clinical psychology, was the first to apply psychologic principles to the treatment of children's behavioral problems. Witmer's clinical focus examined observed behavior versus inferred inner processes (Witmer, 1907). Two decades later, Mary Cover Jones (1924) published her work in treating a child with an irrational fear of furry objects in which she used the principles of respondent conditioning. Although the earliest attempts to apply psychologic principles to clinical problems had taken place with children (Witmer, 1907; Jones, 1924), as late as 1944 there was little published professional literature about behavior therapy with children (Ross, 1964). Most of the work in behavior therapy prior to World War II went unheeded by the psychiatric community. The psychodynamic model, greatly influenced by the work of Sigmund Freud, remained the dominant force in the treatment of children until the mid-1960s (Ross, 1959). Behavior therapy, which gained a legitimate foothold in the 1950s and 1960s, was used primarily to treat adults. The writings of Skinner (1953), Eysenck (1957), Wolpe (1958), Bandura (1961), and Ullmann and Krasner (1965) influenced the growth and acceptance of behavior therapy among clinicians.

The central characteristic of the behavioral approach is a sense of commitment to continuing empiric evaluation of treatment effectiveness (Gelfand & Hartmann, 1984). In addition, the knowledge base of behavior therapy is derived from psychologic research (Ross, 1978). Early behavioral techniques were drawn from learning principles and procedures developed in laboratory research. Pioneering behavior therapists sought to help their clients learn, unlearn, or relearn critical aspects of their response repertoire.

BOX 28–1 • GLOSSARY OF BEHAVIOR MANAGEMENT TERMS AND PRINCIPLES

Chaining—the systematic linking of simple behaviors that have been successfully learned into a complex skill through stimulus contingency management.

Conditioned response—a behavior elicited by a conditioned stimulus achieved by pairing the conditioned stimulus (Pavlov's bell) with a naturally occurring stimulus (food) over a period of time.

Conditioned stimulus—the antecedent to a conditioned response achieved by pairing the conditioned stimulus with a naturally occurring stimulus over a period of time (Pavlov's hungry dog conditioned to salivate by the ringing of a bell).

Consequence—what happens as a result of something else; all behavior has a consequence of positive, negative, or neutral.

Differential reinforcement—a process to decrease the strength of the maladaptive response by reinforcing other behavior that is incompatible with the targeted maladaptive behavior.

Eliciting stimulus—the antecedent to a response.

Extinction—a neutral consequence in which positive and negative reinforcers are withheld, thereby reducing the strength of a behavior.

Fading—a stimulus control process that gradually withdraws the schedule of the presentation of the antecedent event.

Imitation—the act of formulating an identity with another person.

Implosion—a behavioral technique of repeated exposure of an individual to fearful or anxiety-producing stimuli in an effort to decrease the strength of the stimuli.

Modeling—a method of changing behavior through imitation.

Negative reinforcement—the removal of an aversive event, which strengthens and allows adaptive behavior to continue.

Overcorrection—a form of punishment whereby one is held accountable to restore to the original state and improve on the original state that which was negatively impacted by one's behavior (response).

Overt behavior—an action rather than a thought or feeling emitted by an individual that can be measured or counted.

Positive reinforcement—a positive consequence that acts as a reinforcing event.

Premack's principle—for any two behaviors exhibited by an individual, the less frequent behavior can be increased by making access to the more attractive behavior contingent on the emission of the lower rate behavior.

Prompting—cueing to facilitate an adaptive response.

Punishment—a negative consequence, such as the application of an aversive event or the removal of a rewarding event, which serves to suppress maladaptive behavior patterns.

Reinforcing event—a consequence to a response that increases the likelihood of the response recurring.

Reprimand—a verbal rebuke given to a child or individual for displaying maladaptive behavior, which is considered a form of punishment.

Response—an emitted behavior by an individual.

Response cost—a form of punishment used in a token economy system where points are taken away from a child or adolescent when maladaptive behavior is emitted by the individual.

Shaping—an operant behavioral reinforcement principle used to reward successive approximation toward a terminal goal of adaptive behavior.

Stimulus—the antecedent to a response.

Systematic desensitization—the gradual exposure to fear and anxiety-provoking stimuli guided by the individual's ability to apply newly learned counterphobic strategies.

Time out—the time during which a child or adolescent is removed from any positive reinforcement.

Thinning—a gradual decrease in the schedule on which positive reinforcers are presented.

Unconditioned response—the behavior emitted as the result of an unconditioned stimulus.

Unconditioned stimulus—the antecedent that elicits an unconditioned response.

Behavior therapy has continually developed its knowledge base. In recent years, new areas of research, such as social and cognitive psychology, have contributed knowledge that has been successfully integrated into behavior therapy programs. Since the mid-1960s, the scope of behavior therapy has significantly broadened and diversified with ongoing changes in definition, theory, principle, and technique (Werry & Wollersheim, 1989). It is not surprising to note that more clinicians seem to favor the use of pragmatic combinations of viewpoints and therapies tailored to the specific needs of individual clients (Garske, 1982).

The unifying conceptual approach of behavior therapy has arisen from the study of learning in experimental psychology. Contemporary behavior therapy, however, has no single, simple theoretical underpinning (Werry & Wollersheim, 1989). Human development, learning, perception, cognition, and social interaction are relevant in the treatment of psychologic problems. Today's contemporary approach to behavior management stems from four basic principles of behavior therapy: 1) Watson's (1920) respondent conditioning, 2) Skinner's (1938) operant learning, 3) Bandura's (1969; 1977) observational learning, and 4) Meichenbaum's (1979) cognitive behavior modification processing. The basic assumption of each of these approaches is that most behavior is learned and can therefore be changed through a process of learning, unlearning, or relearning.

For more than half a century, the framework for behavior therapy was limited to animal learning (conditioning) principles of Pavlov's respondent conditioning paradigm, and Skinner's conditioning reinforcement technology focusing on overt behaviors. In the middle to late 1960s, researchers began to merge concepts from human-related branches of experimental psychology, such as social and cognitive psychology, into the behavior therapy model dealing with overt behavior and internalized processes (Werry & Wollersheim, 1989). The contemporary behavior therapy model has integrated rational-emotive therapy (Ellis, 1962), cognitive therapy (Beck, 1967), systematic rational restructuring (Goldfried, Decenteco, & Weinberg, 1974), and cognitive behavior modification (Meichenbaum, 1979). The merging of behavior modification, which focuses on overt behavior, and the cognitive–behavioral approach, which focuses on internalized processes, has developed into a unified conceptual approach to contemporary behavior management.

Behavioral Theory

The theoretical approaches to contemporary behavior management are based on a psychologic model of human behavior and committed to the scientific method (Gelfand & Hartmann, 1984). The four most commonly used models are neobehavioristic mediational, applied behavior analysis, social learning, and cognitive behavior modification.

NEOBEHAVIORISTIC MEDIATIONAL MODEL (RESPONDENT [CLASSICAL] CONDITIONING)

The neobehavioristic mediational model is the Pavlovian stimulus-response model of learning that uses conditioning instead of cognition or internal mediating processes. This model's key principle is the linking of conditional stimuli to naturally occurring reflex arcs by means of immediately preceding association (Werry & Wollersheim, 1989). Respondent conditioning uses unlearned or previously established behavior patterns to create stimulus-response links. In Pavlov's hungry dog paradigm, an unconditioned stimulus (food) elicits an unconditioned response (salivation). When a conditioned stimulus (bell) is paired with the unconditioned stimulus (food) repeatedly, the conditioned stimulus (bell) alone will elicit a conditioned response (salivation) similar to the unconditioned response. This paradigm depicts respondent learning.

The neobehavioristic mediational model of behavior therapy is applicable to emotional disorders and particularly to fear and anxiety. Two promising behavior techniques of this model are systematic desensitization and implosion (or flooding) to treat fear and anxiety. These techniques expose the client to the anxiety-arousing stimuli in fact or imagination. Systematic desensitization accomplishes its goal of anxiety reduction through a step-by-step process after the client learns assertion and relaxation tactics as counterphobic devices. Implosion provides repeated, rapid exposure to the fear- or anxiety-provoking stimuli, parallel to the idea of getting back on the horse each time one has been thrown. The use of these techniques in minors has been poorly researched. For the most part, research has focused on the adult; child therapists are not at all attracted to the use of implosion (Werry & Wollersheim, 1989).

APPLIED BEHAVIOR ANALYSIS MODEL (OPERANT CONDITIONING)

Skinner's (1953) operant conditioning approach is axiomatic among behaviorists. The key principle in this model, as the term "operant" suggests, is its assumption that one has some choice and that behavior actively produces a result on the environment. This approach focuses on overt (or observable) behavior, the eliciting stimuli preceding it and the reinforcing events, whether positive or negative, following it. Operant techniques continue to be the most widely used techniques for behavior management.

The applied behavior analysis model systematically manipulates either the events immediately before a behavior (i.e., the eliciting stimuli) or those immediately after (i.e., the reinforcing or punishing contingencies) to influence a change in the target behavior. Operant conditioning techniques can manage a broad span of behaviors, from psychotic and self-mutilating, through simple problems of eating, elimination, and tantrums, to more complex social behaviors (Werry & Wollersheim, 1989). They have been used in a variety of program settings, including parent management programs (Ross, 1981; Patterson, 1982), inpatient (Quay, 1986), school (MacMillan & Morrison, 1986), and community settings (Werry & Wollersheim, 1989) and include positive reinforcement, negative reinforcement, response shaping, extinction, differential reinforcement, and punishment (Table 28-1; see Chapter 6).

MANIPULATION OF CONSEQUENCE

This technique serves to increase desired behavior by rewarding the behavior in a timely fashion (i.e., immediately following the behavior). Rewards or reinforcing events vary from child to child. Also, different stimulus events may serve as reinforcers for a particular child at different times. The child's state of satiation or deprivation plays an important role in determining the momentary strength of a potential reinforcer. Reinforcing events must be individually identified to implement this technique successfully (Gelfand & Hartmann, 1984). Box 28-2 lists the characteristics of a useful reinforcer.

Generalized reinforcers, such as praise or "points," are interchangeable for backup reinforcers rather than primary reinforcers, such as food. Generalized reinforcers are relatively resistant to satiation and do not depend on momentary deprivation states for their effectiveness. In addition, they can be given in tiny parts immediately following the desired behavior (Gelfand & Hartmann, 1984).

Praise is especially effective and is viewed by the child as a description of his or her good behavior rather than as an attempt to change his or her behavior pattern. Praise as a type of reinforcement is notably socially acceptable. Using praise along with material reinforcement may guide the child to deduce that the motivation for his or her satisfactory behavior rests solely in his or her own intrinsic goodness as opposed to a desire to obtain material payment. Vague stereotyped comments, such as "That's a good one!" are not as effective (if at all) as a specific descriptive praise statement (Gelfand & Hartmann, 1984), such as "Billy, I am so proud of you for controlling your temper when Joe broke your Walkman!"

Generalized reinforcers bridge the delay between a performance and the backup reinforcement. These reinforcers can be used flexibly throughout the day. They are able to acquire more incentive value than would a single primary reinforcer because of the generalized reinforcer's association with a number of different backup reinforcers (Kazdin & Bootzin, 1972).

Premack's differential probability principle must be discussed in the study of behavior management and reinforcers (Premack, 1959). This principle holds that for any two behaviors exhibited by an individual, the rate of the less frequent behavior can be raised by making access to the (supposedly) more attractive higher rate behavior contingent on the emission of the lower rate behavior. Parents who use the rule that all homework is finished before the television is turned on use this principle. Thus, a response of higher probability can reinforce a response of lower probability (Gelfand & Hartmann, 1984).

Contingency management programs use techniques not only to facilitate the development of adaptive behaviors, but also to reduce or eliminate

BOX 28–2 • CHARACTERISTICS OF A USEFUL REINFORCER

- Resistant to satiation
- Administered in small units
- Administered immediately following desired behavior
- Exclusively under the treatment agent's control
- Compatible with overall treatment plan
- Practical

REFERENCE

Adapted from Gelfand, D. M., & Hartmann, D. P. (1984). *Child behavior analysis and therapy.* New York: Praeger.

TABLE 28–1 Overview of Common Operant Behavioral Terms

Term	Procedure	Effect on behavior
Positive reinforcement	Application of rewarding event	Increase
Negative reinforcement	Removal of aversive event	Increase
Punishment	Application of aversive event or removal of rewarding event	Decrease
Extinction	Neutral consequence	Decrease
Differential reinforcement	Reinforcement of other incompatible behavior	Decrease

(Adapted from Morin, J. E., & Cutbirth, S. E. (1990). *Behavior therapy program.* Waco, TX: Waco Center for Youth.)

inappropriate or maladaptive behaviors. The key principle in contingency management is the systematic control of the consequences of the target behavior to be changed. Contracts, token economies, points, sticker charts, and so forth are devices of positive reinforcement and tools to reward the client for exhibiting the desired behavior. On the other hand, extinction and punishment techniques are used to decrease undesirable behavior. Overcorrection, response cost, timeout, and reprimands are all subtechniques of punishment. Punishment is the administration of an aversive or unpleasant contingency to undesired behavior. Overcorrection requires extra effort on the part of the child to fix the negative consequence of the undesired behavior (e.g., an enuretic child is required not only to change clothes, but also to wash the wet clothing). Response cost is a variant of fining, which involves the withdrawing of previously acquired rewards contingent on inappropriate behavior (e.g., an adolescent is not allowed to use the family car for a month as a result of going to an out-of-town concert without permission).

Time out means taking away the opportunity to earn rewards. This subtechnique has evolved into the practice of removing the child from the environment to a less attractive environment (i.e., seclusion or isolation) rather than removing the rewards. This procedure is used preferably with younger children rather than with large, strong, resistive adolescents. Excessive time outs may increase a youngster's reputation for courage and toughness (Werry & Wollersheim, 1989). Younger children are less resourceful at entertaining themselves during time out and are less able to recruit peer accomplices in treatment plan subversion (Gelfand & Hartmann, 1984).

A reprimand is used to verbally rebuke the child for an undesired behavior. The manner in which a reprimand is voiced may impact positively or negatively on the child's behavior. A negative impact may result if the child senses anger or feels the reprimand is directed at him or her rather than the behavior. This procedure is easier to use than most other punishment procedures, such as time out or response cost. Punishment should be used only with concomitant efforts to reinforce appropriate behaviors with positive reinforcers (Gelfand & Hartmann, 1984).

MANIPULATION OF STIMULUS

Chaining and fading are two operant techniques that use strategies to manipulate the stimulus. Chaining is a procedure that unifies simple behaviors learned successively into a complex skill through stimulus and contingency management. Fading is a procedure that introduces a stimulus (prompting) to aid in eliciting a difficult to produce, but desired, behavior and then gradually fading (thinning) it out while concurrently maintaining the desired behavior.

Social Learning Model

Albert Bandura (1969; 1977) is the founder of the social learning model. This model is a synthesis of many techniques from other models with a primary focus on building social skills through observational learning (Hops, Finch, & McConnell, 1985; Christoff & Myatt, 1987). Bandura's theoretical model recognizes overt behavior and internal cognitive factors. It stresses the reciprocal interaction among environment, behavior, and internal cognitive processes in psychologic functioning (Werry & Wollersheim, 1989).

Bandura's social learning theory is a useful framework for nurses involved in psychosocial habilitative programs for children and adolescents with disorders that result in or accompany social skills deficits. Child and adolescent psychosocial habilitation programs use the social learning model to teach, individually or in groups, a wide variety of social skills-building topics, such as how to make friends, stress management, cooperation, communication or conversational skills, and how to initiate specified social behaviors. The major concepts of this model include modeling, imitation, reinforcement, modification, and generalization. Motor acts, attitudinal statements, and emotional reactions can be learned from modeling or observational learning (Ross, 1981). Successful imitation is governed by attentional processes, retentional processes, motor reproduction, motivational processes, and if specified, guided practice with corrective feedback. The observational learning paradigm distinguishes between the attainment of a response and its actual performance. In this way the learner can observe the model and obtain the capacity to make a response without actually emitting the response until later.

Guided participation in live performance or filmed demonstrations has proven to be particularly effective in reducing avoidance behavior in fear-provoking situations. The observer watches the model, then gradually imitates the model's performance. Successful experiences are particularly helpful in building self-efficiency expectations, a feeling that one can successfully complete a task. Efficiency expectations and performance skills go hand in hand (Bandura, 1977).

Cognitive Behavior Modification

Meichenbaum's (1977) cognitive behavior modification model is a relatively new development in the field of child behavior therapy. This model attempts to change behaviors and feelings by changing thinking patterns. The approach assesses overt behavior, as do the other models, but it also explores the thinking processes that accompany problem behavior or emotional experiences. According to Ross (1981), all people think, have fantasies, ideas, expectations, memories, and so forth, and these cognitive processes can be put to use in behavior management. This model is essentially derived from Ellis' (1962) rational-emotive therapy, Beck's (1967) cognitive therapy, and systematic rational restructuring (Goldfried et al., 1974). Cognitive behavioral methods for the most part use procedures such as "active instruction in alternative solutions to problems; covert self-instruction; reframing events; challenging maladaptive beliefs; and encouraging children to develop more optimistic or reasonable attitudes about situations that distress them" (Werry & Wollersheim, 1989, p. 3).

Cognitive behavior modification is used to persuade the child to make verbal statements that are self-instructions or that strengthen the uniqueness of the stimuli being presented (Ross, 1981). Verbal self-statements have been shown to improve the task performance of hyperactive, impulsive children (Meichenbaum & Goodman, 1971) and as a basis for developing various forms of self-control (Thoreson & Mahoney, 1974). Self-control takes the form of teaching self-instruction (e.g., teaching a hyperactive child to say to himself or herself, "Stop, look, and listen" or "Stop, listen, and think"), self-monitoring, self-reward, self-punishment, or combinations of these. Self-control, in the context of cognitive behavior modification, can be interpreted as a standpoint where the child has learned to emit responses that help to discriminate or reinforce stimuli for that individual (Ross, 1981). The technique of verbal mediation is an important aspect of any learning and may enter into child behavior management at many stages.

Principles to Practice

To move from principles to practice in behavior management, the nurse takes a contemporary approach using the basic principles of respondent conditioning, operant learning, observational learning, and the operation of cognitive processes. In the planning and implementation of behavior management, the nurse is rarely working with one isolated set of principles, although a given approach to a problem might be formulated in respondent, operant, observational, or cognitive terms. In all likelihood, these frequently occur together and interact in nearly all situations in which behavior is learned (Ross, 1981).

Application of Behavioral Principles Through Nursing Process

ASSESSMENT

Assessment is the first step of the nursing process and is a fundamental step in applying behavior principles. The nursing assessment is a holistic approach in which the nurse gathers both objective and subjective data from all human spheres: psychologic, social, cultural, spiritual, biologic, behavioral, and cognitive (Reakes, 1989). The nurse approaches this step from the window of the presenting problem or problems that lead the child or adolescent to seek treatment initially. These data are obtained by the nurse through interviews, observation, and record reviews (Ziegler, Vaughan-Wrobel, & Erlen, 1986). A sample nursing assessment tool for behavior therapy is shown in Box 28-3.

A functional analysis of behavior is necessary to apply behavioral principles appropriately and effect a change in maladaptive behavior. This analysis is based on the assessment of specific behavior. The maladaptive behavior pattern is studied from the perspective of the relationship between the environmental antecedent and the consequence of the response. It is important to identify the function of a given response in its interaction with the environment. This paradigm can be described as $S \rightarrow R \rightarrow C$, where S represents the antecedent discriminative stimulus, R represents the response behavior, and C represents the consequence. Behavior is generally measured by frequency, latency, magnitude, and duration (Ross, 1981). Frequency is the number of episodes of a specific behavior that has occurred during a certain period of time. Latency is the time from which the antecedent has occurred until the response behavior occurs. Magnitude is a measure of the strength of the response. Duration is the amount of time over which the response behavior occurred.

In assessing behavior, the nurse must differentiate a skill deficit from a performance deficit. A skill deficit generally indicates that learning has not occurred, whereas a performance deficit indicates that one has the skill but finds other activities to be more rewarding (Ross, 1981). During the assessment process, a child's or adolescent's behavior is

(text continues on page 400)

BOX 28–3 • SAMPLE BEHAVIOR THERAPY NURSING ASSESSMENT TOOL

REASON FOR HOSPITALIZATION (Patient/Family Report): ______

I. **Mental/Behavioral Information (Use both objective and subjective data):**

A. Appearance (Objective): (clothing, skin, nails, hair, hygiene) ______

B. 1. Behavior At Interview (Objective): ______

2. Behavior response: ambivalent ______, alert ______, tense ______, sad ______, worried ______, happy ______, angry ______, suspicious ______, impulsive ______,
suicidal (validate) ______
homicidal (validate) ______

C. Speech and Verbal Disturbances:

1. Verbal response Appropriate Inappropriate (validate) ______

2. Speech and verbal disturbances: blocking ______, incoherent ______, repetition ______, rhyming ______, speech defects ______, obsessions ______, flight of ideas ______

D. Orientation: (person, place, time) ______

E. 1. Judgment (recent/past): Good Fair Poor (validate) ______

2. Insight: Good Fair Poor (validate) ______

F. 1. Hallucinations: Auditory, Visual, Olfactory, Gustatory, Tactile (validate) ______

2. Delusions of:
persecution (validate) ______
somatic (validate) ______
grandeur (validate ______

3. Disturbance of Sociability: withdrawn ______, seclusion ______, antisocial ______, nonverbal ______, combative ______, manipulative ______, suspicious ______, destructive ______, profanity ______, verbally aggressive ______
Affective disturbance: depressed ______, agitated ______, euphoric ______, hostile ______, ambivalent ______, anxious ______

GENERAL COMMENTS: ______

II. **Physical and Medical Information:**

A. Vital Signs T______ P______ B/P______ Wt ______ Ht ______ HC ______

B. Known diseases/illnesses/addictions: (also history) ______
(e.g., seizures, diabetes, alcohol/drug abuse) ______

C. Recurrent physical complaints: ______

D. Surgical history: ______

(continued)

BOX 28–3 • SAMPLE BEHAVIOR THERAPY NURSING ASSESSMENT TOOL (*Continued*)

E. Physical disabilities/prostheses/activity limitations: (glasses, hearing aids, handicaps, etc.): ______

F. Neuromuscular symptoms: (e.g., tics, rocking, chronic movements, gait) ______

G. Pregnancy—LMP— ______

H. Current medications and past medications, reason prescribed: ______

I. Allergies (drug/food): (IN RED) ______

J. Sleeping pattern (increase, decrease, changes): ______

K. Eating pattern (appetite, special diet, change): ______

L. Elimination (enuretic/encopretic patterns, changes): ______

M. Skin (bruises, scars, integrity): ______

COMMENTS: ______

III. **Developmental History:**

A. Date and place of birth, complications in delivery and/or early postnatal period: ______

B. Developmental milestones (walking, talking, etc.): ______

C. Males: Age of onset of puberty/sexual activity: ______

D. Females: Age of menarche/sexual activity/birth control: ______

IV. **Psychosocial History:**

A. Family members and relationships: ______

B. Family dynamics (conflict, abuse, divorce, etc.): ______

C. Family illness history (blood relatives, mother, father, siblings, aunts, uncles, grandparents):

Alcohol ______	Drugs ______
Mental illness ______	Cancer ______
Heart disease ______	Hypertension ______
Diabetes ______	Other ______

D. Special Interests (hobbies, pets, etc.): ______

E. Education (grade level, difficulties): ______

(*continued*)

BOX 28–3 • SAMPLE BEHAVIOR THERAPY NURSING ASSESSMENT TOOL (*Continued*)

V. **Plans:**

A. Strengths: ______________________________

B. Weaknesses: ______________________________

C. Patient/Family Needs (educational, support, etc.): ______________________________

D. Environmental Needs (precautions, handicap access, etc.): ______________________________

E. Discharge Planning/Aftercare: ______________________________

always examined through the framework of normal development (Erikson, 1963; Piaget, 1963). Behavior is a primary indicator of a youngster's physical and mental health status.

The nurse uses his or her scientific knowledge, practice wisdom, and ethics of practice in collecting and organizing data systematically to pinpoint a youngster's need for nursing care (Ziegler et al., 1986). During the assessment, the nurse interviews the child or adolescent, family, and when possible the client's siblings and teachers. The nurse may choose to interview the client first to establish an alliance with the youngster and gain his or her cooperation (Clunn, 1991). The framework for the interview process is based on the child's or adolescent's developmental stage, presenting problems, chronologic age, cultural background, and physical health. The nurse may choose to combine the mental health status examination with the initial information-gathering interview.

The initial information-gathering interview includes the reason for admission or referral, fears and worries, self-image, mood, feelings, thoughts, interests, fantasies, aspirations, relationships, peers, school, family, sexual activities, and drug and alcohol use (Clunn, 1991). The nurse uses his or her skill to gather information about these topics while conveying to the client respect for confidentiality and privacy. The nurse interviewer clarifies the procedure while providing support for the client to reduce anxiety and treatment resistance. The three stages of the assessment interview are introduction, working, and termination. In the assessment process, the client–nurse relationship is established, even though the purpose of the interview is information gathering rather than therapeutic intent. Communication strategies used in gathering information during the interview process include the use of descriptive comments, paraphrasing and reflecting, praising, using open-ended questions, and nonverbal gesturing to encourage the client's response (Clunn, 1991).

During the assessment process, data are collected to evaluate adaptive and maladaptive behavior patterns. The client's behavior with parents and separated from parents is addressed, as is the client's behavior with siblings, pets, teachers, and peers. Data also are collected regarding behavior involving activities of daily living, leisure, and schoolwork. Client behavior patterns at home, at school, and in the community need to be captured to identify specific cues to address.

Generally in a treatment facility, the assessment process involves a multiple assessment approach through an interdisciplinary treatment team synergizing a variety of perspectives. In this approach, various disciplines collect data through many tools. Nurses critically analyze the data and identify, prioritize, and target maladaptive behavior patterns.

NURSING DIAGNOSIS

The second step of the nursing process is the formulation of a nursing diagnosis. Ziegler et al. (1986) refer to nursing diagnosis as the pivotal

(text continues on page 403)

CLINICAL EXAMPLE: WINSTON

Winston, age 10.3 years, was referred to a public residential treatment facility from a private psychiatric hospital because his single mother could no longer control him, and her insurance would no longer pay for acute care hospitalization.

According to Winston's mother, school, and MHMR records, Winston's behaviors included hyperactivity, poor impulse control, short attention span, poor appetite, difficulty sleeping, easy distractibility, cursing, property destruction, verbal outbursts, and fighting with peers at school. He also would become physically aggressive with others, need to be physically restrained, and kick, hit, and bite the person attempting to restrain him. The mother also reported that although he didn't actually "run away," he would "lose track" of time and be gone from home for 4 or 5 hours, and she wouldn't know where he was.

Winston had no known allergies or prior surgeries; he had chickenpox when younger and pneumonia at 9 months of age. He had a slight build, weighed 52 lb, and was 4 ft, 3 in tall. His mother reported normal developmental milestones. His appetite was very poor, and according to Winston and his mother, his lack of appetite was caused by his medication. The mother reported she ate only "health foods," and Winston preferred chocolate milk and an occasional cheese sandwich. When admitted to the residential treatment facility, Winston was taking 15 mg Ritalin t.i.d., and 25 mg of Imipramine at bedtime. He also exhibited anxiety in the admission interview by saying "What?" each time he was asked a question. When he appeared to be stressed, he had a small "tic-like" cough and would clear the hair off his forehead with his hand.

Winston was alert and oriented to time, person, and place. His recent and remote memory were intact and his affect appropriate. He denied hallucinations or delusions. He was ambivalent about answering questions, interrupted the interviewer, changed the subject, and had to be redirected frequently. According to records, Winston had a full scale IQ of 129, verbal 125 and performance 128.

Winston's strengths included his intelligence, sense of humor, interest in school, and his mother's verbalization of her intention to work in family therapy and be supportive of his treatment. Patient and family weaknesses were his short attention span and the mother's and client's lack of skills to cope with the symptoms of his illness. The child and his mother had no support, emotional or financial, from his father whom they had not seen in several years and who reportedly was unemployed and living in a park.

Winston stated he "thought" he believed in God, didn't attend church, and thought his mother was a "Buddhist." He shared with the nurse that he had a cat at home and liked to read, play Nintendo, and ride his bicycle.

Winston was admitted to a 10-bed children's unit and into the facility's behavior therapy program consisting of structured environment and daily schedule (Box 28-4), school, individual therapy, group therapy and therapeutic groups, structured activities, behavior therapy point system (token economy), contract system, time outs and cognitive tasks, and special treatment procedures (restraint, seclusion, room or unit restriction).

Every resident of the children's unit had a psychiatric diagnosis of attention-deficit hyperactivity disorder (ADHD) or oppositional defiant disorder.

The following nursing diagnosis and treatment plan were formulated and implemented.

Nursing Diagnosis 1: Ineffective Individual Coping related to impulse control deficit, severe, as evidenced by verbal outbursts, distractibility, physical aggression with peers, and property destruction

SAMPLE NURSING CARE PLAN WITH EXAMPLES OF BEHAVIOR THERAPY TECHNIQUES

Goal: The client will learn alternative behaviors and age-appropriate methods of coping with anger or stress to enable him to live outside the hospital with his family and attend school.

Objectives:

1. The client will accept consequences of his behavior without arguing or screaming.
   Staff will set limits in calm, quiet voice.
   Staff will give consistent consequences for arguing or screaming (e.g., fines, timeouts).
   Staff will reward client with praise or seeking out client to give special attention when he is not arguing or screaming.
2. Client will not exhibit verbal outbursts, screaming, and physical aggression toward others.
   Staff will not address issues with client while he is screaming.
   If a restraint becomes necessary, it will be carried out with a minimum of discussion.

(*continued*)

CLINICAL EXAMPLE: WINSTON (*Continued*)

When the client is calm, the nurse will encourage him to ventilate his feelings and explore with him methods of coping with his anger and frustration.
Staff will praise client frequently when he exhibits positive behavior and ignore negative behavior as much as possible.
After each time out, staff will give the client a short written cognitive task to complete, which references the behavior requiring this consequence (Box 28-5).

3. The client will accept responsibility for his behaviors.
Nurse will implement with client a contract (see end of Clinical Example) to allow him to earn the privilege of riding his bicycle as a reinforcer for adaptive behaviors.
Nurse will develop a sticker chart with client to visually validate his positive behaviors (Box 28-6).
Nurse will spend 10 minutes daily with client to reinforce positive behaviors, successes and expectations.
Nurse will involve Winston in decision making by making choices available to him to gain control over his life.

Nursing Diagnosis 2: Altered Nutrition Less than Body Requirements, related to improper eating habits as evidenced by poor appetite and refusal to eat established appropriate food groups.

Goal: Client will reach ideal body weight and maintain ideal body weight for the duration of his hospitalization.

Objectives:

1. The client will learn healthy eating habits and follow prescribed diet.
Staff will monitor, report to nurse, and document client's food intake each meal.
Nurse will meet with dietitian and client to explore food possibilities and interests.
Nurse will meet with client 10 minutes weekly to educate him in proper food choices and praise him for weight gain and new foods accepted.

Due to his impulsiveness and inability to deal with stimuli from the environment and his peers (agitation of peers being a major obstacle to treatment in a unit with so many ADHD and oppositional children), Winston had difficulty at first in adjusting to the new structured environment. He quickly found he could get attention from the other boys with his sense of humor. He was a leader and tried on numerous occasions to influence the group to rebel against staff.

Winston required restraint and seclusion frequently and time outs often. It was discovered that Winston could only be still and concentrate if he was reading, so he was given reading material of special interest to him to read when in his room at times when he required little or no stimulation. The staff consistently followed the treatment plan, and the nurse spent extra time with Winston to reinforce with him ways of coping with the symptoms of his illness.

During hospitalization, Winston gained some insight into his problems and learned the behaviors necessary to earn points and gain privileges in the token economy system. His medications were changed to 20 mg of Mellaril t.i.d. and 200 mg of Tegretol b.i.d. soon after admission. With ongoing education by the nurse and dietitian, Winston's appetite and choice of appropriate foods gradually improved, and he reached and maintained his ideal body weight. Winston signed up for and attended a community church with a volunteer weekly and expressed an interest in finding a church in his hometown when discharged.

Winston was elected president of his unit patient government, as well as a representative to the campuswide client council, where he was successful in petitioning the facility director to initiate pet therapy on campus. As Winston learned to cope with the frustrations of his illness, his interpersonal relationships with peers and adults improved.

Winston's mother attended and participated in family therapy at least twice a month and took him home or came to visit for holidays and scheduled weekends after his behavior stabilized.

The tools used in Winston's inpatient treatment plan (reinforcers, contracts, cognitive tasks) were explained and demonstrated to Winston and his mother, and she planned to collaborate with MHMR to continue the behavior program after discharge.

Winston was discharged to his mother's care after the treatment team and aftercare coordinator met with the MHMR caseworker, school representative, mother, and client. The mother arranged after-school care for Winston while she worked, and both attended individual and family therapy on an outpatient basis.

Six months after discharge, according to facility quality assurance outcome data, Winston is enrolled in special education in school and living at home, and he and his mother are continuing with individual and family therapy as recommended.

(*continued*)

CLINICAL EXAMPLE: WINSTON *(Continued)*

CHILDREN'S BEHAVIOR CONTRACT

Date: May 1, 1991

This is an agreement between Winston C. (Client) and Sue C., R.N.,C. (Nurse). The contract begins on May 1, 1991 (Date) and ends on May 7, 1991 (Date). The following terms have been agreed upon by both Client and Nurse:

The client will not exhibit: a) cursing, b) property destruction, c) verbal threats, d) screaming, and e) physical aggression to others

The nurse will grant Winston 30 minutes free bicycle time for every 4 consecutive hours he does not exhibit the above behaviors

If the client fulfills his part of the contract, the client will receive the privilege agreed to with the nurse. However, if the client fails to fulfill his part of the contract, the privilege will be withheld.

Client's Signature ____________________

Nurse's Signature ____________________

Adapted from Waco Center for Youth, Waco, Texas. Used with permission.

point for guiding the treatment plan and implementing nursing interventions. The nursing diagnosis identifies the problem, etiology, and symptoms. For example, the client's nursing diagnosis might be "Ineffective Individual Coping related to impulse control deficit, as evidenced by verbal outbursts, distractibility, physical aggression with peers, and property destruction." The treatment goal will focus on the problem (response), while the stair step objectives (predicted outcomes) to achieve the goal will focus on the symptoms (evidence). The client will accomplish these goals and outcomes, which are phrased "The client will. . . ." The nursing intervention focuses on treating the cause of the problem and describes nursing action. The Clinical Examples for Winston and Becky present nursing diagnoses with related goals, objectives, and nursing interventions for a child and an adolescent, respectively, in behavior therapy programs.

Nursing diagnosis provides the caregivers with specific client maladaptive behaviors that need to be changed through the implementation of prescribed behavior management techniques.

PLANNING

Planning is the third step of the nursing process. Ideally, the nurse, client, and parents mutually plan the care based on the nursing diagnosis. The nursing diagnosis identifies the unhealthy behavior response and directs the goal and predicted outcomes for the client. During the planning stage, the nurse prescribes nursing actions and interventions required to move the client toward goal attainment. The nurse targets the client's maladaptive behavior for change through a prescriptive application of behavior management techniques and principles. The planning step of the nursing process is incorporated into a comprehensive interdisciplinary treatment team process in which all treatment team disciplines, along with the client and significant others, develop a comprehensive treatment plan.

IMPLEMENTATION

The fourth step of the nursing process is implementation. This step involves the actual "doing" of a nursing intervention, plus the observation and

BOX 28–4 • DAILY CHILDREN'S UNIT SCHEDULE

MONDAY–FRIDAY
6:30—Wake up
6:30–7:30—Hygiene, room clean up, medications
7:30–8:00—Breakfast
8:00–8:45—Goal group
8:45–11:30—School
11:30–12:00—Lunch
12:00–12:30—Medications or free time
12:30–2:15—School
2:15–245—Individual therapy
2:45–3:30—Rehab: arts & crafts, woodshop, puppets, and so forth
3:30–4:30—Free time—use privileges bought or granted
4:30–5:00—Clean up for supper—quiet time
5:00–5:30—Supper
5:30–6:00—Current events group
6:00–6:30—Problem-solving group
6:30–6:45—Break
6:45–7:45—Individually assigned psychosocial classes
7:45–8:00—Snack time
8:00–9:00—Bath time, hygiene, clean up room
9:00–9:30—Quiet time in room
9:30—Bedtime

WEEKEND SCHEDULE
9:00—Wake up—Medications
9:00–9:30—Hygiene
9:30—Breakfast
10:00–10:45—Goal group
10:45–11:00—Break
11:00–1:00—Unit activity
1:00–1:30—Lunch
1:30–2:00—Medications or free time
2:00–4:00—Campus-wide athletic activity
4:00–4:30—Group
4:30–5:00—Clean up
5:00–5:30—Supper

BOX 28–5 • CHILDREN'S COGNITIVE TASK

Instructions: Mark each one "right" (R) or "wrong" (W).

1. Hitting peers ______
2. Hitting staff ______
3. Screaming ______
4. Tearing up peers' things ______
5. Tearing up your things ______
6. Feeling bad when someone is hurt ______
7. Kicking the dog ______
8. Sharing your feelings ______
9. Respecting your elders ______
10. Following instructions ______
11. Being proud of yourself ______
12. Stealing ______
13. Breaking the rules ______
14. Supporting your peers ______
15. Controlling your temper ______
16. Talking rudely to others ______
17. Making fun of others ______
18. Agitating peers ______
19. Agitating staff ______
20. Ignoring staff questions or instructions ______
21. Making up your bed ______
22. Doing your chores ______
23. Talking in a quiet tone of voice ______
24. Using privileges you don't have ______
25. Cursing adults or peers ______
26. Writing on walls ______
27. Lying to staff or peers ______
28. Telling the truth ______
29. Hurting someone's feelings ______
30. Making racial comments ______

Please write a paragraph about Number ______ above. What is "right or wrong" about it? When you exhibit this behavior, how does it affect others? How does it make you feel? If you are writing about a negative behavior, what could you do instead?

BOX 28–6 • SAMPLE WEEKLY BEHAVIORAL STICKER CHART

Name: ______________________ Date: ______________________

Behavior	Sun	Mon	Tue	Wed	Thur	Fri	Sat
Wake Up							
Hygiene							
Dressing							
Breakfast							
Goal Group							
School							
Lunch							
School							
Rehab							
Free Time							
Activity							
Shower							
Hygiene							
Bedtime							
Bonus							
Total							

This chart is to be posted in a prominent place, such as the door to the client's room or staff office door. A star or sticker is to be placed in each box when a positive adaptive behavior has occurred. Examples: *Wake up*—"The client needs only one reminder to get up in the morning." *Goal group*—"The client participated by staying on subject and needed only minimal redirection when talking out of turn." The weekly behavioral sticker chart has the potential of giving the client the opportunity to visualize his or her positive behaviors, which encourages repeating these behaviors. Negative behaviors should not be incorporated in this chart, but the chart can be used as a companion tool with a behavior contract (i.e., out of possible 15 stickers or stars that could be earned, the behavioral contract would state: 1–5 stickers = no reward; 6–10 stickers = 15 minutes of free Nintendo; 11–15 stickers = 30 minutes bicycle time [individualize the reward to the client's special interest]).

documentation of the client's response to the intervention. Nurses and nursing staff implement the prescribed behavior principle each time the client's targeted maladaptive behavior response is emitted. Staff then observe and document the client's response to the prescribed behavior principle. The implementation of the nursing care plan must be consistent among all nursing staff to facilitate adaptive behavior effectively through the use of behavior principles.

EVALUATION

The last step of the nursing process is evaluation. The nurse compares the actual client outcomes with the predicted outcomes to determine if the desired responses were elicited. Objective behavioral change is measurable. This critical step of the nursing process facilitates the revision of the treatment plan and renews the cycle.

(text continues on page 408)

CLINICAL EXAMPLE: BECKY

Becky, age 15, had been in the custody of the Department of Human Services for 6 months, after she alleged sexual and physical abuse by her father. Prior to her referral to this residential treatment facility, Becky had been living in group homes and foster homes. The behaviors she exhibited toward others appeared to have caused these placements to fail. She had run away on five occasions, made suicidal threats (one with superficial lacerations to an arm), had "temper tantrums" (e.g., throwing herself on the floor and becoming verbally unresponsive), refused to follow instructions or requests of adults, and was physically aggressive to staff and peers.

Becky did not exhibit any of these behaviors during the initial interview but was sometimes flippant and sarcastic, and rather than answer a question, she would say, "You've got my records. You should know the answer to that!" At other times, she was cheerful and cooperative.

Becky had no prior surgeries and had measles, mumps, and chickenpox as a young child. She stated that she had no allergies. Her vital signs were normal. She was $61\frac{3}{4}$ in. tall and weighed 125 lb. She had no physical disabilities or special assistance needs. No information or records were available describing birth and developmental information. According to Becky, her menses began at age 12, were regular, and not unduly painful. She appeared clean and was casually dressed in blue jeans, a black tee-shirt, and a railroad-type denim cap. She wore glasses that had one ear piece missing. When questioned about her spirituality, she said she did not believe in God, and although she didn't practice Satan worship, she felt "those guys probably have the right idea."

Becky was taking 300 mg of lithium p.o. t.i.d., but on admission a lithium level was obtained (below normal range), and the medication was not continued. She was begun on a regular diet; when admission laboratory work revealed a 211 mg/dL cholesterol count, she was referred to the dietitian and started on a low cholesterol diet.

According to psychologic evaluations in Becky's records, WISC/R scores reflected a full scale IQ of 100, performance of 108, and verbal of 103. Her recent and remote memory were intact, and she was oriented to person, time, and place. Her insight and judgment, however, were impaired. She denied hallucinations, delusions, or suicidal thoughts.

Becky was admitted to a 14-bed female adolescent unit with a six-bed, locked stabilization treatment unit. Becky was assigned an open section bedroom and introduced into the facility adolescent behavior therapy program consisting of structured schedule and milieu, school, individual therapy, unit therapeutic groups, behavior therapy point system (token economy), contract system, time outs and cognitive tasks, and restraint, seclusion, and room and unit restriction.

Residents of the female adolescent unit to which Becky was assigned had varying psychiatric diagnoses, including residual attention-deficit hyperactivity disorder, bipolar disorder, oppositional defiant disorder, dysthymia, depression, conduct disorder, and borderline personality disorder.

The following nursing diagnosis and treatment plan were formulated and implemented:

Nursing Diagnosis 1: Alteration in Self-Concept and Disturbance in Self-Esteem, related to lack of positive adult role modeling, creating distrust of authority figures as evidenced by hostility, oppositional, and aggressive behaviors.

Goal: Client will improve self-esteem, incorporate positive adaptive behaviors, and develop coping skills appropriate to her age.

Objectives:

1. The client will develop a therapeutic alliance with the nurse.

   The nurse will meet with Becky two times a week for 30 minutes to focus on exploring ways to cope with frustrations and hurts in a positive manner.

   The nurse will foster trusting, therapeutic relationship with the client by honesty, consistency, and being nonjudgmental of her behaviors or feelings.

(*continued*)

CLINICAL EXAMPLE: BECKY (*Continued*)

2. The client will not exhibit hostile, threatening, or aggressive behaviors.
   Staff will set realistic limits and maintain consistency in rewards and consequences.
   The nurse will encourage and guide the client's use of decision-making skills in gaining control of her behaviors.
   After each verbal or physically threatening episode, staff will meet with the client one on one to elicit cognitive responses and aid her to gain insight to her behaviors.
3. The client will learn to accept responsibility for her behaviors.
   The nurse will discuss maladaptive behaviors exhibited by the client and explore alternative behaviors in weekly individual therapy sessions.
   The nurse and staff will reward acceptance of responsibility with more freedom and less supervision.
   The nurse will advocate for the client to treatment team for privileges (e.g., drivers education, special off campus activities, off campus job when client meets contractual responsibilities) (see end of Clinical Example).

Nursing Diagnosis 2: Increased potential for heart disease, related to knowledge deficit of dietary effect on blood cholesterol as evidenced by blood cholesterol of 211 mg/dL.

Goal: The client's cholesterol level will be lowered and maintained within normal established limits.

Objectives:

1. The client will follow low cholesterol diet and be knowledgeable of reasons for adhering to it.
   The nurse will refer the client to the dietitian for appropriate educational classes to reduce blood cholesterol.
   The nurse will monitor laboratory values and meet with client p.r.n. to share progress toward goal, continue educating, and reinforce importance of following diet.

After a "honeymoon period" of 2 weeks with only minor oppositional behaviors exhibited, Becky ran away from the facility. She was located by the police, returned to the facility, and transferred to the locked stabilization unit for observation. She stayed 1 week and then gave a commitment not to leave unauthorized again.

Becky had considerable difficulty with the unit's structured environment and was hostile and sometimes verbally threatening to staff or peers but was never physically aggressive.

During the first few months in the behavior therapy program, Becky was able to earn only basic privileges due to her refusal to cooperate or follow staff requests. However, once she discovered the correlation between positive adaptive behaviors and freedom to earn privileges, she quickly accumulated large point totals and was able to accept responsibility for her own behaviors with minimal supervision.

Becky attended individual therapy and gained insight into her problems. Her self-esteem improved as she attended drivers education and learned to drive and held an off-campus job at a local thrift store. She was accepted in music therapy class and sang at awards programs and campus chapel services. Although she never chose to attend community church services, she participated in the chapel services and went with the chaplain and other clients to gospel concerts and to community churches to sing with the chapel group.

She remained on a low cholesterol diet during hospitalization and was given education and reinforcement of her diet by the nurse and the dietitian.

Discharge planning was accomplished in collaboration with the treatment team, aftercare coordinator, Becky, and her DHS caseworker. She visited a group home prior to discharge and was agreeable to the placement. According to reports from Becky's caseworker, she is making satisfactory adjustment at the group home, is attending school in regular classes, and has a part time job. She says she is saving money to buy a car.

(*continued*)

CLINICAL EXAMPLE: BECKY (*Continued*)

ADOLESCENT BEHAVIOR CONTRACT

Date: May 1, 1991

I, Becky V (Patient), in collaboration with Sue C., R.N.C. (Nurse) agree to the following:

I will not exhibit the following maladaptive behavior for 1 month: cursing, physical aggression, refusal to follow staff requests

beginning today May 1, 1991 (Date) and ending May 31, 1991 (Date).

If I meet my contractual responsibilities, Sue Cutbirth, R.N.C. (Nurse) will:

advocate for me to the Treatment Team for referral to vocational rehab to get an off campus job.

Signatures:

________________ Patient

________________ Nurse

cc: Treatment Team

Adapted from Waco Center for Youth, Waco, Texas. Used with permission.

Summary

This chapter has discussed the basic principles and theoretical foundations of behavior therapy. Contemporary behavioral management is based on a psychologic model of human behavior and ascribes to the scientific method approach. The neobehavioristic mediational model, applied behavior analysis model, social learning model, and cognitive behavior modification model are the most common behavior approaches. Behavioral principles are applied in clinical examples of child and adolescent psychiatric-mental health care through a nursing process format.

REFERENCES

Bandura, A. (1961). Psychotherapy as a learning process. *Psychological bulletin, 58,* 143–159.

Bandura, A. (1969). *Principles of behavior modification.* New York: Holt, Rinehart, & Winston.

Bandura, A. (1977). *Social learning theory.* Englewood Cliffs, NJ: Prentice-Hall.

Beck, A. T. (1967). *Depression: Causes and treatment.* Philadelphia: University of Pennsylvania Press.

Christoff, K. A., & Myatt, R. J. (1987). Social isolation. In M. Hersen & V. B. Van Hasselt (Eds.), *Behavior therapy with children and adolescents* (pp. 512–535). New York: John Wiley & Sons.

Clunn, P. (1991). Assessment of the Adolescent. In C. R. Hogarth (Ed.), *Adolescent psychiatric nursing* (pp. 133–186). St. Louis: C.V. Mosby.

Ellis, A. (1962). *Reason and emotion in psychotherapy.* New York: Stuart.

Erikson, E. (1963). *Childhood and society.* New York: W.W. Norton.

Eysenck, H. J. (1957). *The dynamics of anxiety and hysteria.* New York: Praeger.

Garske, J. P. (1982). Issues regarding effective psychotherapy. In J. McNamara & A. Barclay (Ed.), *Critical issues, developments and trends in professional psychology*. New York: Praeger.

Gelfand, D. M., & Hartmann, D. P. (1984). *Child behavior analysis and therapy.* New York: Pergamon Press.

Goldfried, M. R., Decenteco, E. T., & Weinberg, L. (1974). Systematic rational restructuring as a self-control technique. *Behavior therapy*, *5*, 247–254.

Hops, H., Finch, M., & McConnell, S. (1985). Social skills deficits. In P. H. Bornstein & A. E. Kazdin (Ed.), *Handbook of clinical behavior therapy with children*. Homewood, IL: Dorsey Press.

Jones, M. C. (1924). The elimination of children's fears. *Journal of Experimental Psychology*, *7*, 383–390.

Kazdin, A. E., & Bootzin, R. R. (1972). The token economy: An evaluative review. *Journal of Applied Behavior Analysis*, *5*, 343–372.

MacMillan, D. L., & Morrison, G. M. (1986). Educational intervention. In H. C. Quay & J. S. Werry (Eds.), *Psychopathological disorders of childhood* (pp. 583–621). New York: John Wiley & Sons.

Meichenbaum, D., & Goodman, J. (1971). Training impulsive children to talk to themselves: A means of developing self control. *Journal of Abnormal Psychology*, *77*, 115–126.

Meichenbaum, D. (1977). *Cognitive-behavior modification: An integrated approach.* New York: Plenum.

Meichenbaum, D. H. (1979). Teaching children self-control. In B. B. Lahoy & E. E. Kazdin (Eds.), *Advances in child clinical psychology.* New York: Plenum.

Morin, J. E., & Cutbirth, S. E. (1990). *Behavior therapy program.* Waco, TX: Waco Center for Youth.

Patterson, G. R. (1982). *Coercive family process.* Eugene, OR: Castalia.

Piaget, J. (1963). *The origins of intelligence in children* (M. Cook, Trans.). New York: W.W. Norton. (Original work published 1952).

Premack, D. (1959). Toward empirical behavior laws: I. Positive reinforcement. *Psychological Review*, *66*, 219–233.

Quay, H. C. (1986), Residential treatment. In H. C. Quay & J. S. Werry (Eds.), *Psychopathological disorders of childhood* (pp. 558–582). New York: John Wiley & Sons.

Reakes, J. C. (1989). Behavioral approaches. In B. S. Johnson (Ed.), *Psychiatric-mental health nursing: Adaptation and growth* (p. 248–267). Philadelphia: J.B. Lippincott.

Ross, A. O. (1959). *The practice of clinical child psychology.* New York: Grune & Straton.

Ross, A. O. (1964). Learning theory and therapy with children. *Psychotherapy: Theory, Research and Practice*, *1*, 102–108.

Ross, A. O. (1978). Behavior therapy with children. In S. Garfield & A. Bergin (Eds.), *Handbook of psychotherapy and behavior change*. New York: John Wiley & Sons.

Ross, A. O. (1981). *Child behavior therapy: Principles, procedures, and empirical basis.* New York: John Wiley & Sons.

Skinner, B. F. (1938). *The behavior of organisms: An experimental analysis.* New York: Appleton-Century-Crofts.

Skinner, B. F. (1953). *Science and human behavior.* New York: Macmillan Co.

Thoresen, C. E., & Mahoney, M. J. (1974). *Behavioral self-control.* New York: Holt, Rinehart, & Winston.

Watson, J. B., & Rayner, R. (1920). Conditioned emotional reactions. *Journal of Experimental Psychology*, *3*, 1–14.

Werry, J. S., & Wollersheim, J. D. (1989). Behavior therapy with children and adolescents: A twenty-year overview. *Journal American Academy of Child Adolescent Psychiatry*, *28*(1), 1–18.

Witmer, L. (1907). Clinical psychology. *The Psychological Clinic*, *1*, 1–9.

Wolpe, J. (1958). *Psychotherapy by reciprocal inhibition.* Stanford, CA: Stanford University Press.

Ullmann, L. P., & Krasner, L. (1965). *Case studies in behavior modification.* New York: Holt, Rinehart & Winston.

Ziegler, S. M., Vaughan-Wrobel, B. C., & Erlen, J. A. (1986). *Nursing process, nursing diagnosis, nursing knowledge: Avenues to autonomy.* Norwalk, CT: Appleton-Century-Crofts.

CHAPTER

29

Psychopharmacology

Geraldine S. Pearson

This chapter focuses on nurses' role in the use of medication to treat psychiatric disorders in children and adolescents. While the use of psychotropic medication with adults has prompted a new era in patient management, the use of these interventions in children often triggers controversy regarding their efficacy, side effects, and long-term impact on development. Nurses must clarify their personal attitudes and feelings regarding the use of psychotropic medication with children. They must understand the relationship between these attitudes, their professional practice, and the treatment philosophy of settings where they are employed.

The philosophic questions about use of medication with children, the wide array of medication available for treatment, and the need to provide ongoing assessment with children treated pharmacologically contribute to the vitality of the psychiatric-mental health nurse's role in holistic care. The nurse in an advanced practice role must collaborate with the prescribing physician and clinical team regarding medication issues. Nurses frequently interpret information about psychotropic medication and provide clinical leadership around medication management to other nonmedical team members.

Nurses teach parents to monitor and manage their child's medication and use self-care models with adolescents independently managing their medication regimens. They participate in communication linkages that provide continuity between disparate parts of the health care system, including school systems, day care facilities, and community health clinics (Hamric, 1989).

Nurses coordinate the psychosocial aspects of the client's life that influence and are affected by pharmacologic treatment. Administration of medication requires a knowledge of the drug's action and potential side effects, along with usual doses, method of administration, and the nursing management role.

This chapter approaches psychopharmacology from the perspective of the nursing process. Medication management in outpatient and inpatient settings is compared. The major categories of psychotropic medications most commonly used with children and adolescents are discussed with regard to function, target symptoms, short- and long-term side effects, and nursing management. Teaching strategies, along with evaluation of efficacy and family and patient compliance, are delineated. The chapter concludes with implications for nursing research and trends in nurses' collaborative roles in medication management.

Historic Perspectives

The nurse's role in medication management of psychiatric disorders has expanded parallel to the development of the nurse's role in other areas of

CLINICAL EXAMPLE: JULIE

Julie, an 18-year-old with a history of bipolar (manic–depressive) illness, was planning to attend an out-of-state university. Her parents were concerned about management of her lithium, which was being used to control her psychiatric illness. The nurse clinician in the clinic who had treated Julie and her family at intervals over several years saw the move to college as an opportunity for greater independence and emancipation from overprotective parents who had difficulties relinquishing control of the medication to their almost adult daughter. The nurse first assessed Julie's feelings about college, independently managing her medication, and leaving home for the first time. Julie and the nurse agreed to collaborate around helping her parents allow Julie to leave home in a positive way.

The nurse made a contact with the student health service at the university and received the name of an intake person for Julie to call and meet with soon after arrival at school. Julie signed a "release of information" form forwarding her health and psychiatric records to the student health service. Julie then established an appointment within days of her expected arrival at school. The nurse arranged for her to have blood lithium levels drawn just prior to leaving and gave her a renewal prescription for her lithium that would allow her to take several weeks of medication to college. Finally, after Julie kept her first appointment, the nurse contacted the intake worker and spoke with the prescribing physician regarding Julie's care and the rationale for her psychiatric management. Her parents were surprised at Julie's independence in managing her own medication and were relieved that the steps toward transfer of care were faithfully followed.

health care. While nurses in the past were viewed as singularly carrying out the physician's orders for administering a particular medication, nurses today perform a much broader function. This newer function includes providing the data necessary for decision making about use of medication; collaborating with the prescribing physician about type, dose, and time of medication administration; and providing follow-up care during the patient's medication regimen.

Nursing practice is progressive, independent, and community oriented. Similarly, nursing roles in pharmacologic management are broad based and vital to the client's total health care.

Nurses teach parents how to manage their children's psychotropic medication. If they do not understand the reasons medication is being used for their child, parents are less likely to be compliant with the treatment. This is especially true when the family is indigent or unsophisticated and needs simplistic and repeated instructions to understand the purpose of medication. Because nurses most often are involved with this population, they are in the best position to gear education to the level of the client and family. Nurses also have the time, patience, and skill to elicit the descriptive nuances of behavior reported by parents that might define the child's response to medication. These skills facilitate the collaboration with the physician prescriber, who often relies on nurses for the information that influences treatment decisions.

Nurses teach self-care activities to adolescents able to oversee their medication independently. Self-regulation of medication is essential if the adolescent is emancipated or expects to require psychotropic medication for a long time (See Clinical Example: Julie).

After medication has been prescribed, nurses often coordinate the function of monitoring the child's behavior. This coordination of care takes place in outpatient and inpatient settings where the nurse is most likely to follow the child and family. For example, the nurse clinician conducting a weekly play therapy group is able to observe the effects of medication on the child during play activities and peer interactions. Observing and interacting with the child or adolescent offer richer data than sitting with the child and parent in an office and asking questions about the child's functioning. In an inpatient setting, the nurse may be involved with one client throughout the shift, conduct group therapies, and participate in the ongoing assessment of the child. All of these opportunities provide the nurse with abundant sources of information about medication response.

Assessment and Planning of Care

The use of medication to manage problematic behavior is a decision that must be carefully considered by the health team. Medication usage has a variety of implied meanings for children and parents. Medication may be viewed as the "cure" to a complex psychiatric and social problem that requires several levels of psychosocial care. Medication is never a cure, in either long- or short-term care; rather, it is an adjunct to other forms of treatment involving the individual and family.

Medication may alleviate problematic symptoms, but the child and family must still cope with the environmental and social problems that either preceded the symptoms or resulted from them. Carefully identifying the symptoms targeted for medication management and understanding them in the context of the child's total functioning provides a holistic framework for care (See Clinical Example: Steven).

While parents may see medication as a cure to perceived problems, it is essential to view the child's problematic behavior from an objective standpoint. The administration of medication should usually be considered after other forms of treatment are in place or as an adjunct to outpatient treatment.

Child's Level of Behavioral Dysfunction

Identifying the symptoms targeted by medication involves a careful assessment of the child's functioning within several spheres. The assessment aims to identify the subtleties of behavior that is biologically motivated versus a response to family dysfunction or some combination of both. The following should be assessed:

- Family. What is the child's role within the family system? What meaning does the child have for the parents? Is the child in a parentified, infantalized, or scapegoated role? Is the child's behavior the same within the family as it is in school or with peers? How does the child relate to adults, including parents or other nonparenting figures?
- School. Is the school identifying a serious behavior problem? Have they articulated what aspects are particularly problematic? Is the behavior deliberate, or does it seem beyond the child's control? Is the behavior inhibiting the child's academic progress even if special classroom services have been provided to facilitate learning?
- Peers. Does the child interact with same-age peers? Do the child's behaviors tend to ostracize him or her from peers? What role does the child tend to take in groups of other children? Are peer relationships within age-appropriate norms? Is the child considered "odd" by same-age children?

The following additional questions about the child's functioning must be considered before using medication:

- How sustained are the symptoms presented by the child? For example, the child with evidence of thought disorder may have seemed odd to others from a very early age, whereas the child exhibiting symptoms of major depression may have shown serious dysfunction for months.
- Do the symptoms carry over into several spheres of the child's life? For example, the child whose functioning at school is socially and academically good but who is disobedient and oppositional at home may be responding to some aspect of the family dynamics that influences behavior. This child may not be a good candidate for medication; however, a child who is actively hallucinating at home, school, and in the neighborhood will likely benefit from antipsychotic medication to alle-

CLINICAL EXAMPLE: STEVEN

Steven, a 7-year-old white boy, had been referred to the outpatient mental health clinic by the school system, who saw his mother, Carol, as enmeshed and overly concerned with her son's normal activity and exuberance. At the time of evaluation, she insisted that he receive medication for his "hyperactivity." The nurse conducting the developmental assessment perceived that Steven's activity level was within normal limits and that his school functioning did not indicate overactive behavior. She began to focus on Carol's fears and worries and discovered that her brother had chronic schizophrenia. She was worried that Steven would "turn out like him." The goals of outpatient therapy focused on helping her understand the normal aspects of her son's behavior, while identifying her own fears and worries as a single parent with psychiatric illness in her immediate family.

CLINICAL EXAMPLE: ROBYN

Robyn, a 7-year-old African-American girl, was referred for an inpatient evaluation by the director of a family support service whose staff was working intensively with her chronically schizophrenic mother to help her maintain daily activities and routines with her three children.

Robyn, the youngest of the sibling group, had reported hearing voices and seeing snakes crawling on her walls. Upon admission, she was anxious, disorganized, somewhat verbally incoherent, and perseverative in her concerns about safety in the hospital. With support from the nursing staff, she settled into her room and began joining milieu activities while initiating hesitant contact with other children. Within 4 days, she began attending school, learning the unit program, and taking more interest in personal hygiene. Within 1 month, she reported no hallucinations and, while her behavior remained odd, she exhibited none of the bizarre behavior seen at admission.

The evaluation team ascertained that Robyn's disorganization was predominantly environmental and that she required a safe, structured, and predictable home. At her mother's request, she was placed in therapeutic foster care where she continued to progress developmentally and make academic gains at school. No medication was used during the hospitalization or outpatient follow-up care.

viate symptoms that negatively affect his or her functioning (See Clinical Example: Robyn).

- Have the child and family been thoroughly assessed before considering medication? Is medication used as an adjunct to other forms of care, such as group treatment or individual and family treatment?
- Have other methods of care been attempted before beginning medication?

Informed Consent

All parents and children are entitled to the process of informed consent when psychotropic medication is being considered. Informed consent provides a basic minimum of control or opportunity for control by the client or in the case of a child, by the legal guardians. The process of informed consent should include an explanation of the purpose and benefits of the treatment, a description of the process (such as duration, procedure, and costs), and an explanation of the involved risks. Explanation of the risks should include those that routinely and less frequently occur.

The health care team must inform the family and child about the alternatives to the proposed treatment, including nontreatment and its possible risks. In addition, the family and child are entitled to a statement describing potential unknown risks of psychotropic medication. This especially applies to children, for whom long-term side effects of many medications are uncertain.

Emotional consent involves a broader parental understanding of the child's problem and the child's "assent" to receiving medication. Children are entitled to an explanation of the process, the target symptoms, and a chance to ask questions or express feelings about the treatment. Piaget would suggest that children can begin to understand the meaning of medication at the stage of concrete operations, around 7 years of age. However, the child's chronologic age may not indicate the stage of their cognitive development, and nurses must remember this when explaining medication to children (Popper, 1987).

Obtaining parental consent to treat a child with medication may involve several interviews and much discussion. To elicit the greatest efficacy of the treatment, the parents must support the medication trial and be realistic in their expectations of the outcome.

Family or Parental Factors in Pharmacologic Treatment

Parents are apt to blame themselves for their child's difficulties. They may attribute the child's difficulties to each other. They may view the child as imperfect. They may see the child as an extension of themselves and their own serious difficulties throughout their childhood or adult life.

Parental ability to understand and accept the use of medication to treat psychiatric illness is related to socioeconomic status, level of education, religious beliefs, and culture. The belief system regarding health care influences parents' degree of compliance in supporting medication management of their child. Parental experience with psychiatric illness in themselves or family members, their own experiences with medication, and their history of addictions or recovery from substance abuse will affect their beliefs about psychopharmacology. Nurses must understand these influences and use them in deciding whether or not medication can be useful in altering a child's behavior.

A thorough family assessment is imperative prior to choosing medication as a method of treatment. The child's positive use of medication will be thwarted if parents are not an active part of the treatment team that recommends this form of intervention. Parents may obstruct the treatment by forgetting to give the child the medication, displaying negative attitudes about efficacy, or withdrawing from treatment. The nurse must engage the family in the child's care prior to giving medication.

Use of Medication in Inpatient and Outpatient Settings

Nursing management of the child receiving psychotropic medication will differ between inpatient and outpatient settings. Within the hospital, the child or adolescent is accessible to nursing assessment throughout the day. Inpatient staff monitor target symptoms on all shifts. The child is apt to receive the medication on a specific and regular time schedule. The milieu tends to support the use of medication as part of a total treatment regimen that usually includes individual, group, and family interventions. Medication is easily changed, doses can be altered, and the child's responses to medication are carefully assessed.

The milieu setting also lends itself to careful discharge planning around medication management. Passes away from the hospital offer a chance for child and family to "practice" managing medication independently. Aftercare planning must occur because the client is most likely to be managed by a private physician or clinic setting in the community. In addition to the child's and family's medication teaching, the community provider requires a thorough explanation of the rationale for using a particular type of medication, dose, and long-term recommendations about care.

Often children leave the hospital and move into residential treatment settings, foster homes, or group home settings where the providers may require education and guidance about managing the child's medication. These individuals must assume the role of parental advocate for the child when parents are unavailable. They must, like parents, understand the child's need for medication, response, side effects, and the necessity for compliance. The child's legal guardian must always give written permission to treat with medication. For children committed to the state welfare system, this guardian might be a court-appointed attorney, a guardian ad litem, or a designated social worker in the welfare department.

Outpatient management of the child on medication poses other challenges to the nurse managing care. Nurses must rely on reports from parents and teachers to assess the child's global functioning. An alliance with parents and schools is essential in ensuring compliance and careful monitoring of the child's target symptoms. Managing medication for a child in outpatient treatment offers more certainty than giving medication in outpatient settings.

The nurse's alliance with parents and teachers becomes crucial if children do not behaviorally respond in a prompt or positive way to the administration of medication. Many drugs require a long trial before ascertaining efficacy, which is difficult for families who want to see immediate response. The nurse's relationship with the family and child can sustain the treatment if progress is not evident.

Children, adolescents, and their families in inpatient and outpatient settings need to understand the time frames of the medication trial (i.e., the amount of time the child may be on the medication). With lithium carbonate or methylphenidate, this time might be months or years. With other medications, such as tricyclic antidepressants, the treatment should be time limited. When the child is likely to take medication on a long-term basis, the nurse or doctor may explore the issue of drug holidays with the family.

Implementation of Medication Management

ANTIPSYCHOTIC (OR NEUROLEPTIC) MEDICATIONS

Antipsychotic medication revolutionized the psychiatric treatment of schizophrenic adults when it was first used in the 1950s. Initially termed tranquilizers, these medications have proven clinically effective in adults in treating thought disorders, hallucinations, delusions, and other kinds of disordered thinking. Their efficacy and superiority over the singular use of psychosocial methods of treatment are well documented in the research literature (Klein, Gittelman, Quitkin, & Rifkin, 1980).

The effectiveness of neuroleptic medication with children and adolescents evidencing schizophrenia or pervasive developmental disorders is not well documented (Campbell, 1985). Certainly, mental health professionals discourage and regard as ineffective the use of these medications as the only method of psychiatric treatment.

Several factors may account for the questionable effectiveness of antipsychotic medication. First, children and young adolescents who evidence disordered thought tend to have more serious deviations in development than their adult counterparts whose first schizophrenic episodes occur in their early 20s. The child with pervasive developmental disorder is unlikely to have negotiated the normal development tasks of early childhood, latency, or early adolescence and therefore is more pervasively disturbed.

The singular use of medication is ineffective in helping the child learn, understand, and use social skills, academic information, or peer relating. Medication may assist the child in becoming more available to achieving developmental tasks by improving concentration or decreasing psychomotor agitation (Campbell, 1985). Medication will not replace or make up for developmental milestones not attained by the psychiatrically disordered child.

Second, development moves along a continuum involving physical, emotional, and cognitive spheres. Achievement of developmental milestones is more difficult to predict in children with thought disorders. Would development have proceeded in a different manner if psychotropic medication had not been used to assist the child in achieving age-appropriate norms? Research in this area is inconclusive. Nurses considering psychotropic interventions must carefully consider this question and hypothesize the risk–benefit issues inherent in the treatment.

Finally, children do not respond to psychotropic medication in the same way as adults. Age, degree of impairment, IQ, and stage of development influence clinical response to medication. Fish, Shapiro, and Campbell (1966) showed that less impaired psychotic children without profound retardation showed clinical improvement on placebo or milieu therapy. More severely disturbed children with a lower IQ responded to high potency neuroleptics, such as trifluoperazine (Stelazine) and haloperidol (Haldol) (Anderson et al., 1984; Cohen et al., 1980).

Response is not always predictable and depends on environmental factors, such as impairment of family, availability of follow-up services, special education, and therapy. Campbell (1985) recommends instituting medication at the onset of psychotic symptoms rather than waiting for other therapies to fail. Although acute symptoms may subside, clients may need long-term treatment with neuroleptics. Equally important are the auxiliary treatments necessary to maintain stabilization (i.e., individual and family treatment and special education).

Neuroleptic medications act on the brain in several ways. They block the uptake of dopamine at receptor sites and have an anticholinergic effect. These actions can pose serious side effects to the individual who takes neuroleptics (Thompson & Schuster, 1968). These side effects depend on the type of neuroleptic, the dosage, the duration of administration, the client's age, the target symptoms, and the presence or absence of organic brain dysfunction. This is especially significant for children if their symptoms require long-term medication management.

Side effects of antipsychotic medication include changes in perceptual and cognitive functions, psychomotor performance, mood, motivation, and interpersonal relationships that interfere with functioning even when doses are within therapeutic range. DiMascio and Shader (1970) called this symptom constellation behavioral toxicity. Also included are sedation, which can interfere with learning, and a worsening of preexisting symptoms (Campbell, 1985).

Other anticholinergic side effects include dry mouth, constipation, and urinary retention. Antiparkinsonian medication is sometimes used prophylactically in individuals receiving neuroleptic medication. While these agents may help prevent the more serious extrapyramidal symptoms, they also can increase the incidence of anticholinergic side effects.

While anticholinergic side effects are unpleasant for the individual receiving neuroleptics, the most serious constellation of side effects involves the central nervous system (CNS). These CNS side effects include dizziness, headaches, insomnia, ataxia, seizures, and sedation (Campbell, 1985). The major CNS side effects are detailed in Table 29-1.

Campbell, Grega, Green, and Bennett (1983a) noted that between 8% and 51% of children and adolescents receiving neuroleptics will develop tardive dyskinesia (TD) and withdrawal dyskinesia (WD). These are abnormal involuntary movements that involve the face, tongue, mouth, upper and lower extremities, fingers, toes, torso, and neck. They are characterized by diaphragmatic and laryngeal muscle involvement and appear as grunts or peculiar vocalizations. The vocalizations may be

TABLE 29–1 Extrapyramidal Side Effects of Antipsychotic Medications

Extrapyramidal Side Effect	Description	Treatment
Acute dystonic reactions	Tonic contractions of muscles in the mouth and torso that can last from minutes to hours; more often associated with high-potency neuroleptics (e.g., haloperidol) Usually occurs after first dose or within first few days of beginning neuroleptic medication; may occur after long-term administration of drug Reactions are painful and frightening and require immediate medical intervention	Intramuscular administration of Benadryl 25 mg
Parkinsonian reactions	Manifested by rigid, mask-like facial expressions, shuffling gait, drooling, finger and hand tremors, or muscular rigidity (cogwheel phenomenon) Rare in preschool children, more common in school-age children and adolescents (Campbell *et al.,* 1984)	Intramuscular or intravenous administration of Benadryl or Cogentin
Akathisias	Evidenced by restlessness or an inability to sit still, excitement, or agitation Usually develops in first 5 weeks of treatment; may be difficult to differentiate from hyperactivity, especially in children Should be carefully noted by nurse	Changing to a different neuroleptic or decreasing the dose may alleviate symptoms
Tardive dyskinesia	Results from prolonged use of neuroleptics Early signs characterized by tongue movement or increased blinking Later signs involve tongue protrusion and unusual mouth movements, such as sucking, smacking lips, or chewing jaw movements (rabbit syndrome).	Most effective treatment is prevention (i.e., regular reevaluation of drug dose and assessment for beginning side effects), along with maintenance on lowest effective dose of medication

Campbell, M., Small, A. M., Green, W. H., Jennings, S. J., Perry, R., Bennett, W. G., & Anderson, L. (1984). A comparison of haloperidol and lithium in hospitalized aggressive conduct disorder children. *Archives of General Psychiatry, 41,* 650–656.

rhythmic, irregular, repetitive, transient, or persistent.

The earliest onset of TD or WD is after 3 months of cumulative drug administration (Campbell et al., 1983a). Recent research suggests that the physical symptoms of TD and WD in children and adolescents are similar to the symptoms in adults (Campbell et al., 1983a; 1983b; Gualtieri, Barnhill, McGimsey, & Shell, 1980). This means that children and adolescents can develop persistent, irreversible TD and WD just like adults do (Paulson, Rizvi, & Crane, 1975).

The child or adolescent taking neuroleptic medication requires careful nursing management. Assessment of the child's daily behaviors will help the nurse identify the target symptoms for medication management. The nurse or parent continually observes for negative side effects of medication. The Abnormal Involuntary Movement Scale (AIMS) test may be used to assess involuntary movement (Psychopharmacology Bulletin, 1985). Many formal checklists also are useful. Box 29-1 is an example of a side-effect index that can be used with children and adolescents taking neuroleptics.

Nurses are particularly sensitive to the nuances of behavioral change that signal the onset of potentially serious side effects. The collaborative efforts of nurses and other members of the clinical team will determine the optimal use of neuroleptics with the seriously disturbed child or adolescent.

ANTIDEPRESSANT MEDICATION

Children and adolescents exhibiting affective disorders, anxiety disorders, and attention deficit disorders may benefit from antidepressant medication. Each of these diagnostic categories will be dis-

BOX 29–1 • SIDE-EFFECTS INDEX

Patient's name and unit: ______________________
Date of examination: ______________ Completed by ______________
Medication(s) and doses currently: ______________________
Pulse: ________ Respiration: ________ BP: ________ Wt: ________

	NO PROBLEM				SEVERE PROBLEM
General:					
Decreased sleep:	0	1	2	3	4
Decreased appetite/wt loss:	0	1	2	3	4
Weakness, fatigue:	0	1	2	3	4
Neurologic:					
Blurred vision:	0	1	2	3	4
Confusion:	0	1	2	3	4
Hallucinations:	0	1	2	3	4
Tics:	0	1	2	3	4
Dizziness:	0	1	2	3	4
Sedation:	0	1	2	3	4
Tremor:	0	1	2	3	4
Cardiovascular:					
Palpitations:	0	1	2	3	4
Hypertension:	0	1	2	3	4
Hypotension:	0	1	2	3	4
Gastrointestinal:					
Nausea, vomiting:	0	1	2	3	4
Constipation:	0	1	2	3	4
Diarrhea:	0	1	2	3	4
Dry mouth:	0	1	2	3	4
Skin:					
Rashes:	0	1	2	3	4

Used with permission of K. E. Towbin (personal communication).

cussed separately because target symptoms, dose, and expected response obviously will depend on the child's problems.

AFFECTIVE DISORDERS. The last decade has witnessed the acknowledgement and treatment of and research into affective disorders in children (Puig-Antich, 1980). The predominant controversy has centered around their etiology (i.e., whether biologically based, related to psychodynamic events that trigger the depression, or both) and their definition (i.e., whether childhood depressions manifest the same symptoms as adult depressions and subsequent treatments). Researchers have emphasized the need for systematic evaluation of symptoms without overattribution of depression to environmental causes. The current literature accepts the similarity of depressive symptomatology between adults and children and acknowledges the use of antidepressant medications in treatment (Puig-Antich, Blau, Marx, Greenhill, & Chambers, 1978). Developmental differences in the manifestation of depressive symptoms have been noted in the literature (Epstein & Cullinan, 1986). Chambers and Puig-Antich (1982) found that children with a major depressive disorder evidence psychotic symptoms, including rare depressive delusions, unlike adults in whom these are common phenomena. The authors suggest that the younger child's cognitive immaturity makes the development of a depressive delusional system unlikely. While bipolar, or manic–depressive, illness occurs rarely in children, they can exhibit symptoms of a chronic, low-grade, protracted depressive disorder (noted in the *Diagnostic and Statistical Manual of Mental Disorders*, 4th ed., Revised [DSM IV] to be dysthymic disorder). It becomes important for nurses to recognize the presence of dysthymia because it has negative implications for successful completion of age-appropriate developmental tasks.

In general, depression in children and adolescents inhibits completion of development tasks and most notably limits social relationships (Puig-Antich et al., 1985). Research is demonstrating that depression that begins in childhood frequently ushers in a chronic course that extends into adulthood characterized by relapse and recurrent need for treatment. Pharmacologic interventions become a necessary adjunct to psychosocial forms of treatment of depression, but they are not without risk or controversy.

Children are developmentally different from adults in the way they biologically metabolize antidepressants. The half-life of this medication tends to be shorter, probably because of children's faster metabolic rate, increased relative liver mass, and lower relative adipose mass (Perel, 1974). However, as with adults, an adequate drug trial of at least 10 to 14 days, and preferably 4 to 6 weeks, is necessary to observe therapeutic changes in depressive symptoms.

Children are more susceptible to cardiotoxic effects of tricyclic antidepressants than adults (Weinberg, Rutman, & Sullivan, 1973). Overdose of tricyclic antidepressants is life threatening and has serious cardiovascular implications. Nurses must ensure that the adults responsible for a child's care understand the issues around safety and management of antidepressant medication. Similarly, children need to be aware of the importance of taking medication as it is prescribed.

Antidepressants most often affect the cardiovascular system. The most common changes in electrocardiograms due to antidepressants involve a slight increase in resting heart rate (no greater than 130 beats per minute), lengthening of the PR interval (to no more than 0.22 second), and widening of the QRS (to no more than 30% increase over baseline). Dosages of tricyclic antidepressants are usually increased every fourth day from 1.5 to 3 to 4 to 5 mg/kg per day. Orthostatic changes in blood pressure are rare (Puig-Antich et al., 1985).

A sudden withdrawal of antidepressant medication can produce adverse effects, including nausea, vomiting, diarrhea, abdominal pain, or flu-like symptoms. To withdraw from antidepressants, the child's dosage should be gradually decreased over several days. Parents managing their child's treatment at home must understand the safest method of medication withdrawal.

ANXIETY DISORDERS. Antidepressants also are useful in treating anxiety disorders. The DSM IV (1994) describes three types of anxiety disorders: social phobia, generalized anxiety, and separation anxiety disorders. The most research attention has focused on separation anxiety disorders and particularly their manifestation as school phobia. The pharmacologic treatment of separation anxiety disorder and obsessive–compulsive disorder is discussed.

Children with separation anxiety disorder present with inordinate fears, ruminations, and compulsions and observable behavior of anxiety (Hershberg, Carlson, Cantwell, & Strober, 1982). While school phobia is the most common manifestation, separation anxiety disorders also can include sleep avoidance, nightmares, and unrealistic worries about family members.

Imipramine hydrochloride (Tofranil) at doses of 100 to 200 mg/day has successfully treated school phobic children (Gittelman-Klein & Klein, 1971). Doses of 1 to 5 mg/kg per day are generally recommended. Pharmacologic treatment alone is not sufficient in dealing with children having separation anxiety disorder, especially if there are notable environmental stressors impacting on the child's behavior. School phobia in particular usually indicates serious dysfunction within the family system and requires intensive family treatment for resolution.

Obsessive–compulsive disorders also represent a variance of anxiety disorders and involve behaviors and thoughts perceived as intrusive, unwanted, and beyond personal control. Compulsions, or repetitive behavior believed to control or prohibit a situation magically, usually occur with obsessions. Compulsions assist the client deal with the anxiety associated with obsessions (Anthony, 1975).

While medications are useful in treating children and adolescents with obsessive–compulsive disorders, no research suggests a primary drug to treat obsessive-compulsive disorder (Towbin, Leckman, & Cohen, 1987). It is recommended that patients receive an adequate trial of medication for at least 12 weeks to determine response (Towbin & Riddle, 1991). Medications shown to be useful in treating obsessive–compulsive disorder in children include

CLINICAL EXAMPLE: TONY

Tony, a 10-year-old male inpatient in a children's psychiatric hospital, was given a consequence for negative behavior while in the unit classroom. When he refused to take a time out, he was escorted back to the unit by two staff. On the return to the unit, a distance of approximately 100 yards, he threatened to run away and began screaming and wailing.

Once on the unit, he went into an unlocked quiet room where he continued crying and began pounding on the walls. The nurse assessed that he could benefit from medication to help him regain behavioral control. She stood at the quiet room door and offered Tony a p.r.n. dose of 25 mg of Benadryl in liquid form mixed with orange juice. He accepted this and quickly settled down, sat in the corner of the quiet room, and was able to process his behavior with staff. After returning to his room, he slept briefly and awakened alert and calm.

clorimipramine (Anafranil) (Insel et al., 1983; Flament et al., 1985) and fluoxetine (Prozac) (Fontaine & Chouinard, 1985; Riddle et al., 1990). These medications inhibit the uptake of serotonin and as with many other pharmacologic agents, are not approved by the Food and Drug Administration for use in children.

Antihistamines or benzodiazepines can successfully treat mild to moderate anxiety states related to developmental issues requiring pharmacologic intervention. Although not well researched, antihistamines and benzodiazepines used with children in inpatient settings offer a short-term intervention for anxiety states. These two categories of medication produce fewer side effects than more potent pharmacologic agents (See Clinical Example: Tony).

STIMULANT MEDICATION

Stimulants have been used primarily to treat children with the diagnosis of attention-deficit hyperactivity disorder (AD/HD) (DSM IV, 1994). These medications act on the CNS and stimulate the reticular activating system, thus improving attention and task performance (Barkley, 1977; Cantwell & Carlson, 1978; Weiner, 1980). Their side effects may include insomnia, poor appetite, headache, and decreased physical growth. Long-term use also can result in tic disorders; discontinuation of the stimulant medication is indicated if a tic disorder emerges.

Not all children diagnosed with AD/HD require stimulant medication. Severity of symptoms, the child's functioning in school, the family's tolerance of the hyperactive behavior, and treatment history should all influence use of these medications. Psychosis and thought disorder preclude the use of stimulant medications. They also are not recommended in children exhibiting a tic disorder. Medications are most often used with latency-aged children.

Target symptoms in the administration of stimulants often are academic and involve the child's ability to concentrate, mood, and motor behavior. Stimulants improve cognitive performance in areas of attention, vigilance, and reaction time (Aman, 1978; Fisher, 1978; Gittelman, 1983).

Research has been unable to predict which children exhibiting AD/HD will respond to pharmacologic management of their behavior. The usual dose for methylphenidate (Ritalin), the most frequently used stimulant, is 5 mg b.i.d. It is usually administered before meals, although administration at meals might prevent the anorexia that can accompany the drug use. If methylphenidate is unsuccessful in improving the child's behavior, the usual progression through stimulant trials involves the use of other medications, including dextroamphetamine (Dexedrine), pemoline (Cylert), or low doses of antidepressants.

Children may discontinue stimulant medication on weekends (termed a drug holiday) when school performance is not essential. It is recommended that all individuals taking stimulant medication discontinue the medication at least once yearly. Sleator, vonNeumann, and Sprague (1974) found that many children do not resume taking the medication after a yearly drug holiday and have shown some improvement in symptoms. Short-term benefits of these medications for children are well documented in the research literature; long-term benefits or changes in behavior are less clearly delineated and require further research.

OTHER MEDICATIONS

LITHIUM. Lithium has been a drug of choice for several decades to treat adult patients exhibiting bipolar disorders, mania, and other types of depression (Goodwin, Murphy, Dunner, & Bunney, 1972; Baron, Gershon, Rudy, Jonas, & Buchsbaum,

1975). The effectiveness of this medication with adults has led several researchers to suggest that similar positive responses might be found in children and adolescents with bipolar illness (Youngerman & Canino, 1978). The highest level of effectiveness of lithium occurs in children and adolescents exhibiting mood disturbance, both cyclic and noncyclic and in those with a positive family history for affective disorder.

Lithium also has been a successful treatment for youngsters exhibiting behavioral aggression or self-mutilative behaviors. Delong and Aldershof (1987) have treated a population of children with these symptoms for 10 years and found that no patient was reported to have serious side effects. They noted dramatic improvement in aggressive males ages 6.8 to 16 years. It is unclear if responders have an associated depression underlying their aggressive behaviors. All researchers emphasize the need for continued longitudinal research to ascertain lithium's long-term response and side effects.

Lithium potentially affects renal, thyroid, and bone systems. Prior to beginning this medication, a physical examination and baseline blood studies are advisable. The usual beginning dose is 150 mg/d in younger children and 300 mg/d in older children and adolescents. Every 5 to 7 days the dose is increased by 150 mg/d (or 300 mg/d) until blood levels reach 0.8 to 1.2 mEq/L. It is best to draw blood for laboratory tests in the morning, 10 to 12 hours after the youngster has received the last dose of the medication. After the therapeutic blood level becomes stable, blood should be monitored at least monthly.

Side effects of lithium may include nausea, diarrhea, polyuria, blurred vision, and excessive thirst. Nurses must instruct parents to withhold lithium if the child has decreased food intake or gastric upset involving vomiting or diarrhea. During salt-depleted states (such as the dehydration following influenza), lithium is poorly excreted by the kidneys, which may result in excessive blood levels.

POLYPHARMACY. Polypharmacy involves concurrently treating a child or adolescent with more than one psychotropic medication. The relative paucity of research concerning the effects of any psychotropic medication with children creates a justified reluctance to practice polypharmacy with children and adolescents unless target symptoms warrant treatment with different pharmacologic agents. Licamele and Goldberg (1989) advise caution when treating childhood disorders with more than one medication. They recommend the administration of more than one medication only when the seriousness of the situation makes the child's personal safety or hospitalization a risk.

The literature provides little information regarding polypharmacy with children. The concurrent use of lithium and methylphenidate (Ritalin) to treat attention deficit disorder accompanied by affective disorder symptomatology (Licamele & Goldberg, 1989) is cited. Similarly, the use of lithium and haloperidol (Haldol) concurrently in an aggressive, thought disordered population has been described (Small & Green, 1984).

Nurses must question the use of polypharmacy with children and adolescents in their care. The diagnosis, target symptoms, side effects, and implications for long-term management must be clear. Nurses can advocate by ensuring that parents and children clearly understand the purpose of using several medications as part of treatment.

Nursing Management of Medication

ADMINISTRATION

Many psychotropic medications can be given in oral, intramuscular, and intravenous forms. The most preferred route of administration is oral because this is least invasive. With some children, an injection, usually administered at a point of behavioral crisis on an inpatient unit, may have psychodynamic meaning beyond the expected psychic and physical discomfort. The injection might, in the most disordered individual, replicate past sexual or physical abuse or might perpetuate a disturbed, albeit unconscious, wish to be hurt, punished, or victimized.

Whenever possible, nurses should choose the least invasive method of medication administration. If a child is "cheeking" a tablet, liquid forms of many drugs are available and can be mixed with juice to ameliorate the taste. Children should be taught to recognize the medication they are taking, noting the color, shape, and size of the tablet or amount of liquid. If they raise questions about the correctness of a medication, the nurse should assess this immediately. In this way, the child begins to take some responsibility for recognizing their medication and participating in the administration.

TEACHING STRATEGIES IN MEDICATION MANAGEMENT OF CHILDREN AND ADOLESCENTS

The first step in teaching families about psychotropic medication involves understanding what medication means to them within the context of their culture, socioeconomic group, health value system, and past psychiatric history. Most parents who pursue psychiatric care for their child will not be knowledgeable about psychotropic medications, yet parents are entitled to this information when medication is used to treat their child. It is essential for the safe management of their child's care and to help ensure compliance with the treatment plan that parents actively participate in learning about psychotropic medication.

In planning teaching strategies, nurses must first assess the family's ability to assimilate information. They must present medication information in an understandable way tailored to the cognitive and emotional strengths and weaknesses of the learners. Nurses must recognize that the level of crisis experienced by the family influences how they comprehend teaching about their child's medication. Families may view medication as a "cure-all" for their child's problems, or they may doubt the value of this form of treatment or try to interfere with a trial. These attitudes influence the success or failure of a medication trial. The nurse must identify and modify these attitudes of families early in treatment planning.

Teaching must be ongoing because people pay attention to information with immediate and personal relevance. For example, parents may be distraught that their suicidal daughter requires antidepressants. They may not comprehend that antidepressants are highly toxic and must be carefully monitored to avoid the possibility of deliberate overdose. They may not realize that antidepressants must be slowly withdrawn when the treatment is completed. The nurse must be prepared to reiterate this information at the time it becomes pertinent to the client's care. Families need clear, concise, written directives about their child's medication to serve as guidelines or reference.

When explaining medications and their uses, nurses must give families permission to ask questions, even questions that appear simple or obvious. Asking parents to repeat directives or explanations will help the nurse assess the depth of their comprehension.

Whenever possible, the nurse should educate the child or adolescent about the medication they are taking, the reasons for taking it, and the potential side effects. While this is at times impossible (e.g., during an acute psychotic episode or if the child is severely depressed), most clients are able to comprehend at least some information regarding their medication. Minimally, children should know the name of the drug they are taking, the target symptoms, the length of time they will take medication, and possible side effects. The depth of this information will depend on the child's cognitive abilities and developmental level. Even the most impaired children and adolescents, however, are entitled to early explanations of this aspect of their care. Nurses should repeat medication information as the child's reality testing or ability to comprehend improves. Parents need to know what their child has been taught about medication and preferably should be present during the teaching.

EVALUATION

Ideally, medication is prescribed to deal with a set of target symptoms presented by the child or adolescent exhibiting psychiatric problems. Evaluation of efficacy of the medication involves assessing change in these target symptoms over time and considering the medication's half-life, therapeutic doses, and the client's compliance with the prescribed regimen.

Clients rarely show complete amelioration of symptoms on medication. Improvement is usually variable and at times difficult to measure. The use of standardized rating scales can objectively determine if symptoms have altered during treatment. Box 29–1 details a side-effects index that can help the care provider ascertain the presence or absence of side effects. The format of the side-effects index, applicable in inpatient and outpatient settings, acts as a guide in assessing the child's negative response to medication. The subjective opinions of others who deal with the child, such as teachers, child care workers, and grandparents, provide additional data in evaluating the effectiveness of medication and in noting side effects.

Nurses are particularly adept at looking holistically at the client and family. Target symptoms may change because of alterations in the environment or child unrelated to medication administration. Parent counseling, a change in classroom, family therapy, or normal developmental changes may assist in the client's improvement. Medication is rarely a singular cure for mental health problems and is most effective in conjunction with other forms of care.

Pharmacotherapy and Implications for Nursing Research

Research involving pharmacotherapy with children and adolescents has increased markedly within the last decade. Specific drug therapies have gained wide acceptance within the psychiatric community and include the use of methylphenidate with hyperactive children, haloperidol for thought disorders, and desipramine (Norpramin) for childhood depression.

Nurses participate in research projects in many ways. As members of the research team, they develop the methodology to measure response to medication. Often, they provide the adjunct care required by clients and families participating in research projects. This adjunct care may include family and individual treatment, education, and acting as a liaison with community agencies who continue care after the client is finished with the research protocol.

Nursing research approaches pharmacotherapy from a holistic perspective that includes, but is not limited to, biologic responses to medication. Nurses are more likely to research the psychosocial aspects of medication management and the child's or adolescent's performance within family and school and with peers.

The following research questions might be posed by nurse researchers:

- What effect does the use of p.r.n. medication have on client groups within the milieu?
- Are medication and adjunct therapy more effective in improving functioning than either treatment given singularly?
- How does parental understanding of medication management affect compliance with pharmacotherapy regimens?
- Can specific pharmacotherapies be related to nursing diagnosis in the same way they currently relate to DSM IV?

Child psychiatric nursing offers a unique perspective to any research involving children and adolescents because it focuses on children and their families in a holistic manner (NIMH, 1990). Research on medication for psychiatric disorders in children or adolescents will continue to expand and answer critical questions about efficacy and response.

Nurses can play key roles in this process, both as colleagues to biologic researchers and through independent nursing research that addresses the psychosocial aspects of medication treatment. Nurses deal with delivery of care within all aspects of the client's life. They are most adept at identifying the subtleties of change occurring outside the laboratory or clinic. These observations provide valuable information about the child's or adolescent's holistic response to pharmacotherapy.

REFERENCES

Aman, G. (1978). Drugs, learning and the psychotherapies. In J. S. Werry (Ed.), *Pediatric psychopharmacology: The use of behavior modifying drugs in children* (pp. 79–108). New York: Brunner/Mazel.

American Psychiatric Association (1994). *Diagnostic and statistical manual of mental disorders* (4th ed.). Washington, D.C.: Author.

Anderson, L. T., Campbell, M., Grega, D. M., Perry, R., Small, A. M., & Green, W. H. (1984). Haloperidol in infantile autism: Effects on learning and behavioral symptoms. *American Journal of Psychiatry, 141*, 1195–1202.

Anthony, E. J. (1975). Neurosis in Children. In A. M Freedman, H. I. Kaplan, & B. J. Sadock (Eds.), *Comprehensive textbook of psychiatry* (Vol. 2). (pp. 2155–2157). Baltimore: Williams & Wilkins.

Barkley, R. (1977). A review of stimulant drug research with hyperactive children. *Journal of Child Psychology and Psychiatry, 18*, 137–165.

Baron, M., Gershon, E., Rudy, V., Jonas, W., & Buchsbaum, M. (1975). Lithium carbonate response in depression. *Archives of General Psychiatry, 32*, 1107–1111.

Campbell, M. (1985). Schizophrenic disorders and pervasive developmental disorders/infantile autism. In J. M. Wiener (Ed.), *Diagnosis and psychopharmacology of childhood and adolescent disorders* (pp. 113–150). New York: John Wiley & Sons.

Campbell, M., Grega, D. M., Green, W. H., & Bennett, W. G. (1983a). Neuroleptic-induced dyskinesias in children. *Clinical Neuropharmacology, 6*, 207–222.

Campbell, M., Perry, R., Bennett, W. G., Small, A. M., Green, W. H., Grega, D. M., Schwartz, V., & Anderson, L. (1983b). Long term therapeutic efficacy and drug related abnormal movements: A prospective study of haloperidol in autistic children. *Psychopharmacology Bulletin, 19(1)*, 80–82.

Campbell, M., Small, A. M., Green, W. H., Jennings, S. J., Perry, R., Bennett, W. G., & Anderson, L. (1984). A comparison of haloperidol and lithium in hospitalized aggressive conduct disorder children. *Archives of General Psychiatry, 41*, 650–656.

Cantwell, D. P., & Carlson, G. A. (1978). Stimulants. In J. S. Werry (Ed.), *Pediatric psychopharmacology: The use of behavior modifying drugs in children* (pp. 171–207). New York: Brunner/Mazel.

Chambers, W. J., & Puig-Antich, J. (1982). Psychotic symptoms in prepubertal major depressive disorder. *Archives of General Psychiatry, 39*, 921–927.

Cohen, I. L., Campbell, M., Posner, D., Small, A. M., Trievel, D., & Anderson, L. T. (1980). Behavioral effects of haloperidol in young autistic children: An objective analysis using a within subjects reversal design. *Journal of the American Academy of Child Psychiatry, 19*, 665–677.

DeLong, G. R., & Aldershof, A. L. (1987). Long term experience with lithium treatment in childhood. *Journal of the American Academy of Child and Adolescent Psychiatry, 26*, 389–394.

DiMascio, H., & Shader, R. I. (1970). Behavioral toxicity, Part 1: Definition; and Part II: Psychomotor functions. In R. J. Shader & A. DiMascio (Eds.), *Psychotropic drug side effects* (pp. 124–131). Baltimore: Williams & Wilkins.

Epstein, N. H., & Cullinan, D. (1986). Depression in children. *Journal of School Health, 56*, 10–12.

Fish, B., Shapiro, T., & Campbell, M. (1966). Long term prognosis and the response of schizophrenic children to drug therapy: A controlled study of trifluoperazine. *American Journal of Psychiatry, 123*, 32–39.

Fisher, M. A. (1978). Dextroamphetamine and placebo practice effects on selection in hyperactive children. *Journal of Abnormal Child Psychology, 6*, 25–32.

Flament, M., Rappoport, J. L., Berg, C. Z., et al. (1985). Clomipramine treatment of childhood obsessive compulsive disorder: A double blind controlled study. *Archives of General Psychiatry, 42*, 977–983.

Fontaine, R., & Chouinard, G. (1986). An open clinical trial of fluoxetine in the treatment of obsessive-compulsive disorder. *Journal of Clinical Psychopharmacology, 6,* 98–101.

Gittelman, R. (1983). Experimental and clinical studies of stimulant use in hyperactive children and children with other behavioral disorders. In I. Creese (Ed.), *Stimulants: Neurochemical, behavioral, and clinical perspectives* (pp. 205–225). New York: Raven Press.

Gittelman-Klein, R., & Klein, D. F. (1981). Controlled imipramine treatment of school phobia. *Archives of General Psychiatry, 25,* 204–207.

Goodwin, F. K., Murphy, D. L., Dunner, D., & Bunney, W. E. (1972). Lithium response of unipolar versus bipolar depression. *American Journal of Psychiatry, 129,* 44–47.

Gualtieri, C. T., Barnhill, J., McGimsey, J., & Shell, D. (1980). Tardive dyskinesia and other movement disorders in children treated with psychotropic drugs. *Journal of the American Academy of Child Psychiatry, 19,* 491–510.

Hamric, A. B. (1989). History and overview of the CNS role. In A. B. Hamric & J. A. Spross (Eds.), *The clinical nurse specialist in theory and practice* (2nd ed) (pp. 3–18). Philadelphia: W.B. Saunders.

Hershberg, S. G., Carlson, G. A., Cantwell, D. P., & Strober, M. (1982). Anxiety and depressive disorders in psychiatrically disturbed children. *Journal of Clinical Psychiatry, 43*(9), 358–361.

Insel, T. R., Murphy, D. L., Cohen, R. M., Alterman, I., Kilts, C., & Linnoila, M. (1983). Obsessive-compulsive disorder: A double blind trial of clomipramine and clorgyline. *Archives of General Psychiatry, 40,* 605–612.

Klein, D. F., Gittelman, R., Quitkin, F., & Rifkin, A. (1980). *Diagnosis and drug treatment of psychiatric disorders: Adults and children* (2nd ed) (pp. 343–370). Baltimore: Williams & Wilkins.

Licamele, W. L., & Goldberg, R. L. (1989). The concurrent use of lithium and methylphenidate in a child. *Journal of the American Academy of Child and Adolescent Psychiatry, 28,* 785–787.

Paulson, G. W., Rizvi, C. A., & Crane, G. E. (1975). Tardive dyskinesia as a possible sequel of long term therapy with phenothiazines. *Clinical Pediatrics, 14,* 953–955.

Perel, J. M. (1974). Review of pediatric and adult pharmacology of imipramine and other drugs. In O. S. Robinson (Ed.), *Report of chairman. Ad hoc committee on tricyclic antidepressant cardiotoxicity* (pp. 1–4). Food and Drug Administration.

Popper, C. W. (Ed.). (1987). *Psychiatric pharmacosciences of children and adolescents: Progress in psychiatry series.* Washington, D.C.: American Psychiatric Association.

Psychopharmacology Bulletin (1985). Special feature: Rating scales and assessment (Vol. 21) no. 4.

Puig-Antich, J. (1980). Affective disorders in childhood: A review and pespective. *Psychiatric Clinics of North America, 3,* 403–424.

Puig-Antich, J., Blau, F., Marx, N., Greenhill, L. L., & Chambers, W. (1978). Prepubertal major depressive disorder: A pilot Study. *Journal of the American Academy of Child and Adolescent Psychiatry, 17,* 695–707.

Puig-Antich, J., Lukens, E., Davies, M., Goetz, D., Brennan-Quattrock, J., & Todak, G. (1985). Controlled studies in psychosocial functioning in prepubertal major depressive disorders: II. Interpersonal relationships after sustained recovery from the affective episode. *Archives of General Psychiatry, 42,* 511–517.

Puig-Antich, J., Ryan, N. D., & Rabinovich, H. (1985). Affective disorders in childhood and adolescence. In J. M. Wiener (Ed.), *Diagnosis and psychopharmacology of childhood and adolescent disorders* (pp. 151–178). New York: John Wiley & Sons.

Riddle, M. A., Hardin, M. T., King, R., Scahill, L., & Woolston, J. L. (1990). Fluoxetine treatment of children and adolescents with Tourette's and obsessive compulsive disorders; preliminary clinical experience. *Journal of the American Academy of Child and Adolescent Psychiatry, 29*(1), 45–49.

Sleator, E., vonNeumann, A., & Sprague, R. (1974). Hyperactive children: a continuous long-term placebo-controlled follow-up. *Journal of the American Medical Association, 229,* 316–317.

Thompson, T., & Schuster, C. R. (1968). *Behavioral Pharmacology.* Englewood Cliffs, NJ: Prentice-Hall.

Towbin, K. E., Leckman, J. F., & Cohen, D. J. (1987). Drug treatment of obsessive compulsive disorder: A review of findings in the light of diagnostic and metric limitations. *Psychiatric Developments, 1,* 25–50.

Towbin, K. E., & Riddle, M. A. (1991). Obsessive compulsive disorder in childhood and adolescence. In M. Lewis (Ed.), *Child and adolescent psychiatry: A comprehensive textbook.* Baltimore: Williams & Wilkins (pp. 685–697).

Youngerman, J., & Canino, I. A. (1978). Lithium carbonate use in children and adolescents: A survey of the literature. *Archives of General Psychiatry, 35,* 216–224.

Weinberg, W. A., Rutman, J., & Sullivan, L. (1973). Depression in children referred to an educational diagnostic center: Diagnosis and treatment. *Journal of Pediatrics, 83,* 1065–1072.

Weiner, N. (1980). Norepinephrine, epinephrine, and sympathomimetics. In L. Goodman & A. Gilman (Eds.), *The pharmacologic basis of therapeutics* (6th ed.) (pp. 138–175). New York: Macmillan.

ACKNOWLEDGMENT

The author wishes to acknowledge the assistance of Kenneth E. Towbin, M.D., and Denise Abbate, R.N., M.S.N., C.S., while preparing this chapter.

CHAPTER

30

Therapeutic Environments

Celeste M. Johnson

The purpose of this chapter is to review the concept of a therapeutic environment and to apply that theoretical framework to nursing interventions within a structured inpatient treatment setting for children and adolescents. This chapter also describes how nursing staff can teach parents to extend therapeutic gains into the home. Critical components of a therapeutic environment for child and adolescent inpatient psychiatric units are identified. The importance of creating a dynamic system, which involves the interdisciplinary team, patient population, and a daily schedule of therapeutic activities, is emphasized. Modalities used in a therapeutic environment are described.

In addition, staff issues and concerns are addressed. The role of staff members is explored in creating and using therapeutic environments as treatment strategies for improving the ego skills and problem-solving abilities of young clients. The importance of maintaining open relationships with colleagues and of modeling effective communication and collaboration is discussed.

Defining Therapeutic Environments

A therapeutic environment, also referred to as a therapeutic milieu or milieu therapy, generally means a particular way of arranging a social environment to promote, facilitate, or accomplish therapeutic goals (Mosher, Kresky-Wolff, Matthews, & Menn, 1986). A therapeutic environment in child and adolescent psychiatric nursing refers to the people and all other social and physical factors in the environment with which the child interacts. The therapeutic environment provides a round-the-clock secure retreat for children whose capacities for coping with reality have deteriorated. Often children encountered in treatment settings come from environments that have not been conducive to their growth and development due to breakdowns in family structure, family boundaries, or communication. The therapeutic environment provides children with opportunities to acquire adaptive coping skills appropriate to their developmental stage. As the 24-hour providers of care, nursing staff have primary responsibility for creating and maintaining the therapeutic environment and helping families create and maintain therapeutic environments at home.

A therapeutic environment enhances the development of the child's adaptive social skills and interpersonal behaviors. DiBella, Weitz, Poynter-Berg, and Yurmark (1982) describe a therapeutic milieu as a supervised group treatment environment that provides a model of the everyday world of reality and maximizes opportunities for patients to benefit from their social and physical surroundings. Devine (1981) and Critchley (1987) describe milieu therapy as an attempt to use the environment as an instrument of treatment. The environment is therapeutic rather than merely a place where traditional therapies occur. Milieu therapy is the organizing therapeutic force of the treatment environment brought about by the interplay of process, content, and time variables of the unit (Rasinski, Rozensky, & Pasulka, 1980).

"A therapeutic environment does not just happen. It must be built systematically and rebuilt daily, the effort itself creating an atmosphere alive with growth in staff as well as patients" (Skinner, 1979, p. 38). Experienced staff engineer the milieu so that each interaction and activity becomes therapeutic. Because client populations constantly change, flexibility and ongoing evaluation are critical to effective milieus. Therapeutic milieus respond to changing variables, creating a dynamic system.

Theoretical Frameworks

Two theoretical frameworks underlie the concept of therapeutic environments: the psychodynamic model and the social learning model. In the psychodynamic model (Daniels, 1975), ego skills are required to function effectively in the environment of the real world. Emotionally disturbed children and adolescents lack these skills as a result of life experiences that have produced overwhelming and unmanageable anxiety, or they have not yet developed these skills. The child experiences a corrective environment in the therapeutic milieu of a structured inpatient treatment setting. This environment must be reality oriented and caring, with opportunities to lower maladaptive defenses and substitute more effective tension-reducing behaviors or coping skills. If successful, the therapeutic environment enhances ego skills by strengthening self-esteem through interpersonal successes and honest expression of feelings and by increasing cognitive problem-solving abilities (Jack, 1989).

In the social learning model (Cummings & Cumming, 1982; Jones, 1953), lack of effective ego skills results from learning that has taken place in environments characterized by unclear, guarded communication patterns; few limits on inappropriate behaviors; poor role models; and discouraged expression of thoughts and feelings. To correct these ego deficits, the inpatient setting uses a therapeutic environment that is purposefully structured to provide situations in which the child is expected to analyze and solve problems as they occur in the everyday activities of the unit. With guidance from healthy role models, the child or adolescent learns and tests new adaptive ways of relating to others and more constructive ways of handling feelings and stressors.

Critical Components of Therapeutic Environments

The following are characteristics or principles of therapeutic environments (Beck, Rawlins, & Williams, 1988; Daniels, 1975; DiBella et al., 1982).

- Every interaction is an opportunity for therapeutic intervention.
- Clients are required to assume responsibility for their own behavior.
- Problems are solved through discussion.
- Community meetings provide an opportunity to discuss information and interactions affecting all staff and clients.
- Inappropriate behaviors are dealt with as they occur.
- Communication is open and direct between staff and clients.
- Clients are encouraged to participate actively in their own treatment and in decision making on the unit.
- The unit remains in close contact with the community. There is frequent communication with family and significant members of the client's social network (e.g., peers, teachers, and youth leaders).

Therapeutic environments can be modified for different treatment settings, including acute inpatient units, day or partial hospitals, and residential treatment centers; however, several program components characterize all therapeutic environments. These include distributed power (Jack, 1989), physical setting, structure, treatment modalities, and therapeutic interactions between clients and staff.

DISTRIBUTED POWER

In therapeutic environments, clients are active, responsive participants who share in the decision-making process. This process conveys to clients that they must help themselves, rather than wait for answers from staff. Clients identify their own problems, set their own goals, and decide on a plan to reach those goals, with the assistance and support of peers and staff.

The therapeutic environment is contrasted to the traditional model in which the physician controls the decision-making process. Clients in the traditional model are dependent on decisions being made for them by someone else; they are passive recipients of treatment. In the therapeutic environment, decision making is shared by clients and staff, with the physician participating in this process. In shared decision making, the milieu must foster open and honest communication and a willingness to allow the group to deal directly with problems as they occur. This concept becomes operational through daily groups, setting and evaluating goals, and weekly community meetings. These groups are attended by all clients and staff members and are a forum for discussing problems that have occurred during the past day or week. Clients may share feelings or concerns about anticipated problems. Milieu staff also can share concerns or identify problems. The group explores the problem, shares ideas about possible solutions, offers emotional support, and when necessary makes a decision to take a particular action. Unit rules can be made, clarified, and enforced through this community meeting.

PHYSICAL SETTING

Another dimension of the therapeutic environment is the physical setting of the unit itself. Because the physical setting is an integral part of the psychosocial climate, it should be given as much consideration as other elements of the treatment program. The value assigned to clients is reflected in the living space planned and prepared for them. A child in crisis cannot be supported in an environment that subliminally and perhaps overtly says, "You are really not that important." Osmond (1959) developed a concept of two different spatial arrangements and their effects on behavior. Sociofugal is the term describing arrangements that discourage human interaction and tend to keep people at a distance. Examples of these arrangements are railroad stations, libraries, and traditional hospital corridors. The term sociopetal describes the opposite arrangement—one that encourages face-to-face interactions among small groups, such as in restaurant booths and family rooms.

Inpatient child and adolescent units should be designed to reflect the special nature of caring for children and to create a home-like environment. Ideally the unit should be arranged sociopetally with all client rooms entering into a family room in the center of the unit. This design not only fosters interaction, but also requires fewer staff members to monitor clients safely. A staff member having a one-to-one talk with one child also can be aware of what is going on around him or her in the environment and is easily available if a situation requires his or her attention.

The family room should include game tables and play materials appropriate for the age and developmental level of the children who live there. Large common areas can be subdivided into smaller conversation pits simply by arranging the furniture. Casual, easily movable furniture encourages informal, flexible behavior and activities by staff and clients. Several activities involving small groups of children or adolescents and staff can occur simultaneously.

Games, puzzles, toys, and books should be geared to the developmental levels of the children or adolescents served on the unit. Colorful carpeting, wall hangings, framed pictures, and live plants contribute to a warm, home-like feeling. In keeping with the goal of a noninstitutional atmosphere, furniture is attractive with ample padding, softness, and wood.

The nurses' desk should be easily accessible and visible. It should be low and open so a small child can approach it without being confronted by a wall or glass barrier. Changing the name of the nurses' station to "communication center" has removed the implied barrier in some settings (Johnston, 1979).

The environment should provide privacy in sleeping and bathing areas. Individual bedside dressers, bookshelves, and desks provide private areas for reading and writing. Semiprivate rooms may be divided by a partial wall to give each patient privacy yet allow visibility at the doorway. Each patient is responsible for the upkeep of his or her own area and shares responsibility for the upkeep of common areas.

Child and adolescent clients may have chores to do just as at home. A work wheel or a calendar may be used to assign chores. Each client takes a unit chore or job for a day or a week. Examples of chores include setting the table for meals, cleaning up after meals, or vacuuming the common areas. Clients may earn tokens or points for completing chores; these can be applied toward increased privileges. For younger children who cannot grasp the abstract concept of points, star charts or sticker charts provide concrete reinforcement when prominently displayed to indicate to everyone that the child has met behavioral expectations.

One norm of a therapeutic environment is active orientation to treatment. Strategic placement of bulletin boards or grease boards containing calendars, schedules, staff names and titles, client names and assignments, current privileges, and primary therapists is important. A bulletin board over each client's bed can display pictures, schedules, and awards. Helpful reading materials, such as newspapers, current magazines, novels, reference books, educational literature, and age-appropriate picture books should be available.

STRUCTURED TREATMENT PROGRAM

Because children and adolescents who require inpatient psychiatric hospitalization often need additional protection, structure, or boundaries, the total environment is consciously structured to provide them. Three basic components make up the overall structure of a therapeutic environment: philosophy; rules, limit setting, and consequences; and treatment level system.

PHILOSOPHY. The philosophy provides the framework against which all client behavior and treatment plans are evaluated. Because the family is an integral part of the child's life, child and adolescent programs are often based on a family systems model with a developmental perspective (Smith & Murphy, 1984). When the child is treated in the context of the family, his or her behavior may be viewed as a symptom of a malfunctioning family system. The child also is evaluated for accomplishment of developmental tasks, and if found to be unsuccessful in completing a developmental task, the focus of treatment becomes helping the child to complete that task.

The inpatient unit becomes a "family" that provides for expression of feelings, effective communication between members, development of coping skills, and positive recreational experiences (Smith & Murphy, 1984). Family relationships are recreated in the milieu. Staff members take on the role of parents, and other clients take on the role of siblings. One advantage of a unit that admits both children and adolescents are the sibling transferences that develop. Children who have conflicts with siblings can learn and practice new skills of negotiating and sharing with peers before testing these skills with siblings. Milieu staff take on a parental role with the child as they pay attention to the child's hygiene, attire, nutritional concerns, and time management.

Family life is simulated with meal preparation, clean up, and other routine activities. Family festivities like birthdays and going away are celebrated on the unit with parties for the child. Transferential feelings of parent to child and sibling to sibling emerge in this atmosphere of closeness. Children often approach discharge with ambivalence, expressing reluctance to leave relationships they have made and expressing pride in their accomplishments. Emphasis is placed on generalizing newly acquired behavioral responses to the home environment by setting and evaluating goals for home visits during hospitalization.

RULES, LIMIT SETTING, AND CONSEQUENCES. Just as in a family, the unit has basic rules to follow and consequences for noncompliance. Consistency in application of rules and consequences is important for children because different consequences for the same behavior can be confusing. Unit rule books or guidelines help the child learn what is expected and help staff members develop consistency. These guidelines provide an objective reference point when clients or staff have questions about the rules. Children and their parents should be oriented to the rules and consequences during admission. Unit rule books and family handbooks are handy references for parents and children after the initial admission process because anxiety often is high during orientation to the unit, and much of what is explained may be forgotten.

A peer or "buddy system" may help older children and adolescents adapt to the milieu culture and learn the rules. Once the child is admitted, a peer may be assigned to explain rules and routines and help the new client get acquainted with the unit culture. The buddy system serves a dual purpose: The new child feels more comfortable with a peer who shares similar problems and is "in the same boat," and the buddy feels needed and important with the responsibility of orienting a new client, resulting in increased competency and self-esteem. The positive changes the buddies have made also are strengthened as they reexperience where they have been, realize how far they have come, and describe where they are now in the treatment and growth process.

Older children and adolescents may be expected to take a basic rules test, which emphasizes their accountability for knowing the rules. The subsequent discussion contributes to relationship building as the staff member and child review the child's answers to the test, discuss the purpose of the rules, and explain the consequences for not following the rules.

The therapeutic environment stresses positive reinforcement rather than punishment. Children are rewarded for following rules and working on their treatment goals. Stickers, stars, or points may be given for following unit rules and routines and for attaining daily goals. On units using a behavioral system, the number of points earned determines the child's level and privileges for the next day. The higher the points, the higher the level and the more privileges earned. Children also may be recognized in community meeting for achieving personal goals; school achievements; specific unit achievements, such as "best routine follower" or "most helpful to peers"; and "most improved" of the week. Clients also may participate in nominating peers for "most improved," which helps them recognize and reinforce a peer's progress in treatment. Special rewards may be given to the "most improved" child based on the child's individual treatment plan, such as a special outing, a walk with a staff member, a special game, a meal off the unit, extra free time, and so forth. Children earning special recognition may be honored by having their names on the unit bulletin board.

The milieu's overall structure must be responsive to each child's individual needs. Limit setting is critical because it reinforces the predictability of the environment; that is, for certain actions, there will be a consequence, and clear feedback is given regarding the results of the behavior. Milieu staff are charged with the daily responsibility of maintaining the therapeutic structure of the treatment milieu by setting appropriate limits. As external limits are set, the child is assisted in developing a functional set of internal controls. In addition, milieu staff are responsible for educating the child or adolescent and their parents about appropriate limit setting so that positive behavioral changes achieved in treatment can be generalized after discharge.

Appropriate behavior and constructive problem solving must be clearly and frequently rewarded. Skills needed to set and maintain appropriate limits without coercion, or force must be mastered by milieu staff who work with children and adolescents. The concept that negative consequences occur when the child does not fulfill his or her responsibilities is consistent with the real world where restrictions or consequences are the results of inappropriate behavior. To make this learning most effective, the consequences must be immediate, logical, appropriate to the child's age and attention span, explained for full understanding, and consistent with the way others are treated. When developing a program, the rewards and consequences should be considered for feasibility in the hospital setting and use in the home setting. The milieu staff also must consider the age and comprehension level of the client and how often or how long the rewards and consequences are in effect. It is important to continually reevaluate rules, rewards, and consequences in light of the philosophy of the program, changing client population, and concern for clients' rights.

Limit setting responses fall on a continuum with positive social interaction at one end of the continuum and time out procedures at the other end (Conley, 1992). Initial attempts at limit setting should be positive and least restrictive. Using positive social interaction, milieu staff can pair smiles, nods, and encouragement when presenting a point or other token to the child for following rules or meeting goals. If the child responds to positive consequences, there is no need to use negative consequences.

Extinction is next on the continuum and is used for mildly inappropriate behaviors that are not disturbing the group. Extinction is simply the process of withholding positive reinforcements or ignoring the behavior. The inappropriate behavior will usually escalate after a period of ignoring before finally extinguishing.

A third type of limit setting is providing direction. Providing direction is a method of prompting or cueing the child while identifying a more appropriate behavior.

Limit setting is a more direct intervention that should be initiated when a direction does not result in an almost immediate behavior change. A limit specifies what the staff member wants the child to do. It also objectively describes the consequences of appropriate and inappropriate behavior.

Next on the continuum is a verbal reprimand or a specific statement that not only informs the child that his or her behavior is inappropriate, but also points out the consequences that will follow if the inappropriate behavior continues. Additionally, a reprimand also includes a description of an alternate behavior and the desirable consequences that will follow when it occurs.

Privilege removal is next on the continuum and should be, if possible, a natural consequence for acting out. For example, acting out at bedtime results in an earlier bedtime for a day or an earlier wake up time.

Time out procedures are the last alternative. Time outs seek to relieve immediate stress and to offer the necessary time for reflection and insight into the feelings involved in the child's behavior. Time outs should not be punitive or a way of controlling the child's behavior, but instead an opportunity for the child to leave the agitating stimulus and regain internal control. It is highly appropriate and desirable for the child to ask for a time out to assist with his or her own internal control over impulses.

As a general rule, time outs should be no longer than 1 minute per year of development. For children functioning at a developmental level less than their chronologic age, their time outs should be adjusted to match their developmental age.

When in a time out, the child is asked to separate himself or herself from peers and to reflect on and revise the behavior. A staff member and the child then review the incident, and the child returns to the routine as quickly as possible. If the behavior continues to escalate, the quiet room may provide clear physical boundaries and a place to punch a bag or yell. The door to the quiet room is left open unless the child has difficulty remaining in the room. Again, control is given to the child (i.e., "the door will stay open if you remain in the quiet room for 2 minutes"). Seclusion is used when all efforts to help the patient control his or her behavior have failed. The goal is to address the incident in a way that is supportive to the child, while making clear the behavioral expectations within the milieu.

Some children may regain control more quickly if left alone in the quiet room. For others, especially very young or developmentally delayed children, solitude may be frightening and may increase anxiety. Because some children self-stimulate and become exhausted before quietening, more humane interventions must be found. Decisions about time out appropriate to the individual child should be made by the interdisciplinary team based on the perceptions of various team members. Variations on the usual time out procedure become a part of the care plan to provide consistency for the specific child.

When using time outs, nursing staff need to observe the following guidelines:

- Remain as calm as possible.
- Be careful not to moralize, lecture, or argue.
- Be consistent. Do the same thing every time, and even more importantly, follow through when a child has been told that a certain behavior would result in a time out.
- Make time outs brief with the understanding that once the child has regained control, time out will end.
- Explain the entire procedure to the child before implementing it.
- Process with the child how his or her behavior led to the time out and that the child is responsible for his or her behavior.
- Specify the behaviors expected when the child leaves time out (Conley, 1992; Johnson, 1991).

Problem solving or "think sheets" may help the child organize his or her thinking during the time out and help him or her identify alternate solutions (Box 30-1). For children who have difficulty processing verbally, asking the child to draw what happened and what can be done the next time is a viable alternative. The child may be asked to talk about the drawing. The staff person can verbalize for the child what he or she is unable to say, thereby helping him or her label feelings. Aids to describing feelings include mood charts with which the child may point to a face depicting a feeling, draw his or her own feelings face, or rate the intensity of his or her feelings on a thermometer.

BOX 30–1 • THINK SHEET

What did you do?

What happened when you did it?

What was going on with you at the time?

How did others react?

What can you do differently the next time this happens?

How are you feeling now about what happened?

The concept of a "freedom room" was originated in Children's Memorial Hospital in Chicago to replace the isolation room traditionally found on an inpatient unit. The room contains mats, a punching bag, and a ball for the child to use to ventilate anger. The child can request to go to the freedom room or can be taken by a staff member. The staff person stays inside the room or directly outside while the child is using it, depending on the child's preference. The room is never locked while in use. Staff members process the child's feelings and behavior with the child after use of the freedom room and explore more appropriate ways to act in similar situations (Smith & Murphy, 1984).

TREATMENT LEVEL SYSTEM. The last component of the overall structure of a therapeutic environment is the level and phase system. This is an organized, concrete way to show a child's progress through treatment. Expectations and privileges increase with advancement to the next treatment level or phase. The phase and level system developed by the child and adolescent psychiatry unit at Children's Medical Center of Dallas provides phases that indicate the client's progress through treatment and levels that reflect daily progress.

The phase system is divided into three treatment phases: A, B, and C. On admission each client is on phase A. While in this phase, the child or adolescent is expected to learn names of staff members and other clients, the rules of the unit, and the daily routine and to accept the need for hospitalization. The interdisciplinary team assists the child to identify the problems for which he or she was admitted to the hospital.

In phase B, the child is expected to demonstrate awareness and the ability to verbalize problems. During this phase, the child begins working on problem-specific goals developed by the child and the treatment team.

During phase C, emphasis is placed on the child taking responsibility for his or her behaviors and using more adaptive techniques in personal relationships with peers, at home, and in the school environment.

Each child moves through treatment phases at his or her own pace. The child also should maintain the expectations of the current treatment phase to remain at that phase. Treatment phase changes are evaluated on a weekly basis in a community meeting. Clients who wish to change phases complete a phase change request with the help of their treatment team and present it to the community of clients and interdisciplinary staff for feedback. The child describes how the expectations have been met for the current phase and discusses goals and plans for the next phase. Staff members and other clients respond to the child's request to change phases by showing their support or stating what they think he or she needs to accomplish before moving to the next treatment phase.

The daily level system is consistent throughout each phase in that the child may earn a set number of points each day. The total number of points earned in a day is 30. The child who earns 25 to 30 points attains level 3; 20 to 24 points, level 2; 19 points or less, level 1. Increased privileges are attached to each higher level. Participation in special outings and activities are contingent on earning level 2 or 3 (Table 30-1).

The level or behavioral program is modified to meet the needs of individual children or adolescents. A star chart or token program are examples of modified behavior programs. A star chart is developed by the child's treatment team and focuses on concrete behaviors. Stars are given to the client to place on the chart when treatment goals are accomplished. Stars are similar to points in that they mark the child's daily progress. The direct communication with the child, helping him or her understand the desired behavior for which stars or stickers are earned, also is therapeutic. Many children find the star chart to be a more visible affirmation of success and therefore more motivating. This approach often is used with younger children. Milieu staff can use their creativity to individualize a star or sticker chart to maximize client motivation and involvement with the behavior plan (Fig. 30-1). A token system provides immediate reinforcement for a child's positive behaviors. Tokens may take the form of beads to make a necklace, checkers, or play money. The child may use the earned tokens to "buy" special privileges (e.g., special walks with a staff member or free time out of the room). The value of this type of behavioral system is its ability to motivate the child to be responsible for his or her behavior and to participate in treatment.

Treatment Modalities

MILIEU THERAPY

The therapeutic environment promotes active involvement in treatment. Each child or adolescent is expected to participate in the daily activities, with clear, appropriate consequences if a child chooses not to participate. Examples of activities include community meeting, goals group, school, group therapy, family therapy, individual therapy, therapeutic recreation, quiet time, free time, and educational and fun field trips (Table 30-2).

CONFRONTATION WITHIN INTERPERSONAL RELATIONSHIPS. Confrontation is a central feature of the therapeutic environment. Sharing experiences and feelings involves forcing the child or adolescent to confront and recognize that his or her habitual responses cause unmanageable problems and possibly deep hurt. Analyzing interactions helps the child see that his or her usual ways of coping are ineffective in getting needs met and that to continue in the same way means more failure and loneliness (Jack, 1989).

Milieu therapy provides the supportive ambiance for the child to apply the new behavioral responses discussed in individual and group therapies. Informal activities provide opportunities for more effective interpersonal relationships as the child is coached to try alternative responses to events he or she has typically perceived as provocative.

COMMUNITY MEETING. A community meeting of all unit staff and clients is held at least weekly. The large circle of clients, nurses, milieu therapists, psychiatric social workers, psychiatrists, psychologists, therapeutic recreation specialists, teachers, and other therapists is led by the program director or designee. Centered on interpersonal issues in the community, the meeting is facilitated for open communication between all members of the therapeutic milieu. The purpose of community meeting is to discuss issues that affect the life of the community and to explore group dynamics of the community. Milieu staff members role model appropri-

(text continues on page 434)

TABLE 30–1 Phase and Level Privileges

	Phase A	Phase B	Phase C
Level 1 (less than 20 points)	Participate in on-unit activities Use computer during class with staff permission	Same as Phase A, level 1 plus the following: Off-ground passes with family as decided by the treatment team	Same as Phase B, level 1
Level 2 (20–24 points)	Level 1 privileges plus the following: Participate in on-ground activities Have on-ground visits during visiting hours Play with unit toys and games Go on swimming field trip Participate at the gym on Fridays, organized activities but not free time Go on educational field trip but not the picnic May watch T.V.	Same as Phase A, level 2 and Phase B, level 1 plus the following: Use the intercom with staff permission Off-unit visits during visiting hours Push elevator buttons with staff permission	Same as Phase B, level 2
Level 3 (25–30 points)	Level 2 privileges plus the following: Go on off-ground field trips Spend money on field trips Conduct room checks with staff Swim on Wednesdays Go on Thursday educational field trip and picnic Free time at gym on Friday Fridays and Saturdays: ½ hour later bedtime if all bedtime points were earned the night before	Same as Phase A, level 3 and Phase B, level 2 plus the following: Go to teen room (ages 11–18) Play Nintendo with staff present Go to vending machines two times per week Participate in special unit activities Spend free time in Jambox with staff supervision Spend money in the gift shop one time per week Use computer during free time with staff supervision Peer visits with parents present May contract for: Special outings with family One late night per week 30 minute later regular bedtime 15–30 minute walk with staff two times per week	Same as Phase B, level 3 plus the following: Go to vending machines three times a week Spend money in gift shop two times a week Spend quiet time in T.V. room Go to Jambox with staff supervision Use computer during free time without supervision Play Nintendo without staff present Use pay phones while off unit alone Go on Phase C field trip Spend quiet time in peer's room with staff approval Help staff write out schedule on board or turn workwheel ½ hour later bedtime on Friday and Saturday if earned all points the night before Peer visits with parents present Fridays and Saturdays: Spend free time in Jambox alone or with peers May contract for: 15–30 minute walk, on grounds with or without staff four times a week

(continued)

TABLE 30–1 Phase and Level Privileges *(Continued)*

Phase A	Phase B	Phase C
		Spend more than $15 in 2 weeks Special outings with family Two late nights per week 1 hour later regular bedtime Sleeping in peer's room Teach or help supervise activities Peer visits without parents present

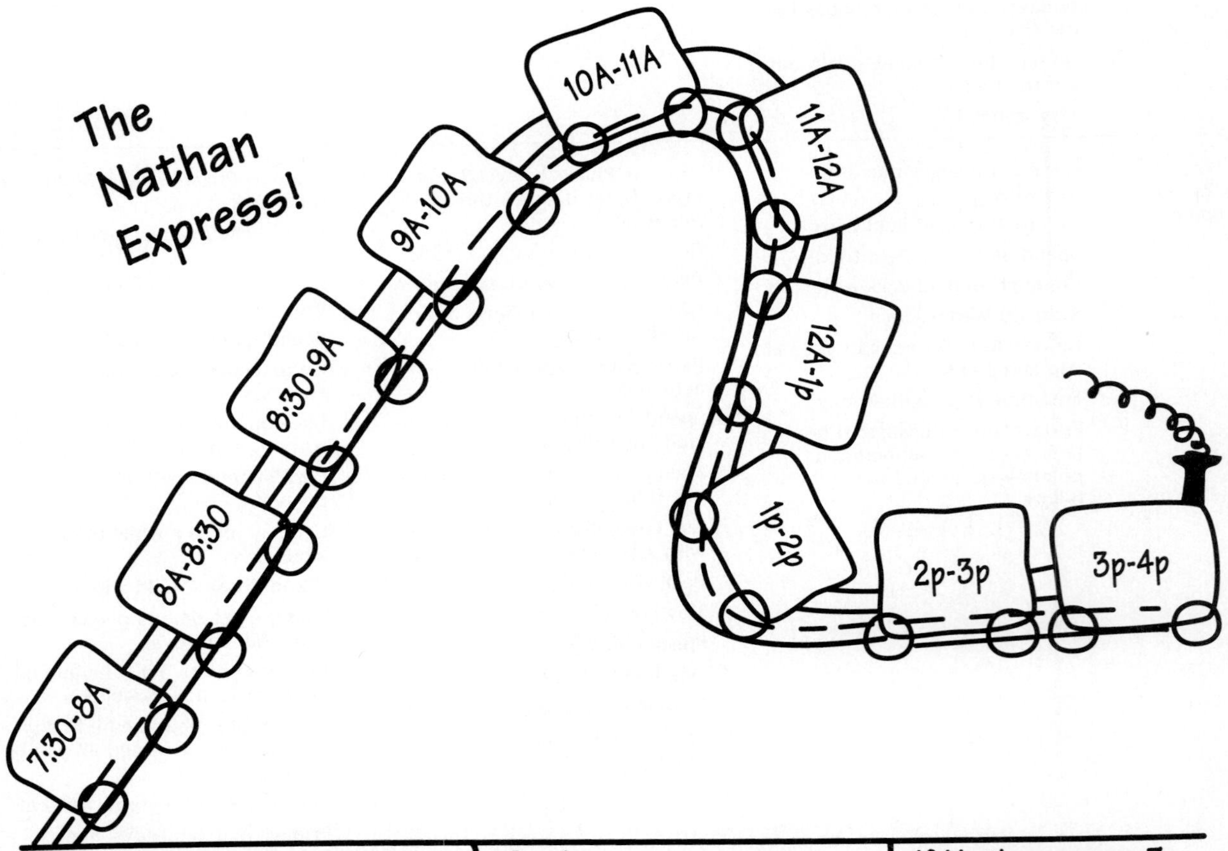
The Nathan Express!
7:30-8A
8A-8:30
8:30-9A
9A-10A
10A-11A
11A-12A
12A-1p
1p-2p
2p-3p
3p-4p
Nathan may earn one sticker per square or time segment. The object is to reward Nathan immediately in an effort to build the "Nathan Express".
Goals:
1) Do as asked with only 2 reminders.
2) Have good sit outs
3) Play nicely with peers
If Nathan earns 7 stickers, he has level 3 for the next shift. Below 7, govern as necessary.

FIGURE 30–1 • Train sticker chart. (Created for a 3-year-old boy by Shelly L. Brody, milieu therapist, at Children's Medical Center of Dallas, Texas.)

TABLE 30–2 Daily Schedule

	Monday	Tuesday	Wednesday	Thursday	Friday	Saturday	Sunday
7:00–8:00	AM care room checks	AM care room checks	AM care room checks	AM care room checks	AM care room checks	Sleep in	Sleep in
8:00–9:00	Breakfast medications	Breakfast medications	Breakfast medications	Breakfast medications	Breakfast medications	Breakfast	Breakfast
9:00–10:00	Goals group exercise	Play group Group therapy	Goals group exercise	Play group Group therapy	Goals group exercise	AM care room checks	AM care room checks
10:00–11:00	School	School	School	Educational field trip	School	Unit cleanup	Chapel service (optional)
11:00–12:00	School	School	School	Educational field trip	School	Therapeutic recreation	Goals group
12:00–1:00	Lunch quiet time	Lunch quiet time	Lunch quiet time	Field trip picnic	Lunch quiet time	Lunch quiet time	Lunch quiet time
1:00–2:00	School	School	School	Field trip picnic	School	Goals group	Therapeutic recreation
2:00–3:00	School	School	School	Values group	School	Music therapy	Outdoor recreation
3:00–4:00	Snacks art activity	Therapeutic recreation	Art therapy	Community meeting	Music therapy	Outdoor recreation	Meal preparation
4:00–5:00	Boys' group girls' group	Music therapy	Therapeutic recreation	Therapeutic recreation	Therapeutic recreation	Meal & activity planning	Meal preparation
5:00–6:00	Dinner journal writing	Dinner journal writing	Dinner journal writing	Dinner off unit	Dinner journal writing	Dinner journal writing	Family style dinner
6:00–7:00	Movie group level 3 field trip	Structured activity	Phase C field trip	Structured activity	Level 3 field trip fun activity	Dance or fun activity	T.V. time or group activity
7:00–8:00	Movie group level 3 field trip	Structured activity	Phase C field trip	Structured activity	Level 3 field trip fun activity	Dance or fun activity	Study time
8:00–9:00	Snacks wrap up group	Snacks wrap up group	Snacks wrap up group	Snacks wrap up group	Snacks wrap up group	T.V. time study time	T.V. time or group activity
9:00–10:00	Get ready for bed	Get ready for bed	Get ready for bed	Get ready for bed	Get ready for bed	Snacks wrap up group	Snacks wrap up group
10:00–11:00						Late night activities	Get ready for bed

ate behavior and rational thinking in the discussion. Issues include introduction of members, clients, and staff and goodbyes to soon-to-be discharged clients or staff who are leaving. Community meetings also are used for treatment level change requests and recognition of clients who have made accomplishments during the week. Children and adolescents are encouraged to bring up their concerns about community living and other significant events affecting life in the community, such as an increase in disruptive behaviors or a discovered elopement plan. Discussion is dynamic and helps to resolve unpleasant feelings.

GOALS GROUP. Goals group is a meeting that includes all clients or a specific group of clients and their treatment team. The group may be held daily or several times a week and may be led by the psychiatrist or another member of the treatment team. Each client has the opportunity in the group to discuss behaviors or concerns and progress toward treatment goals. Upcoming passes, past goals, and plans are presented, and previous passes and activities are explored and evaluated. Goals group helps to integrate new clients into the milieu quickly and provides an awareness of what goes on in the milieu, thereby creating greater group cohesion. Goals group has advantages similar to open report described by Puskar & McAdam (1988). These include encouraging staff–client, staff–staff, and client–client interaction; providing a safe atmosphere for clients and staff to take risks in communicating thoughts and feelings; providing an opportunity for client feedback; making clients more accountable for their behavior; and increasing staff awareness of the process in the therapeutic milieu. Two disadvantages reported by clients include concerns about privacy and discussion of personal issues and initial anxiety about talking in front of other clients and staff. Concerns are diminished with assurance that confidentiality will not be violated, and recognition is made that both clients and staff experience anxiety when speaking in group.

GROUP THERAPY

Group therapy takes on many forms depending on the developmental levels of the children involved and the purpose of the group. For very young children (usually younger than 8 years of age), group therapy is conducted on a play level in a designated play therapy room. The goals and focus of this group are for the children to learn to play cooperatively with one another, to solve simple conflicts with peers, and to begin to view their own behavior and that of their peers (Smith & Murphy, 1984).

Groups also can take on a more structured, directed form in which staff members decide the topics and develop activities to address the topics. Activities may involve puppets, role play, movement, music, art, or story telling. In structured groups, children can learn and practice new ways of dealing with feelings or difficult situations. Social skills group is a special topic group in which children learn to complete social tasks, such as how to make a friend. The child then practices these steps, perhaps while being videotaped, and is given a chance to view the results.

Much of the group activity focuses on honest appraisal of the child's behaviors; surrendering old, ineffective coping strategies; and learning new productive behaviors. A cohesive group of patients works at confronting each other in a supportive environment and then works at the openness, honesty, and trust that lead to improved relationships (Jack, 1989) (see Chapters 23 through 26).

INDIVIDUAL THERAPY

In individual therapy, the child explores feelings, attitudes, and behavior within the safety of a trusting, interpersonal relationship. Personal concerns about peer relationships, family relationships, or intrapsychic conflict are discussed. Often children who have had no experience in treatment prior to entry into the hospital require frequent individual time to allay their fears about hospitalization.

Individual therapy may take place on a verbal or play level, depending on the cognitive functioning and verbal ability of the child. Candidates for play therapy include preschool through latency-age children whose behavior appears regressed from a previous higher level of functioning and children with evidence of intrapsychic conflict interfering with emotional growth (Smith & Murphy, 1984).

FAMILY INVOLVEMENT

Family involvement greatly influences the outcome of treatment. Shorter lengths of stay in the hospital and rapid return to the family environment emphasize the importance of family involvement in the child's treatment and family therapy. The inpatient milieu for children and adolescents must include families because they are integral to the support and maintenance of healthy change. Two traditional avenues for family involvement include family therapy and parent support groups.

BOX 30–2 • FAMILY CONTRACT

To establish a safe and functional family unit, certain rules must be set, followed, and enforced. Failure to abide by these rules will result in negative consequences.

Following the rules and contributing to a peaceful home will result in earning privileges. It is your responsibility to know and follow the rules and to perform your assignments.

If you refuse to abide by this contract, it will be your decision to accept the consequences of your behavior.

You have the right to request a time out if you feel it is needed. You also have the right to call a family meeting to deal with any issue that you feel is important. Meetings will be held as soon as possible.

WHAT WE EXPECT OF YOU:

- Clean up after yourself immediately in the kitchen, bathroom, living room, and at computer.
- Homework must be completed before lights out every night. You are to study for tests at least 1 hour the night before the test is given, not the morning of the test.
- Spend at least 1 hour each day with family.
- Take medication daily.
- Chores must be done on Saturday before any activity. Clean your bedroom and bathroom thoroughly; help with the house and yard as requested. Allowance will be given on Saturday after your chores are completed.
- Do your own laundry.
- Help clean up the kitchen after supper each evening.
- Make your bed each morning.
- Time on phone is limited to 1/2 hour. No incoming or outgoing phone calls after 10:00 PM on weeknights and 11:00 PM on weekends.
- You must be in bed with lights out at 10:30 Sunday through Thursday, 12:15 Fridays, and 11:15 Saturdays.
- Wake up time is Sunday through Friday, in plenty of time to eat and get ready for school or church.
- No profanity, lying, or arguing.
- We must know with whom you are going out, where you are going, and what time you expect to be back.
- You must attend aftercare group each week and all scheduled therapies.

PRIVILEGES YOU CAN EARN:

- Going to a movie
- Going to the mall
- Renting a video
- Having a friend spend the night
- Going to the amusement park
- Increased time on the phone
- Driving the car
- Earning allowance

The following consequences may result if you do not follow the rules or do what is expected.

- Decreased phone time or grounded from phone
- Loss of T.V.
- Loss of radio or records
- Forfeit part of allowance
- No going out with friends
- No stereo, T.V., or Nintendo for 2 days.

We believe that you are responsible for your behavior and that you have a choice in what you do. With this in mind, remember that whether you earn privileges or receive consequences is totally up to you.

I have read and I understand the material contained in this contract. I agree to abide by these rules and responsibilities and accept the consequences.

____
Adolescent's signature/date

____
Dad's signature/date

____
Mom's signature/date

FAMILY THERAPY. Generally, families of child and adolescent inpatients have trouble in two areas: communication and expression of feelings among family members and limit-setting skills. Family therapists use techniques such as role playing to improve communication skills. Parents having difficulty in their roles as parents need help providing structure in the form of rules, consequences, and rewards for the child; learning how to listen to a child's feelings; and learning how to spend positive interactional time with the child. Parents and children can work on developing home programs or contracts for aftercare within the safety of the family therapy session. These programs can be tested on passes and modified as needed through telephone consultation with unit personnel before the child returns. Older children, particularly adolescents, should be involved in the process of establishing family rules, privileges, and consequences. Their involvement increases ownership and likelihood of compliance (Box 30-2).

PARENT SUPPORT GROUPS. Parent support groups are another avenue for involving parents in the treatment process. The expectation is stated prior to admission that parents attend these meetings to become acquainted with other parents. Parents may continue to participate after the child is discharged. Linking support group meetings to family visiting times increases family participation in the group.

In the support group, parents help one another in the therapeutic process as they offer support, reassurance, suggestions, and insight and share similar problems with one another. Often a parent will listen and absorb observations from another parent far more readily than from the group leader. Hearing other parents disclose concerns similar to their own and realizing that they are not unique in their feelings is a powerful source of relief. Parents may feel more in touch with the world and describe the process as a "welcome to the human race" experience (Yalom, 1985).

PARENT TEACHING IN THE MILIEU. Ideally parents are actively involved in the milieu with their child and the child's primary staff. Programs endorsing a family teaching model invite and encourage parents to spend time in the milieu. Parents and staff members learn from each other as they share perceptions of the child's behaviors. Parents may initially shadow milieu staff as the staff person intervenes with the child and explains to the parents the purpose of the action and perceptions of the child's behavior. As the milieu staff teach and role model skills in limit setting, communicating, positive reinforcement, and management of impulsive and aggressive behaviors, parents have the opportunity to practice these same skills with guidance and positive reinforcement from the staff member. Eventually the roles reverse and the staff member is available to assist the parent in changing behavioral patterns of interaction with the child. As the parents practice new skills, they develop confidence in their ability to deal effectively with their children.

School

Because one of the child's primary roles is student, school is an integral part of milieu treatment. Often behaviors that led to admission were first noticed in the school setting and resulted in missed school time and credit. Classroom experiences provide opportunities for achieving success and recapturing lost credits. Educational programs are individualized based on psychologic and educational evaluations of each child. Goals are incorporated into the overall plan of care by the special education teachers who are members of the treatment team. The teacher or an educational coordinator acts as a liaison with the child's local school to guarantee continuity.

Recreational Activities

Recreational and physical outlets are important aspects of the milieu for children and adolescents in inpatient treatment. The increased energy level of children and the need to accomplish developmental tasks, such as jumping and running, make physical exercise and activities a must. Ideally a gym or outside recreational area can provide the space for this release; however, the reality is that not all hospital environments have access to this space. Creative milieu staff can meet the child's need for physical activity through outings to community recreational centers with gyms, swimming pools, playgrounds, roller skating, ice skating, bowling, and modified exercise sessions. Educational field trips to zoos, museums, and libraries and fun field trips to movies, malls, restaurants, and recreational centers also are beneficial. On the outings, many cultural, leisure, and educational experiences are available. Appropriate social skills can be practiced and positive behavioral change reinforced when trips and special activities are used as rewards. Children and adolescents are encouraged to continue their community involvement while on passes with families. Because activities are shared and enjoyed by milieu staff and families, they allow children to view adults as companions in fun, rather than as authority figures only.

Many opportunities for practice in problem solving occur during leisure activities. Milieu staff members have the opportunity to use these relaxed times for observing the usual and habitual responses that demonstrate the strengths or behaviors that have led to trouble for the child. Once identified, strengths are maximized, or new responses are explored, practiced, and evaluated immediately. Thus, the milieu is engineered to provide a safe and supportive environment for learning healthy interpersonal skills.

Staff Concerns

The therapeutic environment works most effectively when the staff is cohesive, and all disciplines work collaboratively. Conflicts between disciplines, shifts, or individuals are easily noticed by clients who try to split the staff or pit one group against another. To maintain staff cohesiveness, milieu staff must be alert to the warning signals and be able to identify and resolve problems among themselves quickly and thoroughly. Open communication is the best antidote for splitting. Staff members need frequent opportunity to discuss and share thoughts and feelings about child and adolescent clients. Avenues for informal and formal communication are essential. A weekly staff group can result in interdisciplinary staff members sharing concerns, expressing feelings related to particular clients or each other, seeking support for working with a particularly difficult child, sharing perceptions, and resolving conflicts.

Conflicts are inevitable within the work group but can be resolved by open and direct communication. Staff must be willing to take the same risks that they expect clients to take: Work on relationships, negotiate, communicate openly and honestly, accept responsibility for their own choices, and be vulnerable and feel "feelings."

Role blurring occurs when members of different disciplines work side by side, often equally involved in group activities with clients. Often the roles staff members fill are based on skills, individuality, and talents, rather than strictly on discipline-based job descriptions. Conflicts may occur when one staff member or one discipline exerts a territorial stance, defining certain tasks as dependent on exclusive educational credentials. Role confusion and territoriality create feelings of anxiety, which can lead to factions of staff isolated from others and covert hostility expressed in undermining the effectiveness of the milieu. Chaos and extremely low morale can result on the unit. These feelings must be handled openly and intrastaff conflict resolved (Jack, 1989).

Because therapeutic environments emphasize a democratic approach to decision making, with clients actively involved in analyzing and solving their problems, one concern for milieu staff is the question of control. Staff members must continually assess the child's abilities to make reasonable decisions if given adequate information and allow the child to assume accountability for the outcome.

Many factors affect the ability of a staff to provide a safe, structured, and supportive environment. The age, level of experience, and personality characteristics of individual staff members influence their effectiveness. Experienced staff members understand systems phenomena, such as the variable levels of unit tension or how acting out can ignite group contagion (Delaney, 1992). Three key factors influence the productivity of milieu staff and shape the tasks of unit leaders: the ability of staff members to accept responsibility, their tolerance for risk and uncertainty, and their need for structure (Bednar, Melnick, & Kaul, 1974). With new staff members, the ability to accept responsibility is low, tolerance for risk small, and the need for structure high. As the staff members develop, competence grows, tolerance for uncertainty increases, and the need for external structure diminishes (Kahn & Fredrick, 1988). Staff members rely less on formal rules as the basis for decision making and may alter some basic norms of the unit to accommodate the needs of a particular child. Because staff must constantly share ideas and negotiate how far a norm will bend, communication and consensus improve. Focus on the rationales underlying routines is sharpened, allowing the structure to move forward (Delaney, 1992).

A parallel process between clients and milieu staff occurs in the therapeutic environment (Kernberg, 1978; Kets de Vries, 1984; Kibel, 1987). Unit leadership affects the milieu staff, which in turn affects the clients. Milieu staff will often create a unit climate that mirrors their own experience of the work setting. If they feel supported by the leaders and have a clear idea of their purpose, then they will approach their clients with confidence, respect, and kind firmness. If milieu staff feel threatened and unsure, they will interact with clients in a way that increases anxiety. If they feel victimized, they will have little to give. Parallelism "often results in vicious circles whereby needy staff withhold, deprived patients demand, drained staff act helpless, abandoned patients become angry, antagonized staff withdraw, leading back to a situation where needy staff withhold, and so on" (Kahn & Fredrick, 1988, p. 137). Leadership must support staff when the milieu becomes stressful, actively listen to staff concerns, recognize what is unique about a staff member's approach to the children, and foster that uniqueness as a means of professional growth. Leadership must care for staff by being supportive and available to them in much the same way that the staff must care for and be emotionally available to the children (Delaney, 1992).

Characteristics of highly effective milieus include unity and clarity of purpose and vision, a strong sense of identity, high levels of interdisciplinary participation and involvement, well-elaborated communication, proaction and willingness to take risks, clear delineation of authority and accountability with freedom to move within these proscribed limits, and effectiveness rather than efficiency as the performance standard (Kahn & Fredrick, 1988). Achieving this type of milieu requires a leadership group that understands the function of the therapeutic environment and how staff members use it to treat clients.

Summary

The environment in which psychiatric treatment occurs is an important influence on the outcome of the client's therapy; that is, the environment itself is an instrument of treatment. The interdisciplinary team working together can effectively create a healing environment in which every interaction and activity is therapeutic for the client. These interactions often take place in the context of group activities, group therapy discussions, community meetings, family therapy sessions, and individual relationships with the staff, other clients, and families. This environment promotes successful social interaction and increases the child's capacity for coping with reality. Open communication between staff members and clients is encouraged. These critical components comprise a therapeutic environment.

REFERENCES

Beck, C., Rawlins, R., & Williams, S. (1988). *Mental health/psychiatric nursing: A holistic life cycle approach.* St. Louis: C.V. Mosby.

Bednar, R., Melnick, J., & Kaul, T. (1974). Risk, responsibility and structure: A conceptual framework for initiating group counseling and psychotherapy. *Journal of Counseling Psychology, 21*, 31–37.

Conley, J. (1992). *In the trenches: The art and practice of setting therapeutic limits with kids who act out.* Paper presented at the Sixth Annual Psychiatric Nursing Symposium. Arlington, TX: The University of Texas at Arlington.

Critchley, D. (1987). Clinical supervision as a learning tool for the therapist in milieu settings. *Journal of Psychosocial Nursing, 25*(8), 18–22.

Cumming, J., & Cumming, E. (1982). *Ego and milieu.* New York: Atherton.

Daniels, R. (1975). The hospital as a therapeutic community. In A. Freedman, H. Kaplan, & B. Sadock (Eds.), *Comprehensive textbook of psychiatry* (Vol. 2). (pp. 1990–1995). Baltimore: Williams & Wilkins.

Delaney, K. (1992). Nursing in child psychiatric milieus: Part I: What nurses do. *Journal of Child and Adolescent Psychiatric and Mental Health Nursing, 5*(1), 10–14.

Devine, B. (1981). Therapeutic milieu/milieu therapy: An overview. *Journal of Psychiatric Nursing and Mental Health Services, 19*(3), 20–29.

DiBella, G., Weitz, G., Poynter-Berg, D., & Yurmark, J. (1982). *Handbook of partial hospitalization.* New York: Brunner/Mazel.

Jack, L. (1989). Use of milieu as a problem-solving strategy in addiction treatment. *Nursing Clinics of North America, 24*(1), 69–80.

Jones, M. (1953). *The therapeutic community: A new treatment method in psychiatry.* New York: Basic Books.

Johnson, C. M. (1991). *Adolescent patients' perceptions of the seclusion experience: A phenomenological study.* Unpublished master's thesis. Arlington, TX: The University of Texas at Arlington.

Johnston, M. (1979). Toward a culture of caring: Children, their environment, and change. *Maternal Child Nursing, 4*, 210–214.

Kahn, E. M., & Fredrick, N. (1988). Milieu-oriented management strategies on acute care units for the chronically mentally ill. *Archives of Psychiatric Nursing, 2*(3), 134–140.

Kernberg, O. (1978). Leadership and organizational functioning: Organizational regression. *International Journal of Group Psychotherapy, 28*, 3–25.

Kets de Vries, M. (1984). Group fantasies and organizational functioning. *Human Relations, 37*, 111–134.

Kibel, H. (1987). Contributions of the group psychotherapist to education on the psychiatric unit: Teaching through group dynamics. *International Journal of Group Psychotherapy, 37*, 3–29.

Mosher, L., Kresky-Wolff, M., Matthews, S., & Menn, A. (1986). Milieu therapy in the 1980s: A comparison of two residential alternatives to hospitalization. *Bulletin of the Menninger Clinic, 50*, 257–268.

Osmond, H. (1959). The historical and sociological development of mental hospitals. In C. Goshen (Ed.), *Psychiatric architecture* (pp. 7–9). Washington, DC: American Psychiatric Association.

Puskar, K., & McAdam, D. (1988). Use of open report as a staff-patient model of communication on schizophrenia research unit: A case report. *Archives of Psychiatric Nursing, 2*(5), 274–280.

Rasinski, K., Rozensky, R., & Pasulka, P. (1980). Practical implications of a theory of the therapeutic milieu for psychiatric nursing practice. *Journal of Psychiatric Nursing and Mental Health Services, 18*(5), 16–20.

Skinner, K. (1979). The therapeutic milieu: Making it work. *Journal of Psychosocial Nursing and Mental Health Services, 17*(8), 38–44.

Smith, C., & Murphy, K. (1984). Developing a children's inpatient psychiatric unit. *Journal of Psychosocial Nursing, 22*(3), 31–36.

Yalom, I. (1985). *The theory and practice of group psychotherapy.* New York: Basic Books.

UNIT

VI

Professional Topics

CHAPTER

31

Legal and Ethical Issues

Jacqueline M. Melonas

Legal and ethical standards are part of the professional framework that underlies the practice of child and adolescent psychiatric nursing. These standards support the decision making of the psychiatric nurse as he or she is faced with the complex clinical situations inherent in this specialty area of nursing. Psychiatric nursing requires a knowledge of the law and how legal standards affect nursing practice. The nurse must understand the difference between law and ethics and how each impacts clinical decision making.

The law regulates professional nursing practice and defines malpractice. It construes the legal relationship between the health care provider and the patient and mandates that patients be afforded certain rights while receiving psychiatric treatment. However, many of the clinical challenges that face the child and adolescent psychiatric nurse cannot be resolved by legal principles, and decision making must then be directed by ethical guidelines.

Child and adolescent psychiatric nurses face a unique challenge because they must not only provide care for the patient, but must also balance the interests and needs of the child, the parent, the health care institution, and the state. The law provides the nurse with the framework for understanding the legal relationships among these entities. It also clarifies the legal duties of the nurse in relation to these individuals and institutions. Nursing ethics provide a basis for decision making that transcends the requirements of the law.

This chapter examines the legal and ethical standards related to specific clinical topics the child psychiatric nurse confronts on a daily basis. These topics are consent to treatment, commitment and involuntary treatment of minors, confidentiality, and child abuse.

Law or Ethics

THE NORMS OF OBLIGATION

Law and ethics struggle to provide guidelines for how human beings can live in relationship to one another with the least amount of conflict and harm (Kjervick; 1990). Figure 31-1 shows one author's conceptualization of the relationship of law and ethics as a circle within a circle, where law is encompassed within the larger circle of ethics (Kjervick, 1990). The sphere of ethics includes matters beyond the scope of the law, but all legal matters contain an element of ethical decision making (Kjervick, 1990).

Fowler (1989) described ethics as "a division of either philosophy or theology that engages in the philosophical study of morality, moral judgments, and moral problems" (p. 956). The American Nurses Association's (ANA) Code for Nurses with Interpretive Statements (1985) states: "When making clini-

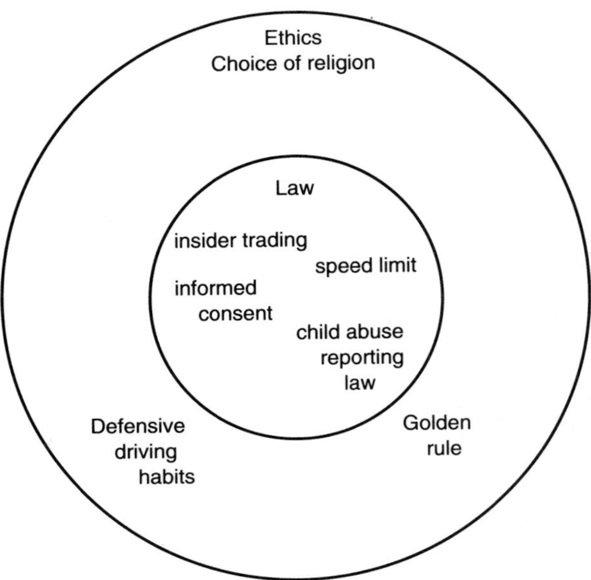

FIGURE 31–1 • A conceptualization of the relationship of law and ethics

cal judgments, nurses base their decisions on consideration of consequences and universal moral principles, both of which prescribe and justify nursing actions" (p. i). The universal moral principles referred to in the ANA Code for Nurses are the ethical duties of the nurse, or "the norms of obligation" (Fowler, 1989, p. 959). The ANA Code for Nurses lists the norms of obligation or universal moral principles as, "respect for persons . . . autonomy (self-determination), beneficence (doing good), nonmaleficence (avoiding harm), veracity (truth-telling), confidentiality (respecting privileged information), fidelity (keeping promises), and justice (treating people fairly)" (p. i). Nurses use these norms of obligation for analyzing clinical situations and making ethical decisions and judgments. Ethical decision making as a process contrasts with the requirements of the law.

SOURCES OF LAW

The law mandates or prohibits behavior. These mandates or prohibitions are supported by the *force* of law. In other words, if the requirements of the law are not followed, one will be sanctioned or penalized (Hall, 1990). For example, the nurse may decide through the process of ethical decision making that reporting child abuse is the right thing to do. However, because child abuse reporting is mandated by law in all states, the nurse must report child abuse or face penalties.

Law is derived from four sources: constitutions (federal and state), statutes, regulations, and case law. The United States Constitution takes precedence over any law that conflicts with it. In health care law, the United States Constitution plays a central role when fundamental liberties are addressed, such as the right to die or abortion cases. State constitutions may provide rights or protections to the citizens of a state in addition to what is provided in the United States Constitution. The second source of law, statutes, is created by the legislative branch. The state Nurse Practice Act is an example of a statute enacted by the legislative branch of a state government. The state mental health code, law, or statute is another example. Statutes usually are written in general language and often must be interpreted by courts or administrative agencies. Administrative agencies are the third source of law. Regulations that affect health care providers often are promulgated by administrative agencies, such as licensing requirements for mental health care institutions. The fourth source of law is the courts. Courts interpret constitutions, statutes, and regulations. The courts also write opinions about trial cases that have been appealed. This law, written by the courts, is *common law* and is developed on a case-by-case basis. The psychiatric nurse will be most interested in case law as it applies to nursing malpractice.

The law is often thought of as a fixed set of rules or decrees that if consulted, will clarify whether the actions or omissions of a person or an institution are "legal" or "illegal." Some areas of the law are well established, so a specific rule of law will almost always be applied to a particular problem. Lawyers call this "black letter law." For example, forcing health care treatment on a patient in a nonemergency situation when that patient has refused such treatment is battery. In general, however, the law is continually evolving as laws are made by courts, legislatures, and administrative agencies.

How should the child psychiatric nurse decide whether the law, nursing ethics, or both should guide his or her actions? First, the psychiatric nurse should be familiar with the Nurse Practice Act in his or her state. The Nurse Practice Act defines the scope and limits of nursing practice, including the practice of advanced nursing practitioners, such as clinical specialists in child and adolescent psychiatric-mental health nursing or nurse practitioners. Second, the psychiatric nurse should be informed about the state mental health statutes. Often the state mental health authority

CLINICAL EXAMPLE: MAGGIE

Maggie, who is 16 years old, is admitted to the psychiatric hospital because of depression and suicidal ideation. She confides in the psychiatric nurse that she was raped 2 years ago by a man who lives in her neighborhood. Maggie begs the nurse not to tell her parents because they would not understand. Further, she states that her father is an unreasonable and difficult person and would blame her for what happened. Ten days after admission, Maggie's parents abruptly decide that she must be discharged from the hospital. They will not discuss aftercare treatment plans with the nurse. Maggie is no longer talking about suicide, but she still exhibits many signs of depression. Maggie states that she wants to continue in treatment. She says she will not leave when her parents come to take her home.

What are the legal responsibilities of the psychiatric nurse in this situation? Are there ethical considerations? What are Maggie's parents' rights concerning making treatment decisions for their child? Does the age of the child matter in this situation? What about confidentiality? Is the nurse legally mandated to report any of this information, and if so, to whom? Is the nurse ethically obligated to appraise anyone of this information? Could the actions or omissions of the nurse injure the patient or her family? What is the potential for liability for the nurse and the hospital? What is the difference between law and ethics, and how does this impact psychiatric nursing practice?

will provide copies of such statutes to mental health practitioners. Some of the areas that state mental health statutes typically govern include the procedures for voluntary and involuntary admissions to mental health facilities, the rights of mental health patients, the parameters of professional–patient confidentiality, and any special procedures concerning minors for consent to treatment or admission to a mental health facility. Third, the psychiatric nurse should stay up to date about case law involving nurses and the nursing standard of care. Professional nursing journals regularly publish legal columns and articles discussing current case law pertinent to nurses. Fourth, the nurse may need to seek the advice of a health care lawyer experienced in mental health law. A health care lawyer may be available through the institution in which one is employed; independent practitioners may need to retain an attorney to provide advice.

The Clinical Example for Maggie is typical of clinical situations that child psychiatric nurses often confront. It illustrates how several of the topics discussed in this chapter may interact. Answering the questions that this scenario poses will clarify some of the legal and ethical standards addressed in this chapter.

Consent to Treatment

WHO MAY CONSENT?

When the patient–nurse relationship is being established, the child psychiatric nurse must consider who may give consent to treatment. Usually, parents present their children to the mental health care practitioner for care. Sometimes other members of the family bring children for treatment, or an unrelated adult may ask the health professional to provide treatment for a child. State agencies, such as Child Protective Services or Juvenile Services, may request that the mental health practitioner provide services to a child under its care. A child may independently seek treatment. It is the nurse's responsibility to ascertain who may legally consent to treatment for a child because treatment without proper consent is battery and may be considered professional negligence (Rosoff, 1981). Statutes and case law provide the legal standards that determine who may consent to mental health treatment for a child.

In general, parents must consent to treatment for their children. The right of parents to make decisions about how to raise their children, including the right to make treatment decisions, has long been recognized by courts under the doctrine of family privacy. The doctrine of family privacy has been established by a line of U.S. Supreme Court cases in which parental decisions about the care and custody of their children were challenged.[1] The Court in *Prince v. Massachusetts* (1944) stated it this way: "It is cardinal with us that the custody, care and nurture of the child reside first in the par-

---

Prince v. Massachusetts, 321 U.S. 158 (1944).
Pierce v. Society of Sisters, 268 U.S. 510(1925).
Wisconsin v. Yoder, 406 U.S. 205 (1972).
Bellotti V. Baird, 443 U.S. 622 (1972).
Parham v. J.R., 442 U.S. 584 (1979).
Meyer v. Nebraska, 262 U.S. 390 (1923).

BOX 31–1 • OKLAHOMA STATUTES §8-201(B)(1)&(2)

B. Upon the application of a parent or legal guardian of the child, a private hospital or other mental health facility may admit the child for inpatient mental health evaluation or treatment if the person in charge of the mental health facility or his designee and a licensed mental health professional deems the child to be clinically eligible for such admission.

1. A child may be deemed eligible for admission for inpatient evaluation when, after a prescreening examination, a licensed mental health professional determines and states in writing that there is a reasonable case to believe that the child may be a child in need of mental health treatment and that such evaluation is necessary to properly determine the condition of the child and the mental health treatment needs of the child, if any.
2. A child may be deemed eligible for inpatient mental health treatment when, after an outpatient or inpatient examination or evaluation, a licensed mental health professional determines and states in writing that in his professional opinion the child is a child in need of inpatient mental health treatment and:
   a. Reasonable efforts have been made to provide for the mental health treatment needs of the child through the provision of less restrictive alternatives and that such alternatives have failed to meet the treatment needs of the child, or
   b. After a thorough consideration of less restrictive alternatives to inpatient treatment, the condition of the child is such that less restrictive alternatives are unlikely to meet the mental health treatment needs of the child.

Oklahoma Statute §8-202(A)(1)

1. Whenever a child fourteen (14) years of age or older who has been admitted to a mental health facility for inpatient mental health treatment notifies the facility of his desire to object to such admission, the facility shall without undue delay assist the child in properly filing such objection with the court.

ents . . . ." The right of parents to make decisions about the care of their children is based on the belief that parents naturally act in the best interest of their children. Further, parents, unlike children, have the maturity, experience, and capacity to make difficult decisions (*Parham v. J.R.*, 1979).

A parent's right to consent or not to consent to treatment is not absolute. The law recognizes that parents do not always act in the best interests of their children. Thus, the state may exercise its powers of "parents patriae"[2] when the mental or physical health of a child is jeopardized.

Parens patriae refers to the role of the state as sovereign and guardian of people under legal disability. (Blacks Law Dictionary, 1979, p. 1003). A minor, one who has not reached the age of majority, is considered to be under a legal disability. The law has recognized that the state has an interest in the welfare and safety of its citizens. Under its parens patriae power, the state may interfere with the constitutional rights of parents to make decisions concerning their children if there is an overriding state interest in the health or welfare of the child. For example, the state may take abused children into its custody for protection or require that school children be vaccinated regardless of the parents' wishes.

STATE LAW REQUIREMENTS FOR CONSENT TO TREATMENT

State mental health statutes spell out who may consent to mental health treatment and under what circumstances. In some states minors older than a certain age may not be admitted to a mental health facility for treatment unless they give voluntary consent along with their parents (Box 31-1). Other states require that minors older than a certain age consent for themselves to voluntary admission (Box 31-2). Several states permit minors who are seeking mental health treatment for substance abuse to obtain treatment without parental consent (Box 31-3).

Most states allow emancipated minors to give consent for medical treatment, including mental health treatment. A state statute or case law may establish the criteria for being considered an emancipated minor. Typically, the minor must be past a certain age and meet one or several criteria for eligibility. These criteria might include being a parent, being married, living separately from parents, and being employed and self-supporting.

BOX 31–2 • FLORIDA STATUTE §394.465 (1986) —VOLUNTARY ADMISSIONS

(1) Authority to receive patients.
  (a) . . . .
  (b) A facility may admit for evaluation, diagnosis, or treatment any individual who makes application by express and informed consent therefor; **however, any individual age 17 or under may be admitted only after a hearing to verify the voluntariness of the consent.** If such individual is under 18 years of age, his parent or guardian may apply for his discharge, and the administrator shall release the patient within 3 days of such application for discharge (emphasis added).

State mental health statutes allow emergency mental health treatment without parental consent when a minor is in imminent danger of hurting himself or herself or others. However, specific statutory procedures may be necessary to protect the interests of the parents and the child when this exception to the rule of obtaining parental consent is applied due to an emergency situation. For example, it may be necessary for a qualified professional to certify that the minor meets the criteria for needing emergency mental health treatment and to file such a document with the state mental health authority or with the court. The statute may require notification of parents as soon as possible and notification to the state mental health authority.

The child psychiatric nurse should be familiar with the statutory requirements for consent to mental health treatment and admission to a mental health facility in the state in which he or she practices. The nurse will participate in meeting the statutory requirements for assessments and documentation to validate the need for mental health treatment. If someone other than a parent requests treatment for a child, they must provide documentation of their legal capacity to consent in the absence of parental consent. This may be in the form of legal guardianship papers, a court order, or other legally valid documentation. Legal counsel may need to be consulted to determine if the documentation meets legal requirements.

BOX 31–3 • NEW HAMPSHIRE REVISED STATUTE ANNOTATED §318-B: 12-A (1989)—TREATMENT OF DRUG ABUSE

Any minor 12 years of age or older may voluntarily submit himself to treatment for drug dependency . . . at any municipal health department, state institution or facility, public or private hospital or clinic, any licensed physician, or other accredited state or local social welfare agency, without the consent of a parent, guardian or any other person charged with the care or custody of said minor.

INFORMED CONSENT

The doctrine of informed consent has ethical and legal dimensions that impact the practice of the child psychiatric nurse. All health care consumers have a basic right to informed consent before treatment is initiated. The right to informed consent for mental health care consumers is often explicitly stated in the state mental health statutes that define the rights of mental health consumers.

Informed consent is based on the strongly held common law concept of the sanctity of a person's bodily integrity. Every person has the right to refuse to be touched or treated. Informed consent means that the consenter has the right to necessary information before consenting to any therapeutic intervention (Rosoff, 1981). In general the information that must be disclosed for the consenter to make an informed decision includes "diagnosis (i.e., the patient's condition or problem), nature and purpose of the proposed treatment, risks and consequences of the proposed treatment, feasible treatment alternatives, and prognosis if the proposed treatment is not given" (Rosoff, 1981, p. 41).

In the health care institution setting the treating physician has the legal duty to obtain informed consent from the patient or the person legally authorized to consent for the patient. The nurse's role is as an advocate and educator for the patient (Weiss, 1990). Additionally, the nurse will be involved in assessing the capacity of the patient to give informed consent (Weiss, 1990). Child psychiatric nurses practicing independently will be responsible for obtaining informed consent before beginning psychotherapy.

The legal requirements of informed consent for mental health treatment usually centers on interventions, such as the administration of psychotropic medications and electroconvulsive therapy. Ethical nursing practice requires a more comprehensive view of informed consent; it encompasses all the decisions that the patient must make about becoming involved and continuing in the therapeutic relationship. The moral principle of respect for autonomy is fundamental to nursing ethics (ANA Code for Nurses, 1985). "Truth telling and the process of reaching informed choice underlie the exercise of self-determination, which is basic to respect for persons" (ANA Code for Nurses, 1985, p. 2). Informed consent also may be useful as a treatment strategy because it builds trust, encourages commitment to the treatment, and can deflect resistance to therapy (Jensen, Josephson, & Frey, 1989)

Who should be informed when the patient is the child, but the parent is the consenter? The parent has the legal responsibility and right to give informed consent unless the minor has the capacity to consent under one of the legal exceptions as enumerated previously. However, all patients have a moral right to participate in their treatment even if they do not have the legal right to do so (Fowler, 1989). The child psychiatric nurse must consider the developmental level and mental status of the child when deciding how much information should be provided to the child. Keeping the child informed and participating in his or her treatment demonstrates the respect that the nurse has for the child's autonomy. It conveys that the child is respected as an individual and that he or she has a responsibility for the therapeutic work.

ETHICAL CONSIDERATIONS

Although the law may provide specific guidelines as to who may consent to mental health treatment, the child psychiatric nurse may be confronted with ethical dilemmas in this area. A situation may arise in which the child psychiatric nurse assesses that a minor needs mental health treatment, but the parents refuse to consent to treatment. The ethical principles of beneficence and respect for autonomy may be in conflict in this situation. If a child is assessed as being at risk for mental health problems, but the exception for treatment in an imminent emergency does not apply, the nurse may feel that it is contrary to nursing ethics to allow the child to go without treatment. The principle of beneficence requires that the nurse do good for a patient even if this involves some risk to the nurse (Fowler, 1989). If the nurse proceeds with treatment contrary to the parents' decision, the nurse is at risk for legal sanctions or a civil lawsuit by the parents.

The ethical principle of respect for autonomy requires that a patient's actions and decisions be respected even if they are contrary to what the nurse believes to be best for the patient (Fowler, 1989). Application of this principle is complicated because the identified patient is the child, but the parents have the legal right to consent to treatment. The patient is not making the autonomous decision but must rely on his or her parents to decide in his or her best interests.

It is possible to use legal and ethical standards to resolve this kind of conflict. Sometimes parents' refusal to provide needed treatment may reach the level of neglect under state child protection laws. Involving the state child protective agency does not put the nurse at legal risk when the reporting is done in good faith and with the best interests of the child in mind. In this way, the nurse is doing good for the patient but avoiding unacceptable risk. Additionally, the psychiatric nurse may be able to persuade parents to reconsider their decision, without violating the principle of respect for autonomy, by maintaining a therapeutic relationship based on respect for the parents' position. Part of the therapeutic work of the child psychiatric nurse involves educating parents about the developmental and mental health needs of the child. Adequately informed parents are in a better position to act in the best interests of their child. Other creative ways may be found to provide services to a child that are less objectionable to parents, such as enrolling the child in an appropriate support group at school.

What should a psychiatric nurse do if a minor independently requests mental health services but does not want his or her parents to know about the treatment? The standards that were applied previously should be followed. A minor may not receive treatment without parental consent unless one of the exceptions apply. The nurse's judgment and clinical expertise is critical in assessing the child's need for treatment. The severity of the child's clinical condition is the major factor in deciding what interventions should be attempted and how much risk the nurse will accept.

Of course, documentation to support the interventions that are provided is imperative for the clinical treatment of the patient and for the nurse who may be required to show justification for particular interventions.

Civil Commitment of Minors

DEPRIVATION OF LIBERTY

Involuntary commitment and confinement to a mental hospital is a severe deprivation of liberty. The Supreme Court has stated "no constitutional basis [exists] for confining . . . persons involuntarily if they are dangerous to no one and can live safely in freedom" (*O'Connor v. Donaldson,* 1975, p. 575). However, children have not been afforded all the constitutional due process rights that adults have in the same situation. Generally, parents have the right and responsibility to consent to treatment for their children. Reformers have argued that minors should have the same or similar due process safeguards as adults who are involuntarily committed (Ellis, 1974) and that parents do not always act in the best interest of their child when they commit him or her to a psychiatric hospital.

BALANCING THE INTERESTS OF CHILDREN, PARENTS, AND THE STATE

The Supreme Court in *Parham v. J.R.* (1979) set the minimum standard for procedural protections to be afforded minors who are presented for psychiatric hospitalization by their parents. In *Parham v. J.R.*, two minors who had been given no choice about being admitted to a Georgia state mental hospital challenged the Georgia law that allowed parents, guardians, or the state to commit people under 18 to mental hospitals. One of these minors had been hospitalized because his parents did not want to care for him and in spite of a recommendation that he be treated in a less restrictive environment. The Supreme Court found that the Constitution does not require a precommitment adversarial hearing for minors; however, an evaluation of the minor by a neutral fact finder is required before hospitalization. The minor's liberty interests and the parents' interests and responsibility for the health and welfare of their child were balanced and considered by the Court.

The Court said that parents should have a substantial role in the decision to admit their children to a psychiatric hospital. To safeguard against the risk of parents acting against the best interests of the child, a neutral fact finder, such as a staff physician, must evaluate if proper admission criteria are met. The fact finder must have the authority to refuse admission of a minor who does not meet admission criteria, and there must be periodic review to decide if continued hospitalization is necessary (*Parham v. J.R.,* 1979, pp. 606–607).

REFORMS AND ADVOCACY

States must provide at least the procedural standards for *Parham v. J.R.* for minors admitted to state hospitals but may provide additional protections. The *Parham v. J.R.* standard also is used as a guideline for admission to private psychiatric hospitals. Many state legislatures have enacted laws that provide more due process procedural safeguards than required by *Parham v. J.R.*.

Commentators continue to call for reforms in the area of civil commitment of minors. It is the responsibility of the child psychiatric nurse to stay current with legislative initiatives in this area and to be familiar with state admission criteria for minors.

The nurse may be confronted with a situation in which parents request admission of their child, but the child objects. Admission of a minor to a psychiatric hospital against his or her wishes involves a loss of personal liberty and self-determination. The psychiatric nurse should act as an advocate using the ethical principles of autonomy (self-determination) and justice (treating people fairly) to see that the hospitalization of a minor patient meets statutory admission criteria.

Confidentiality

LEGAL AND ETHICAL ISSUES

Statutes addressing the rights of mental health patients usually state that a patient has the right to have treatment information maintained confidentially. Nursing ethics protect the patient's right of privacy by preserving confidential patient information (ANA Code for Nurses, 1985, p. 4). Confidentiality is one of the *norms of obligation* of nursing ethics.

Mental health care professionals, by virtue of the nature of their practice, are privy to a patient's innermost thoughts and feelings. This confidential information is the basis for the therapeutic work done by the patient and the professional. The protection of this confidential information builds trust, an essential element of the therapeutic relationship.

State laws related to confidentiality and the care of medical records usually are found among patients rights statutes, medical record statutes, and statutes related to mental health care treatment. Patient treatment records are legal records that must be created and maintained according to state laws. The prudent health care professional is specific in his or her documentation and documents only the information that is necessary for the clinical treatment of the patient. The ethical responsibility of confidentiality related to mental health care is broader than the legal requirements that the health care professional has related to confidentiality of treatment information.

State laws usually provide for parents to consent to disclosure of information about their children. How much information is the child psychiatric nurse required to disclose about the child-patient when parents request treatment information? Parents have a right and responsibility to be involved in the treatment of their child. The child psychiatric nurse is aware that the parents may have strong feelings and fears about what a child may be disclosing about the parents and the family situation.

Parents have a right to know as much information as needed to be involved in treatment decisions concerning their child. They have a legal right to obtain the treatment record. At times the right of the parent to have access to confidential information may conflict with the ethical principles of confidentiality and autonomy of the patient. If possible, the child psychiatric nurse should address these issues with the child and parent before treatment begins. The developmental stages of the child should be considered when discussing with the child and parents how much confidential information will be shared.

Adolescents are often very sensitive about what information will be revealed to their parents. The child psychiatric nurse can use the ethical principles of veracity and justice as a basis for making decisions about dealing with the concern of the adolescent. For example, the child psychiatric nurse can discuss with the adolescent the legal obligations and rights of the parents and nurse related to confidentiality. The nurse can treat the adolescent fairly by telling him or her when confidentiality will be breached (when the adolescent is in danger of injuring himself or herself or others). The nurse can promise to talk with the adolescent prior to talking to the parents about what information will be shared with the parents and why the information is being shared. Anticipating the confidentiality problems that may arise and involving the parents and child in solving any problems provide the parents and child with an opportunity to exercise their self-determination in the treatment situation.

DRUG AND ALCOHOL TREATMENT INFORMATION

The nurse should be knowledgeable about the special protection afforded patient information related to drug and alcohol treatment. The Comprehensive Alcohol Abuse and Alcoholism Prevention Treatment and Rehabilitation Act (1970) and the Drug Abuse Office and Treatment Act (1972) were enacted by Congress to provide protection from misuse of treatment information in this area and thus provide more incentive for people to enter drug and alcohol treatment programs. The regulations, Confidentiality of Alcohol and Drug Abuse Patient Record 1990 (42 CFR part 2), that have been promulgated persuant to the acts provide specific rules regarding disclosure of patient information for drug and alcohol patients in federally assisted programs. Any drug and alcohol treatment program in a clinic, general hospital, provided by a private health care practitioner, and so forth is covered by these regulations. Federal assistance has been broadly defined so that any program that receives direct or indirect federal assistance, including Medicare or Medicaid participation, would be covered by these regulations (42 CFR 2.12).

The child psychiatric nurse should obtain a copy of the regulations governing disclosure of patient information of drug and alcohol treatment. An attorney should be consulted if there are questions as to whether specific information is covered by these regulations and how to comply with the regulations. In general, disclosure of information is prohibited without the written consent of the patient (the consent form must include specific information to be valid, per the regulations) or a court order that has been obtained according to the procedures set out in the regulations. This means that information may not be disclosed to law enforcement authorities, pursuant to a *subpoena duces tecum* or other officials without the patient's consent or a proper court order. Information that is prohibited from being disclosed includes any information about the patient whether or not it is in writing (42 CFR 2.11).

There are exceptions to this general rule. Child abuse reporting under state law is not prohibited. The regulations state that they "do not apply to the reporting under state law of incidents of suspected child abuse and neglect to the appropriate State or local authorities" (42 CFR 2.12(c)(6)).

Under these regulations, minors and parents must consent for release of treatment information regarding the minor (42 CFR 2.14). In some cases, only the minor needs to give consent (42 C.F.R. 2.14 (b) + (c).

Child Abuse

THE ROLES OF THE CHILD PSYCHIATRIC NURSE

In all 50 states, health professionals are mandated to report suspected child abuse. Nurses may be the first health care professionals to suspect that a child has been abused. The role of the child psychiatric nurse may include evaluating whether a child has been abused, providing mental health care treatment to an abused child and his or her family, or advocating for services and resources for abused children and their families. The child psychiatric nurse may be called on to give expert testimony or to support a child victim who is a witness in legal proceedings. The knowledge and the child developmental orientation of the child psychiatric nurse provide a valuable perspective for the roles of evaluator, therapist, advocate, and expert witness.

In 1962, Dr. Henry Kempe and his colleagues published their landmark article "The Battered Child Syndrome" in the *Journal of the American Medical Association*. Kempe's pioneering work, which documented the injuries that children were sustaining at the hands of their parents, forced the health care community, and eventually the larger community, to respond to the problem of child abuse. Twenty years later, sexual abuse was "emerging as one of the major forms of child abuse" (Finkelhor, 1984, p. 1). The number of sexual abuse reports to social service and law enforcement agencies has increased as the public's awareness of the problem has increased. However, a review of several studies shows that the prevalence of child abuse may be greater than even the rapid increase of reports of sexual abuse would indicate.[3]

Considering the magnitude and scope of the problem of abuse, child psychiatric nurses will deal with victimized children and their families and will interface with social and legal systems addressing this problem.

The nurse should be clear about the roles he or she will assume in any professional relationship with a victim or suspected victim of child abuse. These roles have somewhat different goals and at times may be in conflict.

CHILDREN AS WITNESSES

When interviewing victims of child sexual abuse, the techniques mental health professionals use to elicit information differ from those used by police or other investigators (Goodman & Helgeson, 1985; "The Admissibility of Expert Psychological Testimony," 1988). The mental health professional uses the interview diagnostically and for the purpose of obtaining information that can be used in the prosecution of the case. The mental health professional may even use mildly suggestive questioning to "break a frightened or embarrassed victim's silence" (Goodman & Helgeson, 1985, p. 188). The therapist uses inferences from the child's behavior to facilitate communication with the child ("The Admissibility of Expert Psychological Testimony," 1988). Information elicited in this manner may be subject, during legal proceedings, to charges that the mental health professional "coached" the child to manufacture a story. It has been suggested that all such evidence should be preserved by videotape and thus be available for experts representing both sides in a legal proceeding so that the experts can challenge the interpretation of the evidence ("The Admissibility of Expert Psychological Testimony," 1988).

One therapeutic goal in the treatment of the trauma associated with sexual victimization is to help the child achieve some control and understanding of an irrational event (Lamb, 1986). This involves explaining to the child that the abuse did not occur because he or she is different or odd, and that other children have experienced the same thing. The child may join a therapeutic group with other children who have been sexually abused. This educationally therapeutic strategy may result in the child being introduced to correct anatomic terminology, as opposed to the child's personal, idiosyncratic terminology for body parts and for various types of sexual behavior. A child witness who uses the correct anatomic terminology is presumed to have been "coached" in preparing his or her testimony.

The child psychiatric nurse therapist who treats

Russell (1983) reported that his 1978 survey of 930 San Francisco women revealed that 38% of those surveyed had been sexually abused or had experienced unwanted sexual touching before age 18. Twelve percent of the women reporting abuse or unwanted touching had been victimized by a relative (Russell, 1983). A 1980 random survey of adults with a Texas driver's license revealed a reported rate of sexual abuse of 12% for females and 3% for males (Kercher, 1980). Another survey in 1981 of 521 people in Boston found that 15% of females and 6% of males reported an experience of sexual abuse before the age of 16 by someone at least 5 years older (Finkelhor & Hotaling, 1983). It has been estimated that as many as 210,000 new cases of sexual abuse could be occurring each year (Finkelhor, 1984).

victimized children should be aware of how courts view children as witnesses and how the goals of therapeutic process may conflict with the goals of the legal system. As an expert witness, the child psychiatric nurse is in a position to help the court understand and evaluate the testimony of a child. The nurse can provide the court with information about the developmental stage of a child victim and how this may affect the child's ability to provide testimony. The nurse understands and can interpret for the court how a variety of factors can affect the child's ability to testify. Such factors as the child's dependency on the abuser who is a parent, the child's feelings of shame and guilt, the conflictual positive and negative feelings the child may have toward the abuser, and so forth can influence the child's legitimacy as a witness (Stanley, 1989).

In cases of physical abuse or neglect, there is physical or corroborating evidence. In cases of sexual abuse, there is usually no physical evidence, and the child victim and the alleged abuser are usually the only witnesses to the alleged events. This means that the testimony of the child is critical; without it there is no legal case. Unfortunately, the nature of court and legal proceedings is that the emotional problems of the child victim may be exacerbated, and new problems may be produced as a child is plunged into the legal system (Weiss & Berg, 1982).

Child psychiatric nurses who treat victims of child abuse and their families should familiarize themselves with the types of legal proceedings to which the child will be subjected. The nurse can provide anticipatory guidance for the child and families as they are confronted with the unfamiliar actors and procedures of the court. Once allegations of sexual abuse have been disclosed, an official state investigation will proceed, conducted by the police and the state child protective agency. If enough evidence is gathered from this investigation, prosecution of an alleged offender will begin. The child will participate in the court proceedings (Weiss & Berg, 1982). In the role of a therapist or a member of a multidisciplinary treatment team, the nurse will assess the impact that testifying may have on an alleged child victim of abuse. In some cases, the decision not to go forward with legal proceedings is made because of the potentially devastating emotional impact that the proceedings would have on the child.

One of the difficulties for alleged child abuse victims is that they may be subjected to repeated interviews by a variety of professionals involved in investigating and prosecuting a case of child abuse. The child in this situation will be subjected to a variety of investigatory styles, conflicting questions, and interviews by individuals not skilled in interviewing children nor in understanding how a child's developmental stage may affect what answers are obtained. It is no surprise that conflicting stories or even a retraction of the story by the child may result. Some states have developed multidisciplinary teams to respond to and investigate alleged child abuse. This system minimizes the number of times a child is interviewed in the process of evaluating the report or complaint of abuse. In some cases, this evaluation is videotaped for the use of the different players (e.g., police, prosecutor, defense attorney) and may be used in court proceedings (Berliner, 1985).

The child and adolescent psychiatric nurse may function as the evaluator. This evaluation may be the basis for criminal charges against an alleged offender, and the goals of such an evaluation differ from those of the treatment interview. The nurse should be aware of the importance of an objective evaluation. Continuing education about child abuse and techniques for interviewing alleged victims should be pursued. The nurse should be aware of whether the use of anatomically correct dolls in the interview will be allowed to be presented as expert testimony in the jurisdiction. The use of anatomically correct dolls in evaluating sexual abuse in preschool children is used extensively and is the subject of much controversy in the mental health professional community. Some professionals claim that false accusations of sexual abuse have resulted from the use of the dolls to evaluate children (Moss, 1988).

There is a lack of research as to how nonabused children interact with dolls; some preliminary results show that nonabused children play suggestively with dolls (Moss, 1988). Some researchers have developed precise guidelines for interviewing preschoolers with sexually anatomically detailed dolls; precise guidelines are needed to obtain data that are reliable and valid (White, Strom, Santilli, & Halpin, 1986). The nurse testifying about information obtained while using the dolls will be required to demonstrate that an objective method of evaluation was used to illicit the information. In one case, the court ruled that observation of play with the dolls is only admissible if it is demonstrated that the method is accepted in the scientific community (*Amber B. v. Solano County*, 1987).

Additionally, as an evaluator, the child psychiatric nurse should evaluate the child's credibility as a witness. As discussed previously, the mental health professionals are cognizant of the psychologic trauma that may result when a child must

BOX 31–4 • QUESTIONING CHILDREN ABOUT ALLEGED SEXUAL ABUSE

The words and specific language used by adults attempting to get information from alleged child victims of sexual abuse may determine the answers that are given. Preschool children will give literal answers to questions because they interpret words concretely and do not understand nuances in speech. They do not have the verbal ability to express all that they understand and feel in language.

Berliner & Barbieri (1984) give the following examples of a 5-year-old being cross-examined. On direct examination, the child had testified that her father had put his penis in her mouth.

Defense Attorney:	And then you said you put your mouth on his penis?
Child:	No.
Defense Attorney:	You didn't say that?
Child:	No.
Defense Attorney:	Did you ever put your mouth on his penis?
Child:	No.
Defense Attorney:	Well, why did you tell your mother that your dad put his penis in your mouth?
Child:	My brother told me to.

The experienced prosecuting attorney recognized the child's very literal answer and made the child's answer clear on redirect examination.

Prosecuting Attorney:	Jennie, you said that you didn't put your mouth on daddy's penis. Is that right?
Child:	Yes.
Prosecuting Attorney:	Did daddy put his penis in your mouth?
Child:	Yes.
Prosecuting Attorney:	Did you tell your mom?
Child:	Yes.
Prosecuting Attorney:	What made you decide to tell?
Child:	My brother and I talked about it, and he said I better tell or dad would just keep doing it.

REFERENCE

Berliner, L., & Barbieri (1984). The testimony of child victims of sexual assault. *Journal of Social Issues, 40,* 125.

testify and participate in court proceedings related to alleged sexual abuse. Another concern is whether children can be competent witnesses. Even if a child testifies, the effectiveness of such testimony may be negated if a child is confused, contradicts himself or herself, and so forth during cross-examination (Box 31-4). Although the United States Supreme Court has held that "there is no precise age which determines the question of competency" (*Wheeler v. U.S.,* p. 524), several criteria are used to determine a child's competency as a witness:

- Whether the child can understand the difference between the truth and a lie and his or her ability to appreciate an obligation or responsibility to tell the truth
- The child's mental capacity to observe accurately and understand the occurrence
- Whether the child has the capacity to remember independently and recollect the occurrence
- Whether the child is capable of verbally communicating what he or she remembers and can understand basic questions about the event (McComb, 1987–1988, p. 537)

Many states have passed legislation to help reduce the problems related to having children as witnesses and the difficulties in detecting and prosecuting child abusers. Some statutes allow for closed circuit television testimony (Section 9-102, Maryland Courts and Judicial Procedure Annotated Code) among other methods. The constitutionality of some of these statutes is being tested because of the potential infringement on the rights of defendants (Forman, 1989; *Coy v. Iowa,* 1989). The psychiatric nurse should be aware of any statutory protections for child victims in the jurisdiction where he or she practices.

MANDATORY REPORTING

The mandatory reporting of child abuse is based on the state's compelling interest in protecting the health and welfare of abused children. This compelling state interest overrides the confidentiality and the right to privacy (Kermani, 1989). Some state statutes mandating child abuse reporting specifically state that reporting is required notwithstanding mental health care practitioner–patient confidentiality. The health care practitioner is required to report when he or she reasonably suspects abuse. The health care practitioner is not required to be sure or to have proof that abuse is occurring. Even if the allegation of abuse turns out to be false, state mandatory child abuse reporting laws provide immunity from civil and criminal liability for reporters if the reporting was done in good faith and without malice.

ETHICAL ISSUES RELATED TO CHILD ABUSE

Many ethical issues may arise as the child psychiatric nurse meets the legal duty to report child abuse. The conflict between the requirements of the law and ethical concepts is illustrated in the following case study.

Four-year-old Mary, her sister, and two brothers were found wandering in a shopping mall where their mother had abandoned them. Mary was placed in foster care and a preplacement physical examination revealed that she had contracted a chronic venereal disease. Mary began play therapy with the child psychiatric clinical nurse specialist due to her problems in relating to peers, nightmares, and numerous fears. During the course of therapy in the next 8 months, Mary verbalized and demonstrated through play therapy that she had been sexually abused by her mother, two maternal uncles, and possibly other members of the extended family. One uncle was charged and convicted of child sexual abuse of Mary and her siblings. The plan of the Protective Services Agency was to involve the mother and children in therapy and to eventually reunite the family. Periodic court hearings were held to determine if therapeutic progress was being made or if termination of parental rights should be considered.

As Mary developed trust through the therapeutic process with the child psychiatric nurse, she related very violent and bizarre acts to which she had been subjected by her uncle while her mother was present. Mary had very great fears about returning to her mother; she felt she would not be safe or protected by her mother. (She was terrified even during supervised visits with her mother at the Child Protective Agency.)

The child psychiatric nurse was required to make periodic reports to the court about Mary's therapeutic progress so that decisions about custody could be made. During therapy, Mary became frightened after telling the therapist about some of the instances of child abuse and begged the therapist not to tell anyone that she had "tattled." Mary related that her mother told her that Uncle Jack would "boil her bones in a pot" if he knew Mary had told about the abuse.

The child psychiatric nurse knew that the protective agency rarely advocated terminating parental rights. Also, the family therapist working with the mother was of the opinion that this family should be reunited and was strongly advocating this disposition. The child psychiatric nurse believed that the only way to convince the court that this was a situation in which the child should not be returned to the mother was to reveal the enormity of the abuse that had been reported by Mary. However, in the event that the child was returned to the mother, the nurse was convinced that Mary could be in danger because the mother would have access to this information during one of the court hearings. Additionally, the child psychiatric nurse thought that if this information was disputed, it could negate any chance that the child and the mother had to develop a mother–child bond.

The nurse was not legally required to tell the court all the "gory details" of the abuse; however, she was convinced that revealing this information was the only way to draw adequate attention to the situation. The child-patient had requested that this information be kept confidential.

The child psychiatric nurse relied on the ethical concept of "beneficence." The nurse decided that she would make the decision to reveal this information over the objections of the child-patient because the child was not mature enough to weigh all the consequences of withholding this information. Respect for the patient's autonomy was overridden because of the child's immaturity to make this serious decision.

Parental rights were terminated in this case because other evidence was found that corroborated the information the child psychiatric nurse revealed to the court. Further investigation to find this corroborating evidence may not have gone forward if the child psychiatric nurse had not reported this information.

REFERENCES

Amber B. v. Solano County Department of Social Services, 191 Cal. App. 3d 682 (1987).

The admissibility of expert psychological testimony in cases involving the sexual misuse of a child. (1988). *University of Miami Law Review, 42,* 1033–1072.

American Nurses Association (1985). *Code for nurses with interpretive statements.* Kansas City, MO: Author.

Berliner, L., & Barbieri (1984). The testimony of child victims of sexual assault. *Journal of Social Issues, 40,* 125.

Berliner, L. (1985). The child witness: The progress and emerging limitations. *University of Miami Law Review, 40,* 167–179.

Black's Law Dictionary with Pronunciations (5th. ed.). (1979). St. Paul, MN: West Publishing.

Confidentiality of Alcohol and Drug Abuse Patient Records, 42 C.F.R, Part 2 (1990).

Comprehensive Alcohol Abuse and Alcoholism Prevention, Treatment and Rehabilitation Act of 1970, 42 W.S.C. 290dd-3 (1988).

Coy v. Iowa, 108 S. Ct. 2798 (1988).

Drug Abuse Office and Treatment Act of 1972, 42 U.S.C 290ee-3 (1988).

Ellis, (1974). Voluntary children: Parental commitment of minors to mental institutions. *California Law Review, 72,* 840.

Finkelhor, D. (1984). *Child sexual abuse: New theory and research.* New York: Macmillian.

Finkelhor, D., & Hotaling, G. (1983). Sexual abuse in the National Incidence Study of Child Abuse and Neglect. Report to the National Center for Child Abuse and Neglect.

Florida Statutes Annotated 394.465 (1986).

Forman, E. (1989). To keep the balance true: The case of Coy v. Iowa. *The Hastings Law Journal, 40,* 437–456.

Fowler, M. D. M. (1989). Ethical decision making in clinical practice. *Nursing Clinics of North America, 24,* 955–965.

Goodman, G. S., & Helgeson, V. S. (1985). Child sexual assault: Children's memory and the law. *University of Miami Law Review, 40,* 181–208.

Hall, J. K. (1990). Understanding the fine line between law and ethics. *Nursing 90, 20*(10), 34–40.

Kempe, C. H., Silverman, F., Steele, B. Droegemueller, W., & Silver, H. (1962). The battered child syndrome. *Journal of the American Medical Association, 181,* 17–24.

Kercher, G. (1980). *Responding to child sexual abuse.* Huntsville, TX: Sam Houston State University, Criminal Justice Center.

Kermani, E. J. (1989). *Handbook of psychiatry and the law.* Chicago: Year Book Medical Publishers.

Kjervik, D. K. (1990). Legal and ethical issues. *Journal of Professional Nursing, 6,* 138, 185.

Jensen, P. S., Josephson, A. M., & Frey, J. (1989). Informed consent as a framework for treatment: Ethical and therapeutic considerations. *American Journal of Psychotherapy, 43,* 378–385.

Lamb, S. (1986). Treating sexually abused children: Issues of blame and responsibility. *American Journal of Orthopsychiatry, 56,* 303–307.

Md. Courts and Jud. Proc. Code Ann. 9–102 (1985).

McComb, J. S. (1987–1988). Unavailability and admissibility: Are a child's out-of-court statements about sexual abuse admissible if the child does not testify at trial? *Kentucky Law Journal, 76,* 531–567.

Moss, D. C. (1988). "Real" dolls too suggestive. *American Bar Association Journal, 74,* 24–25.

New Hampshire Revised Statutes Annotated 318-B:12-a (1989).

O'Connor v. Donaldson, 422 U.S. 563 (1975).

Oklahoma Statutes Annotated 8–201 & 8–202 (1990).

Parham v. J.R., 442 U.S. 584 (1979).

Rosoff, A. (1981). *Informed consent: A guide for health care providers.* Rockville, MD: Aspen.

Russell, D. (1983). Incidence and prevalence of intrafamilial and extrafamilial sexual abuse of female children. *Child Abuse and Neglect, 7,* 133–146.

Stanley, S. R. (1989). Disclosure of sexual abuse: The secret is out—what now? *Journal of Child Psychiatric Nursing, 2,* 154–160.

Turner, S. A. (1989). Case—Comments. Parham v. J.R.: Civil psychiatric commitment of minors. *Journal of Contemporary Health Law and Policy, 5,* 63–280.

Weis, E. H., & Berg, R. F. (1982). Child victims of sexual assault: Impact of court procedures. *Journal of the American Academy of Child Psychiatry, 21,* 513–518.

Weiss, F. S. (1990). The right to refuse: Informed consent and the psychosocial nurse. *Journal of Psychological Nursing, 28*(8), 25–30.

Wheeler v. U.S., 159 U.S. 523 (1895).

White, S., Strom, G., Santilli, G., & Halpin, B. (1986). Interviewing young sexual abuse victims with anatomically correct dolls. *Child Abuse and Neglect, 10,* 510–519.

Trends, like horses, are easier to ride in the direction they are already going. —JOHN NAISBITT

CHAPTER

32 Trends in Mental Health Care of Children, Adolescents, and Families

Sarah R. Stanley

The practice of child and adolescent psychiatric nursing is in a state of flux. Many nurses are entering the workplace without the skills and educational preparation to deliver quality care in the most effective manner. Nursing positions are being filled with ancillary personnel to control costs. Psychiatric and especially child psychiatric nursing programs have been reduced and splintered and are inaccessible because of location or cost. Legislative and regulatory blockades continue to impact on the child and adolescent nurse specialist who seeks to obtain payment for services to increase access for the many underserved and disenfranchised children and families. Poverty, homelessness, crime, violence, and substance abuse or addictions all contribute to the condition of the underclass and their mental health needs. It is evident that much of the present and future direction for health care will be mandated by economics. The changes in alternate family systems and in the patient/client population will continue. The nurse in psychiatric settings must continue to deal with the complex biologic and psychosocial interface of clients. As the research and knowledge about the neurochemical aspects of adult psychiatric mental disease continue to develop, the child and adolescent components will not be far behind.

Nursing and Health Care Trends

It has been said that "trends tell you the direction the country is moving in and the decisions are up to you" (Naisbitt, 1982). One always has choices. To choose the direction of the trend helps a person along. Even when one decides to go the opposite direction, it is helpful to know what one is up against. As nurses look for trends in nursing and health care, it is important to link the present with the past before moving on. The 1980s presented a stimulating challenge. Society's trends for that decade were predicted to be movement—from an industrial to an informational society, from forced technology to high tech and high touch, from a national to a world economy, from short term to long term, from centralization to decentralization, from institutional help to self-help, from representative democracy to participatory democracy, from hierarchies to networking, from north to south, and finally from either/or to multiple option (Naisbitt, 1982).

The population of the United States grew from 226.5 million in 1980 to 249.9 million in 1990. During that time, 37 million people were born and 20 million died; more than 300 million hospital stays occurred, and the nation's registered nurses (RNs) provided approximately 20 billion hours of patient care (Department of Commerce, 1990). Health care financing; regulatory efforts, such as cost controls and prospective pricing; management actions to restrict staffing; shortages of nursing personnel; lack of agreement on key professional issues, such as education; state regulatory and legislative roadblocks to expanded nursing practice; and many other factors were problematic for all specialty areas of nursing. The forces of conflict within and outside of nursing have not abated. These will certainly be played out as nurses and others struggle for health care reform of the delivery systems so that the 60 million uninsured and underinsured have coverage for essential health services. How the willingness and ability to pay for the improved access is resolved will be a crucial issue for the nursing profession. Pressures to contain costs, despite increasingly complex services for a patient population with more acute and complicated needs, will continue.

IMPACT FACTORS

Health care in the 1990s will be affected by factors such as the following:

- Increased population—a modest projection of 7.2% increase will mean 17.8 million Americans who will require expansion of the present strapped health care delivery system.
- Changed age distribution—the greatest growth in the 1990s will be among the 45- to 64-year-olds, which will increase 31%; the next largest increase will be among those 65 years and older, up 10.5% to 34.9 million individuals. The greatest crunch can be anticipated during the second decade of the 21st century as the baby boom generation reaches age 65 in the year 2010. As the U.S. population continues to age, those attempting to meet the needs will be faced with requirements for more services of higher complexity and expense.
- Health cost increases—the United States spent $604 billion for health care in 1989, an 11% increase. The Health Care Financing Administration (HCFA, 1987) predicts the nation's health expenditures will reach $1,529 billion in 2000. HCFA also estimates that as a proportion of gross national product (GNP), health expenditures will increase from 12% in 1990 to 15% in 2000. These estimates are based on the system as it now exists without any of the significant health care reforms currently proposed factored into the figures.
- Cost control efforts—managed care arrangements in the private sector, the use of an increased proportion of part-time employees who are not provided health insurance, higher copayments and deductibles, and lower benefit limitations will be adopted by more employers (Bryant, 1991).
- Personnel requirements—according to the Bureau of Labor Statistics, health services employment will continue to grow during the 1990s with increased employment of RNs, licensed practical nurses/licensed vocational nurses, and medical assistants. Many believe that the projected nursing increases from 1.6 million in 1988 to more than 2.2 million in 2000 will be impossible to achieve unless more people begin studying for a nursing career, and hospitals and other employers of nurses conduct a major redesign of staff mix and work assignments (AHA, 1990). The economic recession of the early 1990s creates uncertainty and a false picture of the nursing supply and demand picture. Early in the 1990s, a weak economy resulted temporarily in the increased availability of nursing personnel because some employed nurses postponed retirement plans and continued in practice; some employed part-time converted to full-time work or worked more hours to augment family income (e.g., spousal layoffs); and some nurses not employed, particularly those with young children, sought employment for the same reasons. A projected easing of the nursing shortage in the early 1990s reflects temporary responses to economic uncertainty (American Nurses Association [ANA], 1991).

Other serious implications for the 21st century include the following:

- The numbers and costs for care of the human immunodeficiency virus (HIV)-infected persons will continue to grow.
- The severe unmet health needs of special populations, such as the poor, the homeless, and mothers and children, will need to be considered in health-care reform.
- The members of minority groups will constitute a larger portion of the total population. (The present health care system is often insensitive and nonresponsive to their special needs.)
- With health care reform, there will be a move to change the focus on illness and acute care to include aspects of health promotion and disease prevention. Continued lack of a balance between illness care and prevention will continue to only increase costs and decrease effectiveness of the health care system.
- Social problems, such as drug and alcohol abuse and addictions, crime, family violence, ineffective schooling, unemployment, and the possible emergence of a permanent underclass that is effectively cut off from the norms of life in the United States, will have a significant impact on the health care systems and the nurses who work in them.

Nurses and the profession must face difficult questions with prudent strategic planning. A few of the key questions to pose are, can nursing alter how health care is organized and delivered? Which outcomes and issues should nursing choose to influence? Should nursing continue to be a part of broad-based coalitions seeking changes in health care organization and delivery? Whatever the answers, nursing is and must be encouraged to remain a creative viable force in response to the needs of the individuals cared for and the members of the profession (Stanley, 1993). As one evaluates the projections of a concentration of services for an aging population, who are a voting political constituency, with severe and chronic health and mental health needs, the challenges and advocacy work for child and adolescent psychiatric nurses become clearer.

CHILD AND ADOLESCENT HEALTH CARE

The picture of the overall population's health needs and concerns must be applied to the specialty of psychiatric nursing practice and further refined to address the aspects of psychiatric nursing with children and adolescents.

The 1980s saw deterioration in life for the nation's children and adolescents. While infant mortality reported by states improved slightly, still twice as many African-American babies died as white babies, and in 48 states plus the District of Columbia, death rates for children 1 to 14 years only slightly declined. Nationally, 24% of all infants had no prenatal care, 20% of all children lived in poverty, and almost 20% are not covered by health insurance. The reported rate at which children were jailed increased by 41%, the proportion of children living in poverty rose by 26%, the violent death rate for adolescents rose by 12%, and the numbers of unmarried teenagers giving birth rose 10% ("Study finds," 1991). One study on childhood hunger reported that 5.5 million children younger than 12 years old go hungry each day in the United States. These children are twice as likely to get sick and miss school days (Howard & Cerio, 1991).

PSYCHIATRIC AND MENTAL HEALTH NURSES

Psychiatric and mental health nurses became the trendsetters and leaders in the 1970s and early 1980s. They were the first to develop statements on the scope of specialty practice, establish generalist certification, develop a specialty practice structure within the ANA, and develop a system to classify nursing phenomena specific to the specialty (Pothier, Stuart, Puskar, & Babich, 1990). They were among the first specialty groups to have credentialing for clinical specialist (C.S.) in both adult and child psychiatric nursing practice.

According to Peplau (1980), the psychiatric nurse cannot be held accountable for the outcomes of work with a patient, only for the nature of the effort he or she makes in working with patients and their family and for disclosing to those patients the purpose of the work to be done. Being accountable to oneself, nursing peers, colleagues, and the profession at large is important. In public responsibility, the nurse is directed to keep personal accountability and integrity, to sharpen the cutting edge of the profession, and to refine its knowledge and know how (Peplau, 1980).

Early in the development of the nursing specialty, psychiatric nurses placed emphasis on process issues as a basic ingredient to their practice (Fagin, 1981). Psychiatric nurses took the lead to have interpersonal skills incorporated into the overall undergraduate nursing curriculum and developed a subspecialty of psychiatric consultation–liaison nursing to assist medical–surgical nurses with patient behavioral, stress, or anxiety problems. Psychiatric nursing experts believe that the focus on mental health, rather than on psychiatric care, may have been promoted by a need to identify with nursing's health promotion, disease prevention model rather than the medical illness model (McBride, 1990; Drew, 1989).

Because of earlier concentration on health-oriented psychosocial clients, nurses appeared more concerned with the "worried well," than those with serious biologic and neurochemical mental illness. As the National Institute of Mental Health's (NIMH) primary mission became research, nurses lost political impact as a presence there, because their orientation had been clinical rather than research training. In 1976 to 1977, nurses received 1252 NIMH stipends at a cost of $8.1 million; a decade later, only 97 stipends at a cost of $1.2 million were awarded (Pothier et al., 1990).

The psychiatric nurse today finds much uncertainty in the delivery of care as the "decade of the brain" proceeds to the neurobiologic realms of practice. Psychiatry's shift from behavior to the neurosciences has been promoted by the recent breakthroughs in genetics, immunology, and brain function. Biologic, chronic, severe mental illness has gained visibility through the effective activities of consumer groups. There is a concern among some that psychiatric nursing devalues biologic knowledge. This is considered dangerous in light of the increasingly sick clients who require complex care, which includes the combination of physiologic aspects and the environment (McBride, 1990). There are conflicts for nurses as patient advocates. By accepting the responsibility for achieving the balance between the behavioral and biomedical sciences in the prevention or limitation of psychiatric dysfunction, psychiatric and child psychiatric nurses will be engaged in provision of the quality care required for both populations.

The decreased numbers of graduate nurses selecting psychiatry as a specialty steadily continues. In 1968, more than 40% of all who enrolled in specialty master's degree programs were in psychiatric nursing; in 1978, less than 18% selected the field; and by 1988, only 7% of all nurses chose psychiatric nursing (Pothier et al., 1990). It is frequently reported that nurses leaving undergraduate programs are encouraged to work a year or two in medical–surgical nursing before selecting a specialty, such as child or adult psychiatric practice.

In child psychiatric nursing, the decline of programs and content also has been observed as graduate educational programs have been closed. In 1990, only 14 active programs with varied core curriculum content existed. The educational preparation of the child psychiatric and mental health specialist has been debated; however, the national child psychiatric nursing organization established a position statement a decade ago that called for standards reflective of a theoretic background in developmental, intrapsychic, interpersonal, systems, and psychosocial aspects as they relate to children and their families. Graduates of National League of Nursing accredited programs also must demonstrate clinical skill and competencies to practice therapy achieved through a set number of supervised hours (Advocates for Child Psychiatric Nursing, 1980). At the undergraduate level, psychiatric nursing was moved into an integrated model in the 1980s. From an early leadership position, psychiatric nursing has evolved into a specialty practice engrossed in practice, educational, and recruitment challenges.

The child and adolescent psychiatric nursing profession has been progressing each step of the way with psychiatric nurses. One finds that credentialing, standards, payment for services, education, and many other issues and concerns are the same. For child and adolescent psychiatric nurses to retain control of their practice, effectiveness and client outcomes must be recognized. The nurses express need for the following:

- Increased knowledge and skills to meet the health and mental health requirements of the seriously acutely ill child and adolescent and the complex chronic physically ill patients and their families
- Supervision for psychiatric nursing activities
- Increased opportunity for mental health promotion activities and health teaching for patients and families, especially for high risk, disenfranchised people
- Adequate numbers of qualified and trained nursing professionals in the care delivery systems
- Assistance with ethical decision making
- Development and implementation of nursing research studies for improved client outcomes
- Opportunities for clinical career development

Accountability

STANDARDS

Psychiatric nursing took the lead in developing standards for specialty nursing care. In 1973, the ANA appointed a task force to develop the first markers for excellence in nursing care of a specialty area. The Standards for Psychiatric and Mental Health Nursing Practice in 1982 were the first of many determinants for practice and provide criteria for measuring nursing and accountability. In 1985, the Standards for Child and Adolescent Psychiatric Nursing Practice were published and recently the Statement and Standards for specialty practice were rewritten to guide nursing care (ANA, 1994). Thus, quality control continues to be instituted by the profession itself for the nurses performing the care.

CREDENTIALING

Specialty credentials and certification for a nursing specialty practice or role were developed in the 1980s. The majority of nurses report that their credentialing is obtained from a voluntary association rather than from a state licensing agency. Groups and individuals from many sectors of professional and public life are interested in the certification and credentialing results. Legislators, government regulators, professional associations, third-party payers, accrediting agencies, educators, researchers, licensing boards, service sector administrators, practicing professionals from outside nursing, consumers, and nurses are all interested in the process and competency defined by the certification. "First of all, it must be acknowledged that while it is the responsibility of the state to license for entry into nursing practice in order to safeguard the

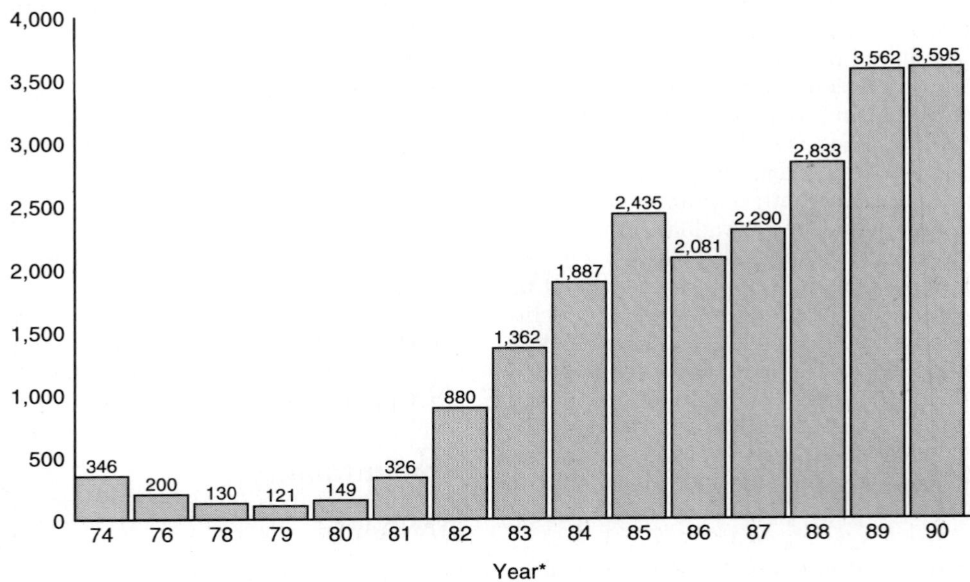

FIGURE 32–1 • Number of nurses tested by American Nurses Credentialing Center in psychiatric and mental health nursing, 1974–1990 (total: 22,197).

public, it is the responsibility of the profession to regulate its specialties as a means of recognizing and promoting advanced knowledge and skills and to ensure orderly development of the field" (Styles, 1990, p. 55).

Specialization credentialing ensures professional competence and quality services and professional satisfaction. The purpose of criteria for nursing practice is to protect the public. Unlike generalist nurses, who upon licensure and entry into practice are expected to be competent to at least a *minimum safe level,* specialists are expected to have *expert competence* (ANA, 1980). Public recognition and knowledge about a nurse's qualifications to provide specialized care increase the consumer's access to a variety of provider options. The consumer also is afforded a higher quality of delivered care.

CERTIFICATION

In 1974, concerned psychiatric nurses led by the Council of Advanced Practitioners in Psychiatric and Mental Health Nursing of the ANA began to assist a volunteer certification board with the development of guidelines for specialist certification of the Advanced Practitioner in Psychiatric and Mental Health Nursing. The first certification examination for Psychiatric and Mental Health Nursing was held in 1974, and 346 applicants successfully completed the examination (Fig. 32-1). This was followed in 1977 by the first certification examination for Clinical Specialist (C.S.) in adult psychiatric nursing (Fig. 32-2) and child and adolescent certification. Certification as a C.S. requires 2 years of clinical practice after completion of a master's degree; documented clinical supervision of practice, including therapy in two modalities; and successful completion of the ANA national examination. At this writing, more than 24,405 nurses have been certified in the specialty of psychiatric and mental health nursing. Of particular interest is that since 1977, 652 child and adolescent C.S.s have been tested, and in 1989, the child and adolescent examination had the highest percentage of increase of all ANA certification examinations (Fig. 32-3). Of the total number of child and adolescent psychiatric nurses ever credentialed, 547 currently hold certification. Recertification occurs on a 5-year basis and depends on evidence of continuing clinical practice, supervision, and education.

In one recent profile of the certified psychiatric C.S., 10% of the sample were child and adolescent. The majority of psychiatric clinical specialists were older than 35 years, female, found in the Northeastern United States, and worked full-time, and less than one fourth receive third-party reimburse-

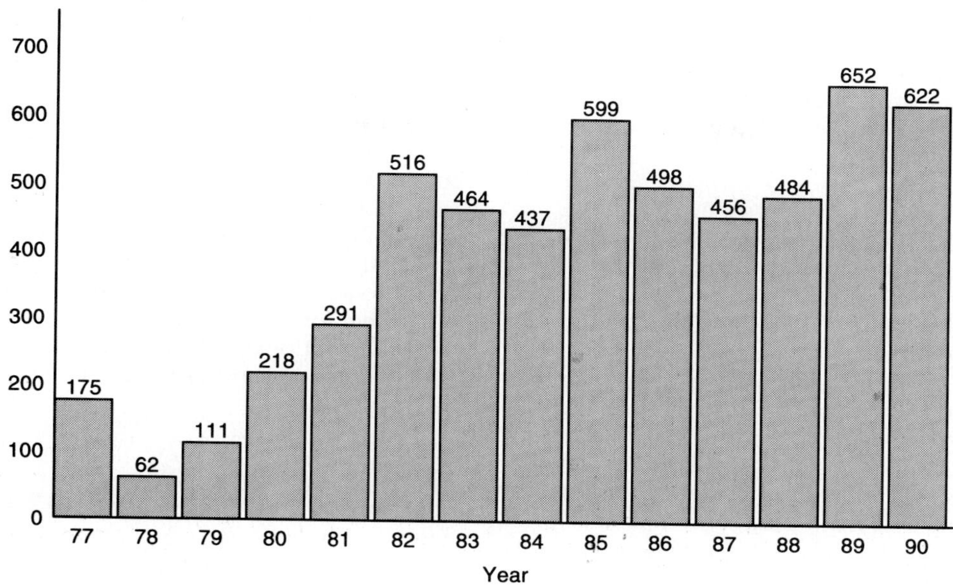

FIGURE 32–2 • Number of nurses tested by American Nurses Credentialing Center for certification as clinical specialists in adult psychiatric & mental health nursing, 1977–1990 (total: 5585).

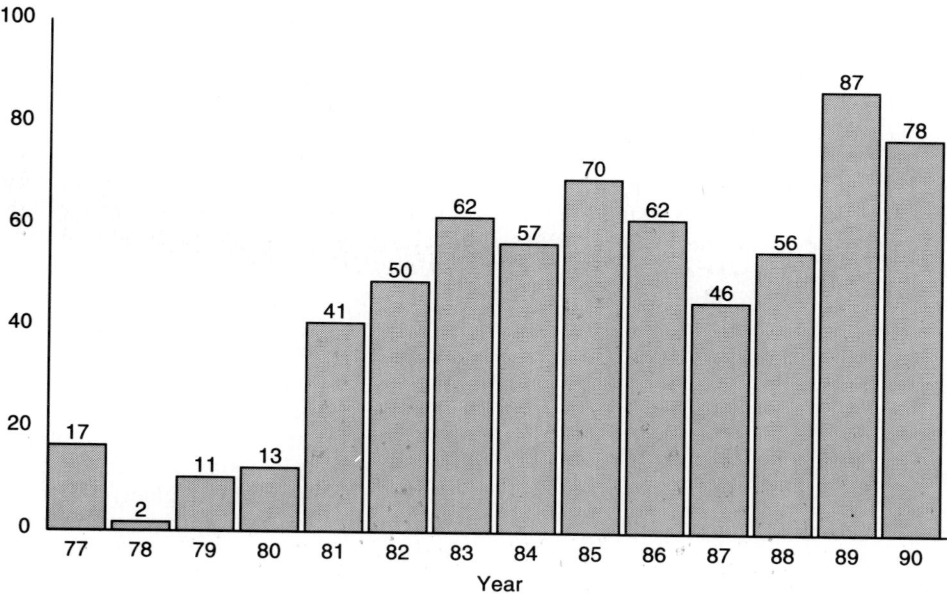

FIGURE 32–3 • Number of nurses tested by American Nurses Credentialing Center for certification as clinical specialists in child/adolescent psychiatric & mental health nursing, 1977–1990 (total: 652).

ment. A third of the respondents worked in two settings, had their primary position in a hospital, and secondary employment in individual or group practice. A few were employed in outpatient mental health clinics (Fox & Merwin, 1990).

SPECIALIZATION

The key words describing trends for specialty nursing are collaboration and coalition building. It has been predicted that the future will see "a powerful coming together of the specialties, and of the specialties with other organizations within nursing" (Styles, 1990, p. 55). Coalitions within the specialty are one place to start. This has begun within psychiatric nursing. Many of the nursing issues are the same for adult and child psychiatric nurses. Reimbursement, legislation or regulation, standards, and practice guidelines emanate from similar principles and precepts. Only the population served is specialized.

ASSOCIATIONS

Currently, four national nursing associations represent the various aspects of psychiatric nursing in the United States: the Association of Child and Adolescent Psychiatric Nurses, the Council of Psychiatric and Mental Health Nursing of the ANA, the American Psychiatric Nurses Association (APNA), and the Society for Education and Research in Psychiatric-Mental Health Nursing. In 1987, representatives of these four groups met to identify common goals, specific areas of commonality, and differences and to explore a collaboration for a united psychiatric nursing image at federal and national levels. This meeting led to the formation of the Coalition of Psychiatric Nursing Organizations (COPNO). Table 32-1 summarizes each member organization's background, purpose, and qualifications for membership.

Representatives of the leadership of each of the organizations meet at least once a year as psychiatric and mental health issues arise that require a united nursing voice or response. Coalitions such as this one increase the visibility and impact in certain areas of nursing, especially specialty practice areas, such as psychiatric and child psychiatric nursing, where there is not a large enough critical mass to influence political or legislative processes working alone. For example, each of the COPNO member groups has a place on the National Mental Health Leadership Forum, established with the support of the National Institute of Mental Health, 1989–1992; it is a significant advancement for the psychiatric nursing field to be acknowledged and to participate fully with other mental health professions and consumer groups.

As opportunities present for nurses to interact with federal agencies for the Alcohol, Drug and Mental Health, the Institutes of the National Institute of Health, especially the NIMH, a unified position representing a larger critical mass of psychiatric child and adult researchers, educators, and clinicians can be most effective. Much work has been done, and must continue, to secure the appointment of psychiatric nurses as members on the NIMH National Advisory Mental Health Council and other federal and national commissions, boards, and panels.

JOURNALS

There are currently three psychiatric nursing journals, the *Archives for Psychiatric Nursing*, the *Journal of Psychosocial Nursing* (sponsored by APNA, formerly the *Journal of Psychiatric Nursing*), and the *Journal of Child and Adolescent Psychiatric Nursing* sponsored by ACPN. The *Journal of Child and Adolescent Psychiatric Nursing* was first published in 1988 and has attracted a wide readership outside of nursing. It has been recommended by health and education professionals for its quality and the fact that the contributions from nurses provide solutions in addition to exploring problems.

Child Psychiatric Nursing Marketplace

POPULATION CHANGE

More than 7 million children, 12% of the total child population, in this country suffer from some sort of mental disorder. One in three children and adolescents with diagnosable mental illness does not receive care or treatment. Many times parents and teachers are unaware of the condition. Many are not receiving treatment, and of those who are getting help, 50% receive care that is inappropriate for their situation. Disorders such as phobias, panic disorder, substance abuse, conduct disorder, or serious depression are more frequently found in younger people today. An increase in negative social factors, such as neglect, abuse, poverty, poor nutrition, lack of regular health care, alcohol or drug abuse, and absence of emotional support at home and school, also contribute to the development of mental illness in the young. The suicide rate for people 15 to 19 years has tripled over the

(text continues on page 464)

TABLE 32–1 Coalition of Psychiatric Nursing Organizations: Member Organizations

Member Organization	Background/Purpose	Membership	Information
Association of Child and Adolescent Psychiatric Nurses (ACAPN)	Organized in 1971 (as the Advocates for Child Psychiatric Nursing), it is the only national group representing child and adolescent psychiatric nurses. *Purpose is twofold:* To recognize the uniqueness of and promote communication among child psychiatric nurses To promote the mental health of infants, children, adolescents, and their families through advocacy, practice, education, and research	Categories are regular and associate: **Regular** Have a master's degree in child and adolescent psychiatric nursing Be a registered nurse with at least 2 years' experience in the field of child and adolescent psychiatric nursing Be a student in an accredited child and adolescent psychiatric nursing program leading to a master's degree **Associate** Be a registered nurse with administrative, clinical, or research interests or be working in child and adolescent psychiatric nursing Be a student in an accredited baccalaureate program in nursing Be a master's prepared child and adolescent mental health professional with clinical or research interests or with 2 years' experience working in child and adolescent psychiatry and have been recommended for membership by an ACAPN member	ACAPN National Office 437 Twin Bay Drive Pensacola, FL 32534-1350 1-800-352-2441
American Nurses Association Council on Psychiatric and Mental Health Nursing	Evolved in 1984 from a merger of the Council of Specialists in Psychiatric and Mental Health Nursing and the Division on Psychiatric and Mental Health Nursing. **Primary objectives:** Increase the impact of psychiatric and mental health nursing on care, professional education, and political systems relative to health care Facilitate advancement of psychiatric and mental health nursing as a significant specialty in nursing and in the mental health field	Open to constituent members of state nurses associations who are generalists or specialists in psychiatric and mental health nursing practice, education, research, or administration	Council Affiliation ANA Fiscal Affairs American Nurses Association 600 Maryland Avenue, SW Suite 100 West Washington, DC 20024-2571

(continued)

TABLE 32–1 Coalition of Psychiatric Nursing Organizations: Member Organizations *(Continued)*

Member Organization	Background/Purpose	Membership	Information
	Specific goals identified by the Council are: To improve psychiatric and mental health nursing practice and meet the mental health needs of the public To influence national, state, and local political and legislative processes To provide mechanisms for communication among psychiatric and mental health nurses with the ANA organizational units and with outside groups To provide for professional development and networking of council affiliates		
American Psychiatric Nursing Association (APNA)	Organized in 1986 to provide a forum for psychiatric nurses working in psychiatric settings. Charter includes but is not limited to programs that will advance the professionalism of its members. Major emphasis placed on continuing education for psychiatric nurses. *Purposes:* Learn new clinical strategies Dialogue with peers Compare approaches Apply research findings in own settings Build networks and alliances with individuals and groups Consider new careers and patterns	Open to registered nurses who are interested or engaged in psychiatric and mental health nursing practice, education, and research	APNA P.O. Box 89 Thorofare, NJ 09086 (609) 848-1000
Society for Education and Research in Psychiatric/Mental Health Nursing (SERPN)	Organized in 1986 by vote of members of former Council of Directors of Graduate Programs in Psychiatric/Mental Health Nursing, with expanded mission "to support the generation and transmission of knowledge specific to the promotion of mental health and to the nursing care of the mentally ill and those at risk for mental disorders . . . (and to) provide a forum to advance the scientific basis of the specialty of psychiatric/mental health nursing and to shape its future direction."	Open to all professional registered nurses who have a minimum of a master's degree in psychiatric/mental health nursing education or research. Associate membership is available to students who are enrolled in graduate programs that have psychiatric/mental health nursing as their major area of concentration.	SERPN National Office 437 Twin Bay Drive Pensacola, FL 32514 (904) 479-9024

(continued)

TABLE 32–1 Coalition of Psychiatric Nursing Organizations: Member Organizations *(Continued)*

Member Organization	Background/Purpose	Membership	Information
	Stated functions of SERPN are to: Articulate the essential components of psychiatric/mental health nursing in undergraduate and graduate education Promote the advancement of psychiatric/mental health nursing research Critically evaluate extant and emerging theories, findings, and practice in psychiatric/mental health nursing Foster the use of research findings in the delivery of care, education, and social policy related to psychiatric/mental health nursing Develop and promote social policy that emanates from psychiatric/mental health nursing education and research Articulate the role of psychiatric/mental health nursing in meeting the needs of the mentally ill and those at risk Create systems for the sharing of knowledge and resources among nursing and other psychiatric/mental disciplines		

past 3 decades with a figure of 1979 completed suicides in that age range for 1990. According to the National Advisory Mental Health Council, NIMH (1990), mental disorders in young people cost our nation more than $1.5 billion in treatment costs each year. However, less than one fifth of these receive appropriate treatment, and many do not recover because their disorders are not adequately understood (NIMH, 1990). The factor of lost lifetime productivity, independent living, and consistent work capabilities adds significantly to the personal and family loss and to society's loss.

The earliest nonfamily settings for care of children were the group homes for orphans in colonial times. These were followed by residential schools for education and rehabilitation of the mentally deficient in the second half of the 19th century. At this time, reform schools also developed to contain delinquent children. By the 1920s and 1930s orphanages and reform schools provided only detention and custodial services. Many were less than humane settings. These settings developed into therapeutic residential centers in the 1930s and 1940s. The services involved the daily life needs of the child. Hospital psychiatric units first appeared following World War II and evolved to deal with the complexities of developmentally oriented milieu programs that promoted individualized goals for each child. There was to be dynamic care that included group psychotherapy, occupational therapy, recreational activities, specialized education, and concentrated work with families or caregivers.

Changes in families have been a contributing factor to the mental health needs and ability of caregivers to seek help. There are more single parents, foster parents without knowledge of the developmental background of the child, abusive home situations, dramatic increases in homeless families and children, parents with poor parenting skills, and children exposed to alternate sexual orientation situations. There are undeniable changes in outpatient mental health care, such as poor compliance, court-mandated service, declining numbers of qualified professionals in the public sector, unavailable resources, disjointed and uncoordinated services from various agencies, and little or no research on patient or family outcomes.

Progress on research into the role of risk factors and protective factors for children has provided child psychiatric nurses with some data and basis for clinical plan development. The current and future decades will see more focus on the psychobiology of parent–child interactions, the role of risk and protective factors, and contributions of genetic factors. The challenge continues to be determining the extent to which a child's or adolescent's mental disorder results primarily from a disturbed environment, a genetic predisposition, or the interaction of both (NIMH, 1990). The crucial infant psychobiologic factors of temperament and attachment have been found to be critical to the child's social and emotional development. The affectionate bond of attachment between the infant and the caregiver, the innate differences of the child, the quality of bonding, and responsive caregiving are all developing fields of research and study in which nursing can have a key role. The results will contribute significantly to the improvement of care.

ECONOMICS

The fiscal impacts on hospitals and health care in the 1970s resulted in a direct cut in funding and support for residential treatment. Third-party payers would finance acute care but not in a nonmedical setting, and the number of psychiatric units within hospitals increased dramatically in the public and private sectors. An additional factor in the reduction of residential sites was the lack of evidence to support long-term care as the solution for severely disturbed children (Jemerin & Philips, 1988).

Some authors report that inpatient child and adolescent psychiatric hospitalization is revenue driven and at times unnecessary (Lewis, 1989; Carbray & Pitula, 1991). Reasons for increased hospitalization include insurance companies and other third-party payers offer better coverage for inpatient care because costs are more controllable, and the way in which costs are reimbursed has fostered strong profit incentives. Because psychiatric services generally are reimbursed based on the actual cost retrospectively, providers can charge whatever payers will pay (Lewis, 1989; Geraty, 1989; Schwartz, 1989).

As a backlash to the soaring cost of health care, and especially psychiatric and mental health care, outcomes and effects are not always easily captured. Many employers and companies have taken drastic cutback positions on mental health benefit packages. The average annual mental health and substance abuse benefit cost per employee continues to rise, and inpatient benefits are being limited on maximum payable over the employee's lifetime, maximum days of care per year, or maximum payable per year. For outpatient coverage, more than two thirds of employers have limitations on maximum payable per year, and one third of all employers have maximum number of visits per year and maximum payable per visit (Ruffenach, 1991). The economic theory that with increased access to services and decreased costs for the user, more services will be used has been detrimental for nurses seeking provider recognition. It is difficult to establish whether mandated mental health benefits will increase use or simply be a substitution of one benefit or service for another that has been previously covered. Insurers are resistant to mandate benefits for health care in general and especially for mental health care. However, nurses have begun to express what constitutes a basic mental health package for children and adolescent mental health care at national and local levels (Stanley, 1990, 1993; Finke, 1990).

INTERVENTIONS

Psychotherapy, pharmacotherapy, behavioral therapy, cognitive therapy, and preventive interventions remain the core aspects of psychiatric care. Health promotion and preventive efforts have been and continue to be the hallmark of nursing care, especially child psychiatric care. Nurses continue to believe that preventive activities are cost-effective and relieve individuals, families, and society of great burdens and suffering. Intensive and consistent intervention with sensitivity to the special needs of the family concerning health care, education, child-rearing practices, and child development strengthen the ability for parents and the child to live and grow in a productive and supportive manner. A reported 230 psychotherapeutic techniques can be conducted with individuals, groups, or families in the treatment of children and adolescents with mental disorders (NIMH, 1990). These focus on various psychologic processes, behaviors, or family interactions. Clients may be treated in a variety of settings, such as schools, offices, homes, clinics, other community settings, and hospitals.

The multidisciplinary approach is being promoted as desirable and efficient. Inpatient teams that include nurses and nursing input are required in some facilities. The NIMH has included nursing as one of the four core mental health disciplines since the mid-80s.

CONSUMERISM

One of the fastest growing and most effective consumer and patient advocacy groups has developed in the past decade. The mental health advocacy organization, the National Alliance for the Mentally Ill (NAMI), has helped obtain recognition of the needs of the mentally ill in this country. This group has 1005 affiliate local chapters in the United States, Puerto Rico, and the Virgin Islands. In over a decade, the organization has developed from 284 members to over 130,000. The association's purpose is to eradicate mental illness; improve of the quality of life of those who are affected by serious, no-fault brain disease; and conduct activities of family support, public education, research, and advocacy.

At one time it was common to blame parents for a child's mental disorder. New information, however, has lead mental health professionals to acknowledge abnormalities in the chemistry and structure of the brain of a child with a mental disorder. The supporters of NAMI believe that these disordered conditions are not directly related to the parents' interactions with the child or parenting. The organization supports substitution of encouragement for parents who seek help for their child in place of blaming the parents for the child's condition. The NAMI Child and Adolescent Network is comprised of numerous local chapters whose goal is to work for adequate and appropriate services for children and adolescents (Box 32-1).

Advocacy and consumer groups supply written and media materials that are specific to mental health and mental illness. Handbooks, reprints, videotapes, and so forth are available through the local and national offices of many of these organizations. The lobbying efforts of the larger consumer groups have been effective in assisting some budget processes at the federal level to seek and gain increased funding for mental illness treatment and research. The inclusion of consumers on national forums and as a visible and viable expression of needs to legislators and others making decisions about scarce resources is a trend that will continue.

LEGISLATION AND REGULATION

For nursing and other health care providers, legislative issues continue to focus on increasing access to adequate and appropriate mental health treatment for individuals across the life span. Nursing as a profession has worked diligently to secure legislation and produce regulation that preserves and enhances the quality of health and mental health care, protects access to that health care, and promotes the rights of the men and women in the health care profession. Many nursing groups have accepted the challenge to fight for quality care and safe, healthful, and equitable work places.

Nurses have developed strong effectiveness at

BOX 32–1 • NATIONAL ALLIANCE FOR THE MENTALLY ILL—CHILD AND ADOLESCENT NETWORK (NAMI CAN)

MISSION STATEMENT

The mission of NAMI CAN is to advocate for improved systems of care for children and adolescents with serious brain disorders or mental illnesses, including serious emotional disturbances.

THE GOALS

1. To embrace and provide family support, education, and training to families of children and adolescents with serious brain disorders or mental illnesses, including serious emotional disturbances
2. To impact local, state, and federal special education programs mandated to provide appropriate educational opportunities according to Public Laws 94-142 and 99-457
3. To ensure that no family in the United States be forced to relinquish custody of a child to obtain needed services and treatment
4. To ensure that a comprehensive, community-based system of care is available to every child in need of such services
5. To eliminate stigma regarding children and adolescents with serious brain disorders or mental illnesses, including serious emotional disturbances, and to eliminate stigma regarding their families, through educating the nation's citizens with factual, research-based information
6. To challenge public policy makers and leaders to place the needs of children and adolescents with brain disorders or mental illnesses, including serious emotional disturbances, and the needs of their caring families, at the top of the national agenda
7. To actively support research initiatives that promote the understanding and ultimately the cures of these disorders or illnesses
8. To insist on equality of medical coverage by insurance and health policies regarding the care and treatment of children and adolescents with these disorders or illnesses
9. To ensure family participation in the individual planning process for the child's treatment
10. To ensure family participation in systems planning processes at local, state, and national levels
11. To collaborate with all other family and professional organizations representing mutual concerns and needs of NAMI CAN

NAMI CAN RESOLUTIONS

I. In many states, parents must relinquish custody of their child for the child to receive any services. This is a deplorable practice that is devastating to the families.

Be it resolved that NAMI CAN endorses a strong national advocacy campaign to end this tragic practice.

II. Most private insurance policies have lifetime limits or other restrictions regarding psychiatric coverage. This is a discrimination that results in severe financial hardships on families, often leaving them without the ability to pay for desperately needed services and care for the child.

Be it resolved that NAMI CAN endorses a strong national advocacy campaign to cover Mental Illness as any other disease or illness is covered.

III. Families around the country have had major problems obtaining appropriate educational services for their mentally ill or severely emotionally disturbed children.

Be it resolved that NAMI CAN endorses a strong national advocacy effort to ensure that these children are properly served by the educational system in all states.

Reprinted with permission of the National Alliance for the Mentally Ill.

the grassroots level where the constituents speak for their issues to the elected official either at the local, state, or federal levels directly to members of the U.S. Congress. Child and adolescent psychiatric nurses have been appointed and elected to groups, committees, or coalitions that focus on child and adolescent health, mental health, and safety concerns.

The 101st Congress demonstrated substantial health care and mental health gains for children. Some of the broad health accomplishments were the following:

- Increased federal funding for care of HIV-infected children and adults
- Comprehensive civil rights protection for the disabled, including the mentally disabled
- Direct funding for child and elder care services and authorized day care centers in the Department of Veteran's Affairs' health facilities
- Reauthorization of health care programs for the homeless
- Increased funding for nursing education and federal funding for nursing research and clini-

cally based research on patient outcomes in rural and underserved areas
- Reauthorization of health worker shortage programs for recruitment and retention programs to increase the number of practicing nurses
- Direct reimbursement for nurses

The direct reimbursement for nurse services encompassed several areas: Medicaid reimbursement for clinical specialist and nurse practitioners in rural areas, direct payment for nurses who provide services to employees and beneficiaries of the Federal Employees Health Benefits Program, Medicaid reimbursement for services provided by family and pediatric nurse practitioners, and Medicare payment of services for nursing home residents by nurse practitioners.

Nurses and nursing organizations have been actively seeking to improve health care for Americans of all ages and situations (Krauss, 1993). The need remains for legislation and regulation to deal with the blockades and barriers to adequate mental health and preventive mental health actions for those who are poor or who live in underserved rural and metropolitan areas. The commitment continues to seek parity for psychiatric and child psychiatric nurses as care providers and to support efforts to facilitate the organization of comprehensive coordinated health, mental health, and education services for children (Krauss, 1993). Health and mental health care services must remain in the most convenient and accessible settings, such as schools and the workplace.

Summary

The future trends for child and adolescent psychiatric nursing will be with the continuation of specialization, standard setting, and credentialing. Economic reshaping will result in major adjustments in the practice marketplace. Residential and long-term treatment become the first choice selection less often. Community based operations will increase to serve the chronic and severely long-term mentally ill of all ages.

Psychiatric nursing's balance of the decade of the brain and the neurobiologic thrust of psychiatric research and education is critical for this and future decades. The following are challenges for child and adolescent psychiatric nursing:

- To produce highly qualified, skilled, competent nurses for every level of care
- To reach greater numbers of children, adolescents, and families in need of care
- To forge a place for nursing's effectiveness
- To measure outcomes of nursing interventions
- To improve the quality of care provided
- To develop a cadre of child and adolescent psychiatric nurse researchers to provide solid data on which the profession and specialty can move forward
- To develop and maintain collaboration with the core mental health disciplines (psychiatry, psychology, social work) at the federal, state, and local levels
- To continue advocacy for children and adolescents' rights and needs
- To assure reimbursement for psychiatric nursing services delivered by qualified providers

For now, psychiatric nursing will take place more often in the general hospital setting treating acute situations and an increasing number of complex medical cases. Then a shift to community-based care will occur to reduce high cost and high tech inpatient care. Managed care systems, day treatment, partial hospitalization, preadmission screening, and outpatient services will take on a new meaning in delivery of care.

Prevention efforts must be a priority in light of the limited dollars available for overall health care. Mental health lobbying and advocacy for disenfranchised children, homeless, HIV-infected people, women, and the poor must remain in the forefront. Systems model-based treatment, predicated on collaboration between professionals and agencies, is critical to the comprehensive care of children.

REFERENCES

Advocates for Child Psychiatric Nursing, Inc. (1980). Position Statement: Child Psychiatric-Mental Nurse Clinician.

American Hospital Association (1990). *Bureau of Labor Statistics data, hospitals*. Washington, D.C. p. 16.

American Nurses Association (1980). *Nursing: A social policy statement*. Kansas City, MO: Author.

American Nurses Association (1991). *Nursing and health care in the 1990s: An environmental assessment working paper*. Kansas City, MO: Author.

American Nurses Association (1985). *Standards of child and adolescent psychiatric and mental health nursing practice*. Kansas City, MO: Author.

American Nurses Association (1982). *Standards of psychiatric and mental health nursing practice*. Kansas City, MO: Author.

American Nurses Association (1994). Statement on Psychiatric Mental Health Nursing Clinical Nursing Practice and Standards of Psychiatric-Mental Health Clinical Nursing Practice. Washington, D.C.: Author.

Appelbaum, P. (1989). Admitting children to psychiatric hospitals: A controversy revived. *Hospital and Community Psychiatry, 400*(4), 334–335.

Bryant, M. (1991). Are rising mental health costs driving you crazy? *Business & Health*, January, 36–43.

Burgess, A., & Burns, J. (1990). Partners in care. *American Journal of Nursing, 6*(June), 73–74.

Carbray, J., & Pitula, C. (1991). Trends in adolescent psychiatric hospitalization. *Journal Child and Adolescent Psychiatric and Mental Health Nursing, 4*(2), 68–71.

Center for Study of Social Policy (1991). *Kids count.* Washington, D.C.: Author.

Dalton, R., Bolding, D., Woods, J., & Daruno, J. (1987). Short-term psychiatric hospitalization of children. *Hospital and Community Psychiatry, 38*(9), 973–976.

Dalton, R., Muller, B., & Forman, M. A. (1989). The psychiatric hospitalization of children: An overview. *Child Psychiatry and Human Development, 19*(4), 231–244.

Drew B. J. (1989). Devaluation of Biological Knowledge. *Image: Journal of Nursing Scholarship, 20*, 25–27.

Fagin, C. (1981). Psychiatric Nursing at the Crossroads: Quo vadis. *Perspectives in Psychiatric Care, 19*(3), 99.

Finke, L. (1990) Public-Private Sector Coordination, Testimony, "Mental Illness in America," Public Hearing on Child and Adolescents. Los Angeles: National Institutes of Mental Health.

Fox, J., Merwin, B., Dial, T., Tebbut, R., Pion, G., Kohout, J., VandenBos, G., Johnson, M., Schervish, P., & Whiting, L. (1990). Human Resources. In Mandeischeid R. W. and Sonnenschein M. A. (Eds.), *Mental health, 1990.* chap. 4 United States, USDHHS, 196–215.

Geraty, R. (1989). Administrative issues in inpatient child and adolescent psychiatry. *Journal of American Academy of Child and Adolescent Psychiatry, 28*(1), 21–25.

Health Care Financing Administration (1987). National health expenditures, 1986–2000. 8(4).

Howard, L., & Cerio, G. (1991). Millions of hungry kids. *Newsweek.* April, 1991.

Institution of Medicine (1989). *Research on Children and Adolescents with Mental, Behavioral and Developmental Disorders.* Washington, D.C.: National Academy Press.

Jemerin J. M., & Philips I. (1988). Changes in inpatient child psychiatry: Consequences and recommendations. *Journal of the American Academy of Child and Adolescent Psychiatry, 17*(4), 397–403.

Krauss, J. (1993). Health care reform: Essential mental health services. Washington, D.C.: American Nurses Association.

Krauss, J. (1991). Put the community back in mental health. *Archives of Psychiatric Nursing, V*(1), 1–3.

Lewis, J. E. (1989). Are adolescents being hospitalized unnecessarily? The current use of hospitalization in psychiatric treatment. *Journal of Child and Adolescent Psychiatric and Mental Health Nursing, 2*(4), 134–138.

McBride A. B. (1990). Psychiatric Nursing in the 1990s. *Archives of Psychiatric Nursing, IV*(1), 21–29.

Naisbitt, J. (1982). *Megatrends: Ten new directions transforming our lives.* New York: Warner Books.

National Advisory Mental Health Council, NIMH (1990). *National plan for research on child and adolescent mental disorders.* Washington, D.C.: DHHS Pub. no. (ADM) 90–1683.

Oda, D. (1989). The imperative of a national health strategy for children: Is there a political will. *Nursing Outlook, 37*(5), 206–208.t

O'Toole, A., & Loomis, M. (1989). Classifying human responses in psychiatric-mental health nursing in classification systems for describing nursing practice: Working papers (pp. 20–30). Kansas City, MO: American Nurses Association.

Peplau, H. (1980). The psychiatric nurse-accountable? To whom? For what? *Perspectives in Psychiatric Care, XVIII*(3), 128–134.

Pothier, P. (1987). The future of psychiatric nursing revisited. *Archives of Psychiatric Nursing, 1*(5), 299.

Pothier P., Stuart G., Puskar K., & Babich K. (1990). Dilemmas and directions for psychiatric nursing in the 1990s. *Archives of Psychiatric Nursing, IV*(5):284–291.

Puskar, K., Lamb, J., & Martsorf, D. S. (1990). The role of the psychiatric/mental health nurse clinical specialist in an adolescent coping skills group. *Journal of Child and Adolescent Psychiatric and Mental Health Nursing, 3*(2), 47.

Ruffenach, G. (1991). Slashes in mental-health benefits start to hurt patients, medical officials say. *Wall Street Journal*, B, 1.

Schwartz, I. M. (1989). Hospitalization of adolescents for psychiatric and substance abuse treatment: Legal & ethical issues. *Journal of Adolescent Health Care, 10*(6), 473–478.

Stanley, S. (1993). Nursing's involvement with the American health security act of 1993. *Journal of Child and Adolescent Psychiatric and Mental Health Nursing, 6*(4), 35–38.

Stanley, S. (1990). Review of the Institute of Medicine report on children and adolescents. *Journal of Child and Adolescent Psychiatric and Mental Health Nursing, 3*(2), 62–64.

Study finds 80's saw deterioration in life for U.S. children. (1991, February 2). Baltimore Sun.

Styles, M. (1990). Eyes on the future: Will the profession unite? *American Journal of Nursing, 10*, 83, 55.

U.S. Department of Commerce (1990). *Statistical abstract of the U.S.* (pp. 20 and 24).

Wallen, J., & Pincus, H. A. (1988). Care of children with psychiatric disorders at community hospitals. *Hospital and Community Psychiatry, Feb. 39*(2), 167.

APPENDIX

Statement on Psychiatric-Mental Health Clinical Nursing Practice and Standards of Psychiatric-Mental Health Clinical Nursing Practice

STANDARDS OF CARE

"Standards of Care" pertain to professional nursing activities that are demonstrated by the nurse through the nursing process. These involve assessment, diagnosis, outcome identification, planning, implementation, and evaluation. The nursing process is the foundation of clinical decision making and encompasses all significant action taken by nurses in providing psychiatric-mental health care to all clients.

Standard I **Assessment**

The psychiatric-mental health nurse collects client health data.

Standard II **Diagnosis**

The psychiatric-mental health nurse analyzes the assessment data in determining diagnoses.

Standard III **Outcome Identification**

The psychiatric-mental health nurse identifies expected outcomes individualized to the client.

Standard IV **Planning**

The psychiatric-mental health nurse develops a plan of care that prescribes interventions to attain expected outcomes.

Standard V **Implementation**

The psychiatric-mental health nurse implements the interventions identified in the plan of care.

Standard V-A **Counseling**

The psychiatric-mental health nurse uses counseling interventions to assist clients in improving or regaining their previous coping abilities, fostering mental health, and preventing mental illness and disability.

Standard V-B **Milieu Therapy**

The psychiatric-mental health nurse provides, structures, and maintains a therapeutic environment in collaboration with the client and other health care providers.

Standard V-C **Self-Care Activities**

The psychiatric-mental health nurse structures interventions around the client's activities of daily living to foster self-care and mental and physical well-being.

Standard V-D **Psychobiologic Interventions**

The psychiatric-mental health nurse uses knowledge of psychobiologic interventions and applies clinical skills to restore the client's health and prevent further disability.

Standard V-E **Health Teaching**

The psychiatric-mental health nurse, through health teaching, assists clients in achieving satisfying, productive, and healthy patterns of living.

Standard V-F **Case Management**

The psychiatric-mental health nurse provides case management to coordinate comprehensive health services and ensure continuity of care.

Standard V-G **Health Promotion and Health Maintenance**

The psychiatric-mental health nurse employs strategies and interventions to promote and maintain mental health and prevent mental illness.

Advanced Practice Inverventions V-H to V-J

The following interventions (V-H to V-J) may be performed only by the certified specialist in psychiatric-mental health nursing.

Standard V-H **Psychotherapy**

The certified specialist in psychiatric-mental health nursing uses individual, group, and family psychotherapy, child psychotherapy, and other therapeutic treatments to assist clients in fostering mental health, preventing mental illness and disability, and improving or regaining previous health status and functional abilities.

Standard V-I **Prescription of Pharmacologic Agents**

The certified specialist uses prescription of pharmacologic agents in accordance with the state nursing practice act, to treat symptoms of psychiatric illness and improve functional health status.

Standard V-J **Consultation**

The certified specialist provides consultation to health care providers and others to influence the plans of care for clients, and to enhance the abilities of others to provide psychiatric and mental health care and effect change in systems.

Standard VI **Evaluation**

The psychiatric-mental health nurse evaluates the client's progress in attaining expected outcomes.

STANDARDS OF PROFESSIONAL PERFORMANCE

"Standards of Professional performance" describe a competent level of behavior in the professional role, including activities related to quality of care, performance appraisal, education, collegiality, ethics, collaboration, research, and resource utilization. All psychiatric-mental health nurses are expected to engage in professional role activities appropriate to their education, position, and practice setting. Therefore, some standards or measurement criteria identify these activities.

While "Standards of Professional Performance" describe the roles of all professional nurses, there are many other responsibilities that are hallmarks of psychiatric-mental health nursing. These nurses should be self-directed and purposeful in seeking necessary knowledge and skills to enhance career goals. Other activities—such as membership in professional organizations, certification in specialty or advanced practice, continuing education, and further academic education—are desirable methods of enhancing the psychiatric-mental health nurse's professionalism.

Standard I **Quality of Care**

The psychiatric-mental health nurse systematically evaluates the quality of care and effectiveness of psychiatric-mental health nursing practice.

Standard II **Performance Appraisal**

The psychiatric-mental health nurse evaluates his or her own psychiatric-mental health nursing practice in relation to professional practice standards and relevant statutes and regulations.

Standard III **Education**

The psychiatric-mental health nurse acquires and maintains current knowledge in nursing practice.

Standard VI **Collaboration**

The psychiatric-mental health nurse collaborates with the client, significant others, and health care providers in providing care.

Standard VII **Research**

The psychiatric-mental health nurse contributes to nursing and mental health through the use of research.

Standard IV **Collegiality**

The psychiatric-mental health nurse contributes to the professional development of peers, colleagues, and others.

Standard V **Ethics**

The psychiatric-mental health nurse's decisions and actions on behalf of clients are determined in an ethical manner.

Standard VIII **Resource Utilization**

The psychiatric-mental health nurse considers factors related to safety, effectiveness, and cost in planning and delivering client care.

INDEX

Page numbers followed by *f* indicate figures; those followed by *t* indicate tabular material; those followed by *c* indicate charts.

B

C

D

E

O

P

R

S

T

ISBN 0-397-54832-X

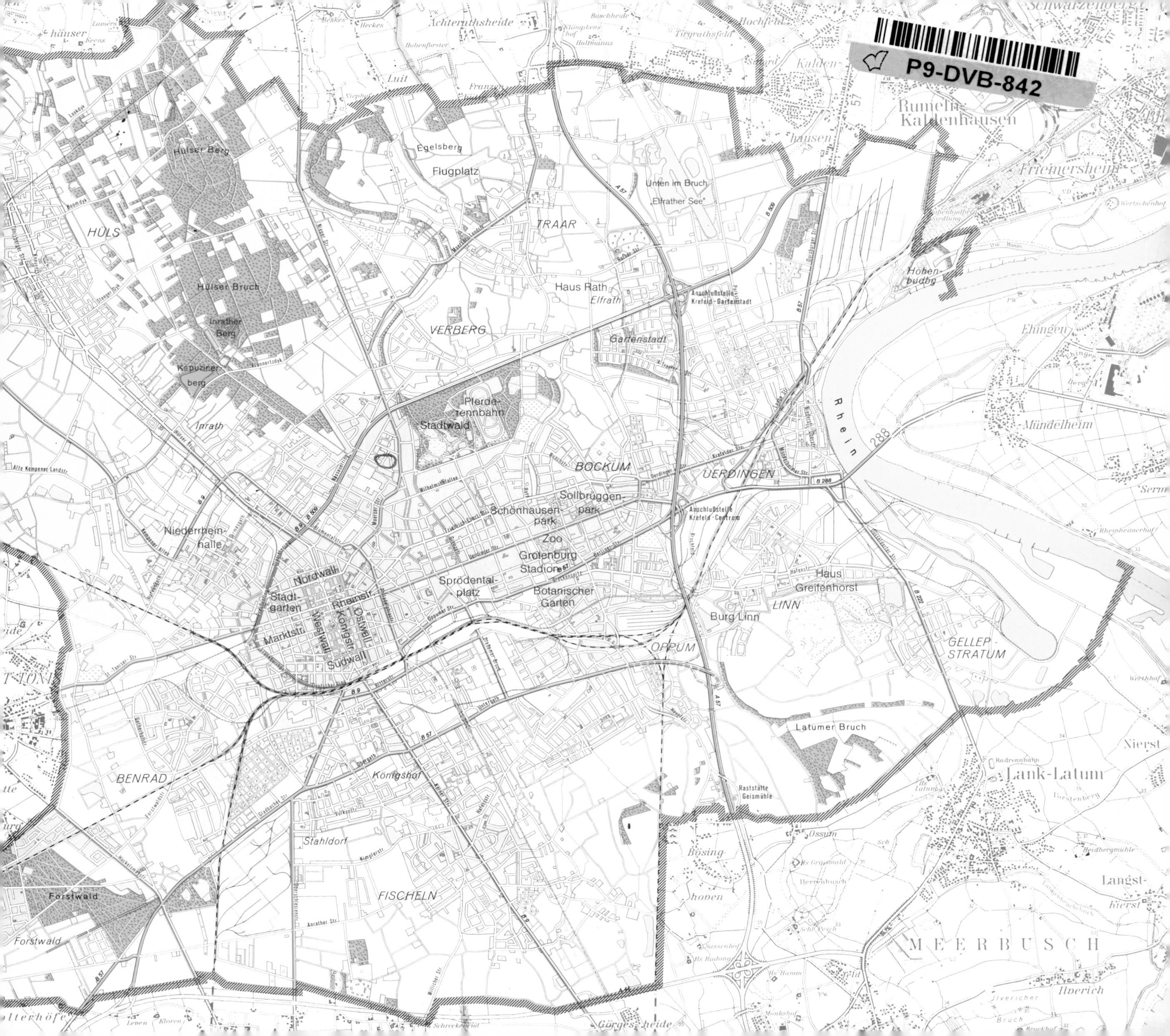
Achterathsheide
Egelsberg
Flugplatz
Hülser Berg
HÜLS
Hülser Bruch
Inrather Berg
Kapuzinerberg
Inrath
TRAAR
Unten im Bruch
"Elfrather See"
Haus Rath
Elfrath
VERBERG
Gartenstadt
Pferderennbahn
Stadtwald
BOCKUM
UERDINGEN
Rhein
Sollbrüggenpark
Schönhausenpark
Zoo
Grotenburg Stadion
Niederrheinhalle
Nordwall
Stadtgarten
Rheinstr.
Ostwall
Westwall
Königstr.
Marktstr.
Südwall
Sprödentalplatz
Botanischer Garten
Haus Greifenhorst
LINN
Burg Linn
OPPUM
GELLEP-STRATUM
Latumer Bruch
BENRAD
Königshof
Stahldorf
FISCHELN
Forstwald
Lank-Latum
MEERBUSCH
Rumeln-Kaldenhausen
Friemersheim
Hohenbudberg
Mündelheim
Ehingen
Ossum
Bösinghoven
Langst-Kierst
Nierst
Ilverich
Gördesheide
Raststätte Geismühle
Anschlußstelle Krefeld-Gartenstadt
Anschlußstelle Krefeld-Centrum

ZIETHEN-VERLAG
5000 Köln 50, Unter Buschweg 17
Telefon (02236) 61028

1. Auflage

Redaktion und Gestaltung:
Horst Ziethen in Verbindung mit
dem Verkehrsverein Krefeld e.V.

Fotografie: Holger Klaes u.a.

Gesamtherstellung:
ZIETHEN-Farbdruckmedien GmbH,
D 5000 Köln 50

Printed in Germany

Bildnachweis siehe letzte Seite

ISBN 3-921268-39-7

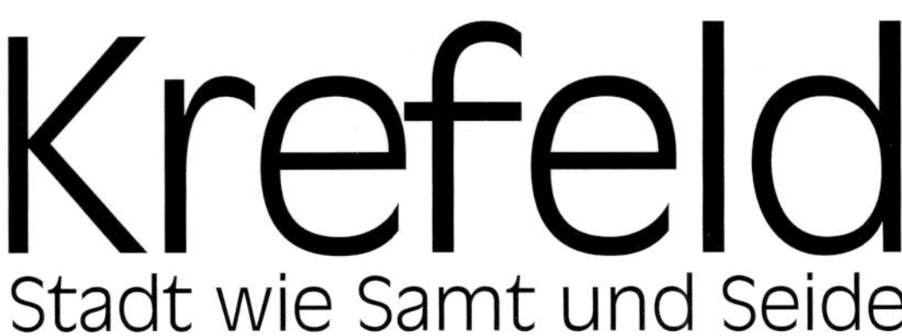

Krefeld

Stadt wie Samt und Seide

Krefeld, eine junge Stadt

Das Jahr 1607 ist das entscheidende Datum in der Krefelder Geschichte. Die Stadt, rund 2000 Hektar groß, liegt acht Kilometer vom Ufer des Rheins entfernt an einer der ältesten Nord-Süd-Straßen des Rheinlandes, auf der schon die Römer ihre Legionen bewegten, der heutigen Bundesstraße 9. Die 5000 Einwohner, meist Bauern und Leineweber, haben sich soeben von dem großen Brand erholt, der ihr Städtchen vernichtete, und ihre Fachwerkhäuser neu aufgebaut. Seit dem Jahr 1600 ist die „Herrlichkeit Crefeld" im Besitz des Hauses Oranien und gehört damit als Exklave zu den befreiten Niederlanden, die sich anschicken, ihr „Goldenes Jahrhundert" zu erleben. Im Jahr 1607 erklärt der neue Landesherr Krefeld zur religiösen Freistatt. Inmitten der buntgefärbten Kleinstaaterei, aus der sich die Landkarte jener Jahre zusammensetzt, wird Krefeld zu einer Insel der Religionsfreiheit. In den folgenden Jahrzehnten wird das neutrale Fleckchen zum Magneten für Glaubensflüchtlinge aus der Umgebung, so auch für Mennoniten, die die Kunst der Seidenherstellung beherrschen.

Für Historiker ist dieses Ereignis der Beginn der modernen, kapitalistischen Wirtschaft im Rhein-Ruhr-Raum und darüberhinaus. Die neuen Bürger bringen nicht nur das exklusive „know how", sondern auch Geld in die Stadt. Sie nehmen Weber unter Vertrag, die von ihnen einen Webauftrag, gesponnene Seide und oft auch den Webstuhl erhalten. Die fertigen kostbaren Stoffe werden dem Auftraggeber, dem „Verleger" gebracht, der die Arbeit entlohnt.

Die Geschäftsbeziehungen der „Verleger" sprengen den Rahmen des bis dahin stillen Städtchens. Sie reisen nach China, um dort die Rohseide einzukaufen. Sie schiffen sich nach Amerika ein, um dort ihre Ware zu verkaufen. Die Stadt beginnt zu wachsen. 1692 muß sie zum erstenmal erweitert werden. Es ist der erste einer ganzen Serie von Wachstumsschüben.

Im Jahre 1703 tritt ein Erbfall ein. Krefeld wird preußisch. 28 Jahre später lassen sich die Brüder Friedrich und Heinrich von der Leyen in Krefeld nieder. Sie gründen eine neue Seidenfabrikation die in wenigen Jahren einen weltweiten Ruf und ausgreifende Verbindungen begründet. Preußens König Friedrich Wilhelm I hat viel Verständnis für die Wechselbeziehungen zwischen einer florierenden Wirtschaft und seiner Steuerkasse. Er besucht im Jahre 1738 die Stadt Krefeld, ist Gast im Haus von der Leyen und räumt den Seidenwebern und der Stadt Krefeld einige Privilegien ein.

City of Velvet and Silk

Krefeld – A Youthful City

The year 1607 is a crucial date in the history of Krefeld. The city, covering an area of approximately 2000 hectares, is situated about eight kilometres from the banks of the Rhine along one of the oldest north-south routes in the Rhineland – the State Route No. 9 of today – a road along which Roman legions once passed. The 5000 inhabitants, mostly peasants and linen weavers, had just recovered from a big fire which destroyed their town and had rebuilt their half-timbered houses. Since 1600, the "Domain Crefeld" had belonged to the House of Orange, being an enclave of the Free Netherlands, whose "golden century" was just about to begin. In 1607 the new sovereign declared Krefeld a religious "free state". Amidst the many small states which at that time made the map of Europe a myriad of small colourful dots, Krefeld became an oasis of religious freedom. In the succeeding decades, the neutral hamlet attracted religious refugees from the whole of the region, including the Mennonites, who were masters of the art of silk weaving.

For historians, this was the beginning of the modern capitalist economic system in the Rhine/Ruhr region and beyond. The new citizens brought not only technical "know how" but also money to the town. They employed weavers under contract and supplied them with spun silk, a weaving commission and often also a loom. The finished costly fabrics were then returned to the contractors who paid for the labour.

The business concerns of the contractors reached well beyond the limits of this hitherto quiet small town. They travelled to China in order to purchase raw silk. They sailed to America to sell their goods there. The town began to grow and in 1692 it had to be enlarged for the first time. This was the beginning of a whole series of expansionist activities.

In 1703, hereditary claims resulted in Krefeld becoming a part of Prussia. Twenty-eight years later, the brothers Friedrich and Heinrich von der Leyen settled in Krefeld. They built a new silk factory, establishing international fame and a worldwide network within a short time. The Prussian King, Friedrich Wilhelm I, had a perfect understanding of the inter-relationship between a healthy economy and his tax revenue. In 1738 he visited the town of Krefeld, was a guest in the house of the von der Leyen's and at the same time granted privileges to the silk weavers and to the town.

Under his son Frederick II the Great, the economy began to flourish. For Frederick the Great and his court, the Krefeld silk weavers guaranteed that many sumptuous local goods could be purchased within the

Sein Sohn Friedrich II, der Große, führt die preußische Wirtschaft zu großer Blüte. Für Friedrich den Großen und seinen Hof sind die Krefelder Seidenweber die Garanten dafür, daß man mit Seidentapeten, Stoffen, Bändern, Tressen und anderen Posamentierwaren einigen repräsentativen Glanz im eigenen Land einkaufen kann. Friedrich der Große besucht Krefeld zweimal. Er sorgt für bessere Postverbindung. Er verbietet, in Krefeld Soldaten zu werben. Unter dem besonderen Schutz der Majestäten gedeiht das Gewerbe. Die Krefelder „Seidenbarone" führen zeitweise Regie über mehr als 50 000 Handwebstühle, die in Krefeld und in der Umgebung der Stadt in den Häusern der Weber stehen. Diese Weber sind es aber auch, die mit Beschäftigungsüberdruck oder totaler Flaute das Auf und Ab der Mode oder der wirtschaftlich günstigen oder hemmenden politischen Zustände risikoreich durchleben.

Eine Entwicklung von außerordentlicher Dynamik setzt ein. Sie wird schließlich im 19. Jahrhundert auf die Spitze getrieben, als die Erfindung von Dampfmaschine und Elektrizität dazu führt, daß Maschinen und Arbeitskräfte in Fabriken zusammengefaßt werden. Der häusliche Arbeitsplatz der Weber verliert seine Daseinsberechtigung. Krefeld wird zur schnellwüchsigsten Stadt Deutschlands. Es ist zugleich die steuerkräftigste, also in Relation zu seiner Größe die reichste Stadt im Lande. Der Glanz der großen Vermögen und die Armut der aus der alten Arbeitswelt herausgerissenen Bevölkerung existieren in allen denkbaren Erscheinungsformen nebeneinander.

Diese Zeit prägt immer noch das Krefeld von heute. Als Nachbarn der Textilindustrie und als deren Zulieferer sind ein hochentwickelter Maschinenbau und große chemische Werke entstanden. Immer neue Stadtviertel werden gebaut. Schließlich greift die Dynamik in die Umgebung der Stadt ein. Ein ganzer Kranz von umliegenden Gemeinden, darunter die traditionsreiche Handelsstadt Uerdingen und auch das winzige Gellep, in dem vor 2000 Jahren die Römer lagerten, werden in die Stadtgrenzen einbezogen. Krefeld wird eine Stadt am Rhein.

Der Wohlstand verlangt nach Darstellung. Die durch anspruchsvolle Tätigkeit und weite Reisen gebildete Gesellschaft hat kulturelle Bedürfnisse. Stadttheater, Sinfonieorchester, Museen für bildende Kunst, Textiles, Archäologie, Volkskunde, Schulen für Ingenieurbildung und Gestaltung werden gegründet, die bis heute Bestand haben und sich zu einer kulturellen Ausstattung summieren, wie kaum eine andere Stadt gleicher Größenordnung sie vorweisen kann.

state: silk tapestries, fabrics, ribbons, decorative trims and other haberdashery. Frederick the Great visited Krefeld twice. He improved postal services. He prohibited the drafting of soldiers in Krefeld. It is no wonder then that trade soon boomed under the protection of the monarchy. The Krefeld "silk barons" for a time became lords over more than 50,000 hand looms which stood in the weavers' houses in Krefeld and its surroundings. The weavers themselves, however, were the people who had to bear the brunt of economic change, excessive demand for labour on the one hand or total stagnation on the other, due to the economically favourable or unfavourable political situation or the vagaries of fashion.

Business expanded tremendously, peaking in the 19th century, when the invention of the steam engine and electricity brought machines and the workforce together into the factories. The weavers' traditional workplaces at home lost their importance. Krefeld became the fastest growing city in Germany. It also paid the most in taxes, i.e. in relation to its size it was the richest city in the state. The splendour of vast fortunes and the poverty of a populace torn from its traditional world existed side by side in every imaginable form.

That period has left its mark on the Krefeld of today. The textile industry was supplemented and complemented by a highly developed machine manufacturing industry and huge chemical plants. The town continuously expanded. After a time, development also spread to the surrounding areas. The independent communities around the town were integrated into the city of Krefeld, among them the old mercantile centre of Uerdingen and tiny Gellep, which was a Roman camp 2000 years before. Krefeld had become a city on the Rhine.

Wealth demands expression. Society, well-educated, sophisticated and widely travelled, develops cultural needs. Municipal theatres, symphony orchestras, museums for the pictorial and visual arts, textiles, archaeology and folk art, engineering and design schools were established and still exist today. Thus today hardly any other city of the same size can compete with Krefeld insofar as the range of cultural activities is concerned. Even before the modern welfare state took over responsibility, its citizens were engaged in establishing homes for the elderly, hospitals, children's homes and other welfare institutions to compensate for social inequalities. This tradition, too, lives on. The development of sports facilities mirrors the dynamic development of the city and sports too enjoy great popularity today.

Ehe der moderne Sozialstaat die Verantwortung an sich zieht, bemühen sich Bürger mit der Gründung von Altersheimen, Krankenhäusern, Kinder- und Wohlfahrtsheimen um die Glättung krasser sozialer Defizite. Auch das ist lebendige Tradition. Die Entwicklung des Sports entspricht der Dynamik der Stadtentwicklung und findet massenhaften Zulauf.

Aus dem Geschilderten ergibt sich die Summe, daß Krefeld bis heute eine junge Stadt ist, die sich mehr um die Dinge kümmert, die Glanz, Erfolg und Prosperität versprechen, als um die Wahrung von Traditionen. Ein gewisser Bürgerstolz belebt immer neu das Bewußtsein, daß die Stadt ihre Entwicklung nicht dem lenkenden Willen eines Fürsten oder Bischofs verdankt, sondern der Unternehmungslust und dem Fleiß ihrer Bürger. Aufbauend auf diesem Fleiß ist aus dem abseits liegenden Landstädtchen eine Stadt mit einer Viertelmillion Einwohnern geworden, die am Rande des Ballungsraums an Rhein und Ruhr selbstbewußt mit dem prägenden Signum „Stadt wie Samt und Seide" ihr eigenes Profil wahrt.

Das Krefeld von heute ist wieder einmal dabei, sich mit Hilfe seiner dynamischen Eigenschaften von einer einschneidenden Krise zu erholen. Die Ursache dieser Krise läßt sich mit wenigen Zahlen illustrieren: Zur Zeit Friedrichs des Großen konnte ein Handweber in der Minute etwa 45 Schußfäden ins Gewebe einbringen. Heute wird der Schußfaden von Druckluft oder mit Hilfe eines Wassertropfens durch die Kette geschossen, und zwar 1350 mal pro Minute. Früher bediente ein Weber einen Webstuhl. Heute überwacht ein Weber 30 oder auch mehr Webmaschinen. Die Textilindustrie ist von der personal- zur kapitalintensiven Industrie verwandelt. Zusätzlich kam die Auswanderung der Arbeit ins lohngünstigere Ausland. Der Stadt gingen 30 000 Arbeitsplätze verloren, annähernd ein Viertel des gesamten Bestandes. Aber Innovationskraft und Kapitaleinsatz haben großen Wirtschaftszweigen die Zukunft neu erobert. Das gilt auch für die Textilindustrie, die mit neuen Technologien und neuen Produkten Märkte erschloß. Krefelds Wirtschaft ist weltläufig geblieben. Fast die Hälfte der hier erzeugten Industriegüter wird exportiert. Das gibt es in keiner anderen Stadt Deutschlands.

Geübt darin, mit Krisen umzugehen, und ebenso darin, das Leben zu genießen, bestimmen für den Krefelder Optimismus und rheinische Lebensfreude, nachbarschaftliche Geselligkeit und unstillbare Reiseneugier ebenso wie Anspruch an kulturelle Vielfalt das Klima seines betriebsamen Lebens. In diese Atmosphäre bezieht die Stadt ihre Gäste gern ein.

It follows then that Krefeld is to this very day a young city, a city that puts more stock by activities promising glory, success and prosperity than by adhering to old traditions. Its inhabitants maintain a certain pride and awareness that the city does not owe its development to the dominant will of a sovereign or bishop but to the enterprising spirit and diligence of its citizens. This very diligence transformed this previously obscure country town into a bustling city with a quarter of a million inhabitants. Bordering on the urban and industrial areas of the Rhine and the Ruhr, it self-confidently keeps its own identity, justifying its slogan "city of velvet and silk".

The Krefeld of today, with its dynamic skills, is once more able to recover from a deep crisis. The reason for this crisis can best be illustrated with a few statistics: in the time of Frederick the Great, a weaver at a manual loom could introduce about 45 weft threads per minute into the fabric. Today, the weft threads are shot into the warp with pressurised air or with the help of water droplets which fall at the rate of 1350 per minute. In the past, one weaver operated one loom. Today a weaver supervises 30 or more weaving machines. The textile industry was transformed from a labour-intensive to a capital-intensive industry. Furthermore, production shifted to foreign countries with lower wages. The city lost 30.000 jobs, almost a quarter of the total workforce. Innovation and capital investment have, however, opened up new opportunities for a large sector of the economy. This is equally true in the textile industry, which has conquered new markets with new technology and new products. The economy of Krefeld has always been export-oriented. Unlike any other city in Germany, almost half of the industrial goods produced here are exported.

Accustomed to overcoming crises but also to enjoying life, the busy inhabitants of Krefeld live in an atmosphere of optimism and joie-de-vivre, typical of the Rhineland. They have an open, sociable disposition, an unquenchable thirst for travelling and a penchant for diverse cultural activities. No wonder then that the city welcomes its guests with open arms.

Als monumentalen klassizistischen Bau errichtete der „Seidenbaron" Conrad von der Leyen 1794 sein Stadtschloß. 1860 übernahm die Stadt es als ihr Rathaus.

The monumental neoclassical building was erected in 1794 as a town residence for the "silk baron" Conrad von der Leyen. It has been used as a city hall since 1860.

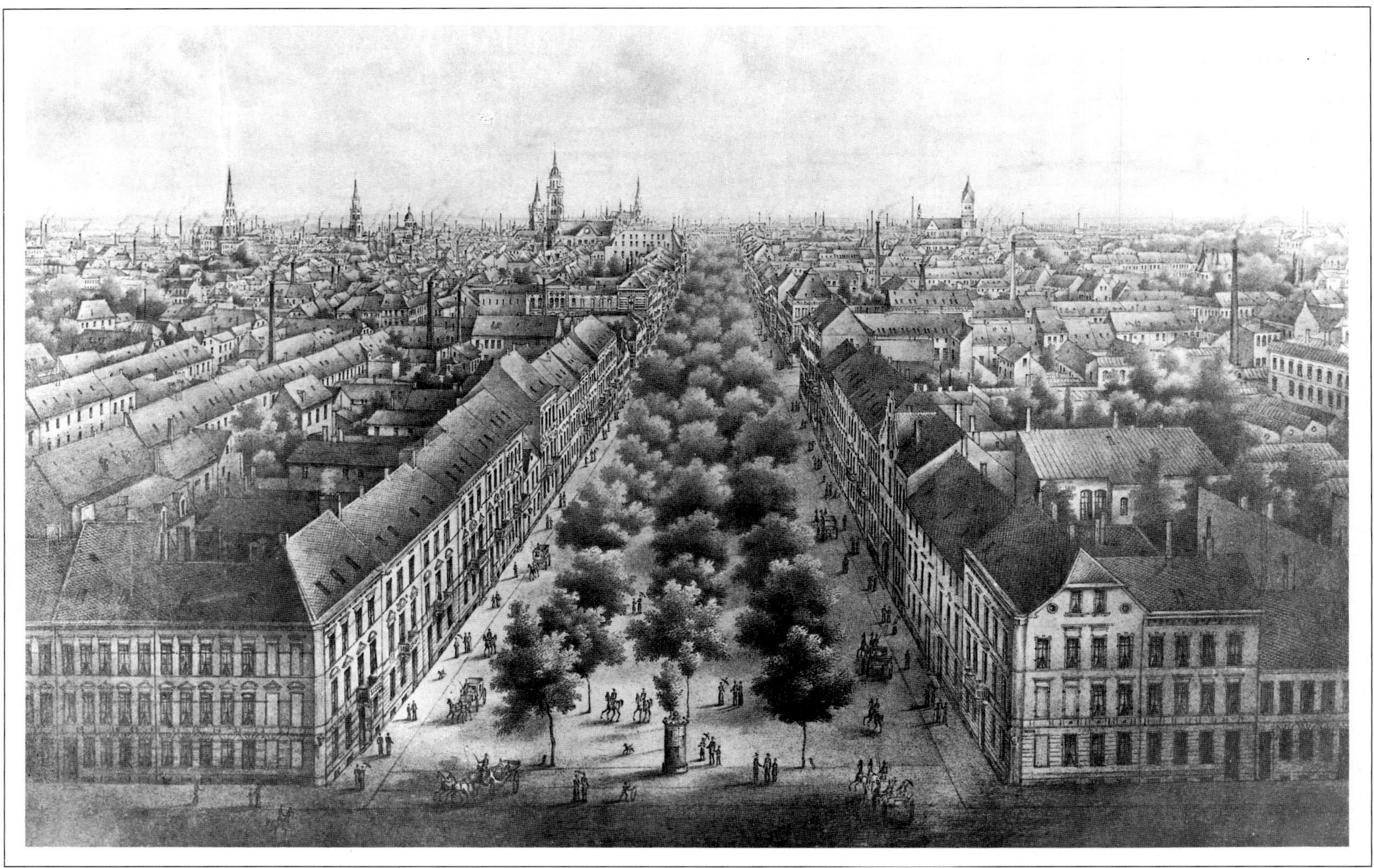

Krefeld, Westwall im Jahre 1894
Blick von der Liebfrauenkirche nach Süden

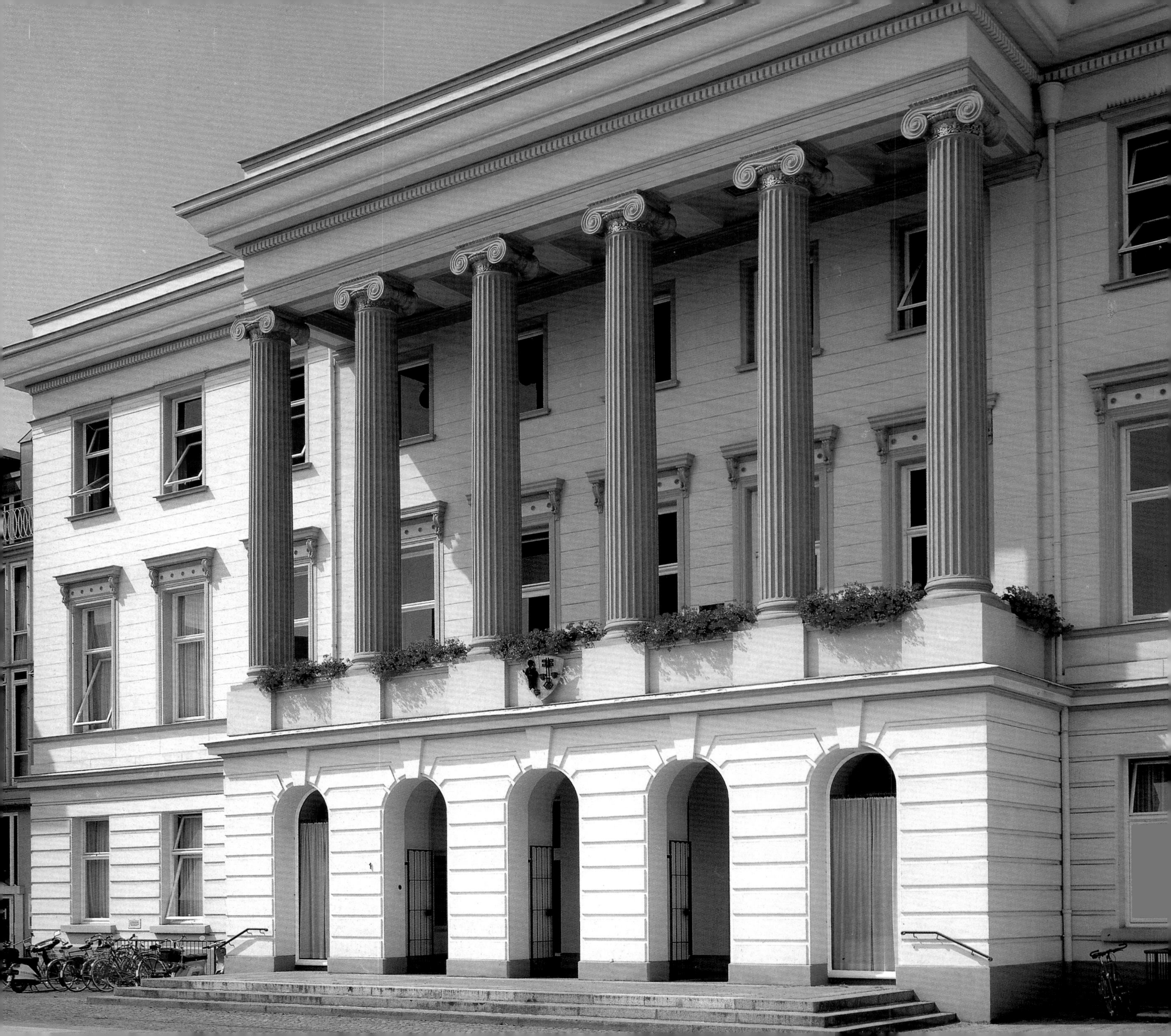

6 Pottbäckermarkt auf dem Theaterplatz / Pottbäcker Market at Theatre Square

Krefelds Theatertradition ist über hundert Jahre alt. Der Bau des Architekten Graubner aus dem Jahr 1963 ist hier Kulisse für den beliebten niederrheinischen Töpfermarkt.

Krefeld's theatrical tradition is more than a hundred years old. Built by the architect Graubner in 1963, the theatre here serves as backdrop for one of the popular pottery markets of the Lower Rhine Area.

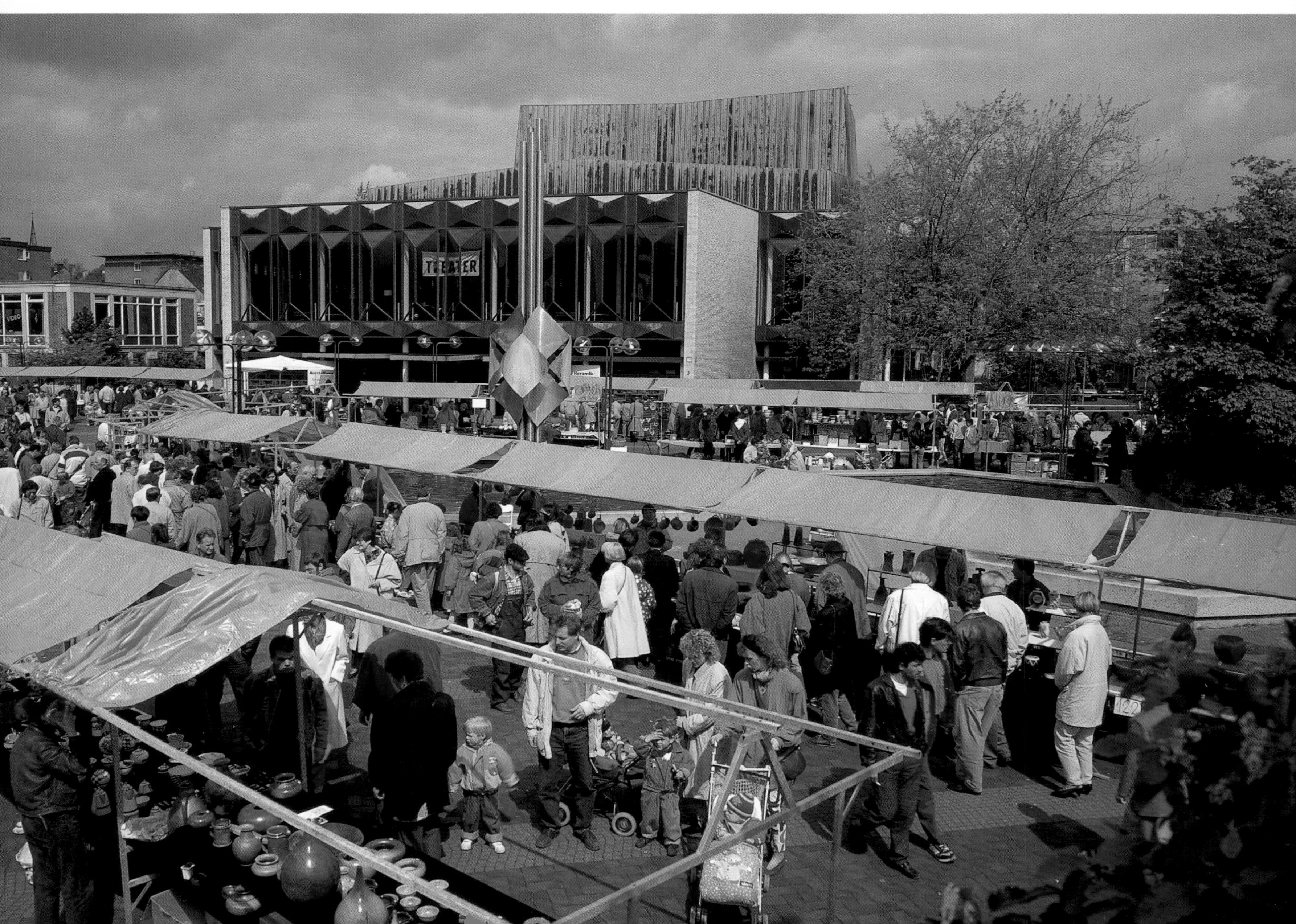

STADTTHEATER/Municipal Theatre

Schauspiel, Oper, Operette, Ballett, Musical und ein Sinfonieorchester leisten sich die Städte Krefeld und Mönchengladbach gemeinsam. Das Publikum fordert internationales Niveau.

Plays, operas, operettas, ballet, musicals and a symphony orchestra are supported jointly by the cities of Krefeld and Mönchengladbach. The audience demands international standards.

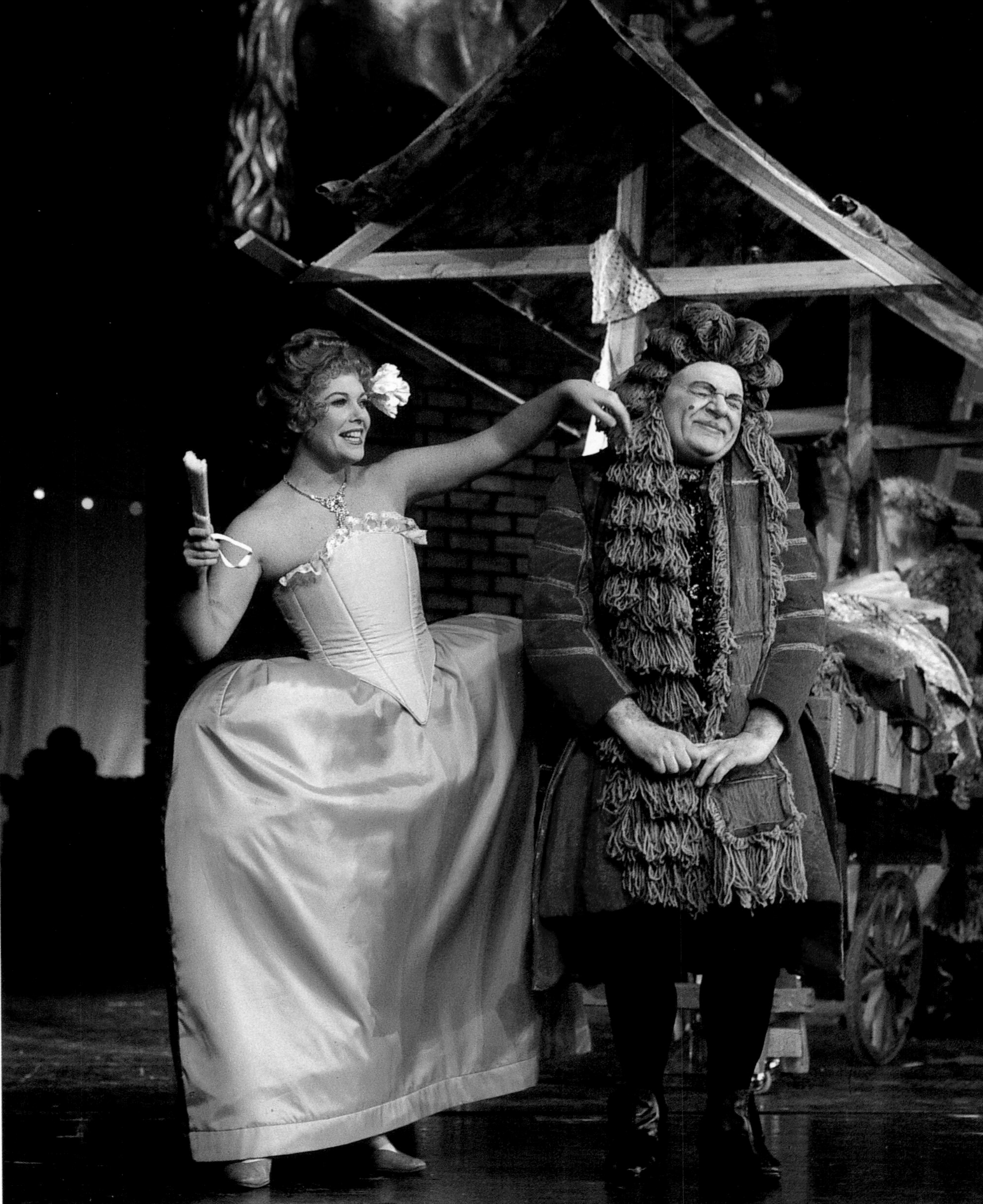

Zentrum für Tagungen, Kongresse und große Geselligkeiten ist das Seidenweberhaus am Theaterplatz. Im Erdgeschoß finden Krefelder und Gäste Information und Kartenverkauf.

Der große Saal des Seidenweberhauses dient nüchternen Ärztekongressen ebenso wie glanzvollen Konzerten oder Gala-Veranstaltungen, insbesondere Präsentation immer neuer Mode.

The silk-weavers' house at Theatre Square serves as a centre for conventions, congresses and large festive events. The ground floor houses a tourist information office and a box office for Krefeld's inhabitants and visitors.

The great hall of the silk-weavers' house hosts such sober events as doctors' conventions as well as splendid concerts or gala events showcasing the latest fashions.

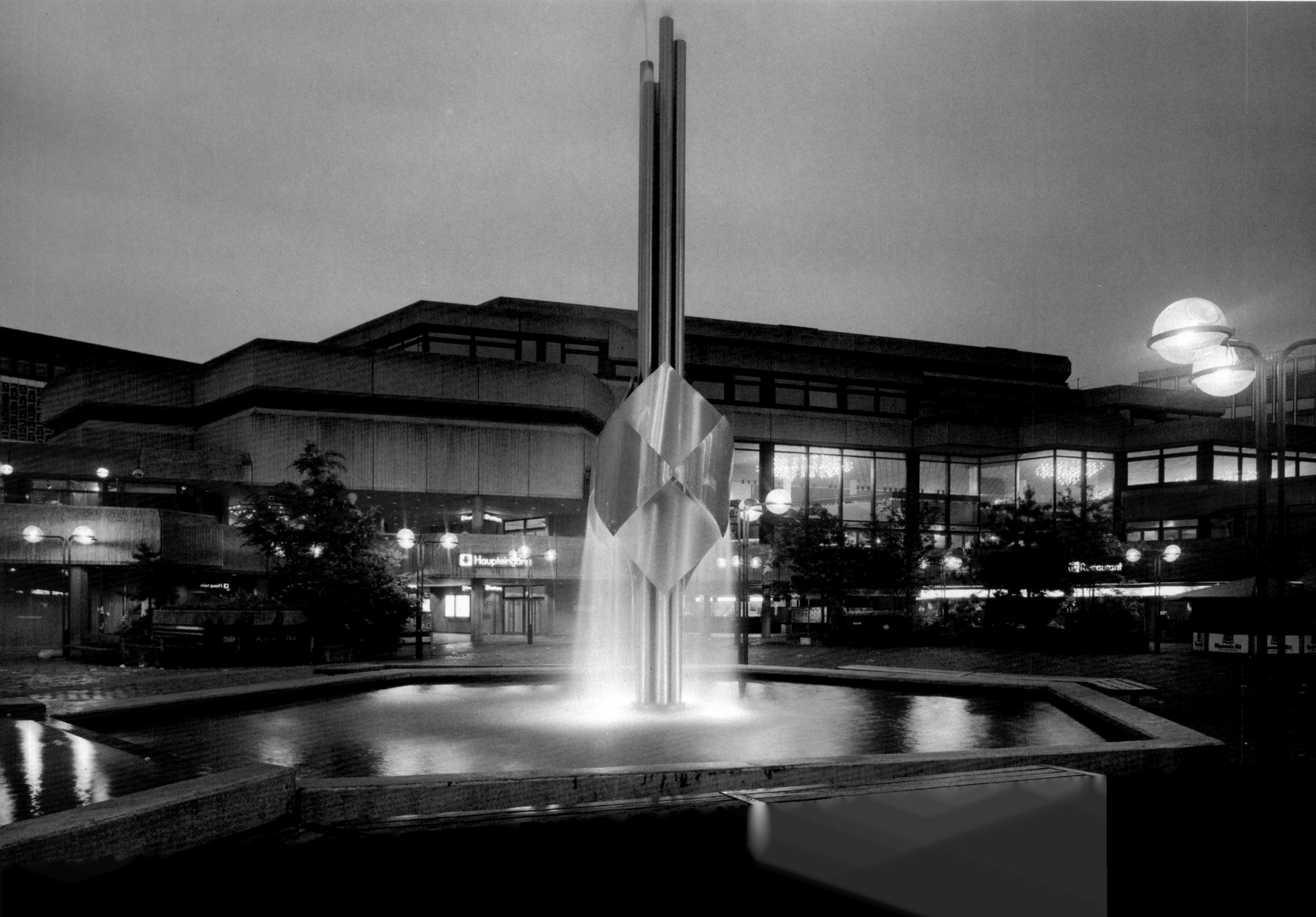

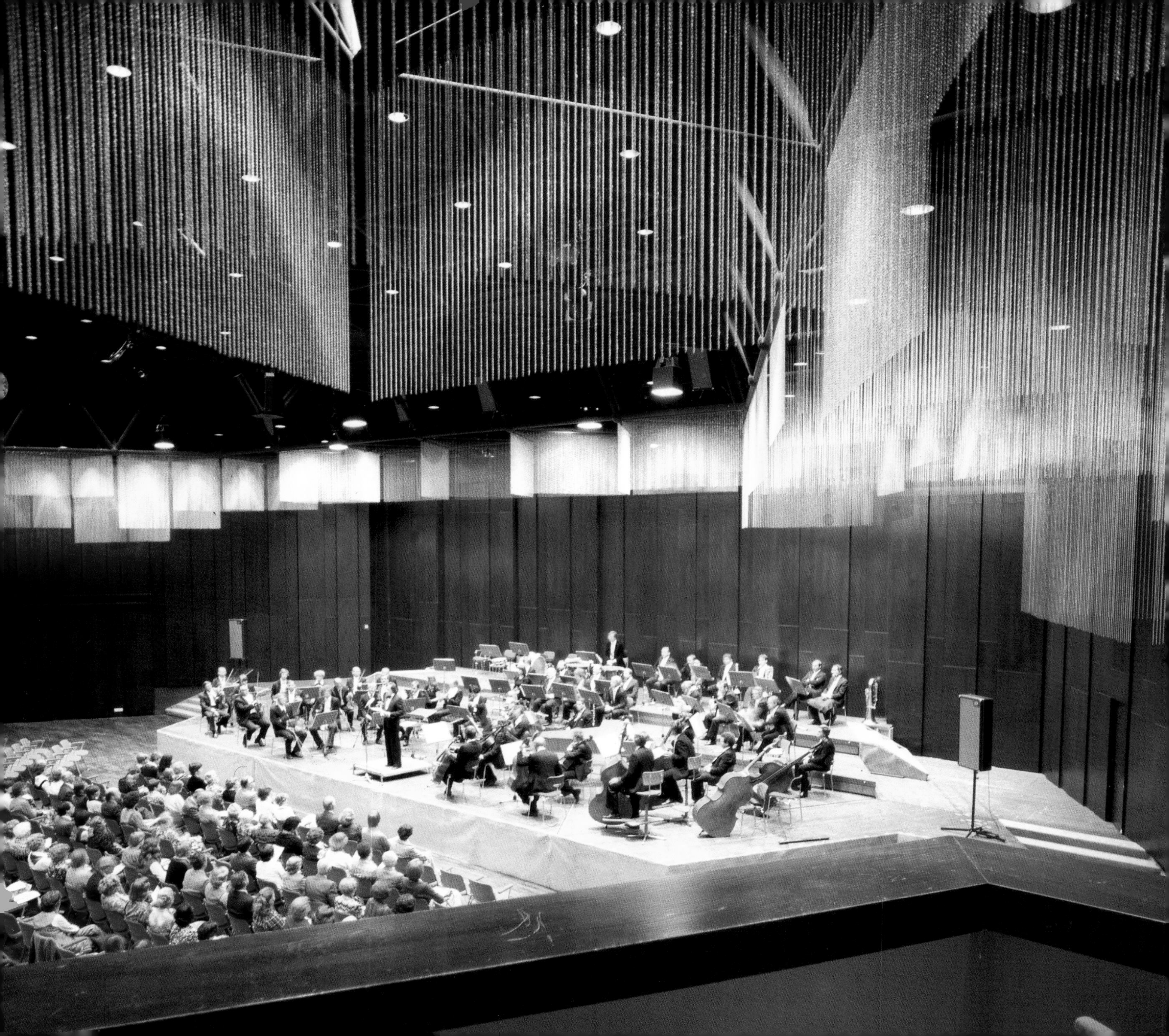

Dem Zentrum der dynamisch wachsenden Stadt gab der preußische Baumeister Adolph von Vagedes Fasson mit dem Viereck der repräsentativen „Wälle". Unser Bild zeigt den Ostwall.

Ein Liebling des Stadtpublikums ist der „Puppenbrunnen" am Südwall. Die beweglichen Bronze-Figuren lassen Gestalten aus der Geschichte der Stadt lebendig werden.

The centre of this rapidly growing city with its distinctive "walls" was designed by the Prussian master builder Adolph von Vagedes. Our picture shows the eastern wall.

The "puppets' well" at the southern wall is a favourite with the city dwellers. The moving bronze figures recreate life from the historical past of the city.

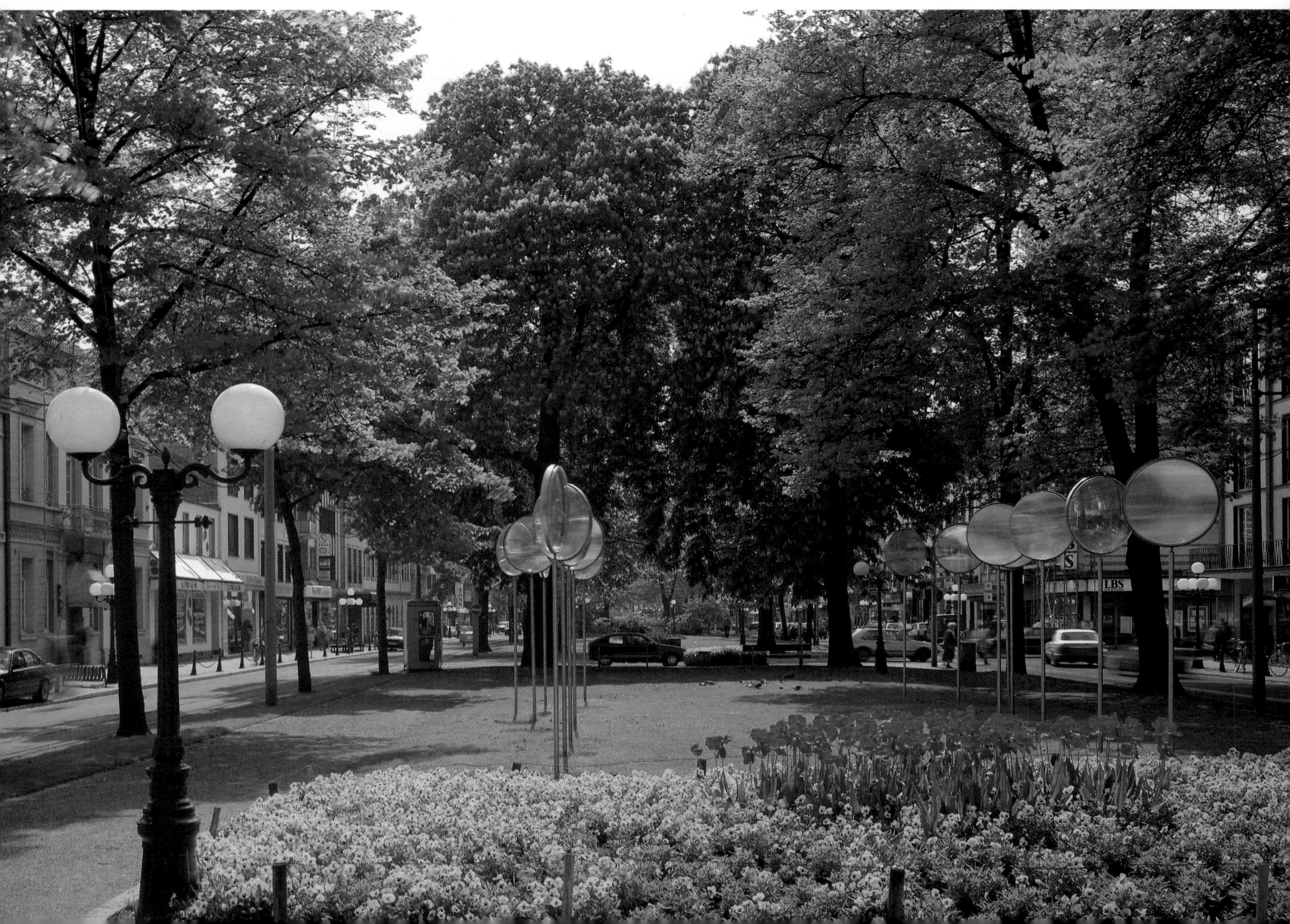

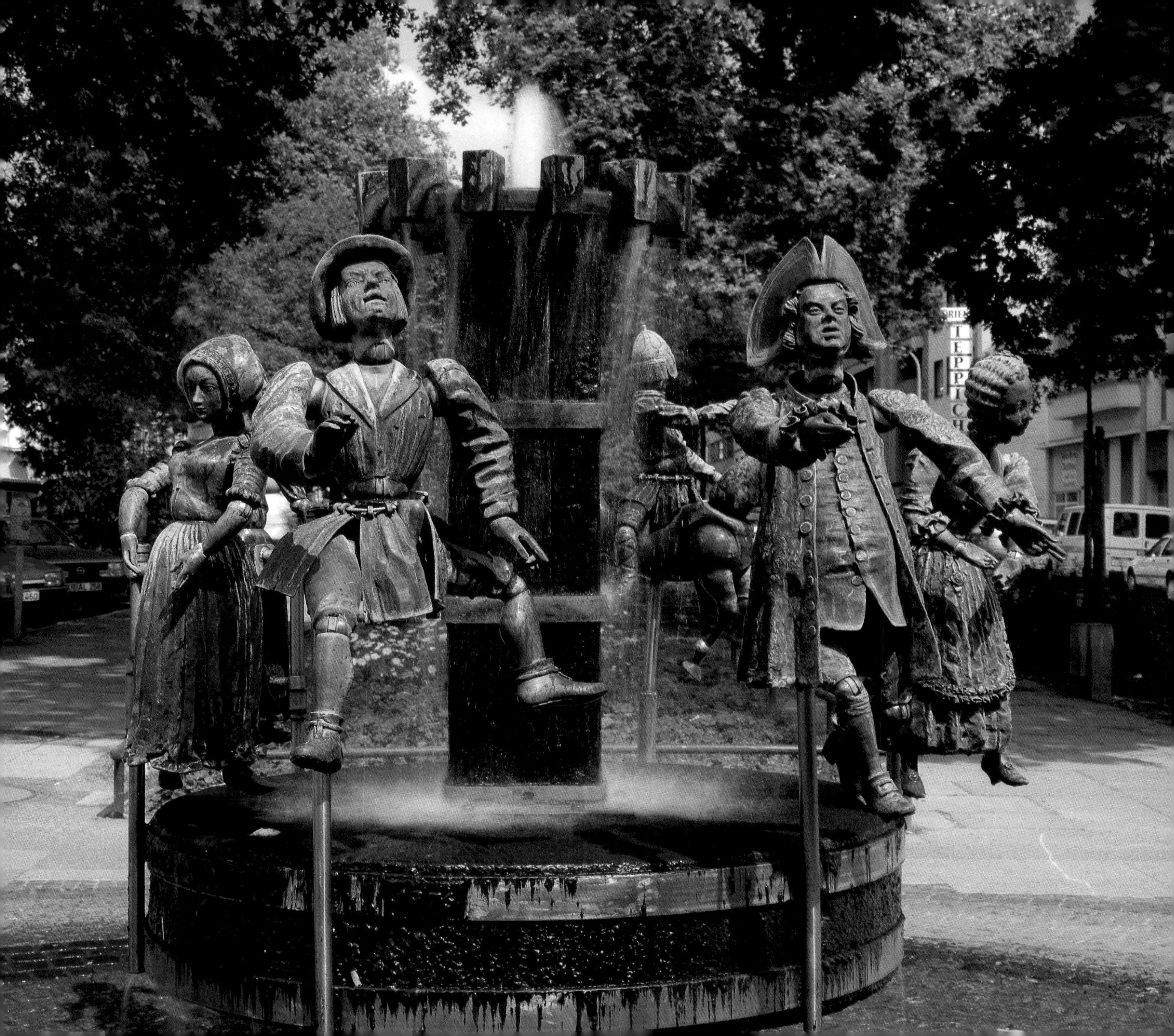
TEPPICH

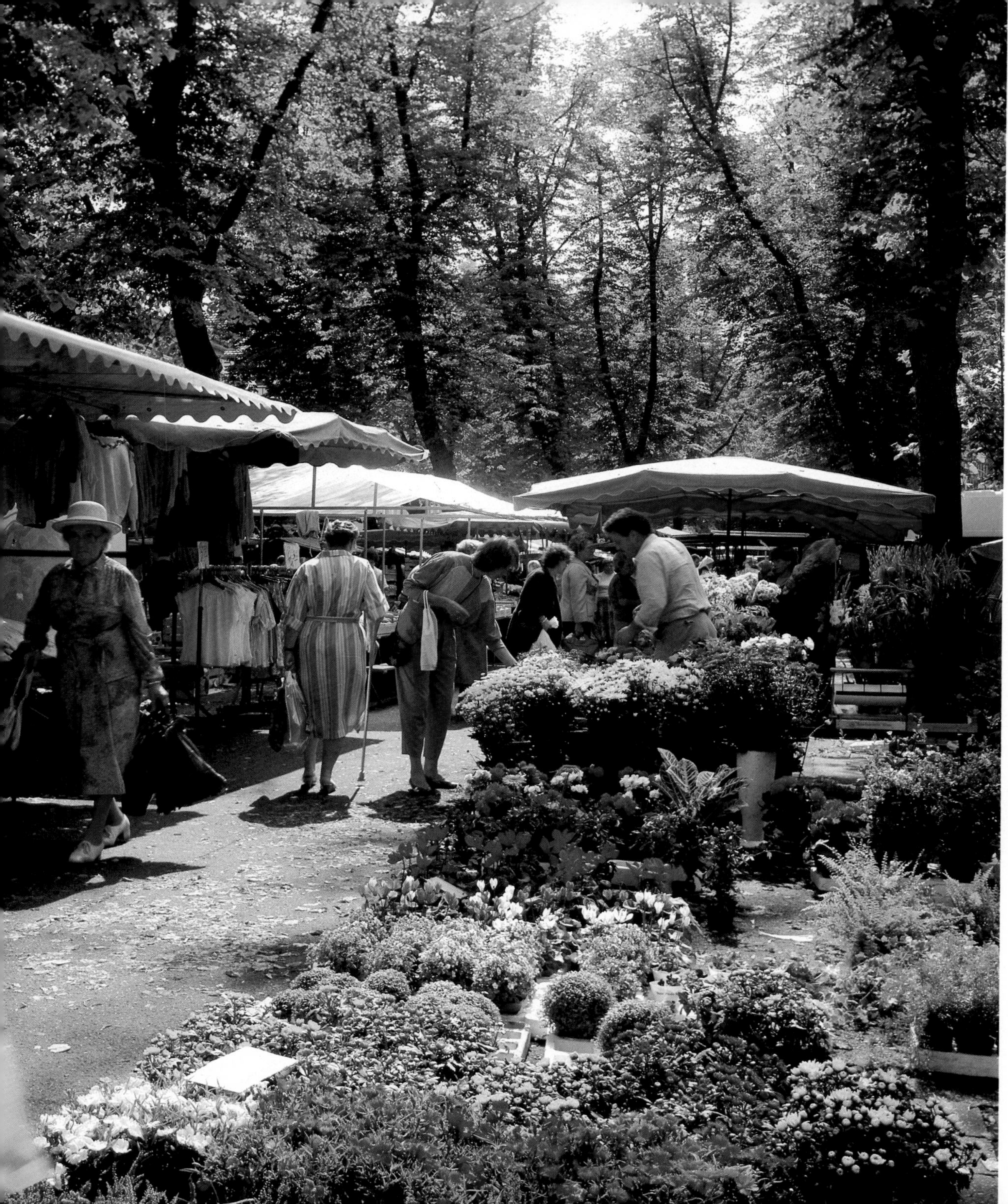

WESTWALL / Western Wall Market

Zweimal in der Woche – und das seit hundert Jahren – treffen sich Bauern, Gärtner, Händler und ihre Kunden auf dem Wochenmarkt zu einem Bild freundlicher Buntheit.

For more than a hundred years peasants, gardeners, merchants and their customers have met at the farmers' market twice a week – a friendly scene of vivid colours.

KAISER-WILHELM-MUSEUM ▷

Ihrem Kaiser zu Ehren, ihren Mitbürgern zur Geschmacksbildung bauten die Krefelder um 1900 ihr Kunstmuseum. Heute ist das Haus eine erste Adresse der internationalen Moderne.

The people of Krefeld built their art museum as early as 1900, both in honour of the emperor and to cultivate the tastes of their fellow citizens. Today the museum houses modernist works by artists known all over the world.

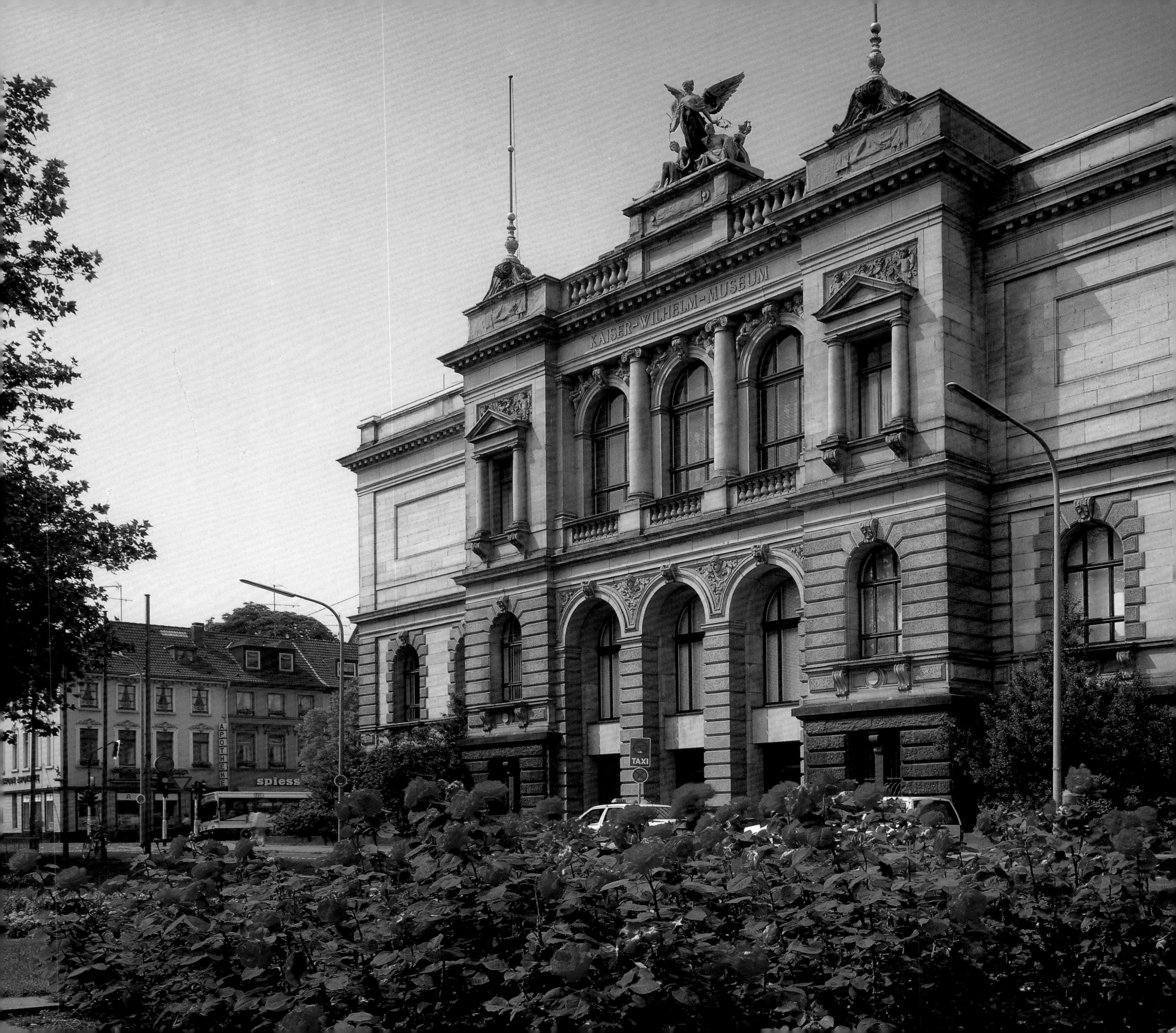
KAISER-WILHELM-MUSEUM
APOTHEKE
spiess
TAXI

Der durch Samt und Seide geschulte Geschmack hat die Krefelder zur Kunst gebracht. Private und öffentliche Sammlungen haben Weltruf. Hier ein Blick ins Kaiser-Wilhelm-Museum.

In Krefeld, people cultivated a love of the arts through their taste for velvet and silk. Private and public collections enjoy international fame. Here a view into the Kaiser-Wilhelm-Museum.

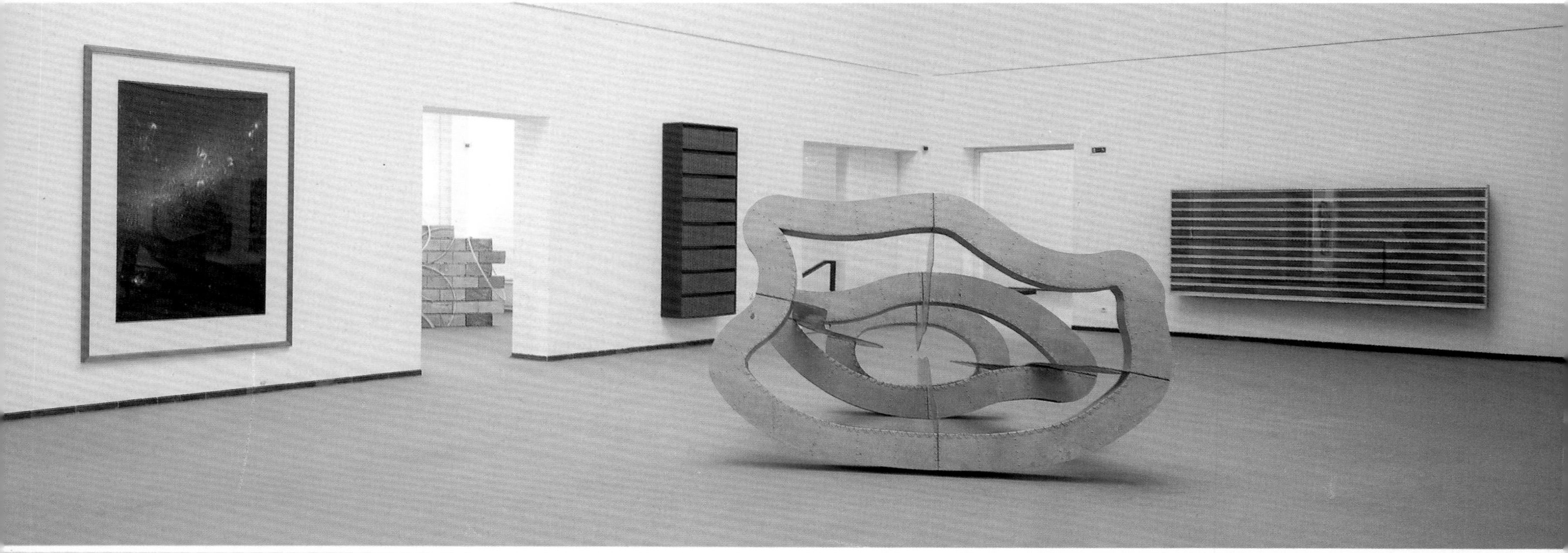

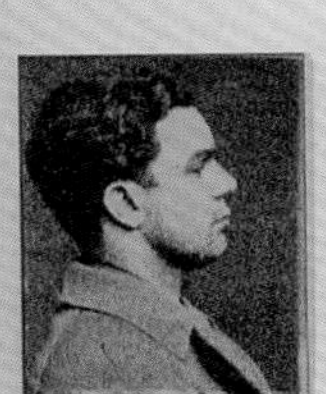

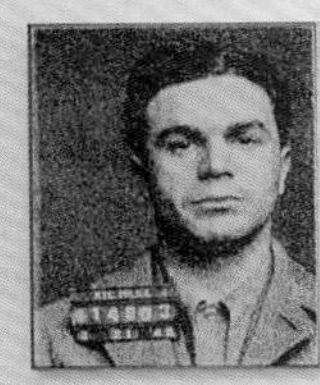

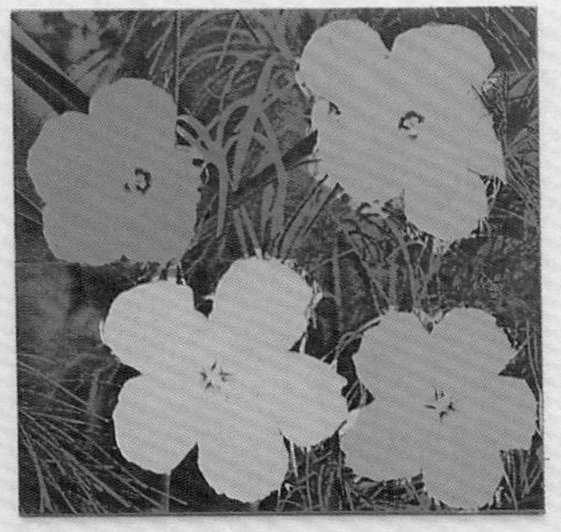

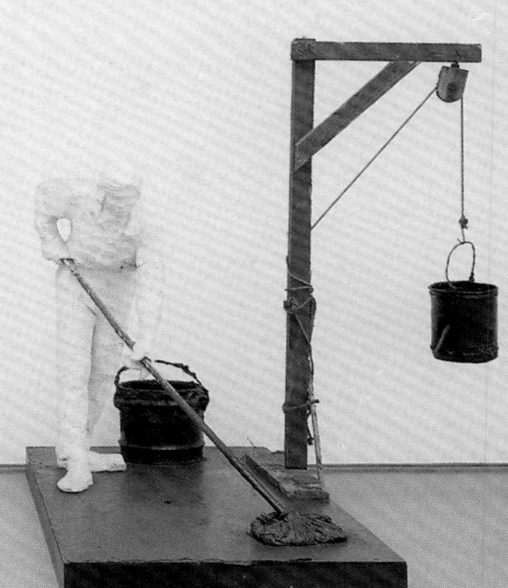

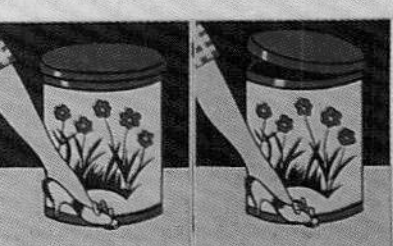

Mies van der Rohe baute für den Textilfabrikanten Lange das Wohnhaus, das später Museum der Moderne wurde. Claes Oldenburgs Plastik signalisiert einen Ort der Kunst-Avantgarde.

Mies van der Rohe built the residence of the textile entrepreneur Lange which was later to become a museum of modern art. Claes Oldenburg's sculpture indicates that avantgarde art, too, has its place here.

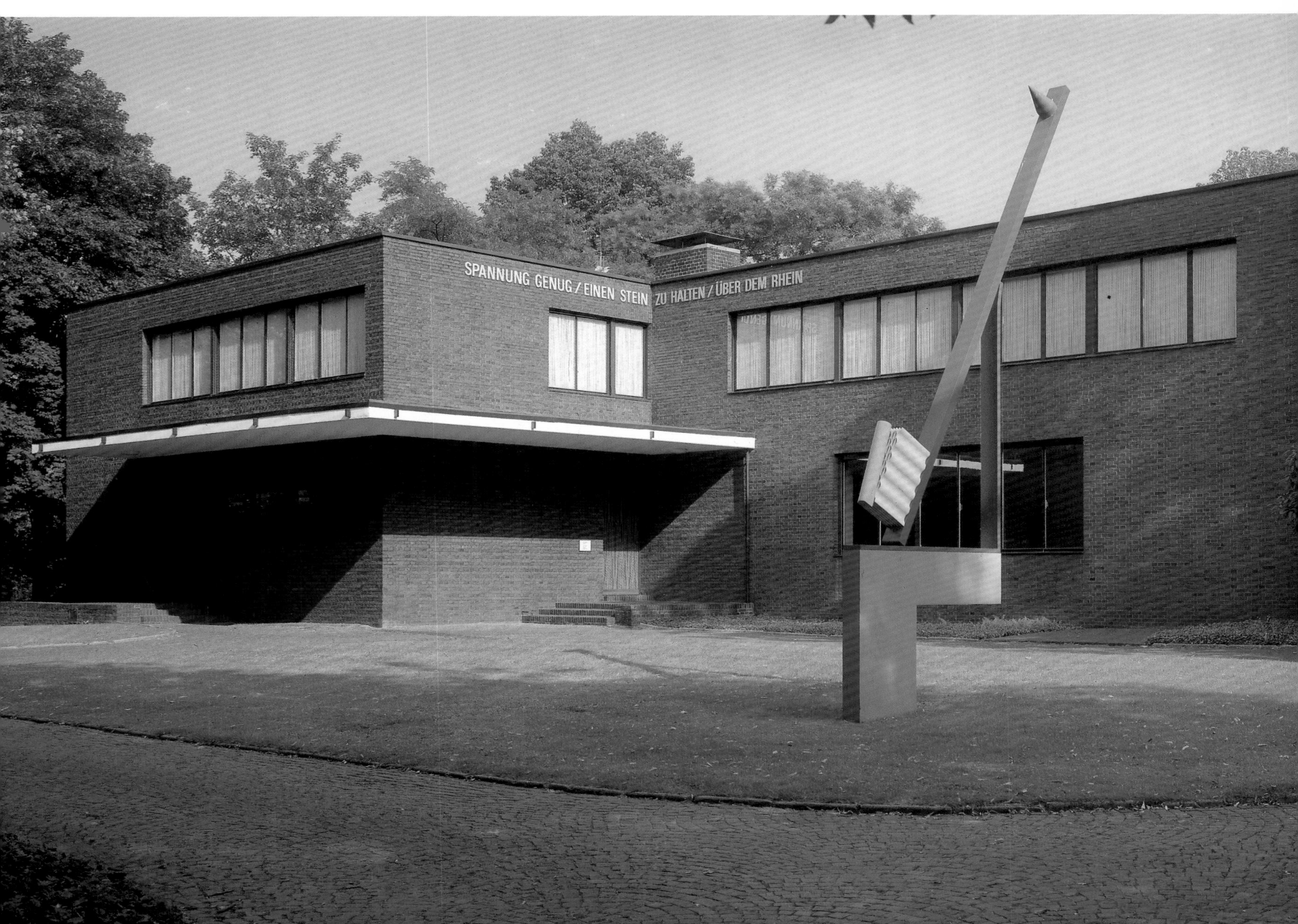

Stiftungen der Bürger an ihre Stadt haben in Krefeld Tradition. Am nördlichen Tor zur Innenstadt, dem Friedrichsplatz, kam Krefeld so zu einem attraktiven Fontänen-Brunnen.

There is a long tradition of endowments to the city by its citizens. Friedrichsplatz, or "Square", at the northern end of the city centre, received its attractive fountain in this way.

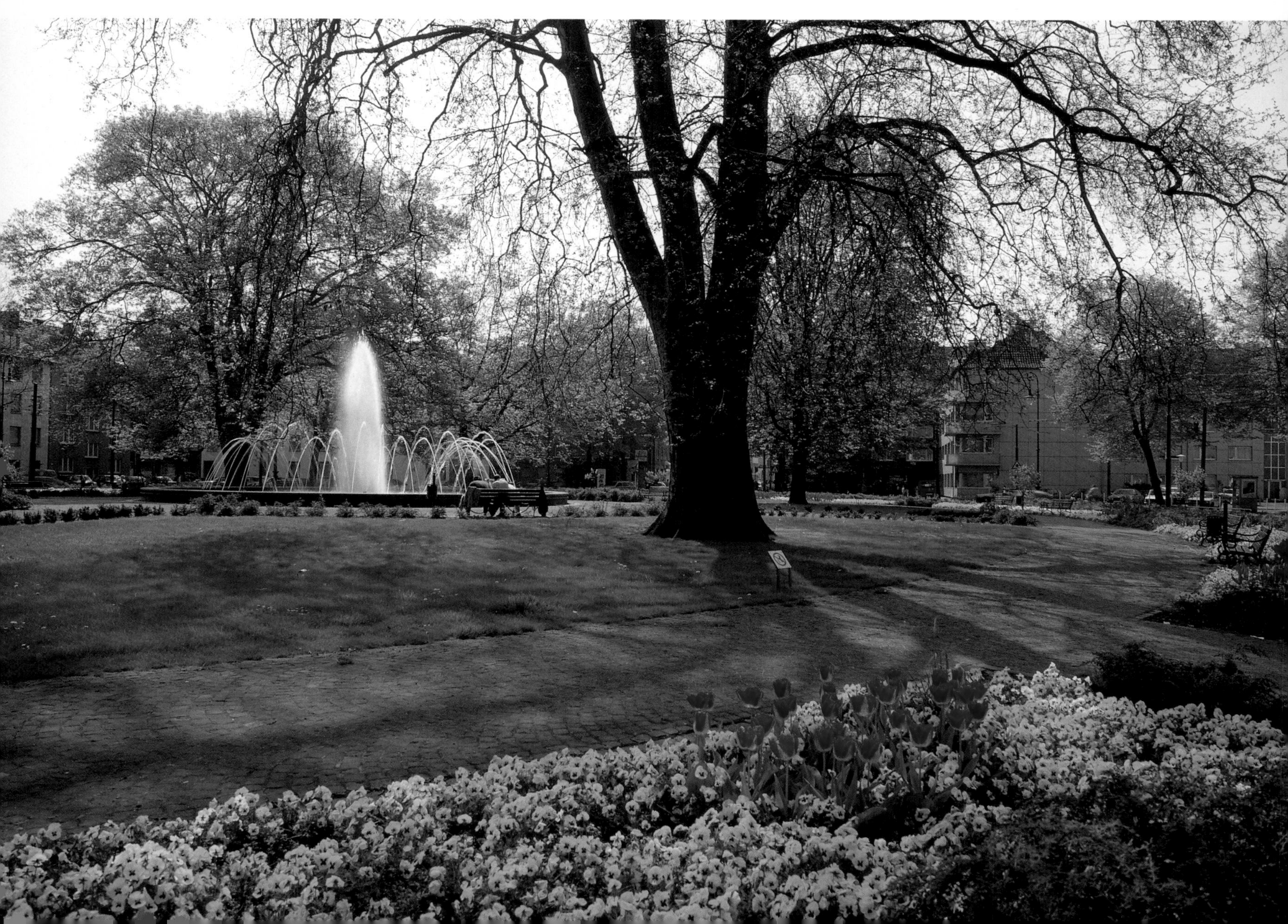

Die Zahl 100 weist mit vielen Jubiläen zurück in die „Gründerzeit", die auch Krefeld prägte. 100 Jahre alt ist der repräsentative Bau von Land- und Amtsgericht.

Krefeld, too, profited from the fantastic economic boom of the last century. The distinctive courthouse building also dates back to that time.

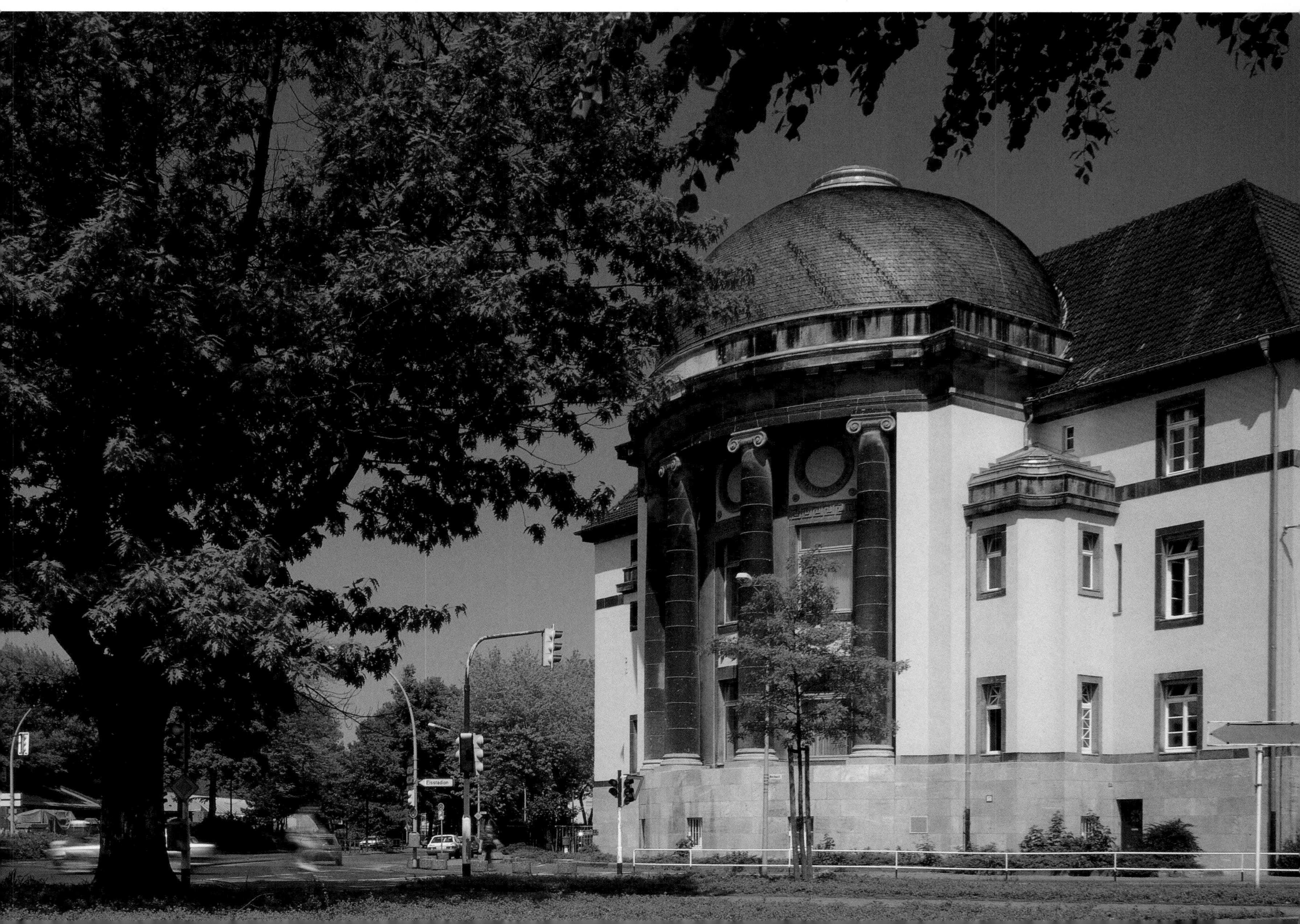

Mode und aktueller Zeitgeist gehen Hand in Hand. Die jeweils neue Architektur fand deshalb in Krefeld immer ihren Bauherrn. Dieser ansehnliche Schulbau überstand den Krieg.

Die Pläne zu diesem Haus und dem Teil der Innenstadt, in dem es steht, genehmigte Friedrich der Große höchstpersönlich. Das Haus der Familie Floh wurde wieder aufgebaut.

Fashions and the spirit of an age go hand in hand. Modern architecture therefore quickly found its supporters in Krefeld. This attractive school building survived the war.

Frederick the Great himself approved of the plans for the House and for the part of the city centre in which it stands. The house has been reconstructed.

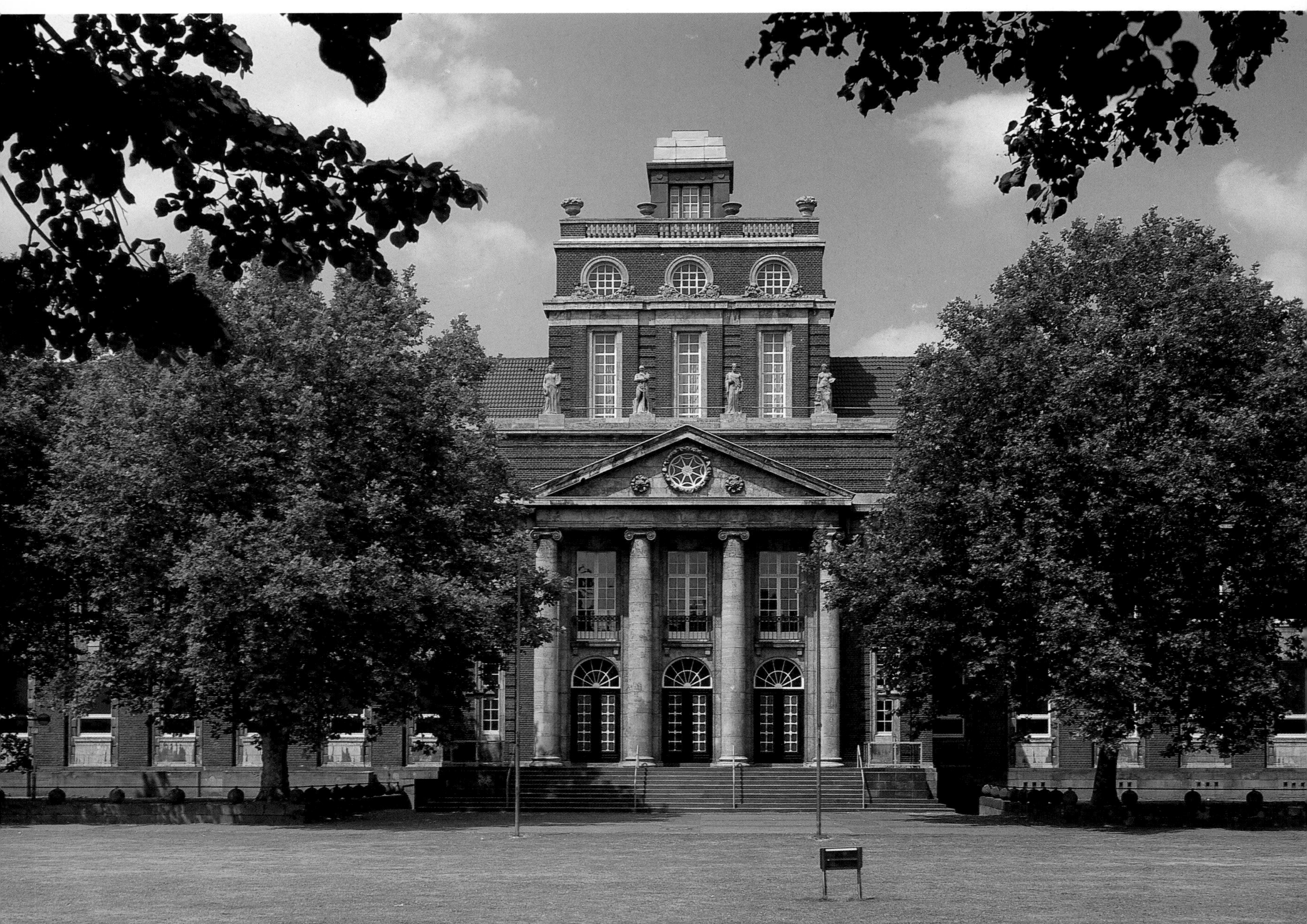

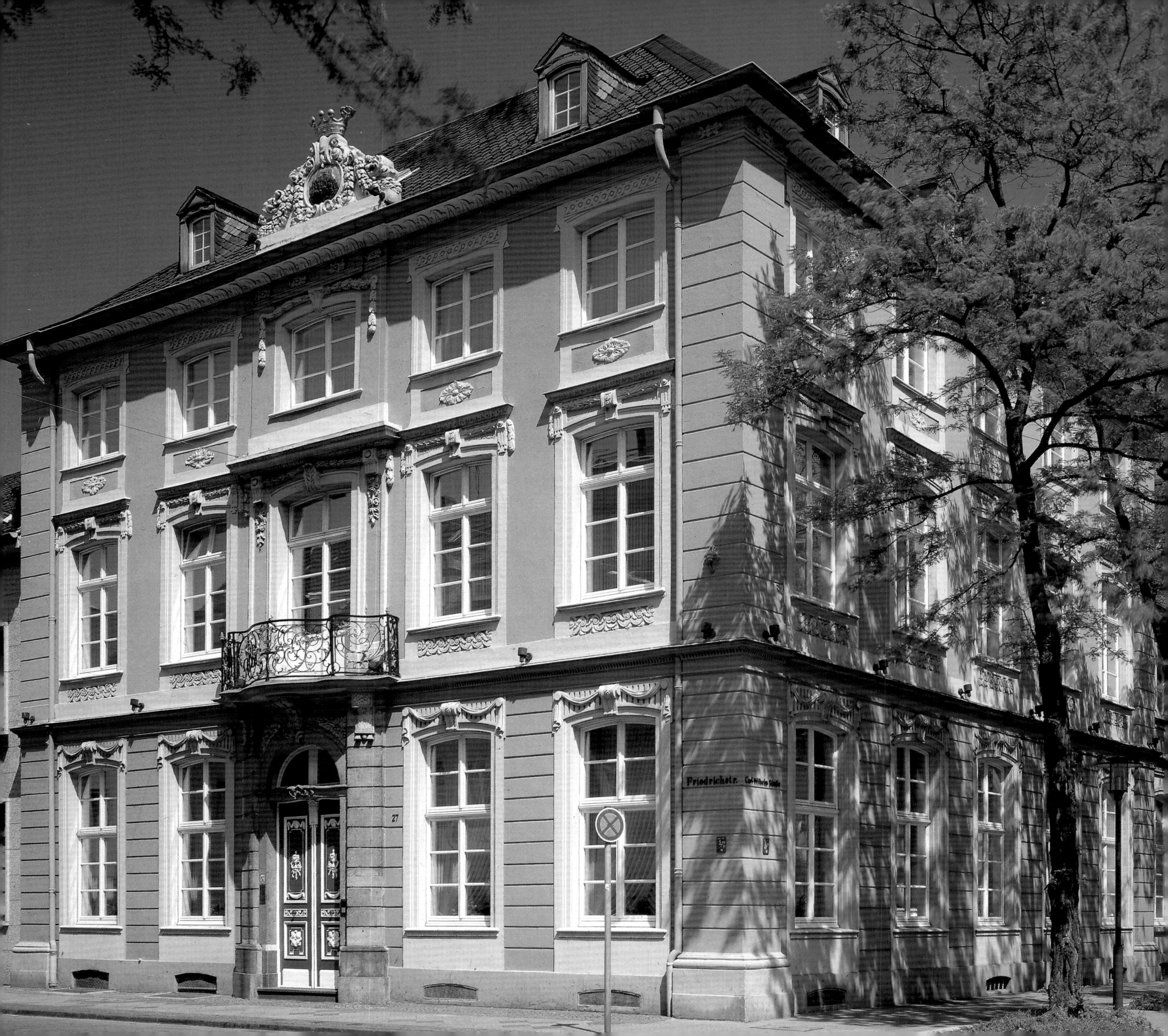
Friedrichstr.
27

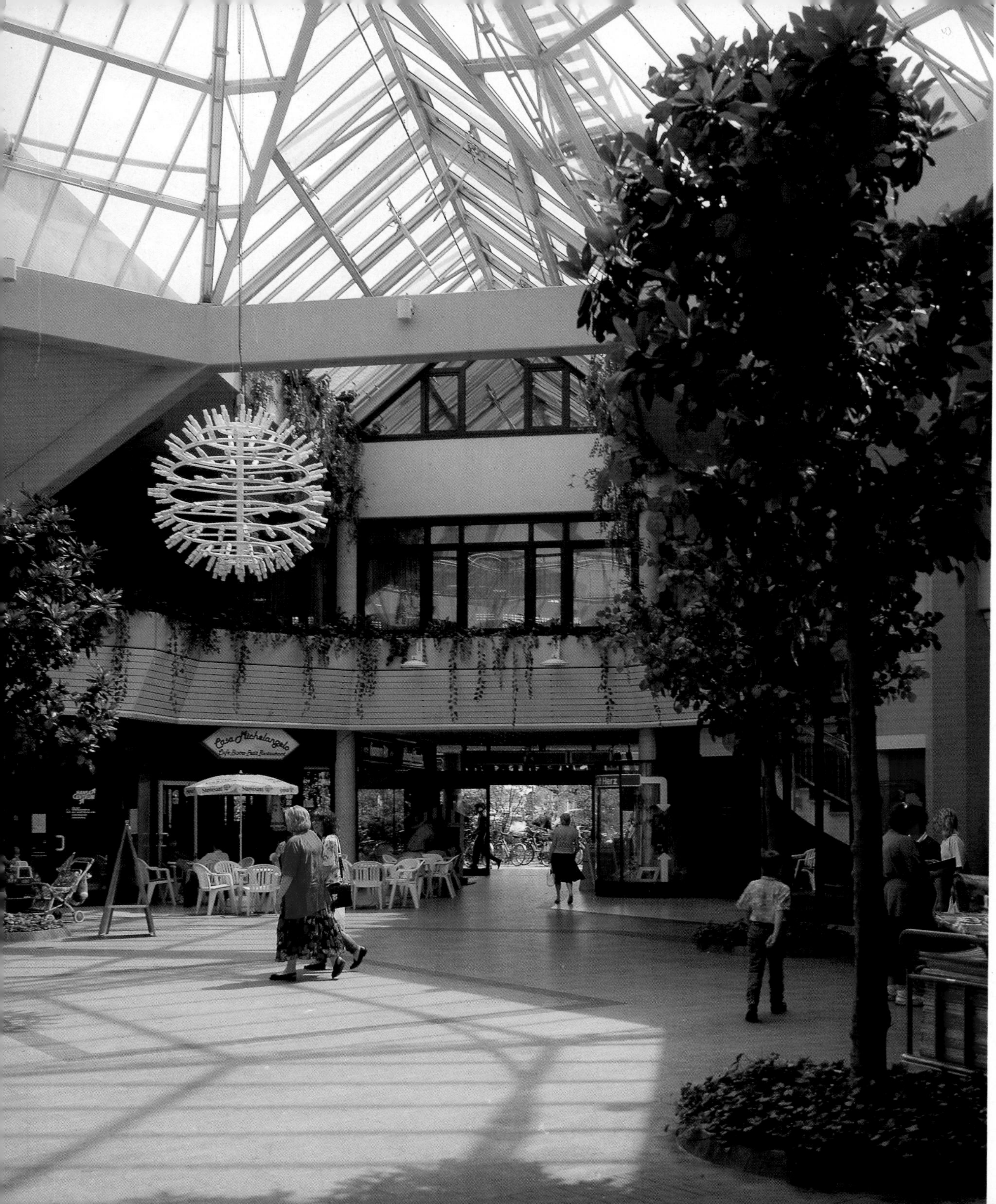

Hansazentrum / Hansa Centre

An der Schnittstelle zwischen südlichen Stadtteilen und City begegnet man sich unter der Glaskuppel des „Hansa-Zentrums", das geschäftliche Vielfalt zusammenfaßt.

Where the southern suburbs and the city centre meet, people gather under the glass cupola of the "Hansa Centre", which houses a wide range of businesses.

ET BRÖCKSKE ▷

Das Bier alter Brauart, das Altbier, ist das Regionalgetränk des Niederrheins und der Krefelder. In deftigen Brauereigaststätten fließt es zum Wohle der Geselligkeit.

Beer brewed according to an ancient tradition, the so-called "Altbier", is the regional favourite of the Lower Rhine Area and the people of Krefeld. In the rustic brewery inns it is guaranteed to enhance sociability.

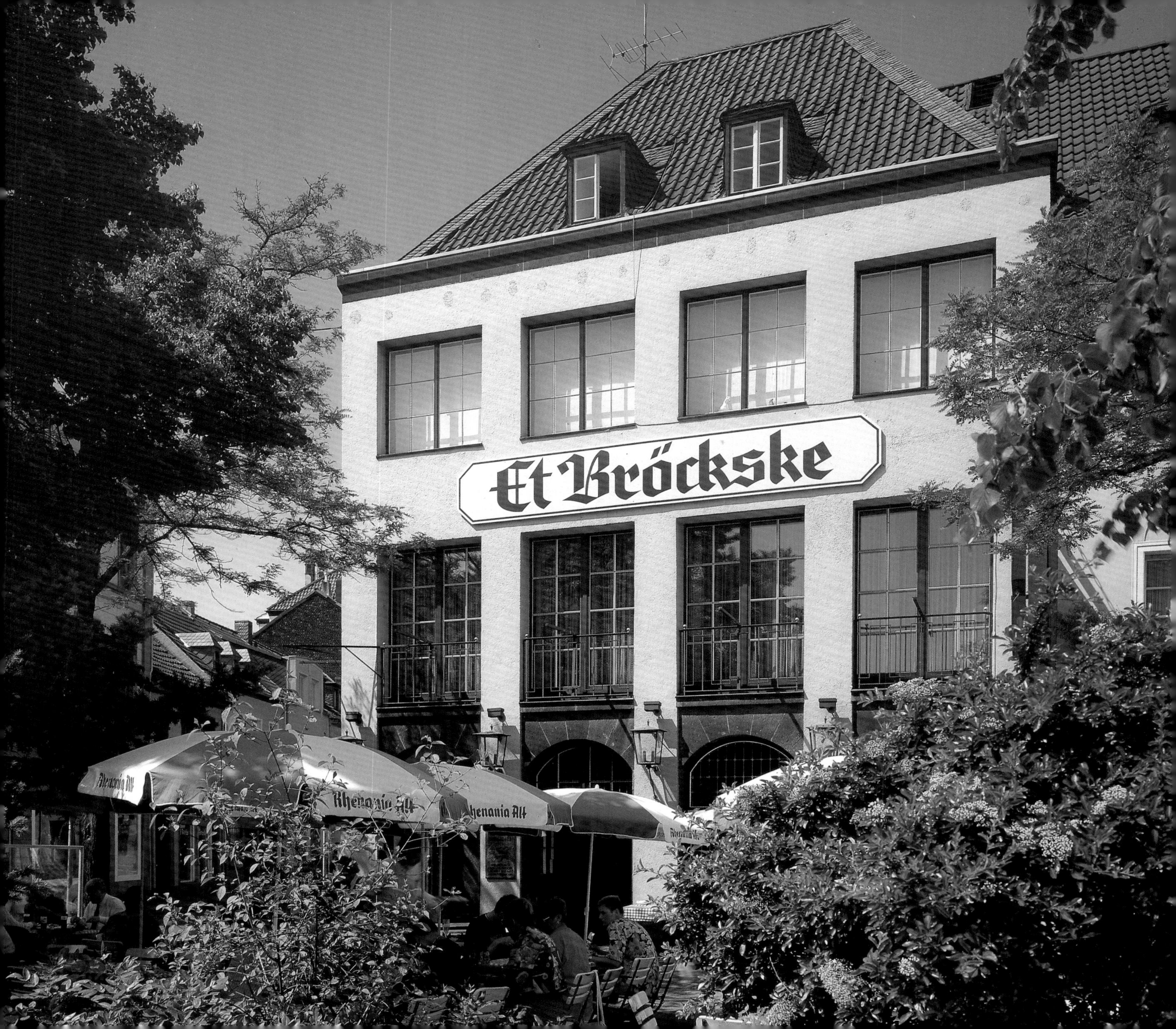
Et Bröckske
Rhenania Alt
Rhenania Alt
Rhenania Alt

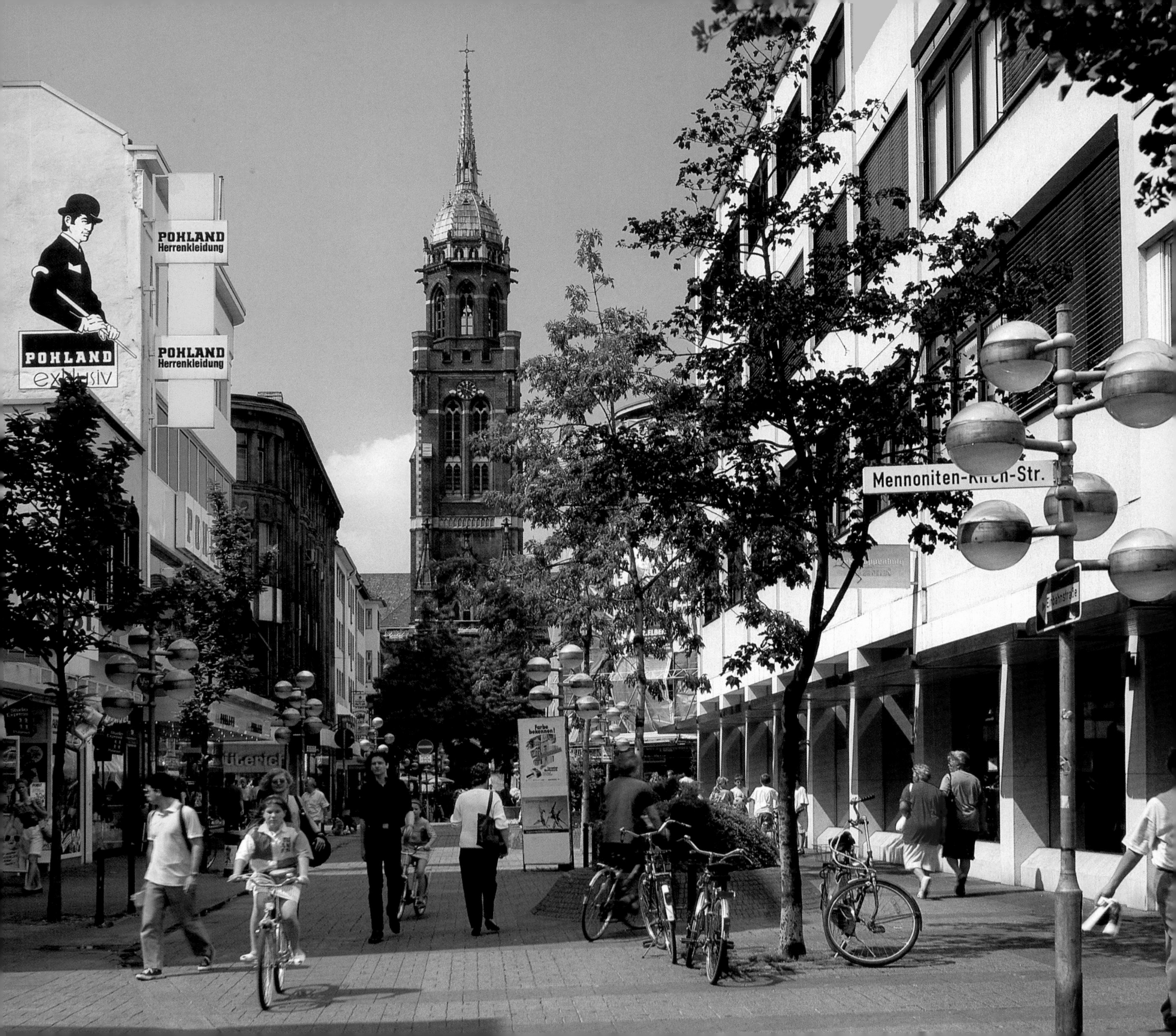

POHLAND
Herrenkleidung
POHLAND
Herrenkleidung
POHLAND
exklusiv
Mennoniten-Kirch-Str.
Farbe bekennen!

Als Wahrzeichen der Stadt steht der Turm der St.-Dionysius-Kirche über der geschäftigen Rheinstraße. Für den Bau votierte und zahlte am Ende des 19. Jahrhunderts der Stadtrat.

Ernst Fiedrich Zwirner, Baumeister am Kölner Dom, gab der Dionynisius-Kirche 1844 spätklassizistischen Ausdruck. Moderne Restaurierung unterstrich dies auf noble Weise.

The steeple of St. Dionysius Church above the busy street Rheinstrasse serves as a landmark in the city. The building was erected and paid for by the city council at the end of the 19th century.

St. Dionysius Church received its late neoclassical exterior in 1844 from Ernst Friedrich Zwirner, the master builder of Cologne Cathedral. It was successfully enhanced by modern restoration.

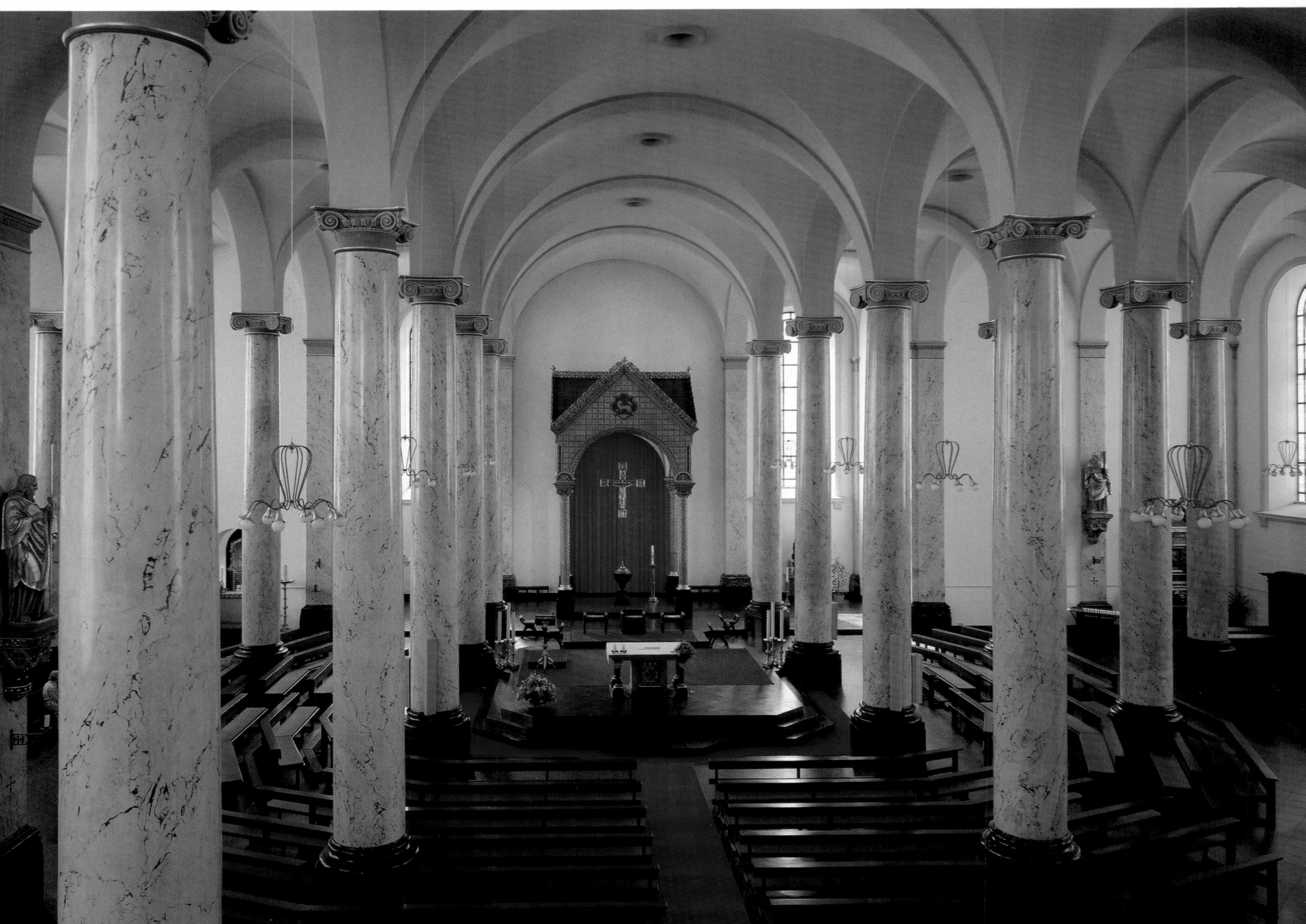

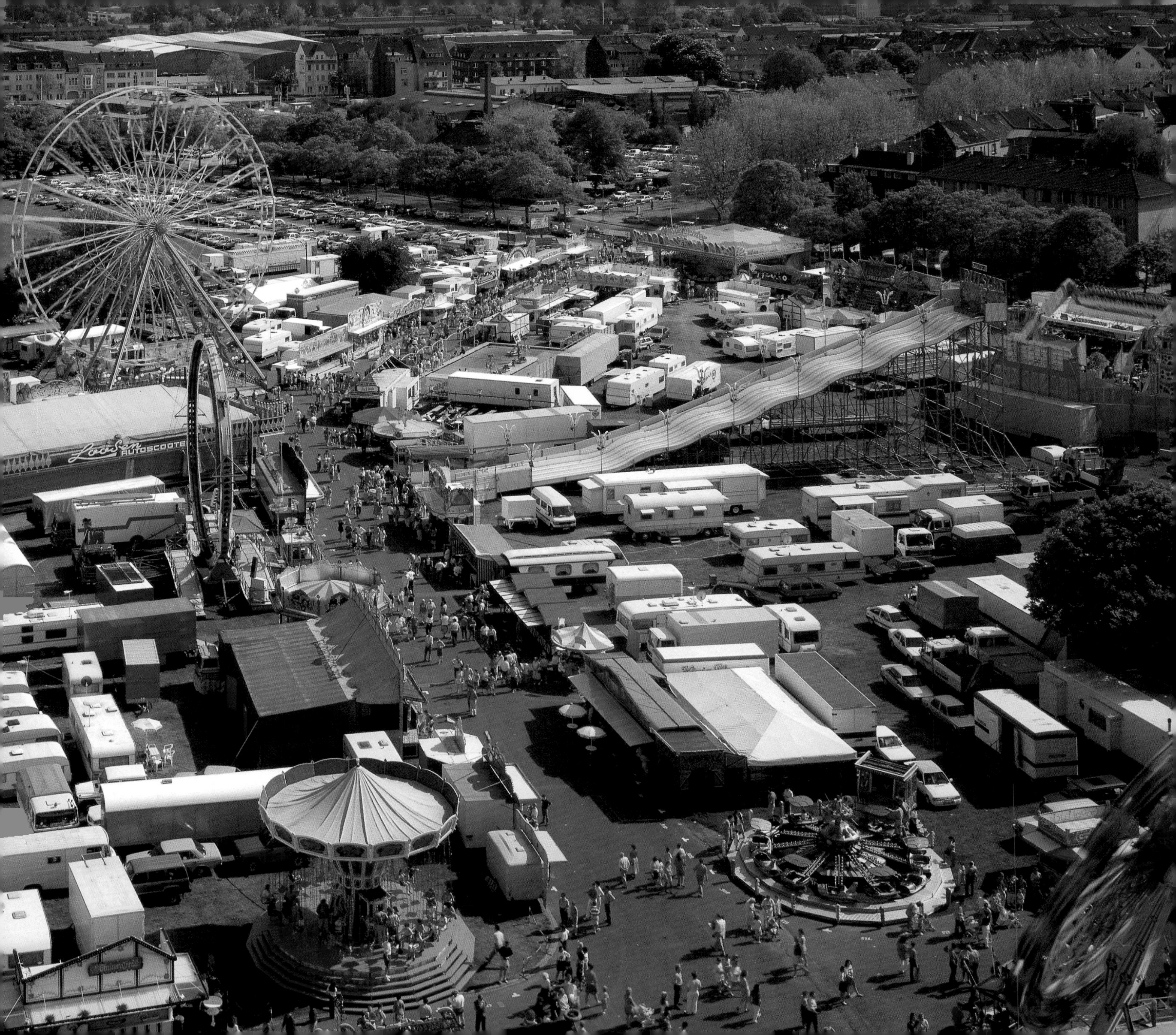
Loosen
AUTOSCOOTE

Zum Jahreskalender einer rheinischen Stadt gehören unverzichtbare Volksfeste wie der Karneval oder die Kirmes. Für letztere ist zweimal im Jahr ein großer Platz reserviert.

Für eine Stadt im flachen Land sind Kirchtürme unentbehrliche Profildetails. Napoleons Ingenieure bauten die Achse der Uerdinger Straße, die schnurgerade ins Zentrum führt.

No city on the Rhine can do without the traditional annual festivals such as its carnival or fairs. This square is the site of a fair twice a year.

For cities built on level ground, steeples are indispensable landmarks. Napoleon's engineers built the crossroads at Uerdinger Strasse which lead directly into the centre.

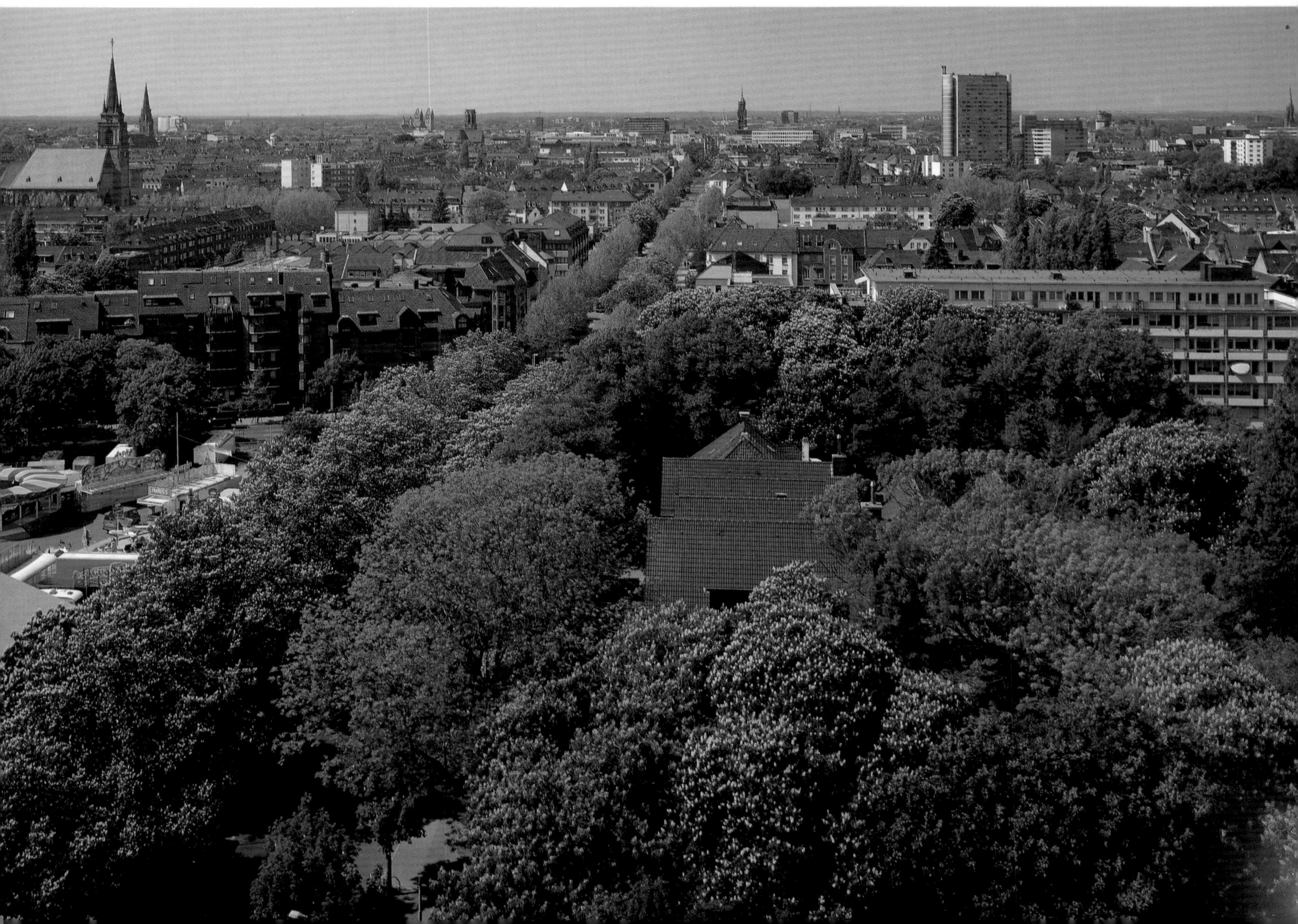

Im Rahmen eines weitläufigen Parks gedeihen im Botanischen Garten 3000 Blumen- und Pflanzenarten. Neben allerlei Exoten kommt der niederrheinische Bauerngarten zur Geltung.

Alle Krefelder und Gäste lieben den Zoo. In einem alten Park wurden 1200 Tiere unter den Kronen großer Bäume heimisch. Vögel und Affen residieren in gläsernen Tropenhäusern.

Set within an expansive park, the botanical gardens house 3000 flower and plant species. Here, the traditional farmers' garden of the Lower Rhine Area receives the same attention as the exotic plants.

Inhabitants of Krefeld and visitors alike love the zoo. In an old park, 1200 animals have found a home under a canopy formed by tall trees. Birds and monkeys reside in tropical glasshouses.

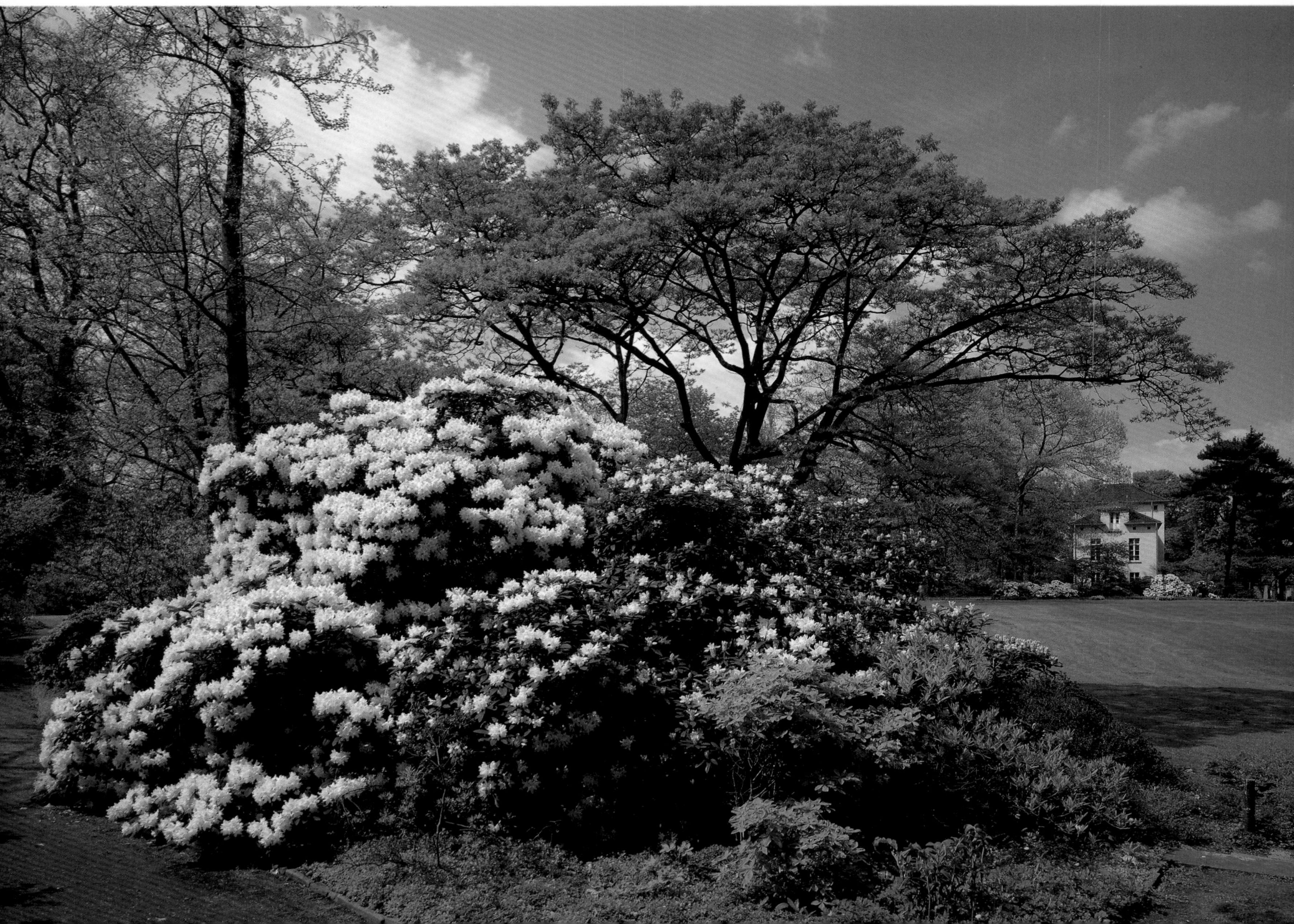

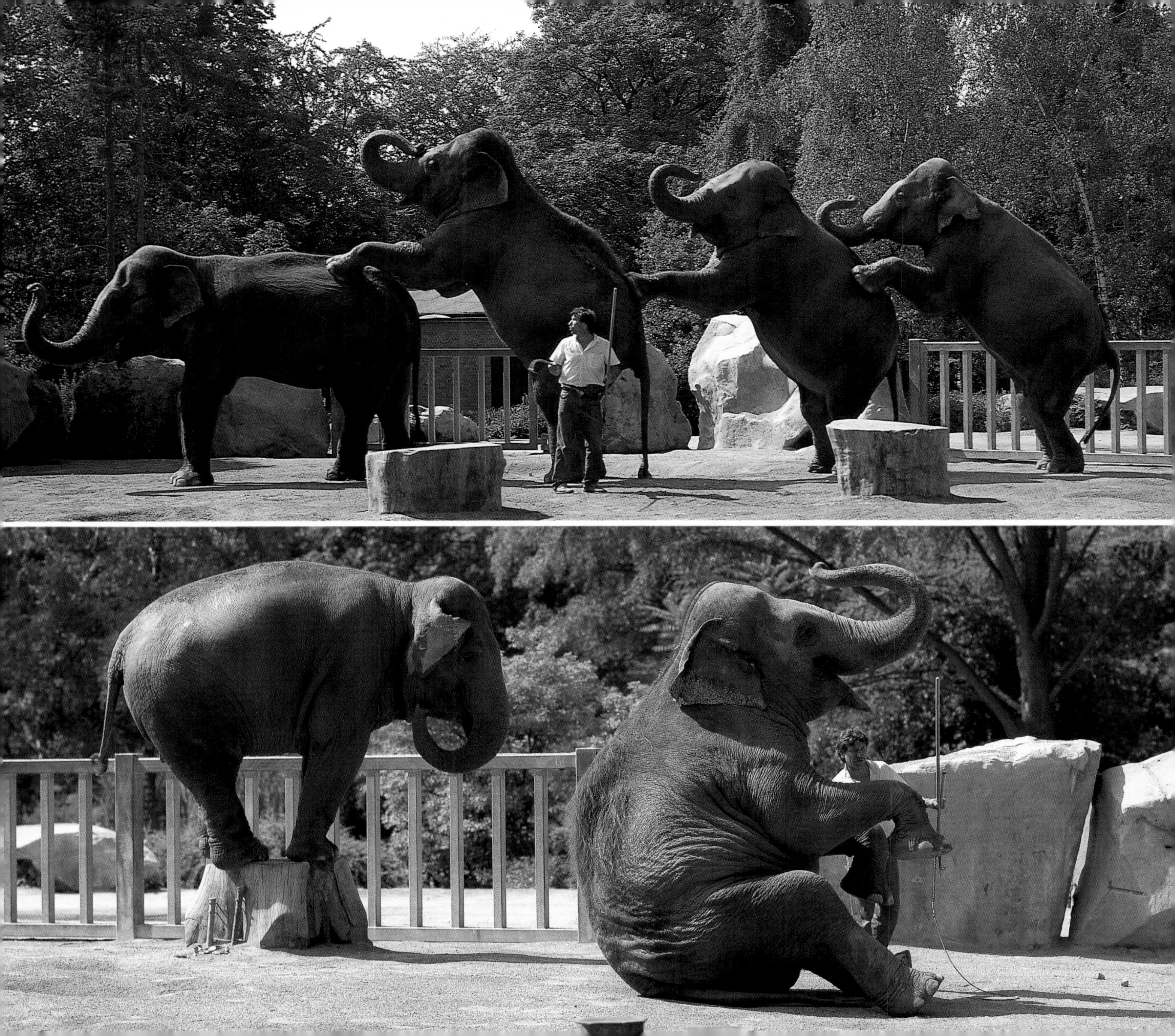

Mit der Anlage einer großzügigen Parkanlage beschäftigte Oberbürgermeister Dr. Johansen in den 20er Jahren arbeitslose Mitbürger. Die Notlösung schmückt nun die Stadt.

In the twenties, Mayor Dr. Johansen had this generous park built in an effort to create jobs for the unemployed. Although it once met a different need, it now graces the city like a jewel.

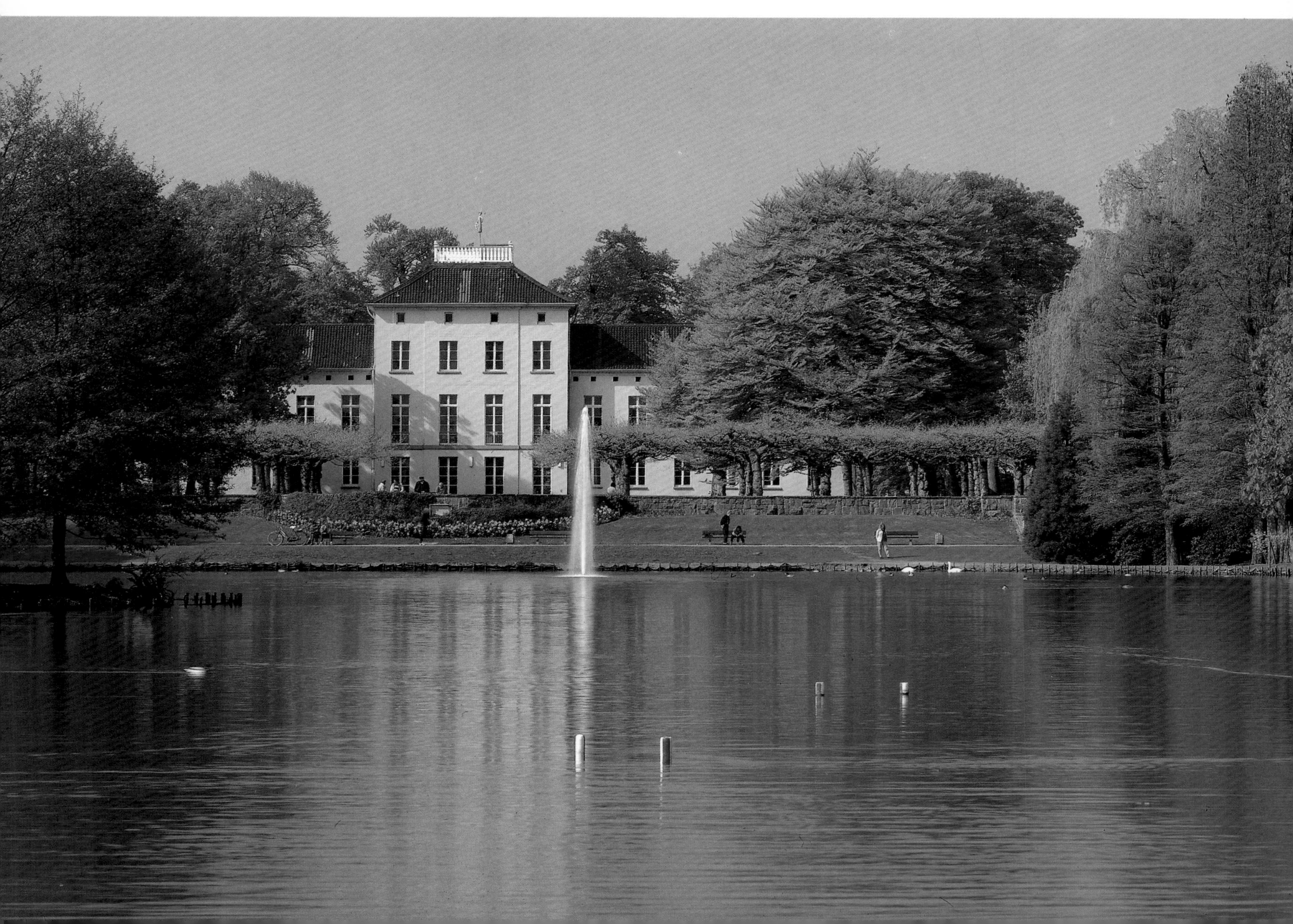

Die „Seidenbarone" traten das Erbe des niederrheinischen Landadels an. Haus Sollbrügen, ehemals ein kleiner Rittersitz, wurde Landhaus von beinahe italienischer Prägung.

The "silk barons" followed in the footsteps of the gentry of the Lower Rhine Area. House Sollbrüggen, once a small knight's keep, became an Italian style country house.

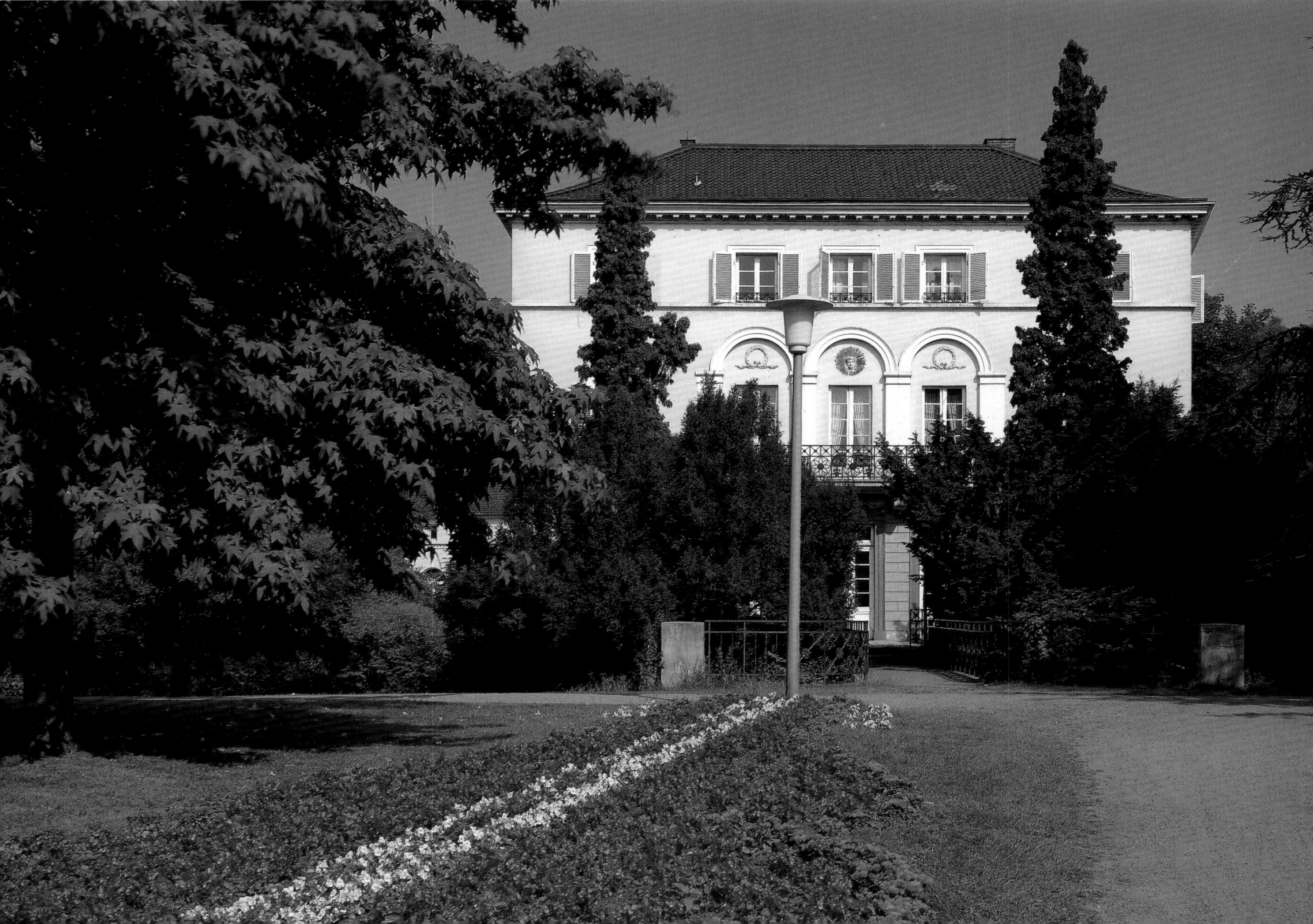

Maximilian Friedrich Weyhe, der Schöpfer des Düsseldorfer Hofgartens, fand in Krefeld viele Auftraggeber. Sein Schönhausenpark umgibt als englischer Garten heute die Musikhochschule.

Das kurkölnische Lehnsgut Neuenhofen bekam sein gefälliges Aussehen als Landsitz der Familien Floh und de Greiff. Heute ist es als Zentrale des Deutschen Roten Kreuzes nützlich.

Maximilian Friedrich Weyhe, who created the Hofgarten in Düsseldorf, also found sponsors in Krefeld. Nowadays, his English-style Schönhausenpark surrounds the Music School.

The former fiefdom of electoral Cologne, Neuenhofen, received its charming looks when it served as a country residence of the Floh and de Greiff families. Today it houses the headquarters of the German Red Cross.

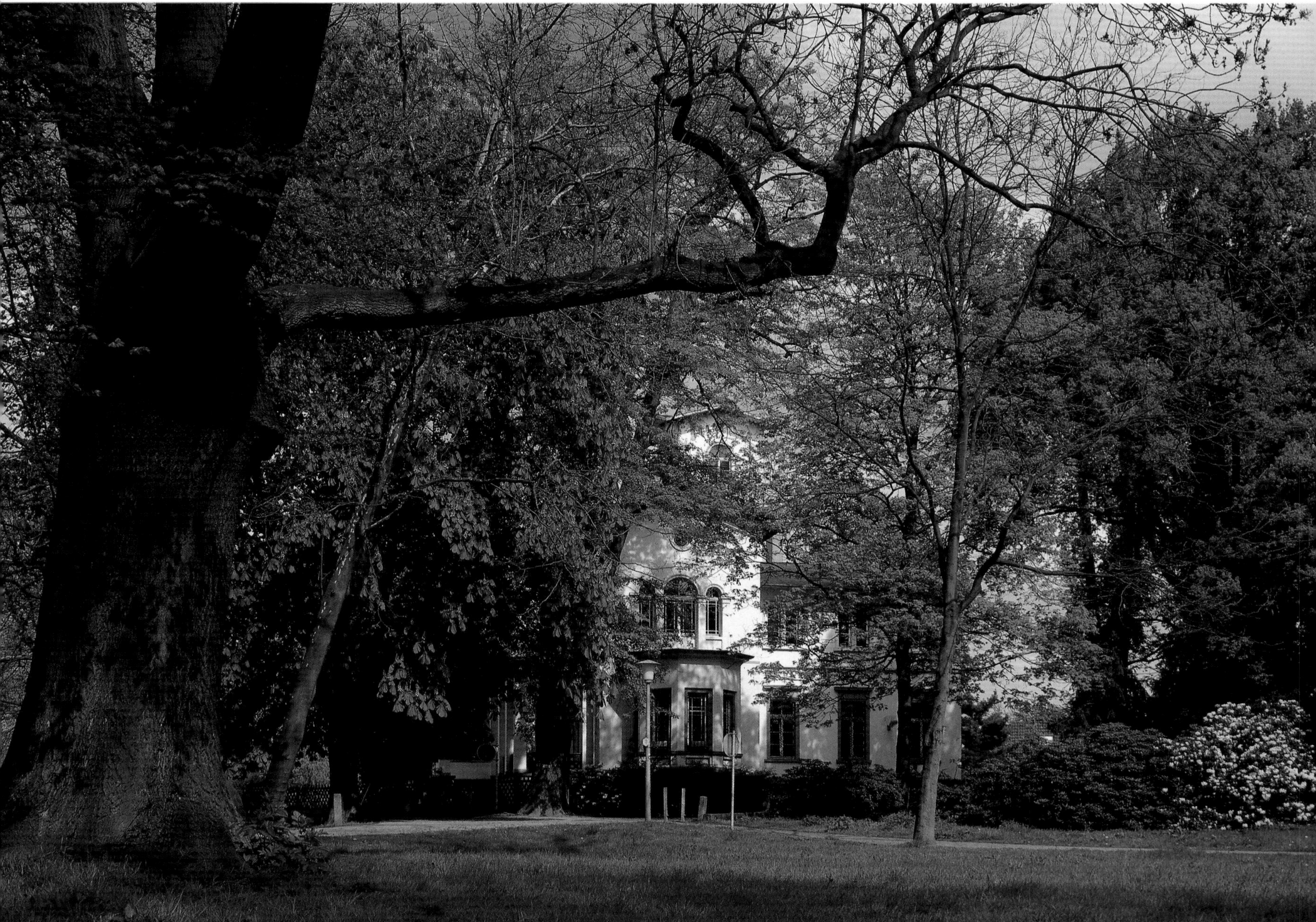

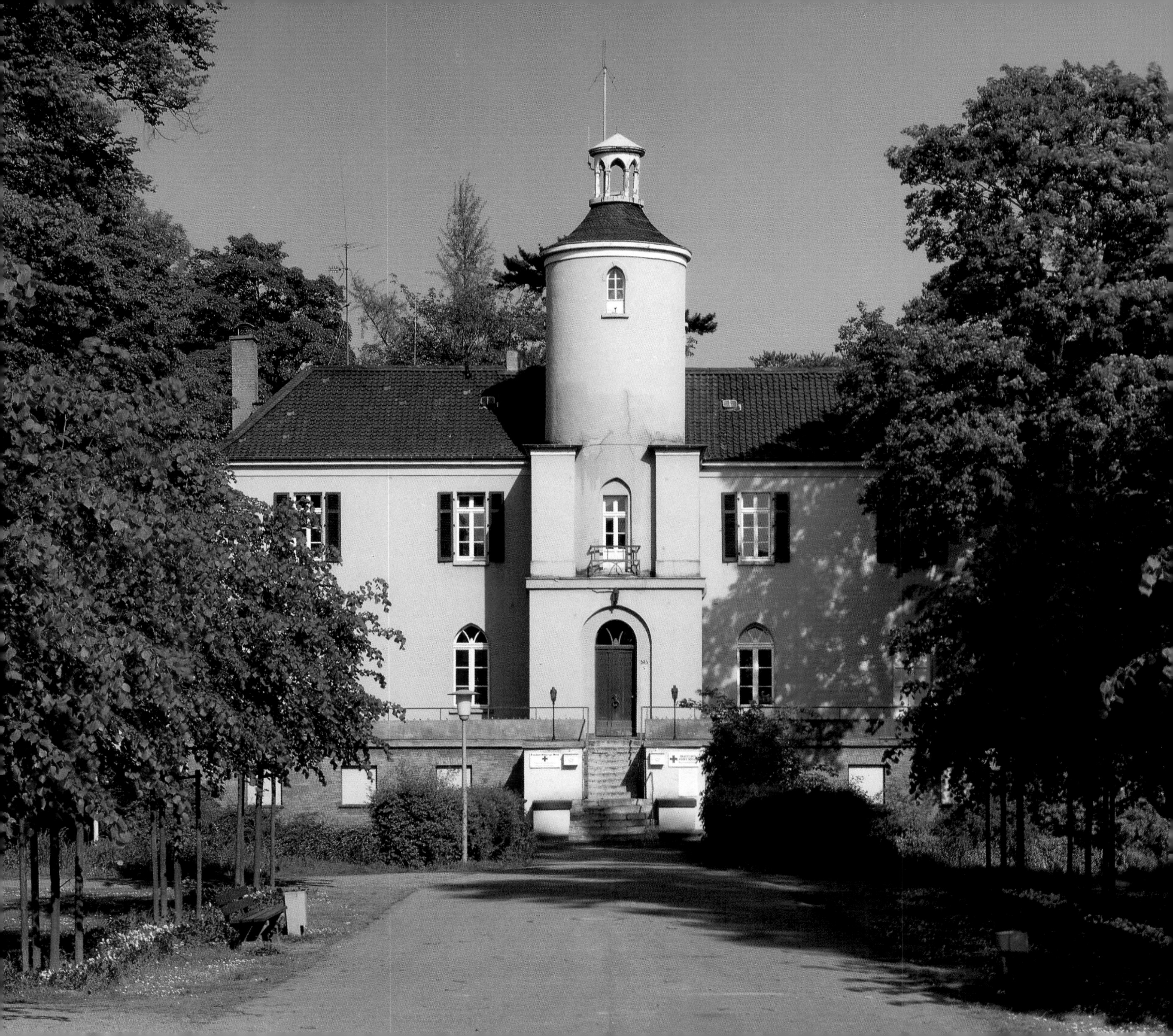

Ins Grüne zog es die Krefelder als frichgebackene Großstädter schon um die Jahrhundertwende. Bis heute ist das Stadtwaldhaus mit seinem Biergarten Ziel der Spaziergänger.

Even at the turn of the century, the people of Krefeld, having just become citizens of a big city, appreciated a little fresh air. The Stadtwaldhaus with its beergarden is still a popular place for Sunday outings.

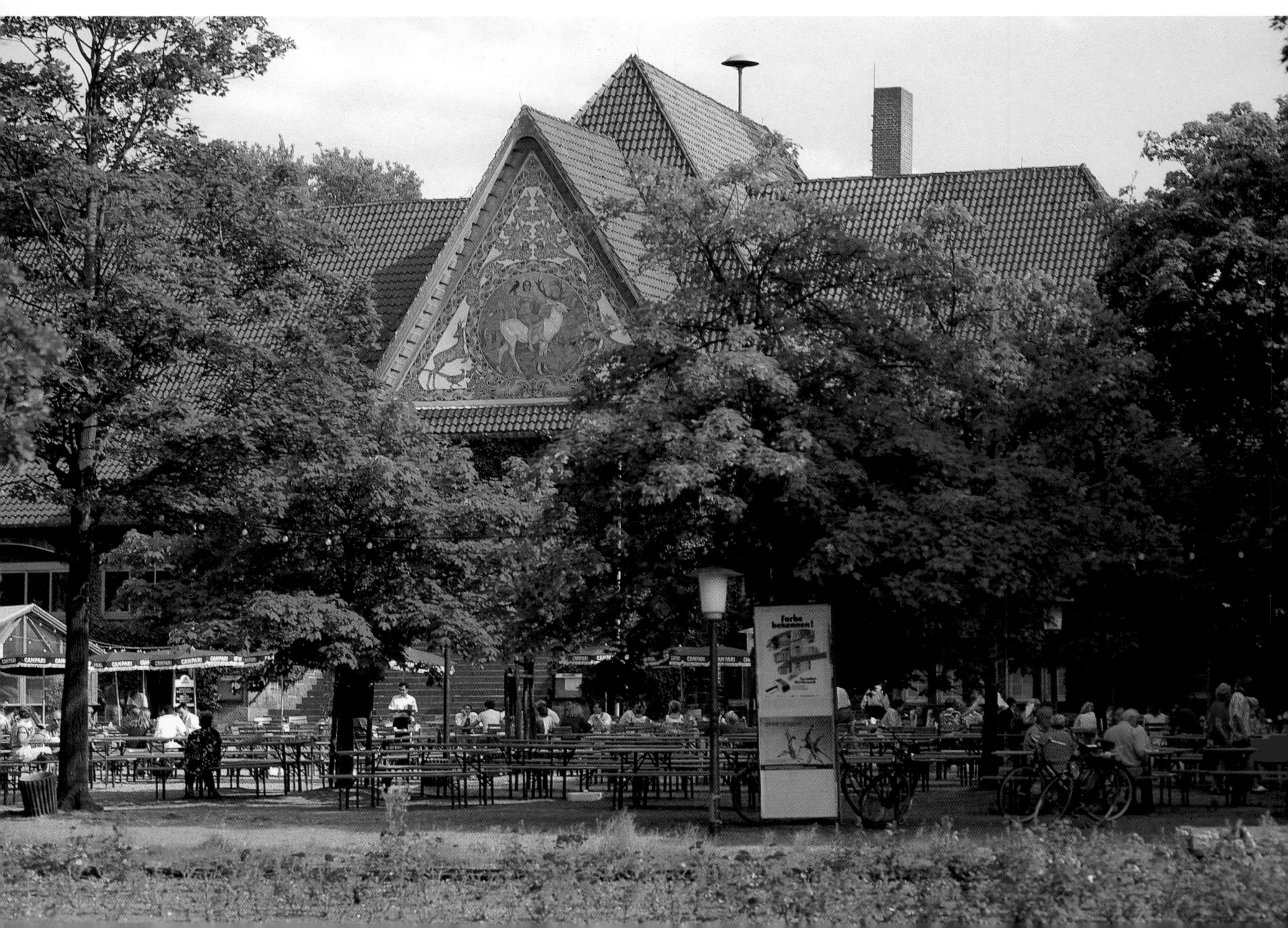

Der Seidenfabrikant Deuß schenkte seiner Heimatstadt einen Wald. Um 1900 war daraus ein 119 Hektar großer Park mit weitläufigen Wiesen, Galopprennbahn und Weiher geworden.

The silk manufacturer Deuss left a forest to his native city. By the year 1900 it had developed into a park of 119 hectares, encompassing expansive meadows; race track and ponds.

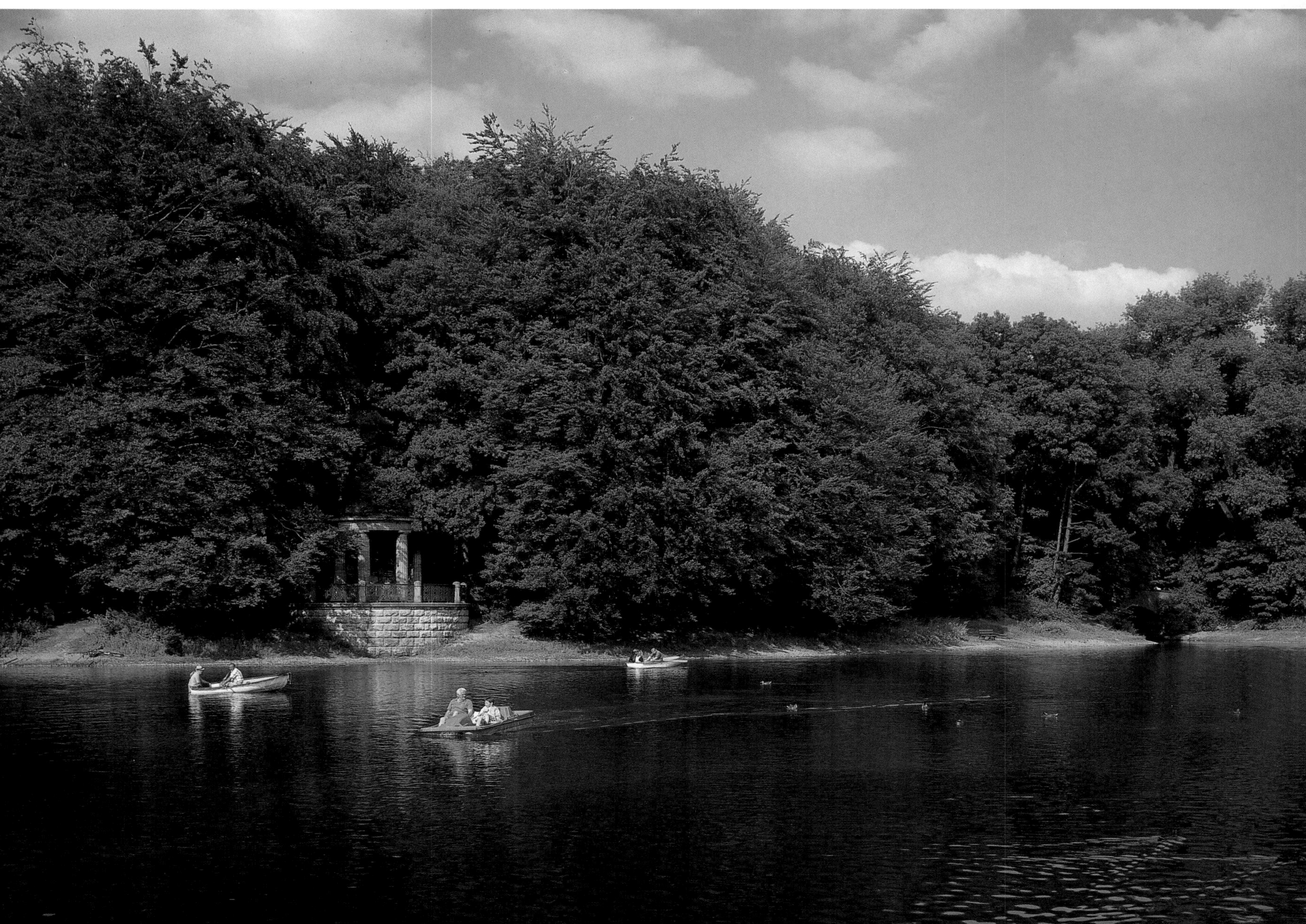

Eingebettet in die Kulisse des Stadtwaldes ist die Krefelder Galopp-Rennbahn eine der schönsten im Lande. Die Rennen werden von großem Publikum mit Interesse verfolgt.

With the municipal forest in the background, the Krefeld race track is one of the most beautiful in the country. The races draw large crowds and are watched with great interest.

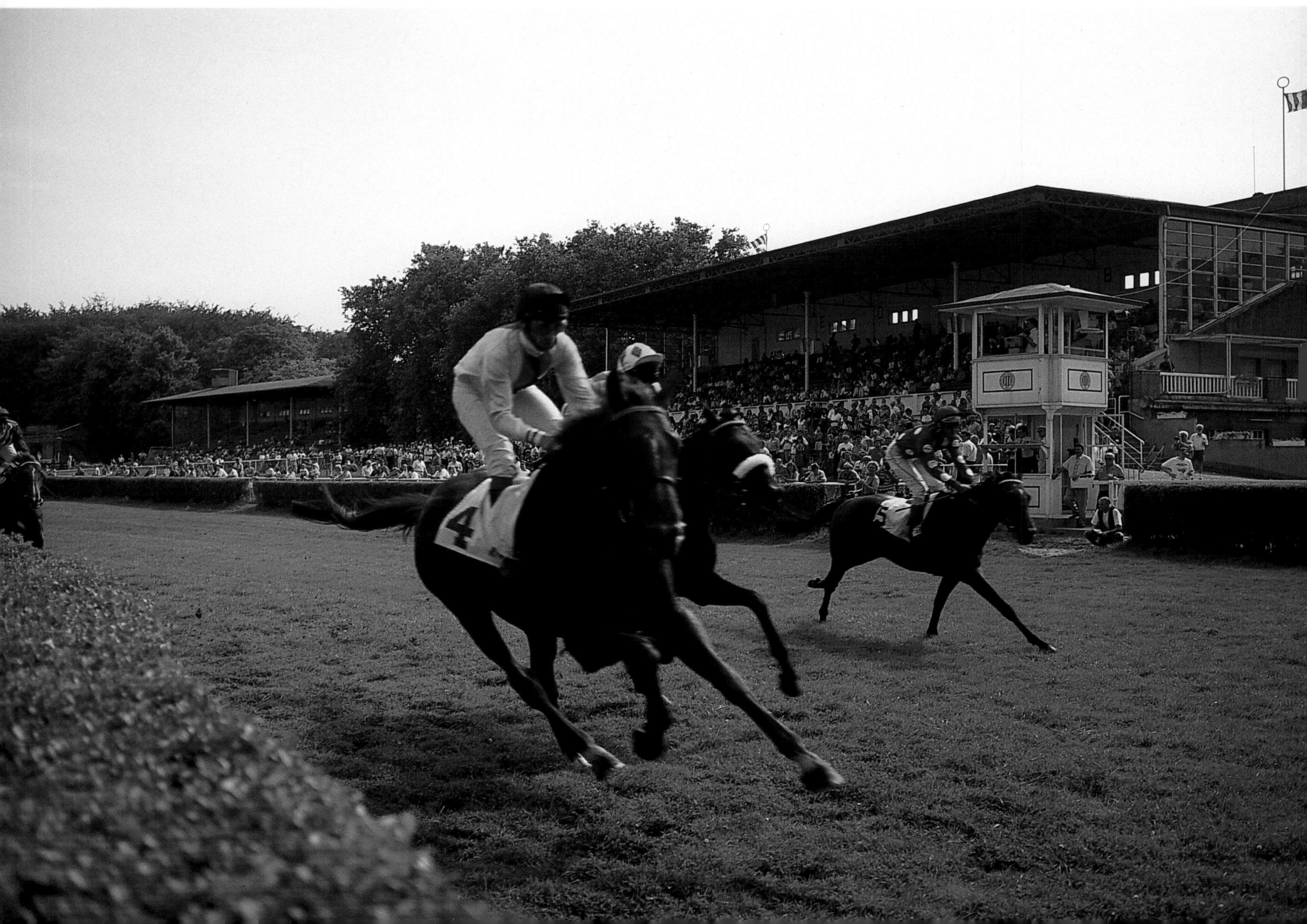

Auf dem städtischen Großhüttenhof unterhält die Landwirtschaftskammer Rheinland ihre Lehr- und Versuchsanstalt für Obstbau und Geflügelzucht, die auch Vermarktungskonzepte erprobt.

The Chamber of Agriculture of the Rhineland operates its academy and research institute for fruit-growing and poultry farming on the city-owned Großhüttenhof. New marketing concepts are also tried out here.

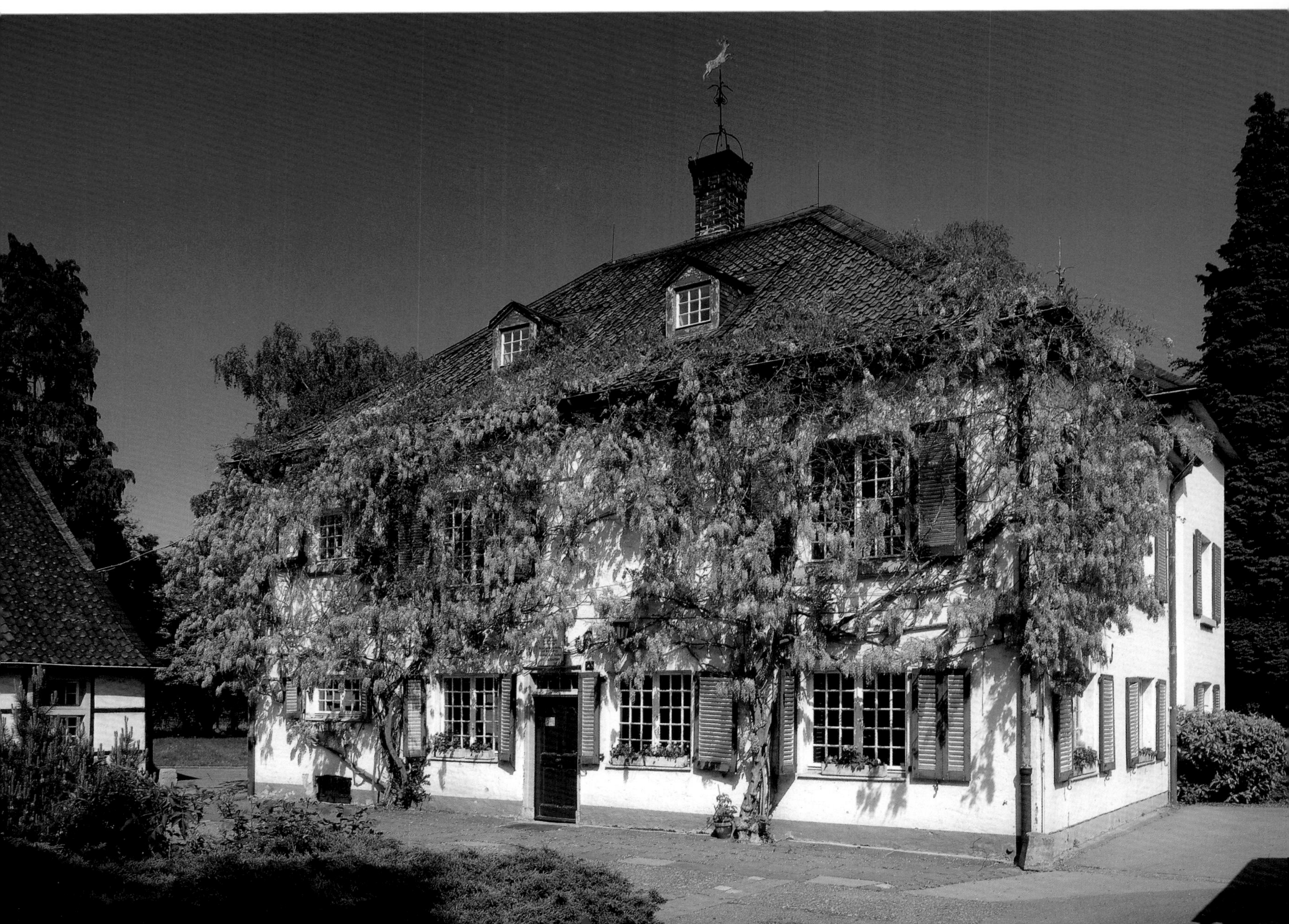

Den Kennern der Eishockey-Szene ist die Rheinlandhalle ein Begriff. Temperamentvoll stärken die Krefelder „ihrem" KEV bei Bundesligaspielen den Rücken.

The Rheinlandhalle is a byword among ice hockey enthusiasts and the Krefeld fans never fail to provide ardent support for their home team in league matches.

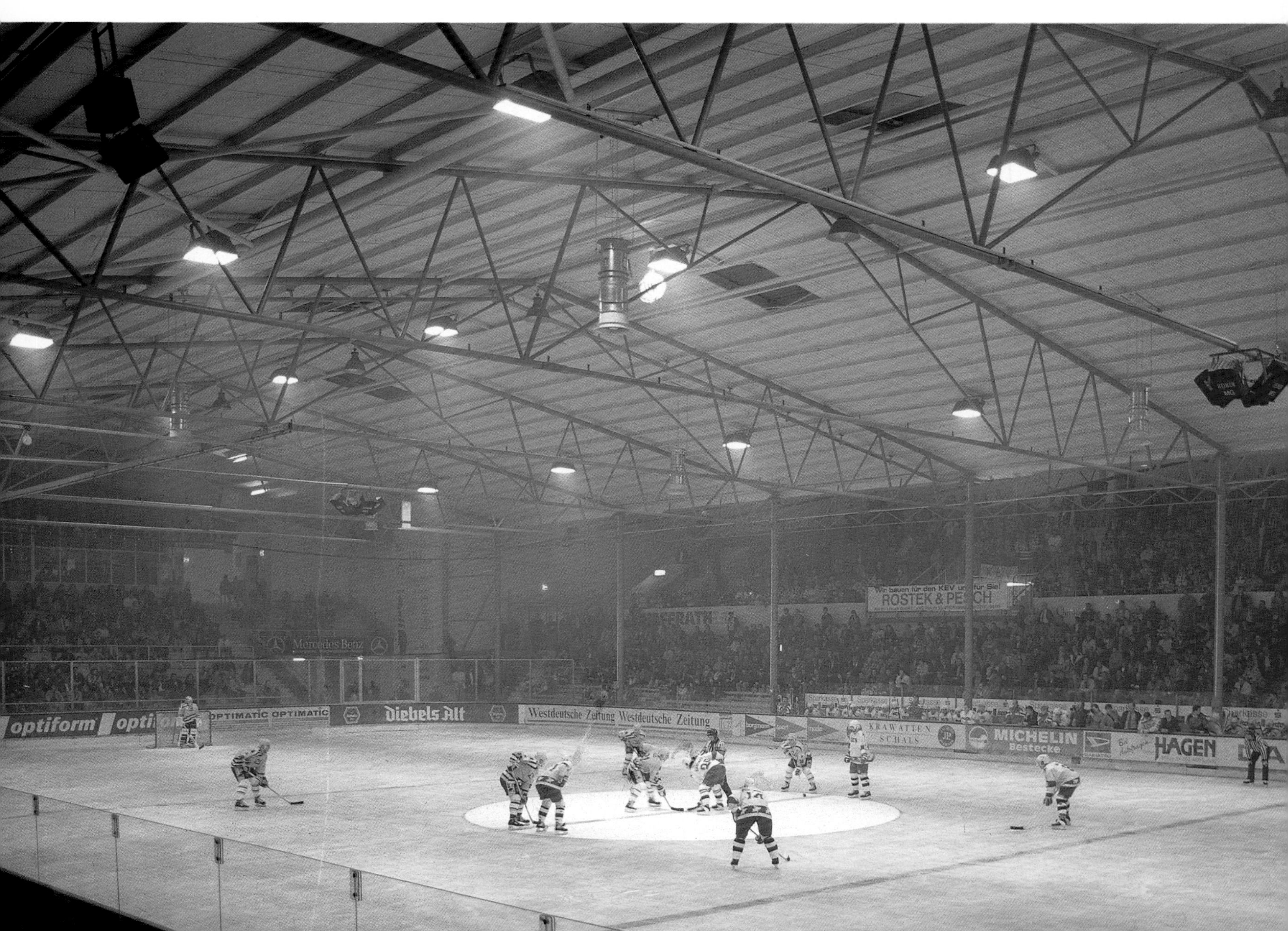

Ein Drittel aller Krefelder ist sportlich aktiv. Soviel Bewegungsdrang gipfelt im Bundesliga-Fußball mit der Mannschaft des FC Bayer 05 Uerdingen bei Begegnungen im Grotenburg-Stadion.

A third of Krefeld's population participates in some kind of sport. For many, one of the highlights of the sporting year will be a hard-fought German league football match in the Grotenburg stadium.

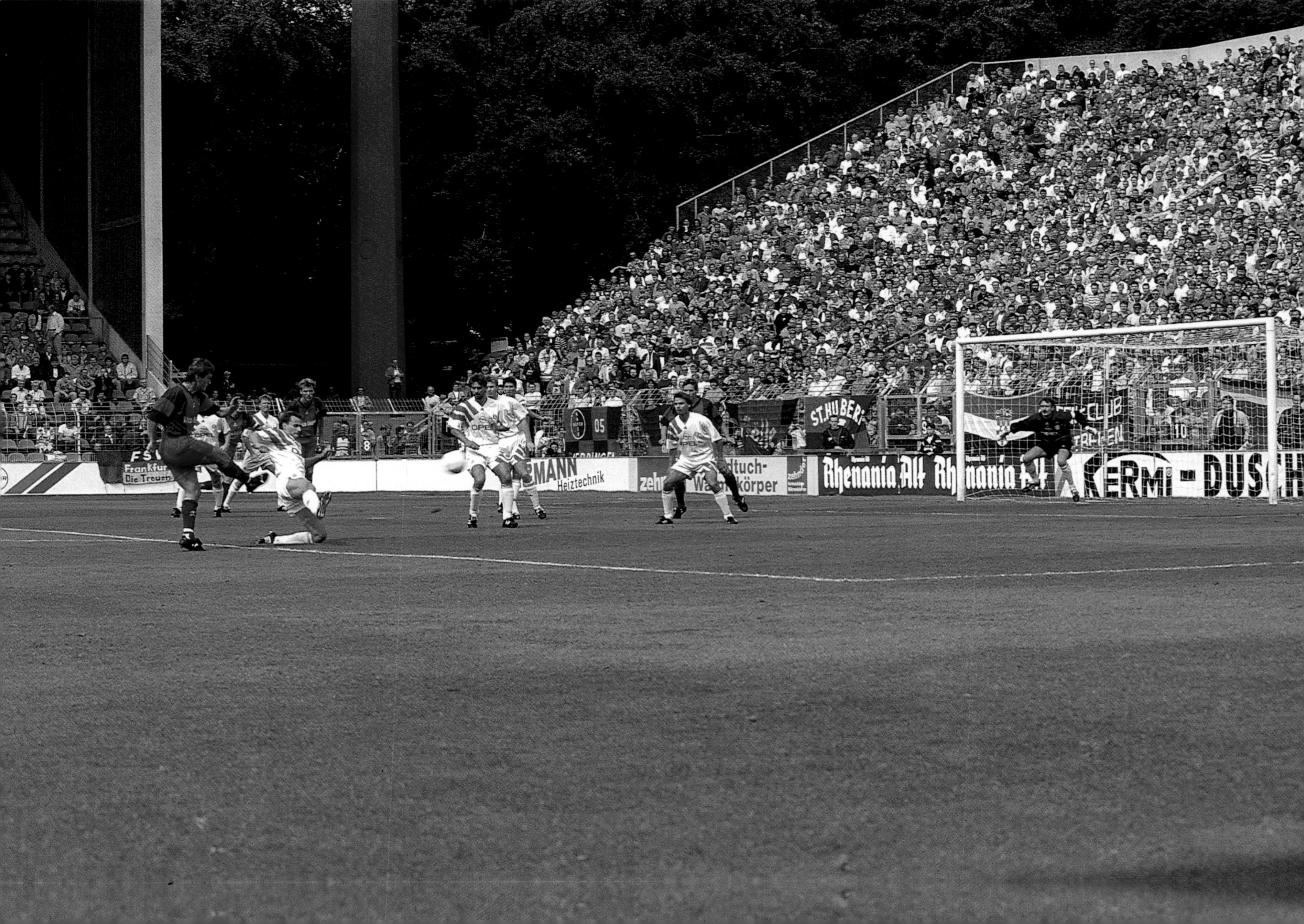

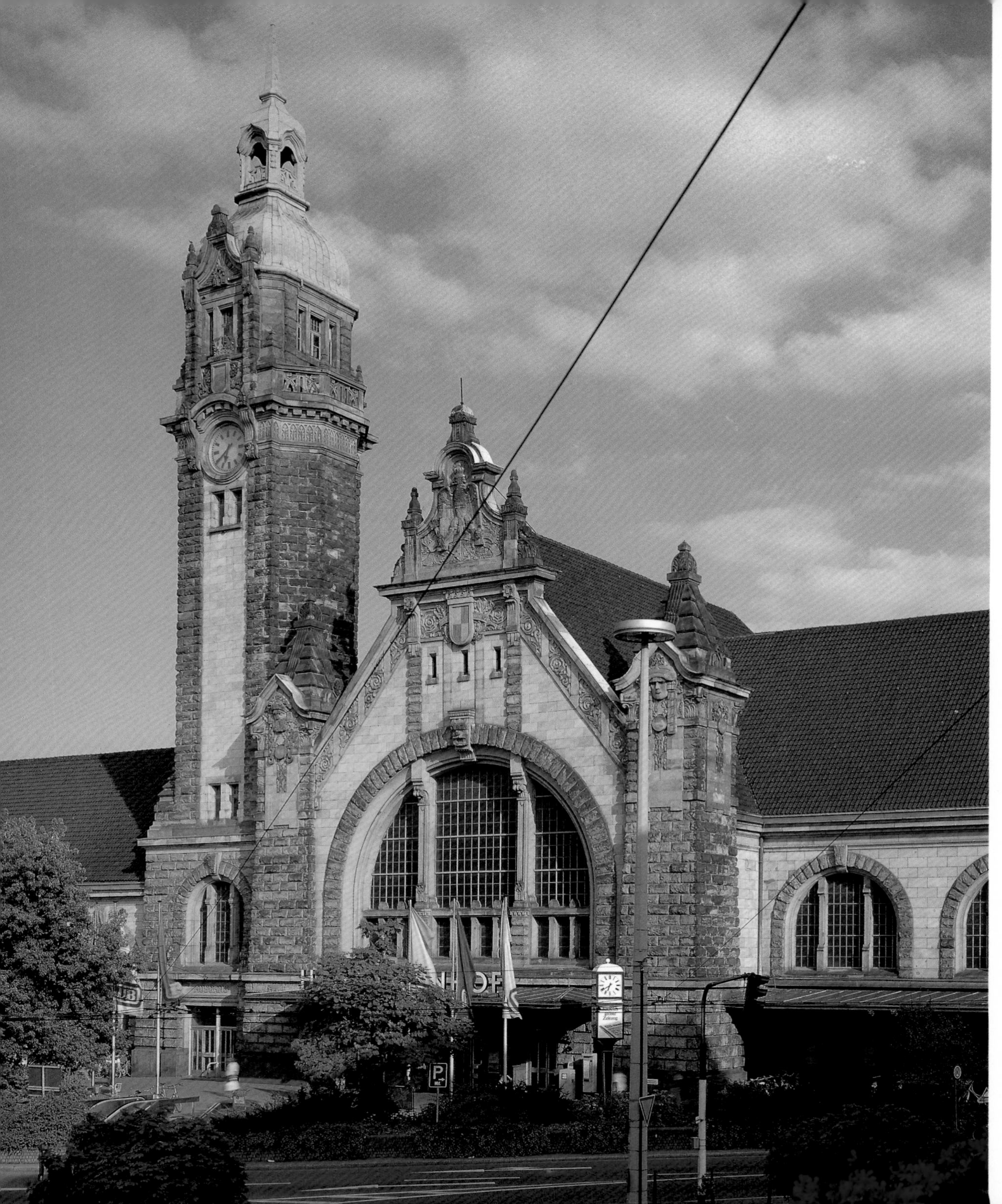

HAUPTBAHNHOF / Central Station

Die Krefelder Bahnanlagen krönte der preußische Staat im Jahre 1906 mit einem repräsentativen Bahnhofsbau, zu dem auch das gläserne Gewölbe der Gleishalle gehört.

The Krefeld rail facilities were "crowned" with a distinctive railway station, including the glass vault, in 1906, sponsored by the Prussian State.

Die malerische Handelsstadt Uerdingen wurde vor hundert Jahren zur Industriestadt. Nur eine kurze aber liebevoll gestaltete Anlage unterbricht die Fabrik-Kulisse am Stromufer.

The picturesque mercantile centre of Uerdingen became an industrial city a hundred years ago. The long row of factories is broken up only by a small but beautifully laid-out park.

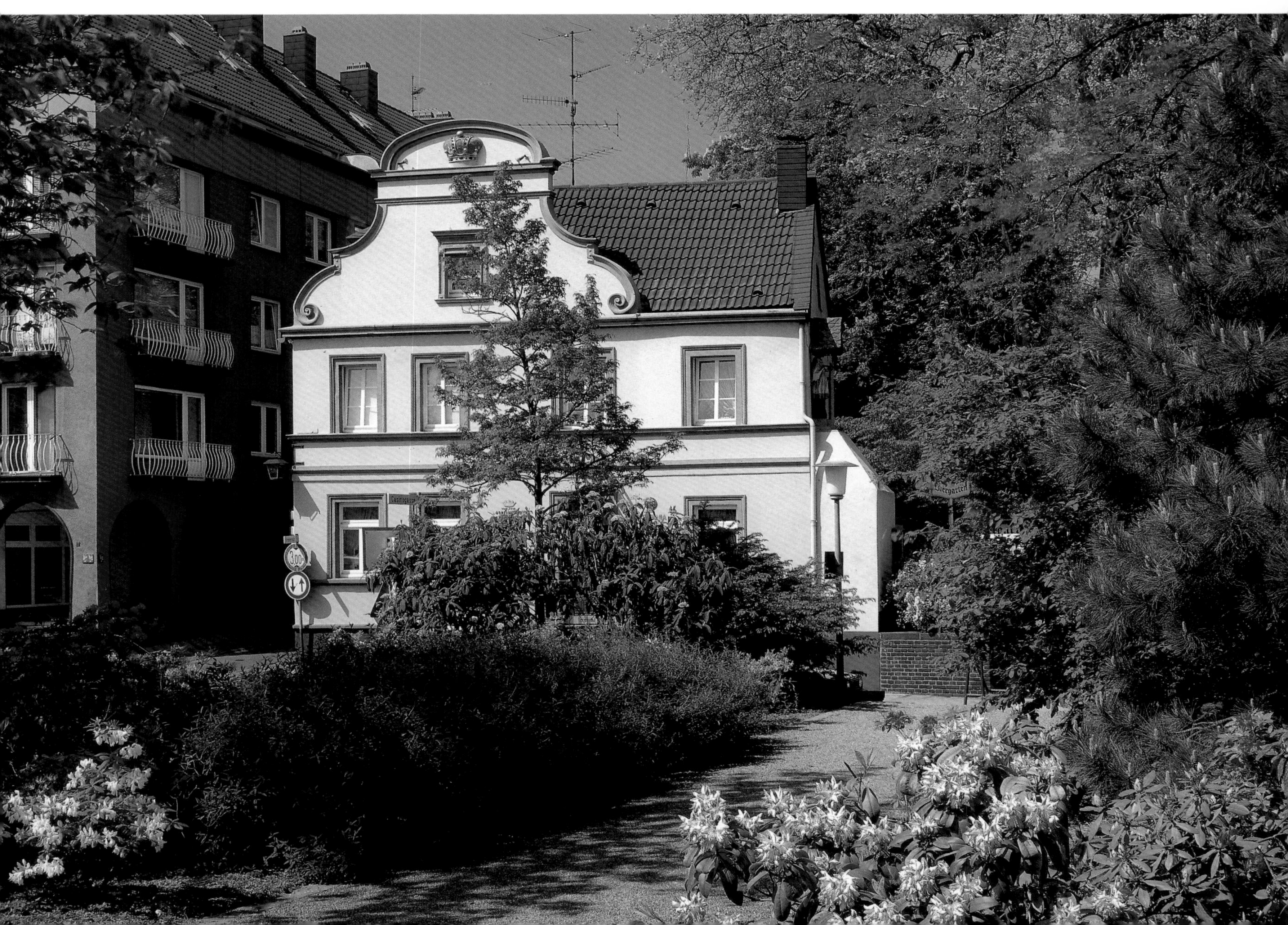

Die Rheinufer von Krefeld und Duisburg verbindet seit 1936 eine Brücke. Die Stahlkonstruktion vereint auch nach dem kriegsbedingten Wiederaufbau Technik und Schönheit.

The banks of the Rhine at Krefeld and Duisburg have been connected by a bridge since 1936. The steel construction combines both technology and beauty, even with its reconstruction after the war.

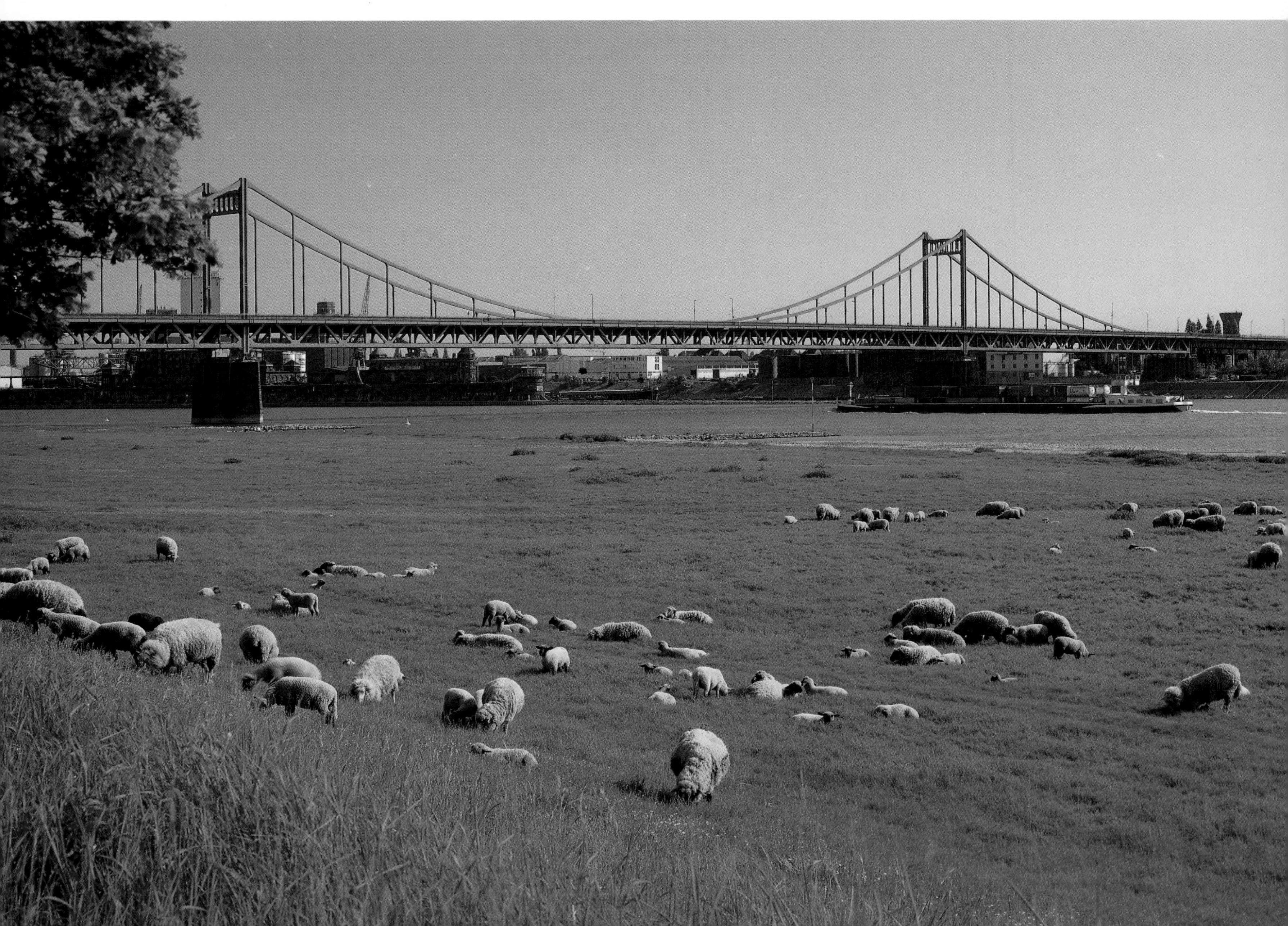

Den Krisentälern der textilen Monostruktur versuchte die Stadt 1902 mit der Eingemeindung des Städtchens Linn und dem damit möglichen Bau des Rheinhafens zu entkommen.

Das Bild auf der folgenden Doppelseite zeigt einen Überblick über die imponierenden Uerdinger Industriekulisse mit dem größten Betrieb der Stadt, den Bayer Werken.

In 1902 Krefeld tried to counter the doldrums of its textile monoculture by incorporating the small town of Linn into the city. Thus, the building of a harbour on the Rhine became possible.

The picture on the following two pages shows the impressive industrial skyline of Uerdingen with the town's largest firm, the Bayer works.

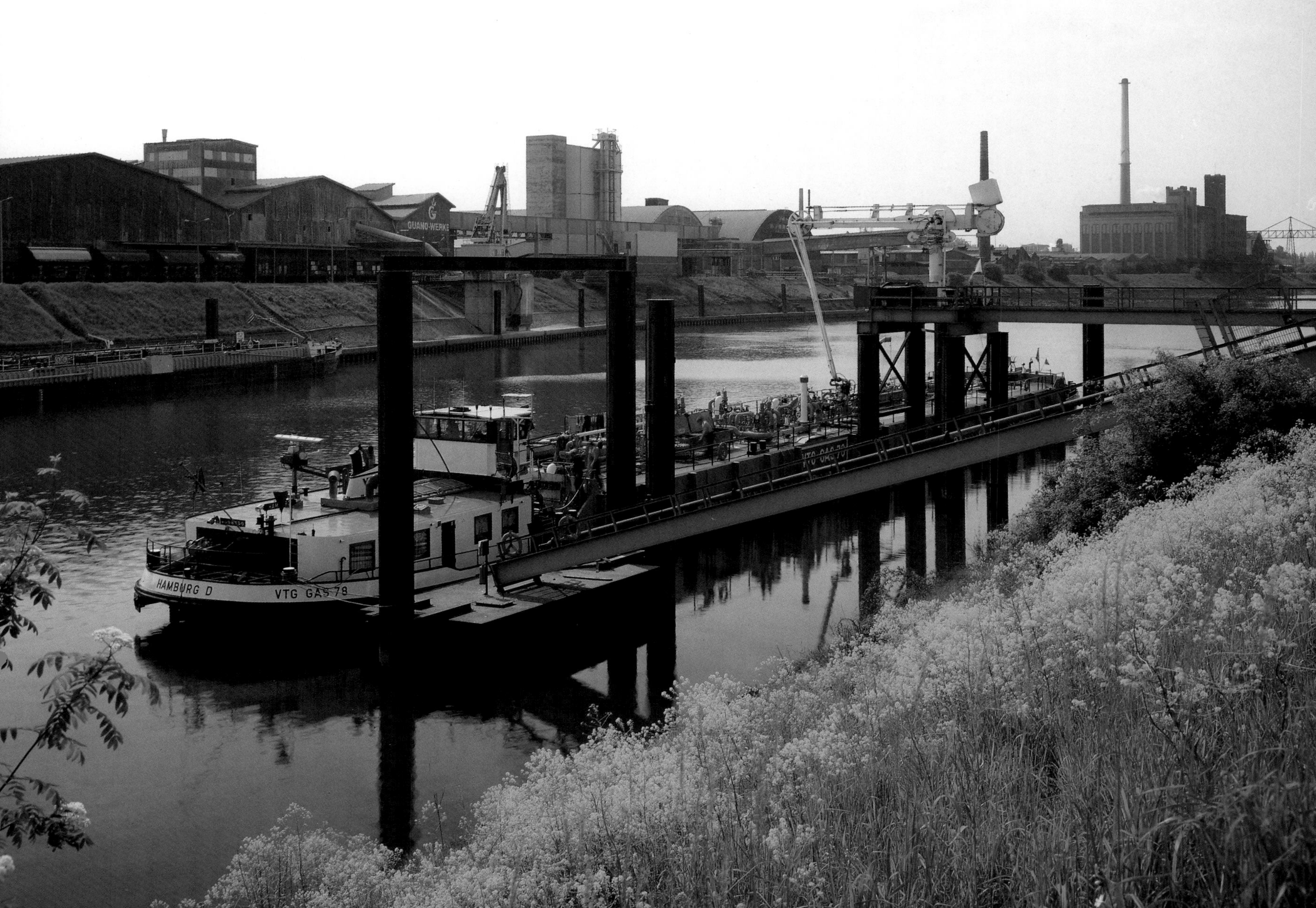

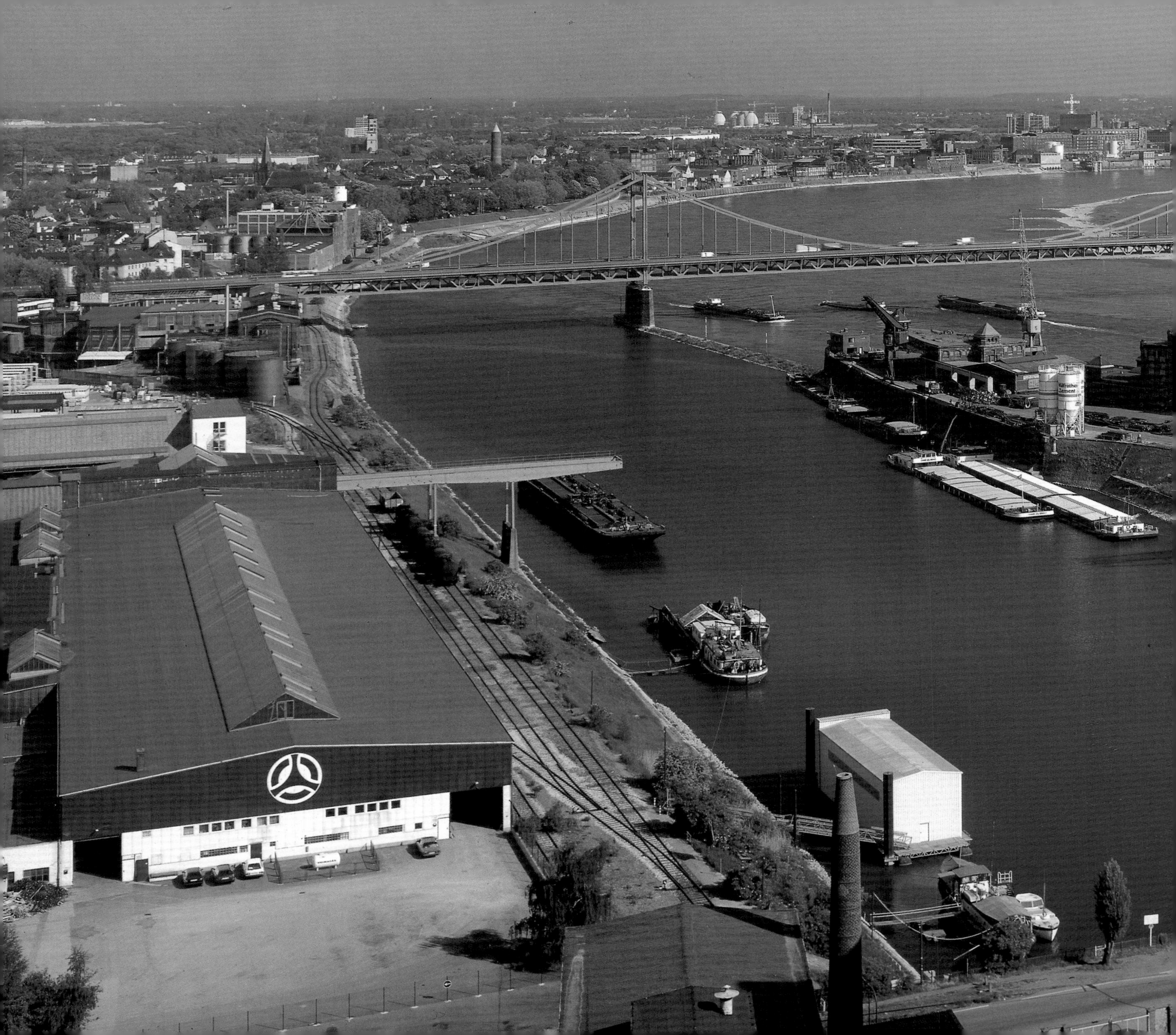
5
Zement

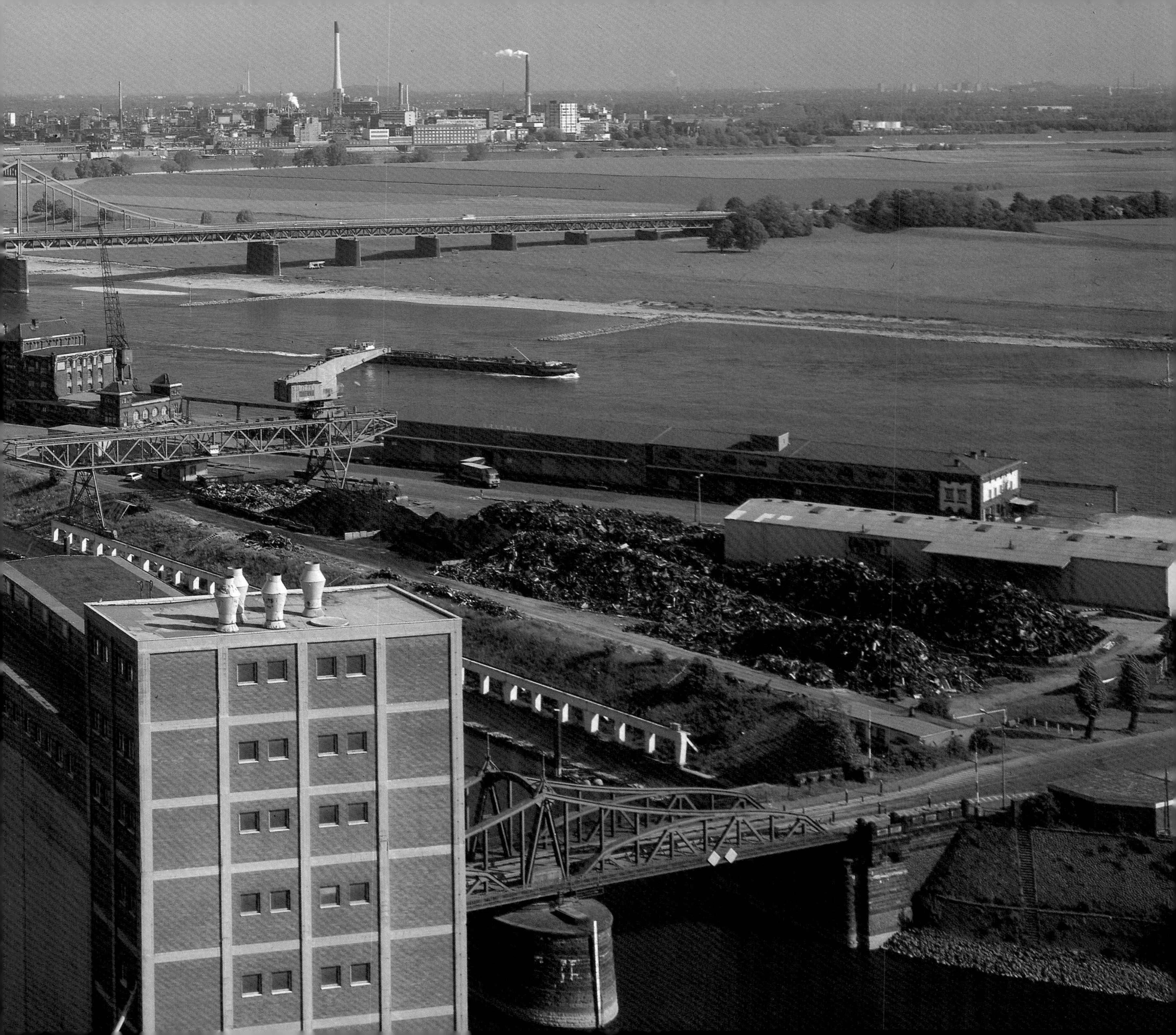

Der Kaufmann Balthasar Herberz baute für sich und seine Brüder die drei Häuser, die als Westfront des Uerdinger Marktes das Bild des schönen Platzes maßgeblich bereichern.

The merchant Balthasar Herberz built three houses for himself and his brothers. They constitute the western front of the market square of Uerdingen, contributing significantly to its picturesque appearance.

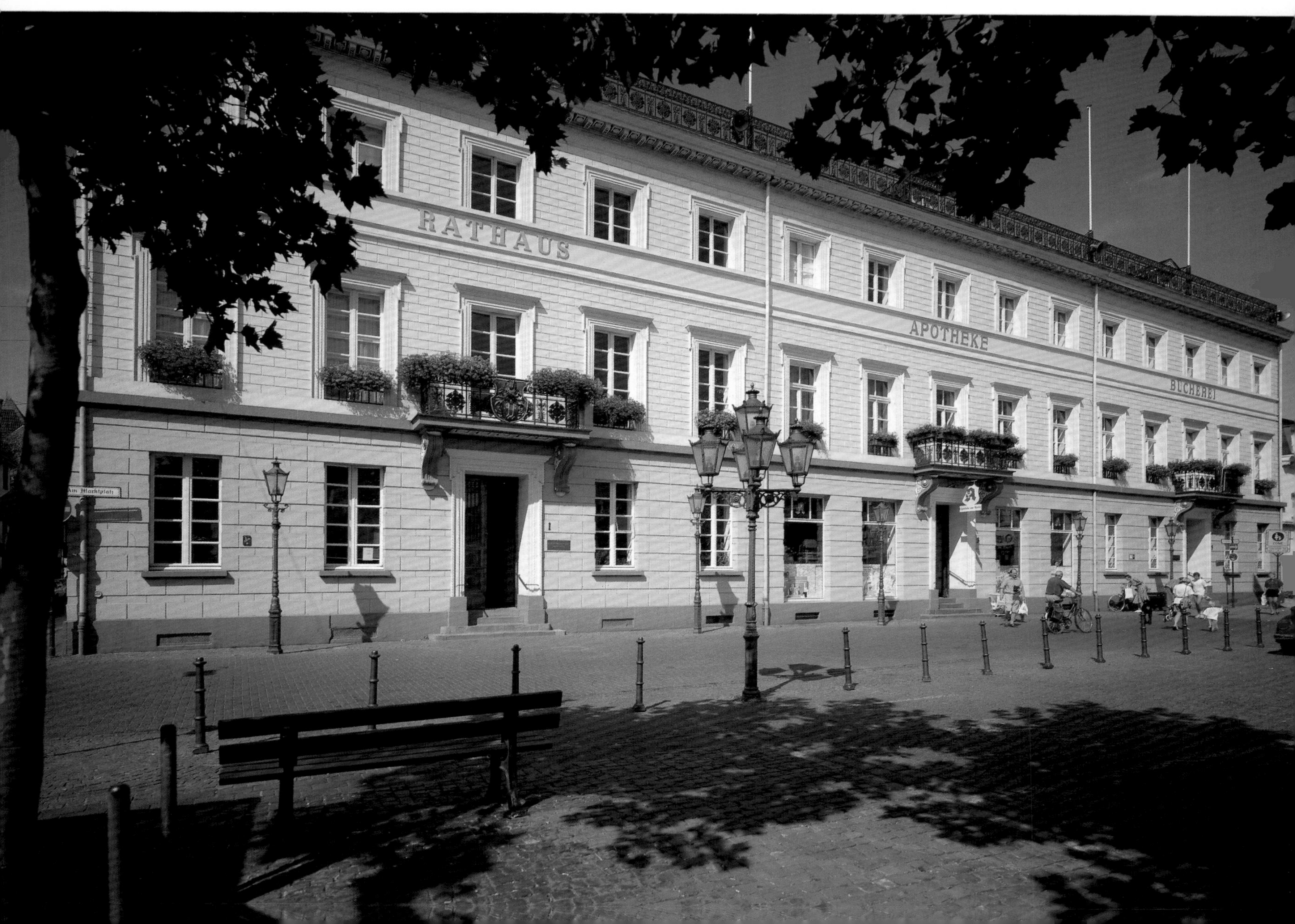

Balthasar Herberz ließ seinen Salon im Stil der Spätrenaissance ausmalen. Das Haus ist heute Bezirksrathaus, der schöne Saal bei Brautpaaren als Rahmen der Trauung beliebt.

Balthasar Herberz had the hall painted in the late Renaissance style. The building now serves as a district city hall. This beautiful room is sought after by couples as a setting for their wedding ceremonies.

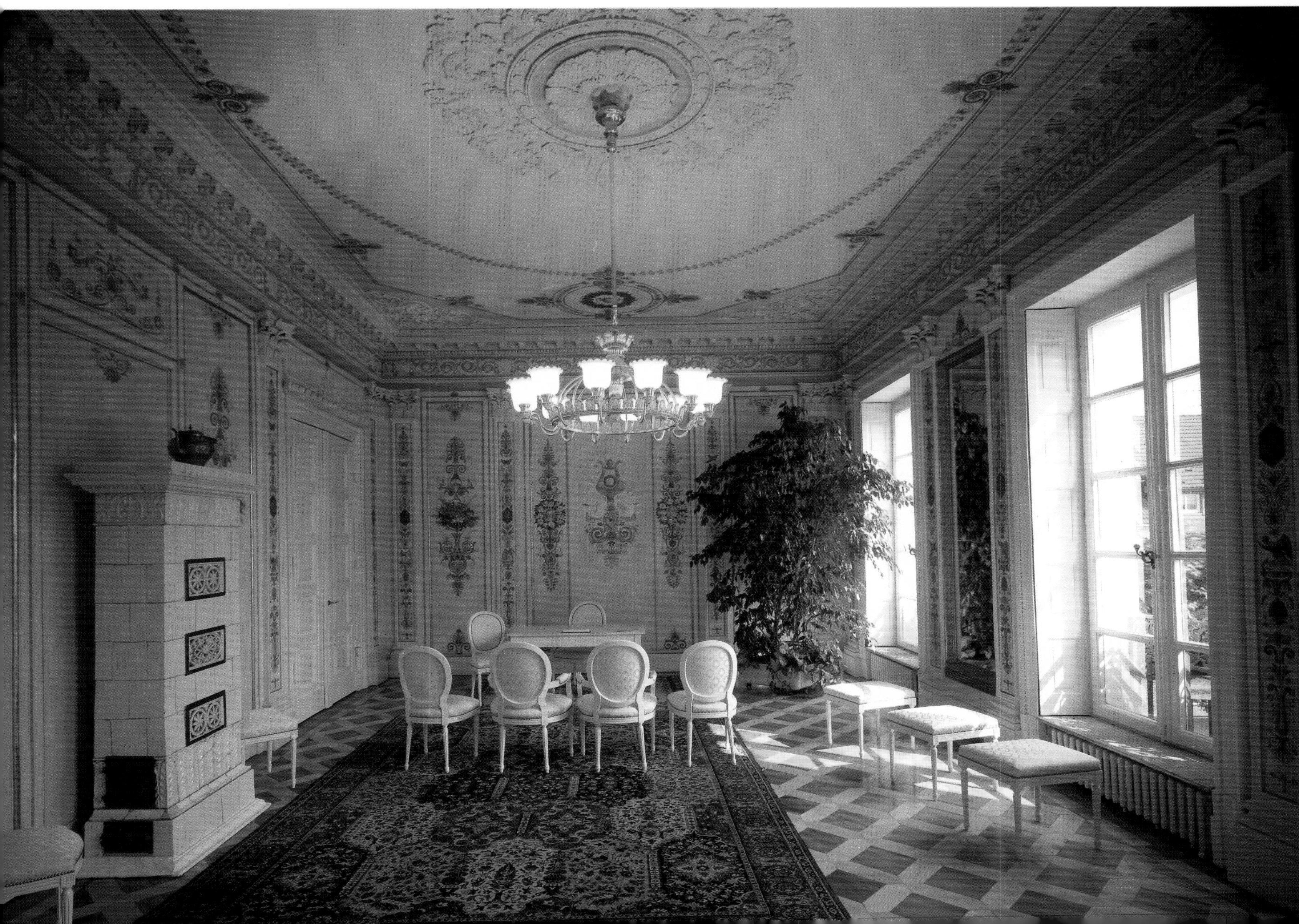

Die historische Nachbarschaft von kirchlicher und weltlicher Mitte einer alten Stadt ist in Uerdingen erhalten. In der Mitte der südlichen Häuserzeile des Marktes steht das alte Rathaus.

In Uerdingen the historical proximity of clerical and secular centres, typical of old towns, is preserved. The old city hall stands in the centre of the row of houses at the southern end of the market square.

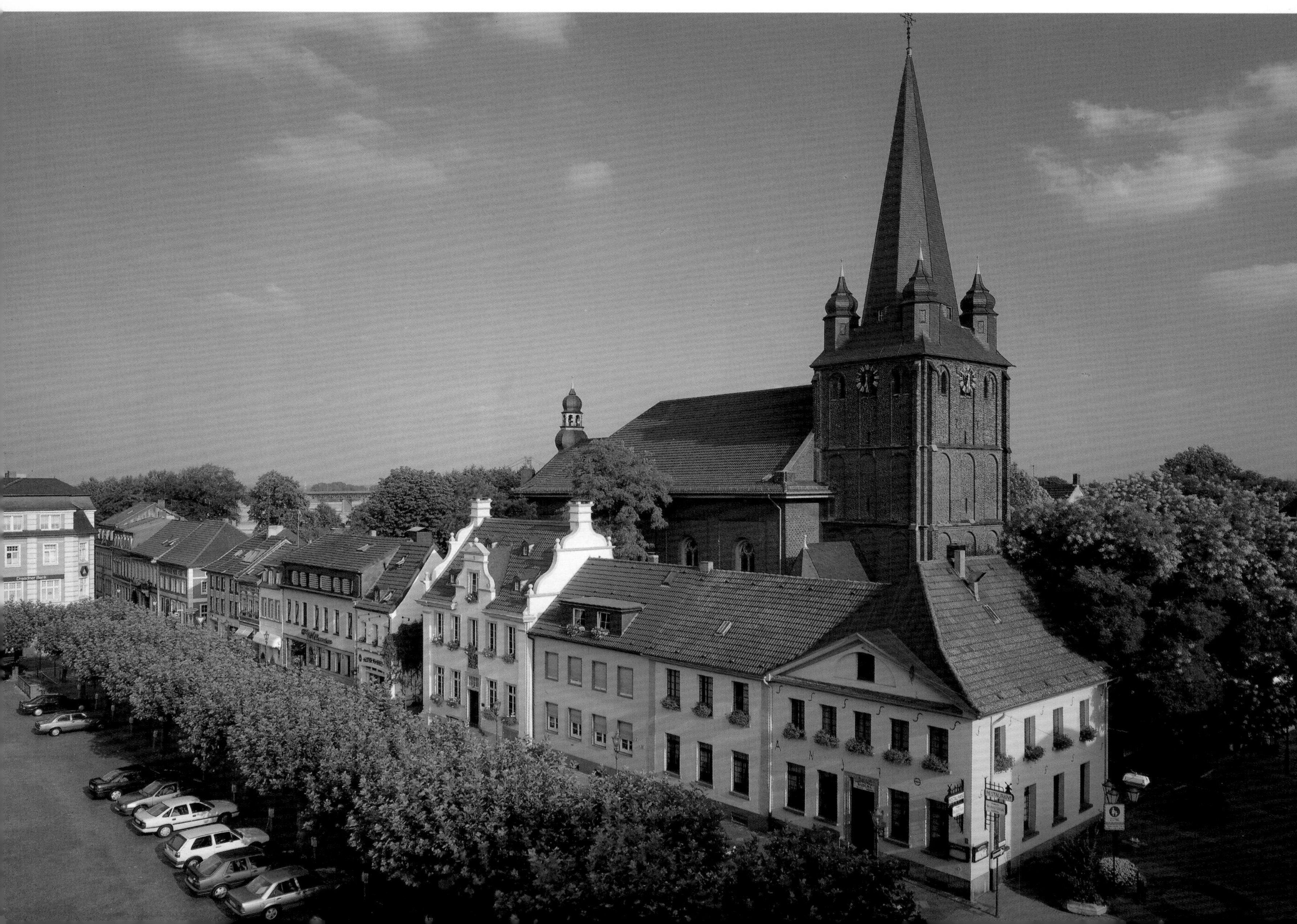

Fränkische Stammesfürsten, klevische Grafen, Kölner Erzbischöfe und Kurfürsten, Krefelder Seidenbarone und schließlich die Stadt besaßen die Burg, die jetzt Museum ist.

Franconian chiefs, counts of Kleve, archbishops and electors of Cologne, silk barons of Krefeld and, finally, the city have all owned the castle, which now serves as a museum.

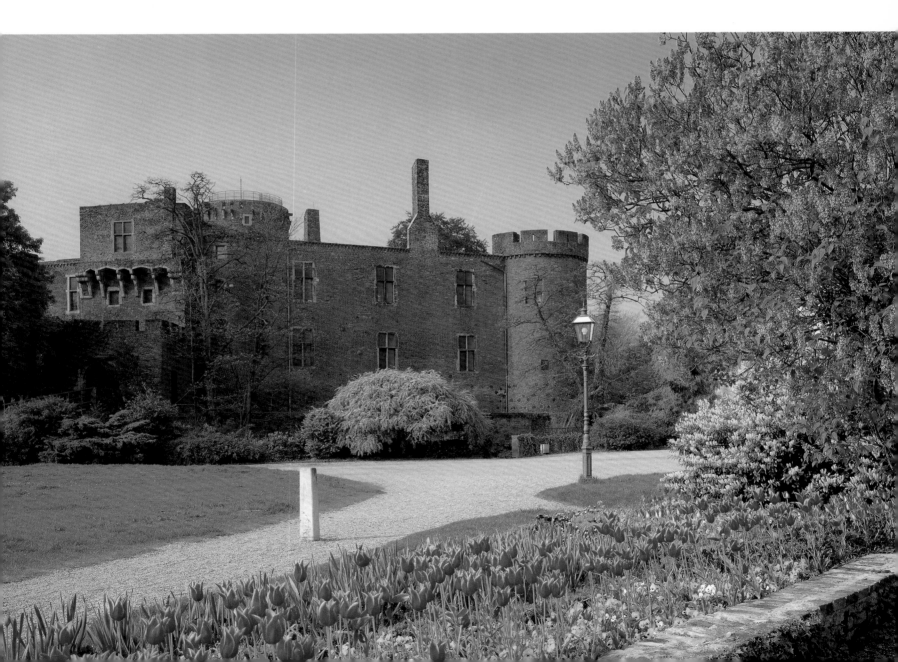

Mechtild von Geldern, verwitwete Gräfin von Kleve, übernahm im 14. Jahrhundert Burg Linn als Witwensitz. Einigen Glanz höfischen Lebens verbreitete sie in den Rittersälen.

Alle Jahre zu Pfingsten lebt rund um die Burg der Flachsmarkt wieder auf. Deutschlands größter Handwerkermarkt könnte keine schönere Kulisse finden und lockt viele Besucher an.

Mechthild von Geldern, widowed countess of Kleve, took over Linn Castle in the 14th century as her widow's seat. She endowed the knights' hall with the splendour of courtly life.

Every year at Whitsun the flax market comes to life around the castle. The biggest artisans' market in Germany could not find a nicer backdrop and attracts a great deal of visitors.

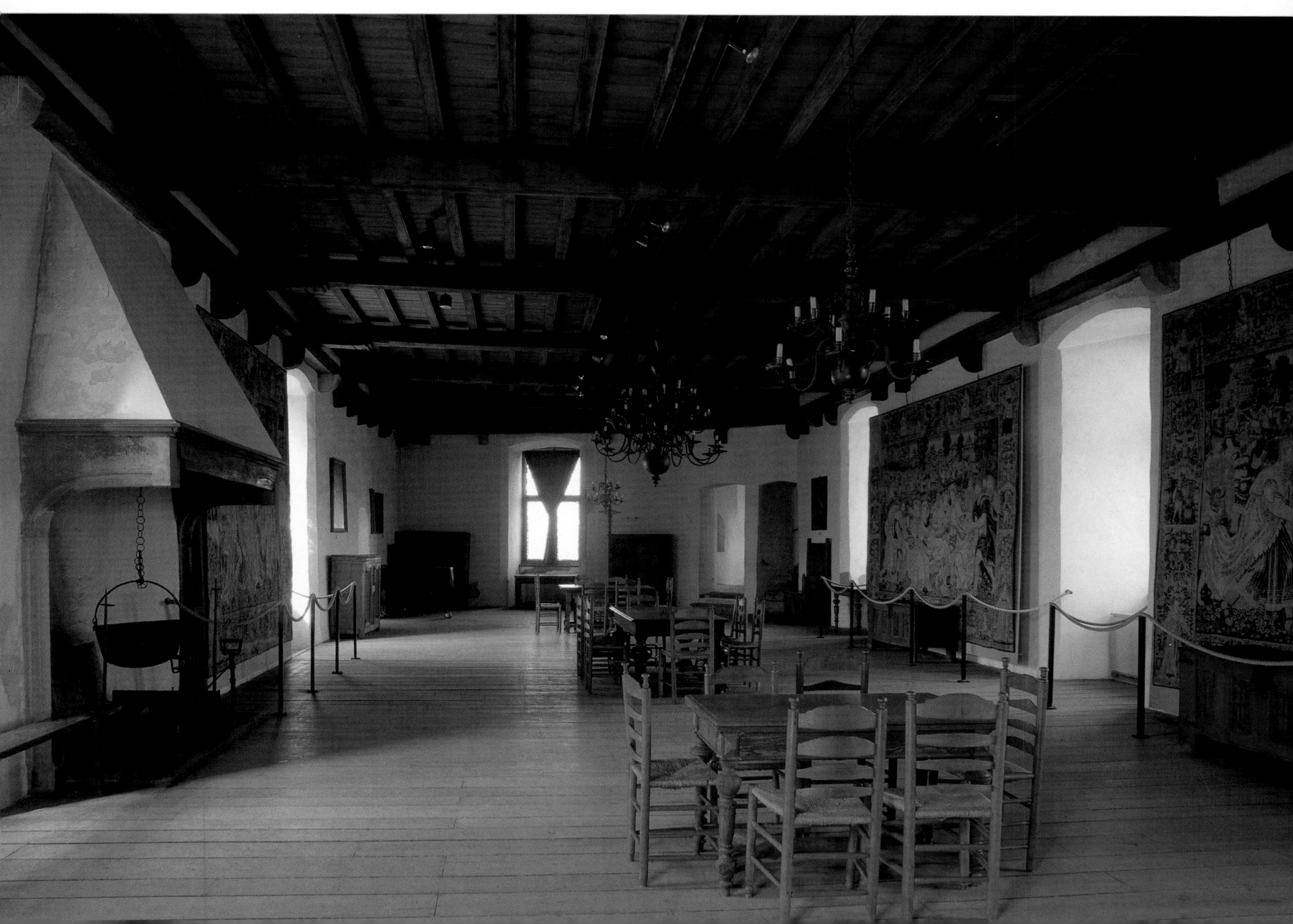

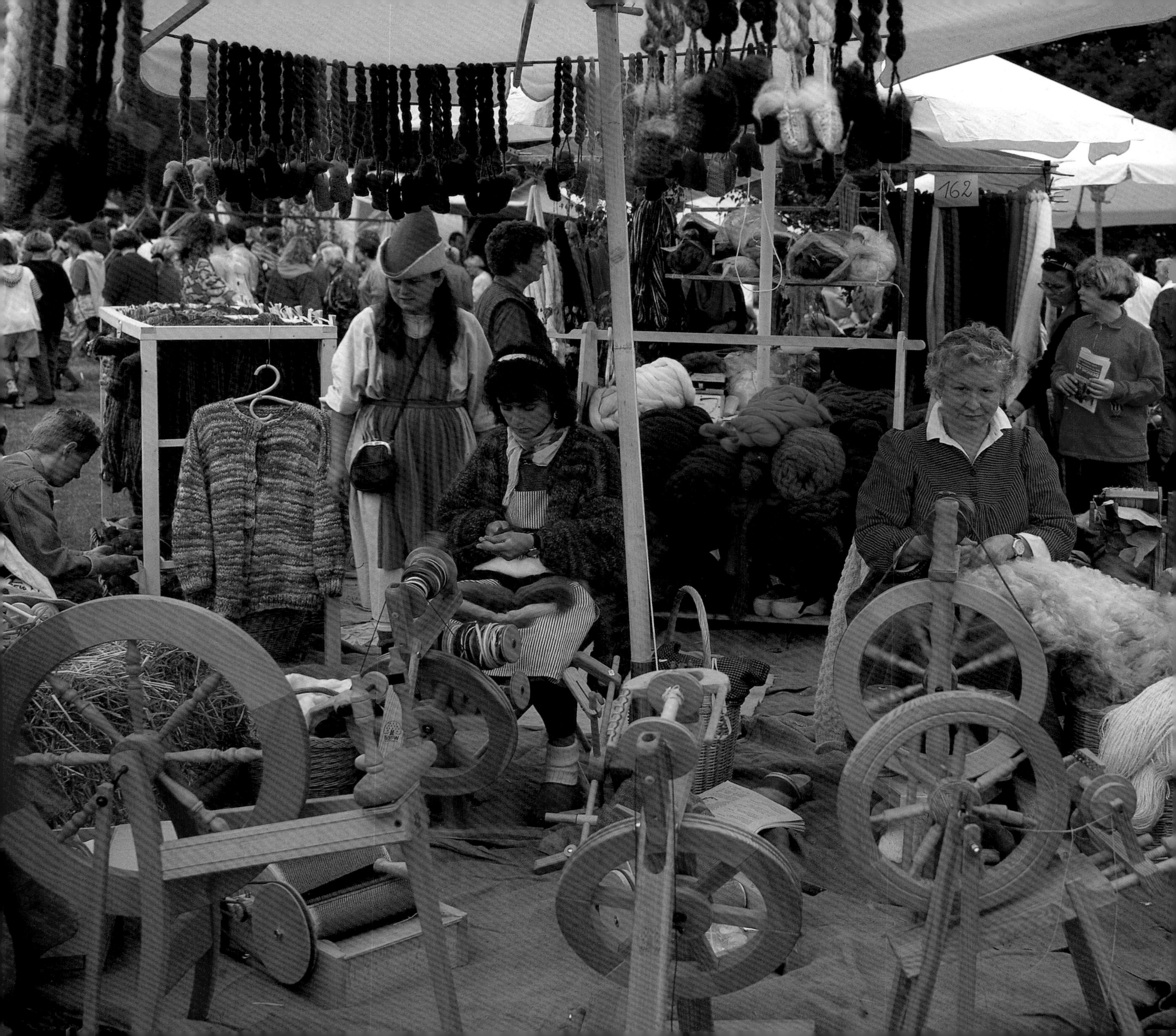
162

Das Jagdschloß im Vorhof der Burg Linn birgt als besonderen Schatz eine Küche, in der Gegenstände aus dem 18. und 19. Jahrhundert zu einer kompletten Ausstattung versammelt sind.

The hunting lodge in the front court of Linn Castle houses a special treasure, a kitchen equipped with a complete selection of objects from the 18th and 19th centuries.

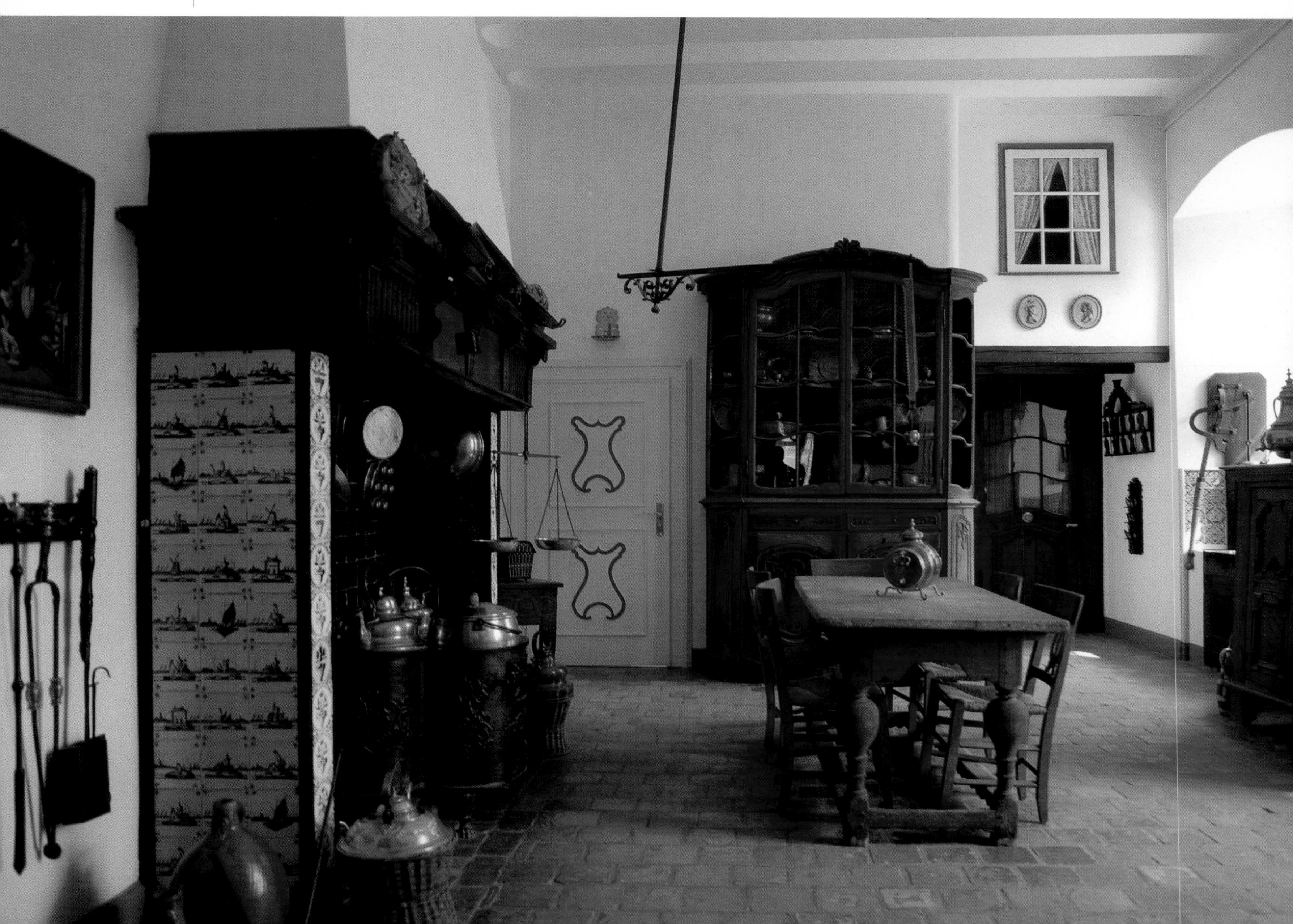

Marianne Rhodius, letzte Erbin der „Seidenbarone" de Greiff, wohnte im Linner Jagdschloß und empfing hier ihre Gäste. 1926 kamen Burg und Jagdschloß in den Besitz der Stadt.

Marianne Rhodius, the last heiress of the "silk barons" de Greiff, lived in the hunting lodge of Linn castle and received her visitors there. In 1926 the castle and hunting lodge passed into the city's ownership.

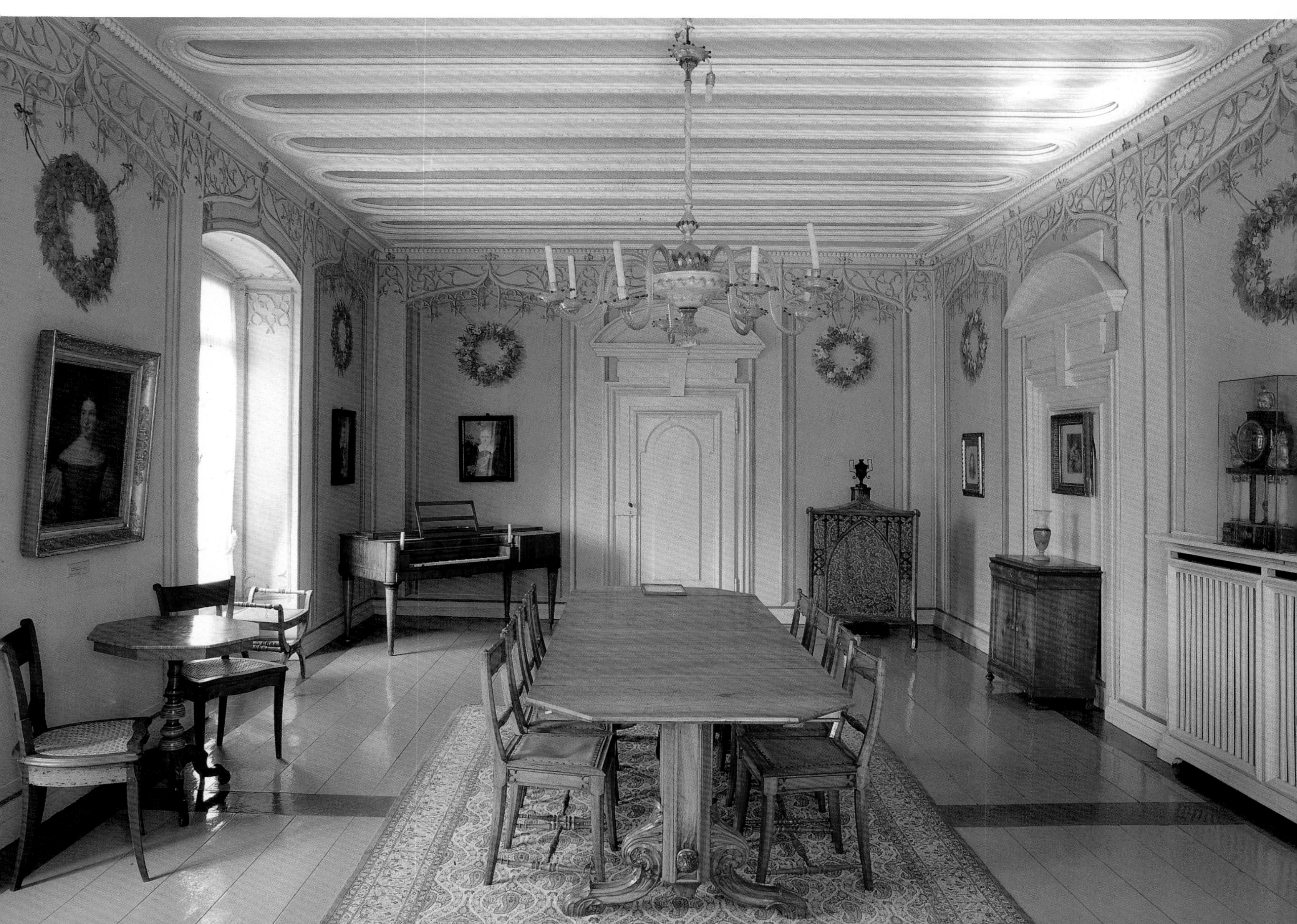

ITAL.
EIS
Adria

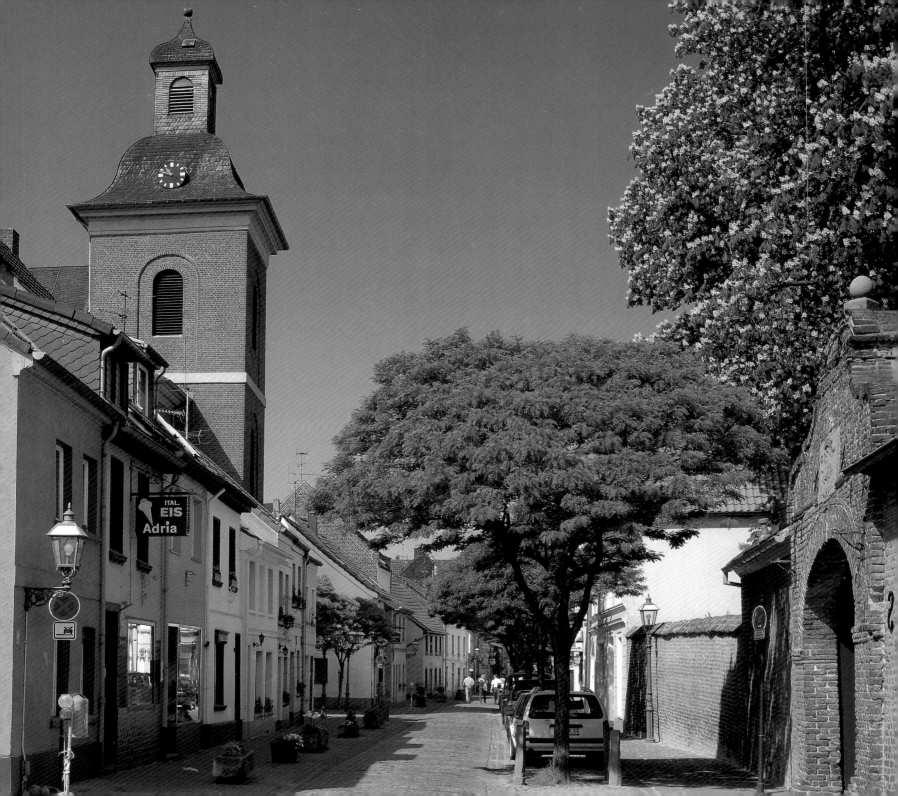

Burg und Städtchen Linn sind gemeinsam gewachsen und gehören zusammen. Die Stadtmauer blieb erhalten. 1901 schloß sich das Städtchen Krefeld an und machte den Hafenbau möglich.

In Gelduba, dem heutigen Stadtteil Gellep-Stratum, siedelten jahrhundertelang Römer und Franken. Ihre Spuren sichern Archäologen, die ihre Funde im Museum Burg Linn zeigen.

The Castle and the town of Linn have grown together and belong together. The city wall has been preserved. In 1901, the town was swallowed up by Krefeld, thus enabling the city to build a harbour.

Gelduba, the suburb Gellep-Stratum of today, was for centuries a settlement of the Romans and the Franks. Archaeologists have preserved the traces they left. Their findings are shown in the museum at Linn Castle.

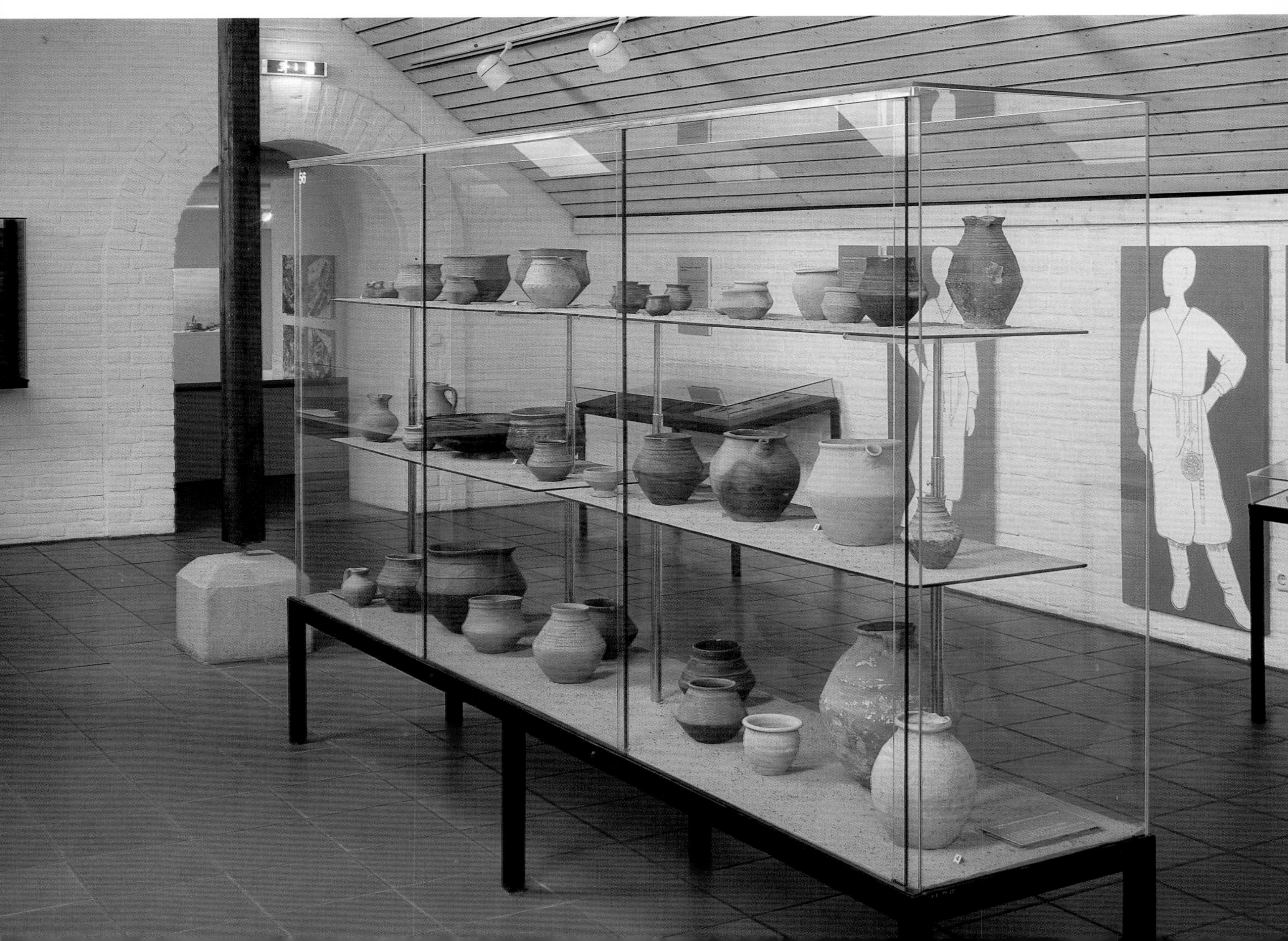

20 000 Textilien aus 2000 Jahren hütet das Deutsche Textilmuseum im Stadtteil Linn. Wechselnde Ausstellungen zeigen in immer neuen Themen die Vielfalt textilen Schaffens.

Das mittelalterliche Burgstädtchen Linn mit seinen malerischen Perspektiven ist für viele Besucher eine Überraschung. Viele Häuser aus dem 17. Jahrhundert werden liebevoll erhalten.

The German Museum of Textiles at Krefeld-Linn houses 20 000 textiles spanning 2000 years. Changing exhibitions with ever new topics show the diversity of textile production.

The medieval castle town of Linn with its picturesque perspectives is a surprise for many visitors. Many houses from the 17th century are being preserved with tender care.

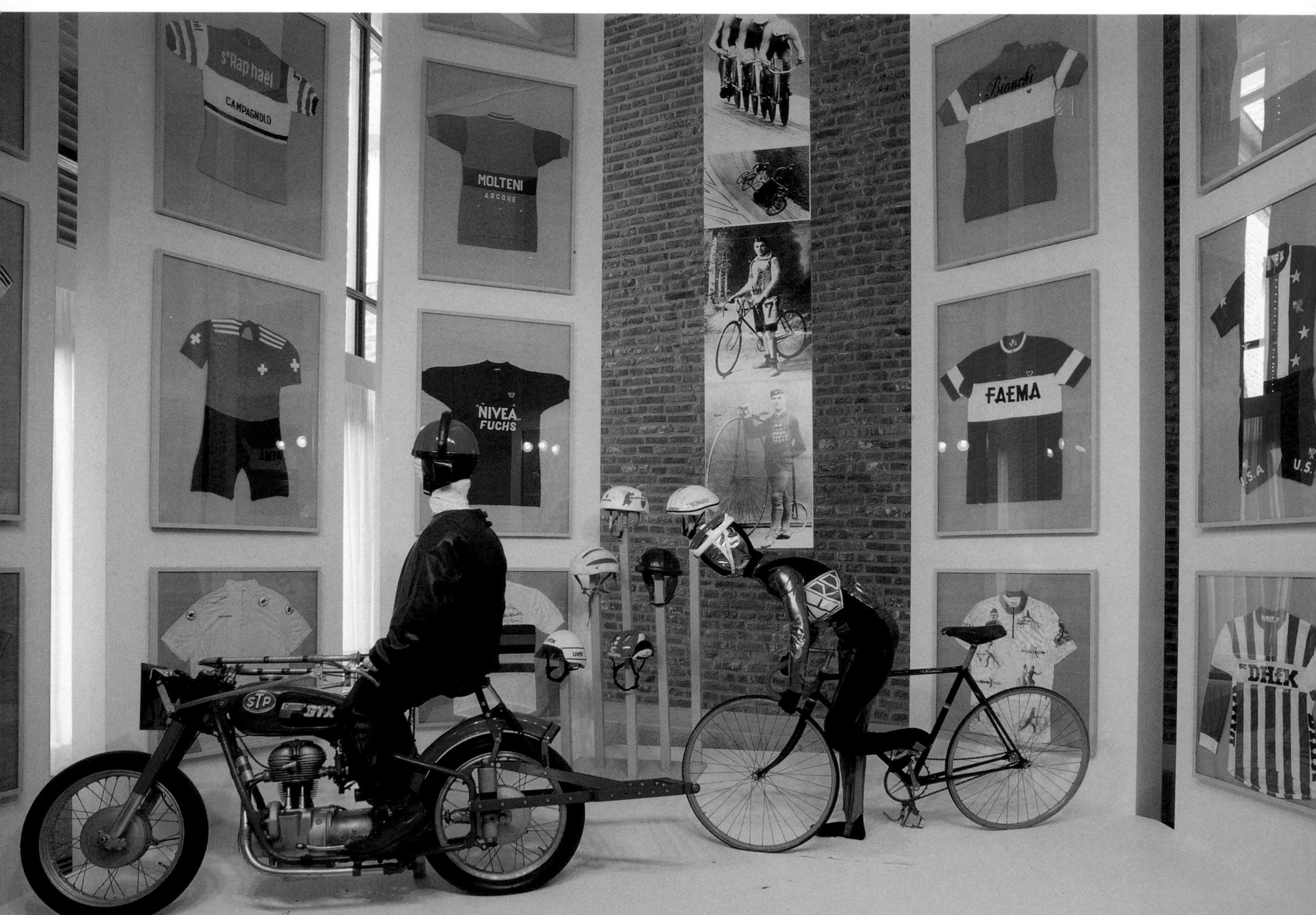

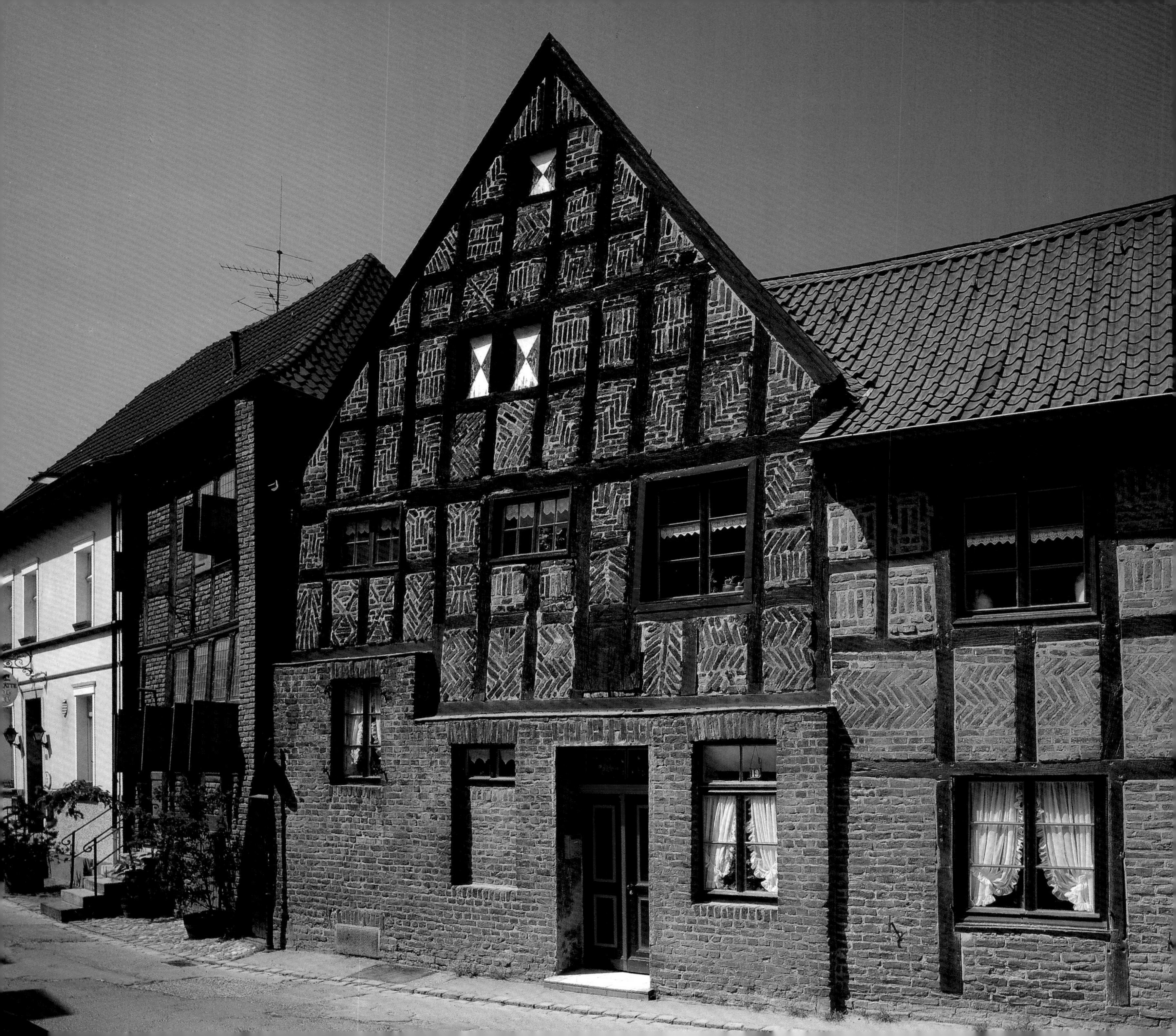
19

1843 konnte der Seidenfabrikant Cornelius de Greiff zum erstenmal eine Kaffeegesellschaft in sein neues Gartenschlößchen einladen, das er als Architekturjuwel in einen Park baute.

In 1843 the silk manufacturer Cornelius de Greiff was able to invite guests to a coffee party at his new garden palace for the first time. This architectural jewel was built in a park.

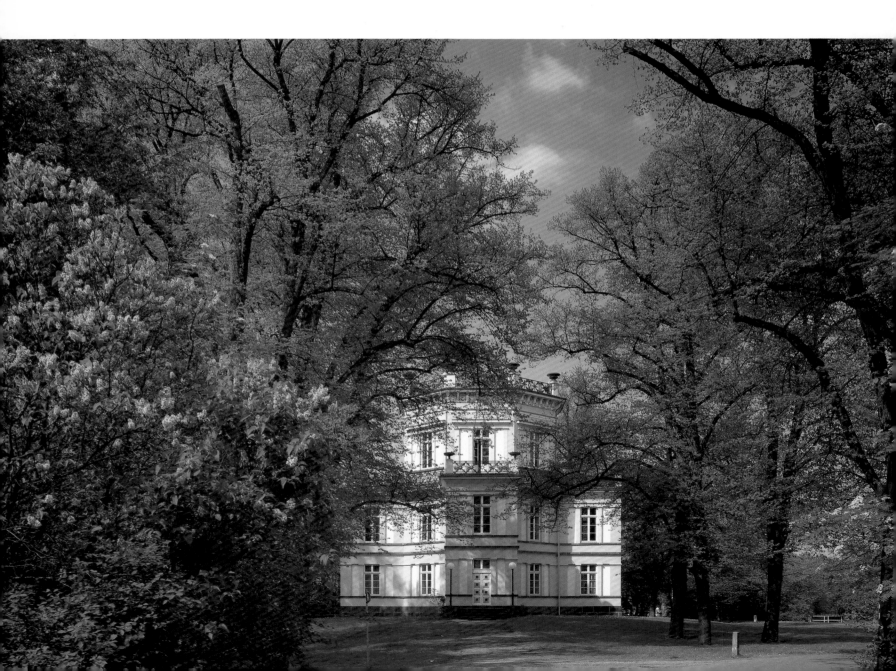

Nachts von Scheinwerfern beleuchtet, grüßt die Geismühle die Autofahrer auf der Nord-Süd-Passage der Autobahn 57. Sie und weitere drei Windmühlen weisen auf das nahe Holland hin.

On motorway 57 the windmill Geismühle, lit up by floodlights, greets travellers by night. Together with three other windmills it is a reminder of nearby Holland.

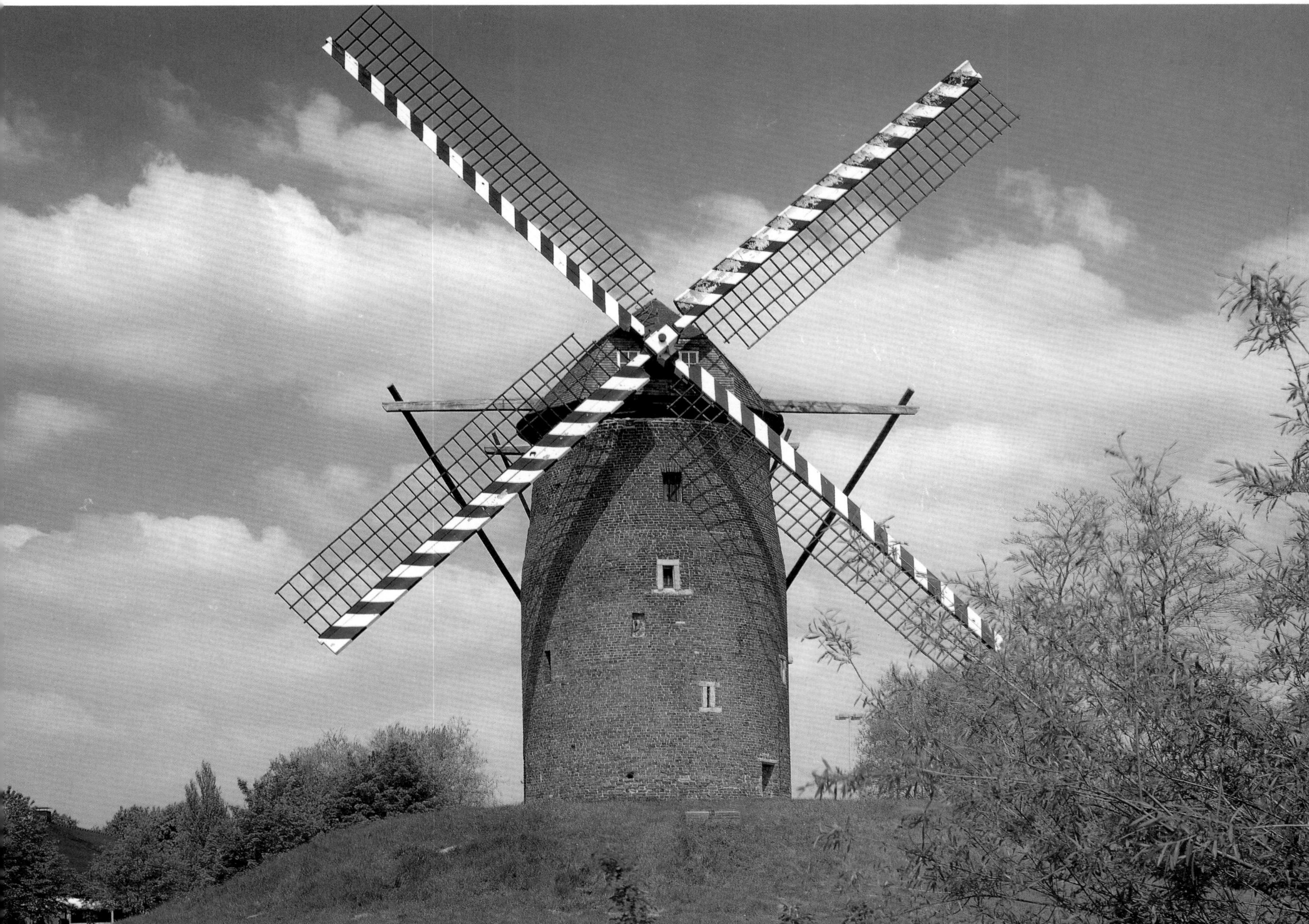

Das Selbstbewußtsein der Krefelder Stadtteile wird in ausgeprägtem Eigenleben deutlich, so auch in großen Schützenfesten. Unser Bild zeigt den Schützenzug im Stadtteil Fischeln.

The different parts of the city of Krefeld proudly maintain their own identity, both in their daily lives and in greater events like the big riflemen's festivals. Our picture shows the riflemen's parade in the suburb of Fischeln.

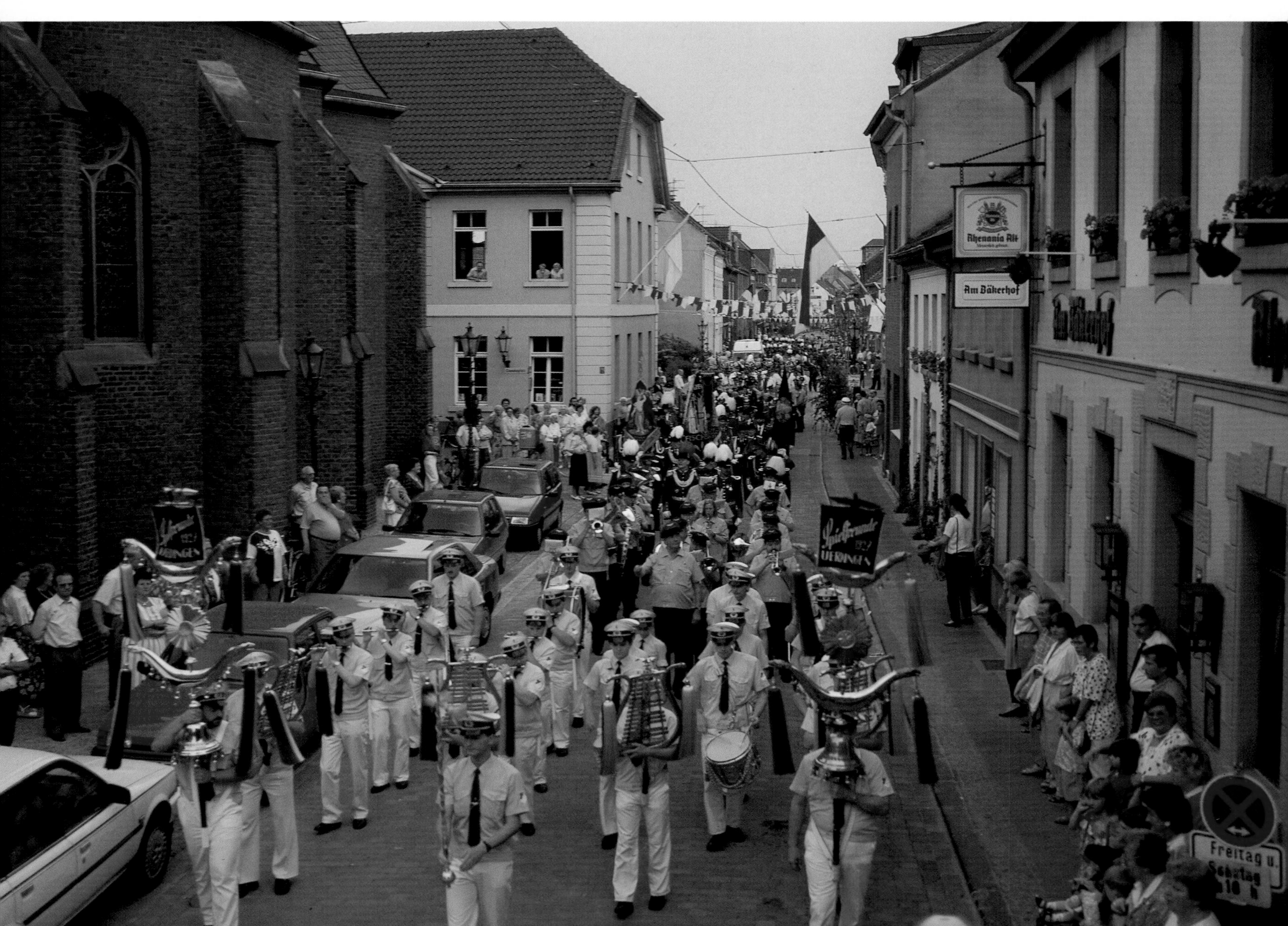

Das älteste Bauwerk in Krefeld ist der Turm der Fischelner Clemens-Kirche. Der schöne Kirchenraum wurde in gotischer Zeit gebaut und 1867 durch einen Kapellenkranz ergänzt.

The oldest part of Krefeld is the steeple of St. Clemens Church at Fischeln. The beautiful nave was built in the Gothic period and extended in 1867 with a circle of chapels.

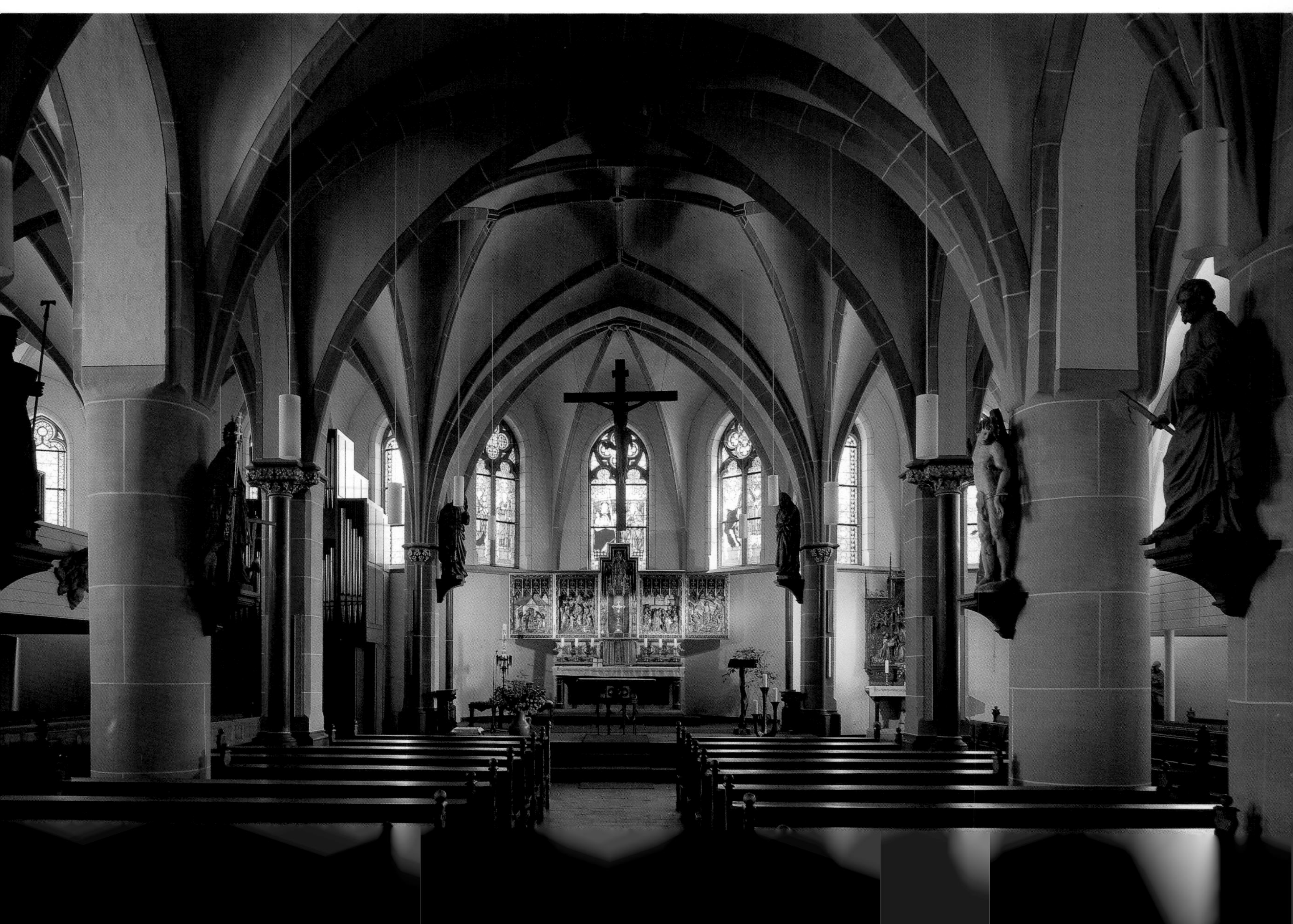

Mit Spenden und städtischen Zuschüssen leisten die Krefelder sich das Vergnügen, sonntags mit dem „Schluff" ins Grüne zu fahren. Am „Nordbahnhof" tanken Bahn und Gast.

Donations and municipal sponsorship maintain the historic train "Schluff", providing the people of Krefeld with the chance of a Sunday ride into the countryside. Train and guests "tank up" at the "Northern Station".

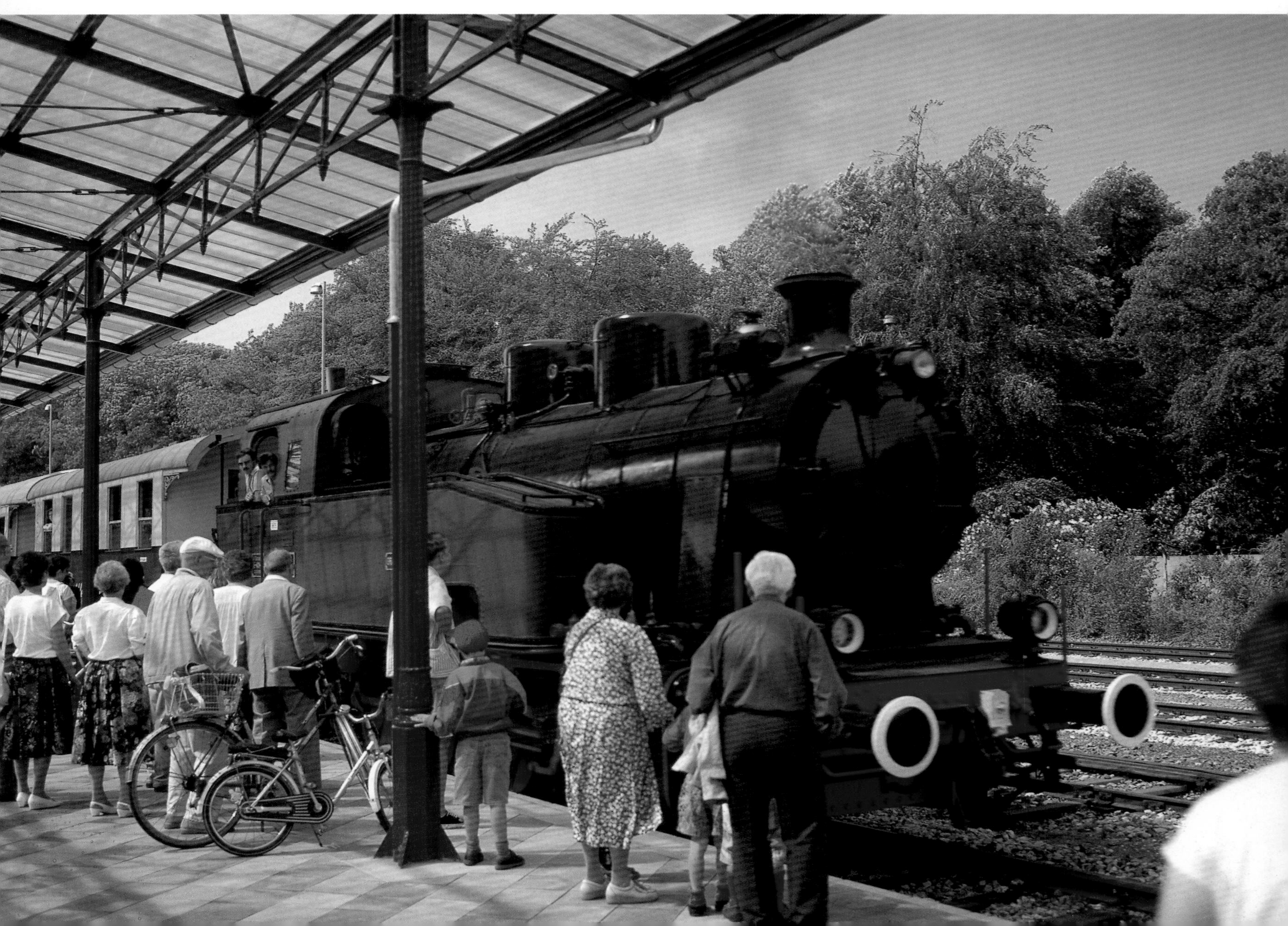

Seit 60 Jahren ist die Gaststätte der Brauerei Gleumes unverändert. Hier wird bei Altbier und Muscheln jeder Gast sofort in die Runde der Krefelder Geselligkeit aufgenommen.

The Gleumes brewery has remained unchanged for 60 years. Over special dark beer and mussels, every guest is received with the customary friendliness of the people of Krefeld.

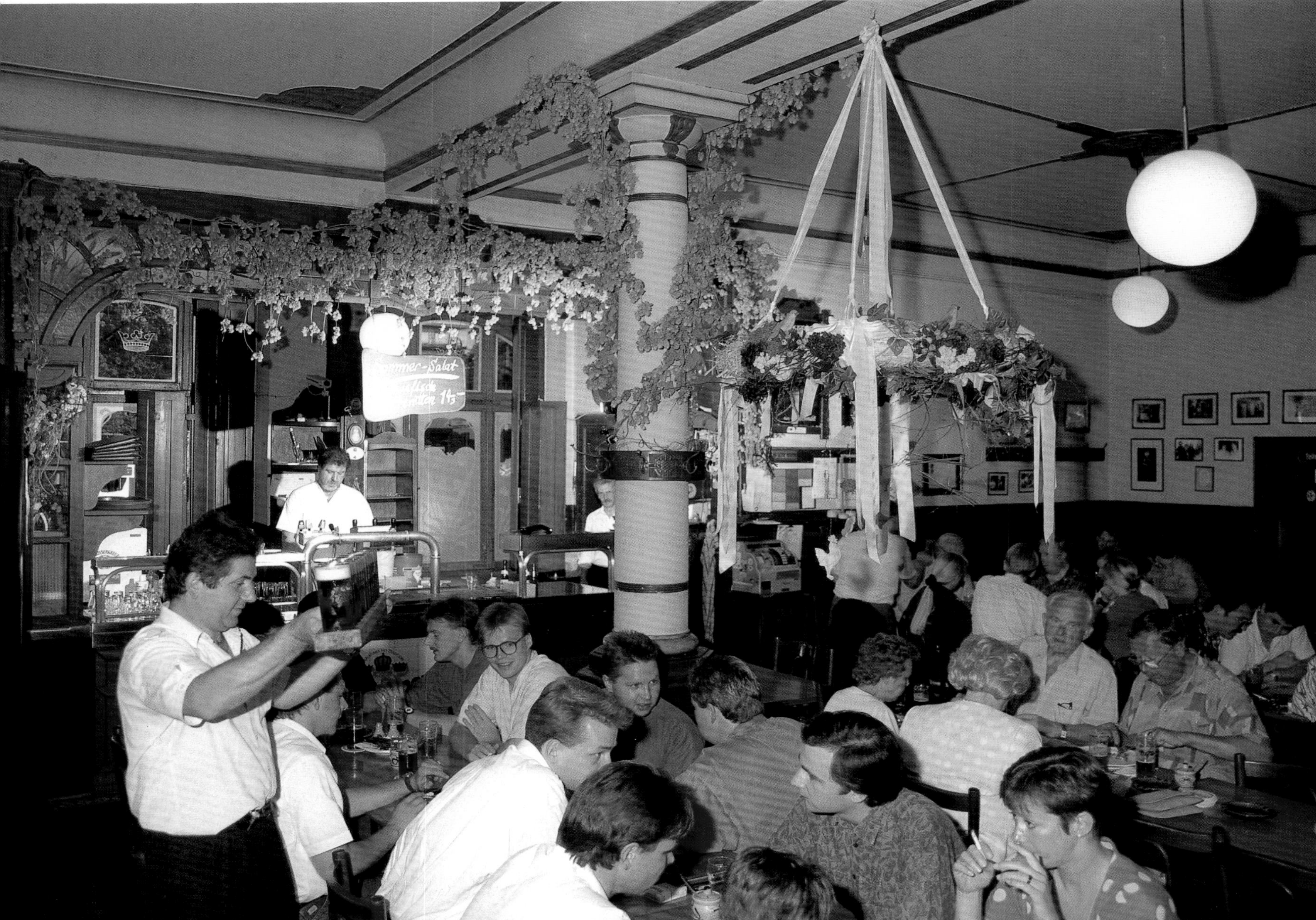

Viehzucht und -mast am Niederrhein sind international berühmt. In der Krefelder Niederrheinhalle wechseln die Tiere den Besitzer. Sie ist der größte Viehversteigerungsplatz im Lande.

Im Osten und Süden grenzt Krefeld an das Ballungsgebiet von Rhein und Ruhr. Im Norden und Westen öffnet sich die Landschaft so wie hier im Krefelder Stadtteil Hüls.

The Lower Rhine Area is famous for its farming and raising of cattle. Cattle are bought and sold in the Niederrheinhalle at Krefeld – the greatest cattle auction in the state is held here.

In the east and south, Krefeld borders on the densely populated industrial areas of the Rhine and the Ruhr. In the north and west, the landscape opens up, as here in the suburb of Hüls.

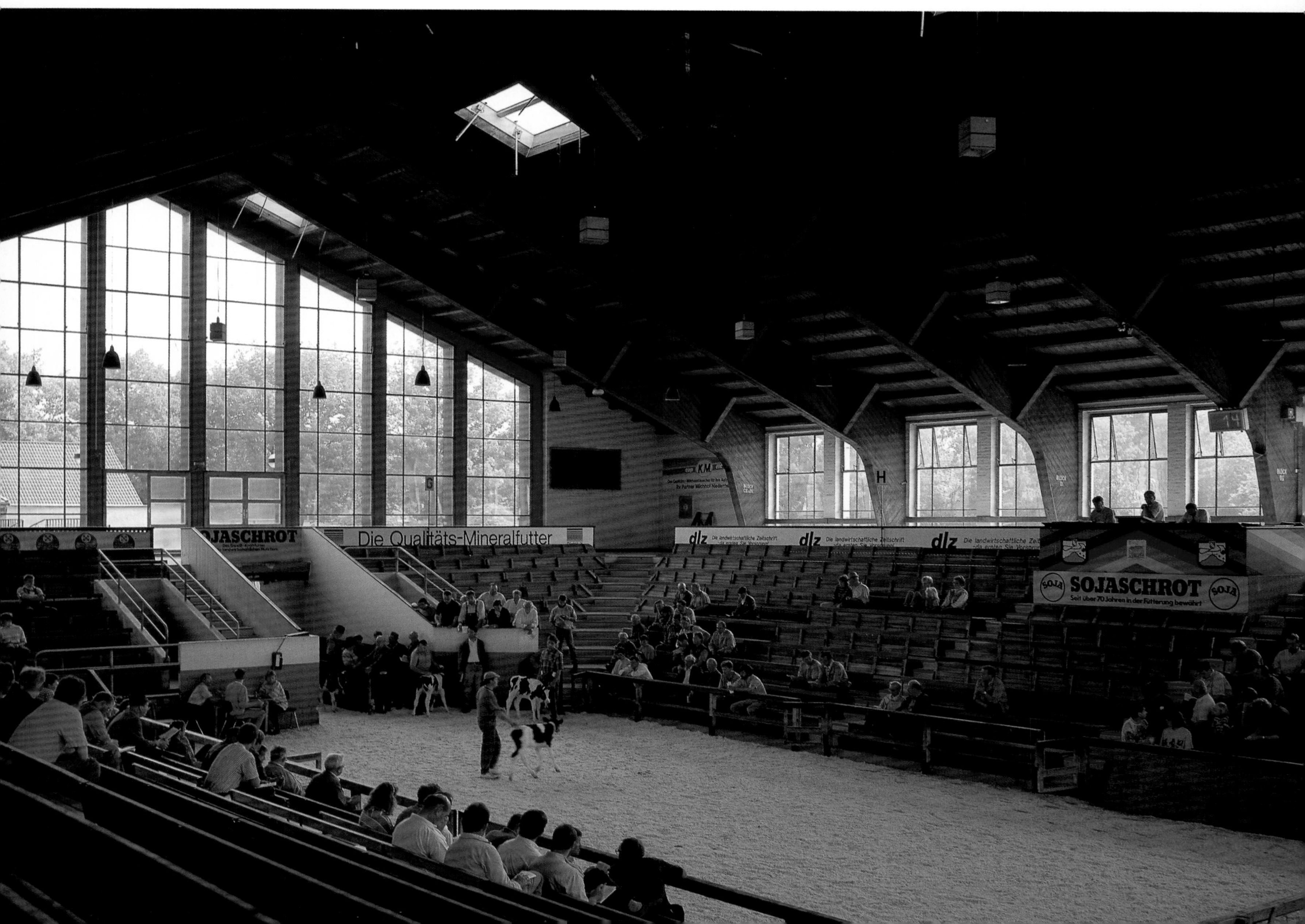

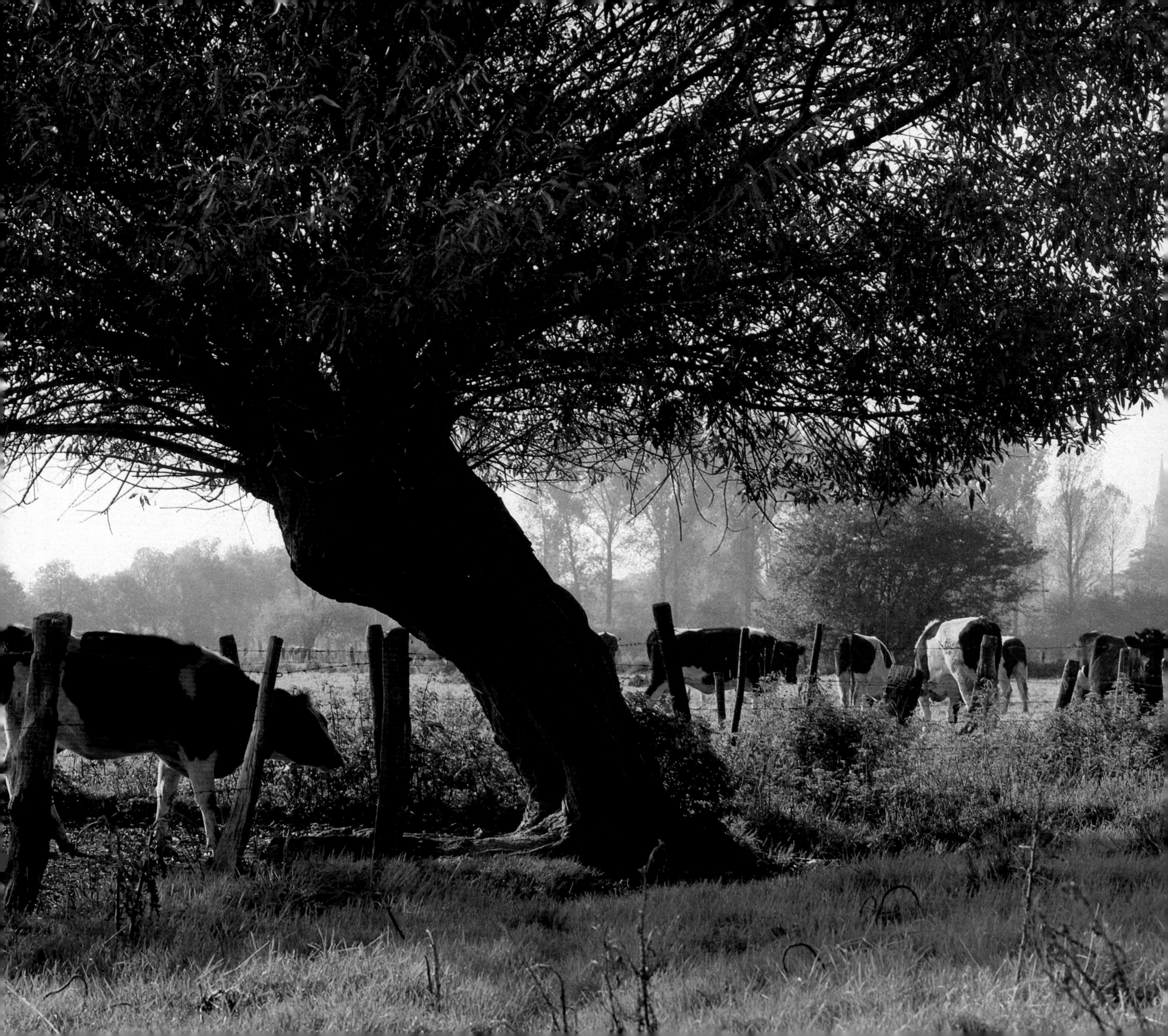

Umgewandelt in Eigentumswohnungen besteht das Beginenkloster „Klausur" mit seinen reizvollen Fachwerkhäusern fort. Der Turm der Cyriakus-Kirche krönt den Stadtteil Hüls.

The Beguine monastery "Retreat" with its charming half-timbered houses lives on, having been turned into condominiums. The church steeple of St. Cyriakus towers above the suburb of Hüls.

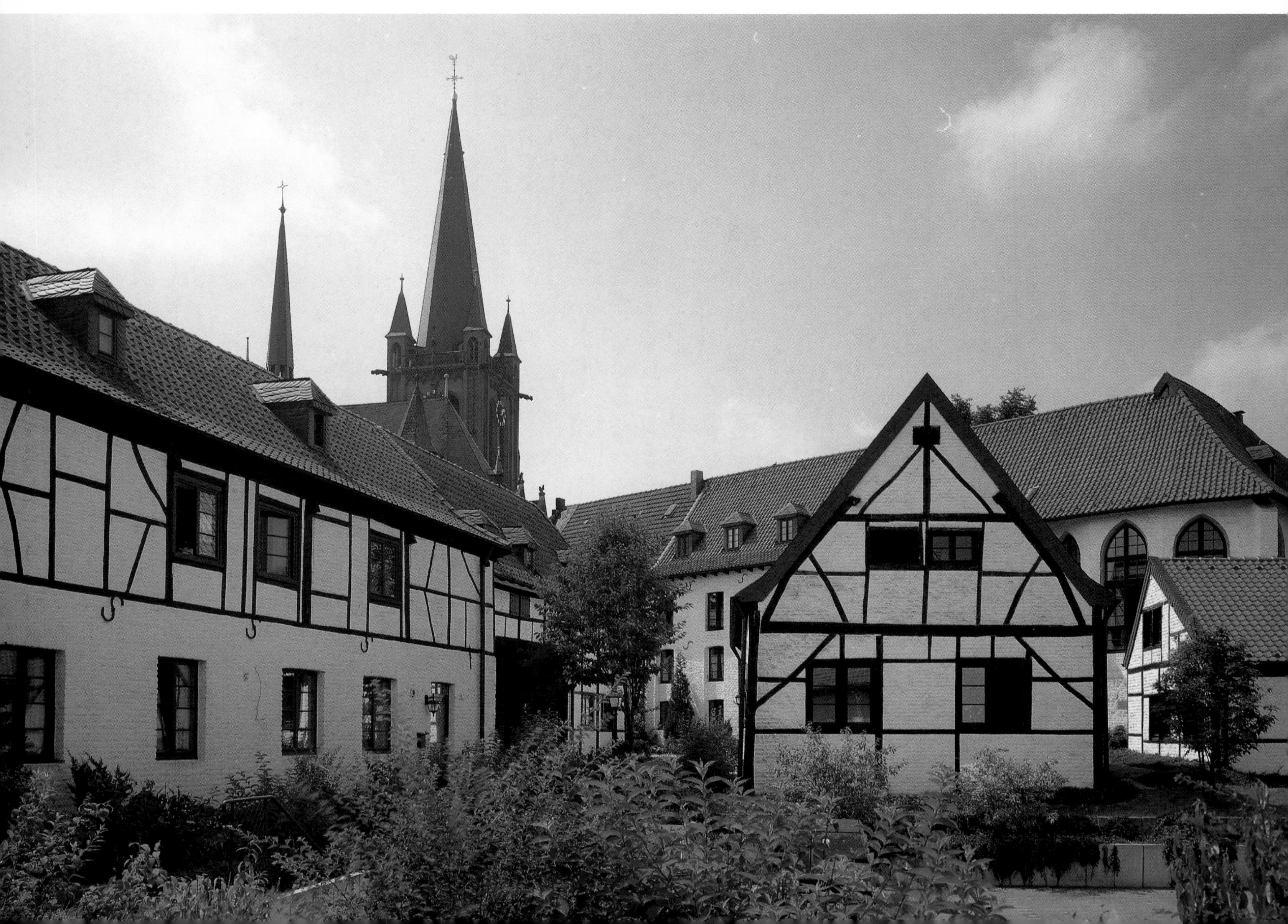

HÜLSER MARKT / Market at Hüls

Der Hülser Markt liegt auf halbem Weg an der alten Straßenverbindung zwischen Köln und Kleve. Hier spannten die Fuhrleute nach einer Tagesfahrt aus.

The market-place of Hüls lies on an old route half way between Cologne and Kleve. Here, drivers would unwind after their day's journey.

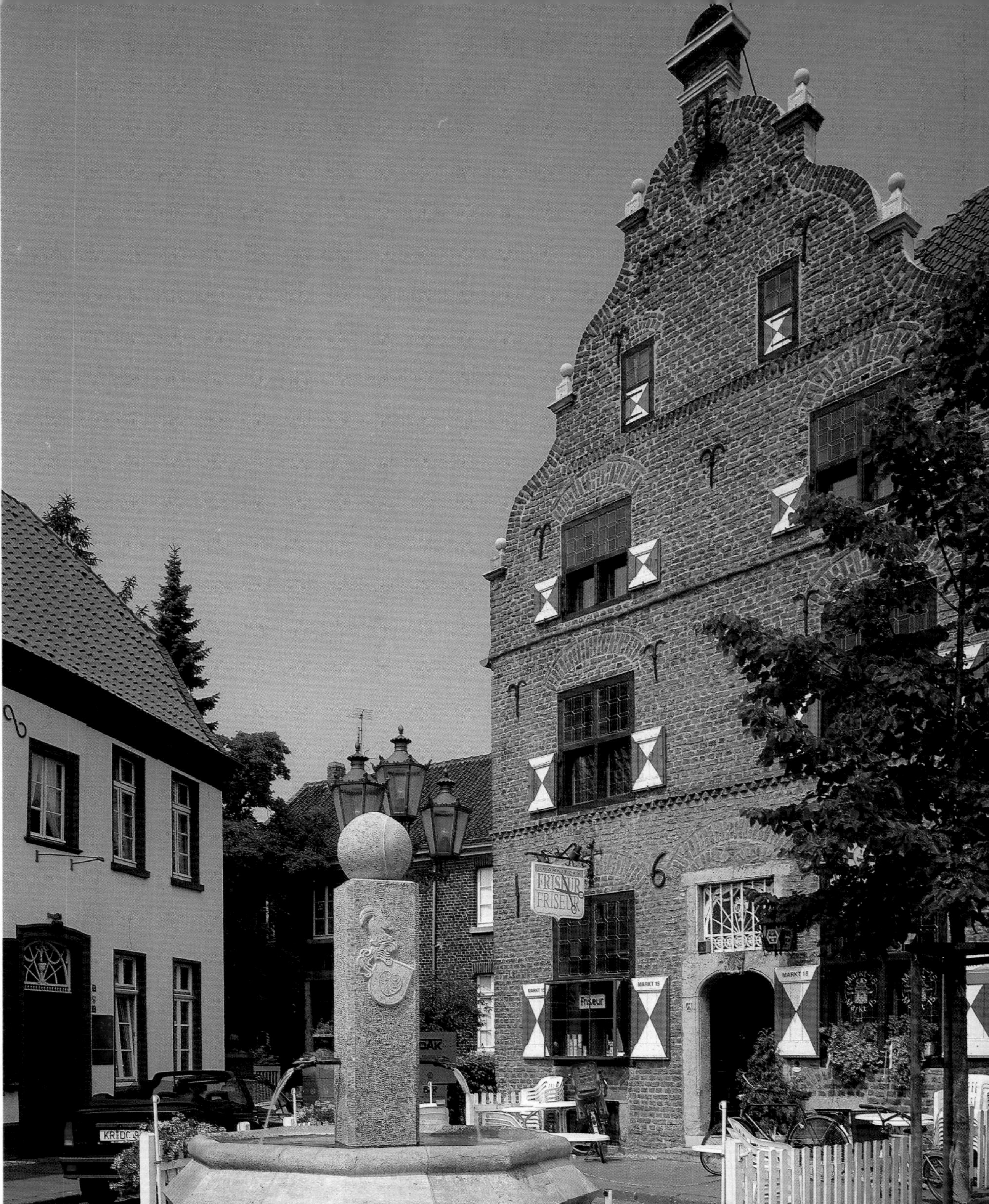

Eine Reihe von Baggerseen wurde in den 70er und 80er Jahren zu einer 2000 Meter langen Regattastrecke ausgebaut. Segler, Kanuten und Surfer haben sich an den Ufern niedergelassen.

In the seventies and eighties a series of gravel pits was turned into a regatta course. Sailors, canoeists and surfers have found their way to its banks.

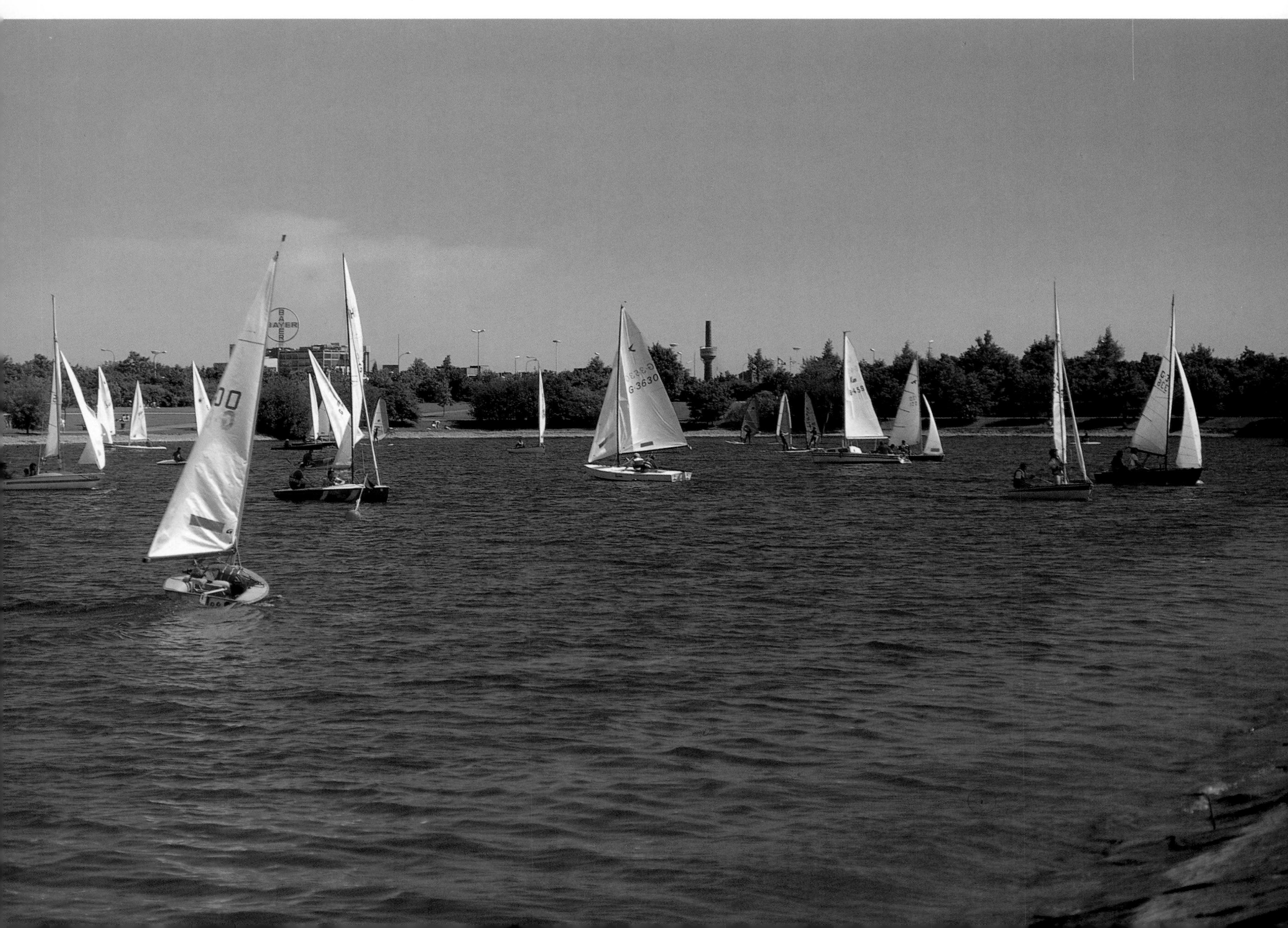

Eine 1000jährige Eibe in der Nachbarschaft von Haus Rath weist auf das Alter des ehemaligen Herrensitzes hin. Das strapazierte Gemäuer wurde als Wohnhaus neu belebt.

A 1000 year old yew-tree in the neighborhood of Rath House testifies to the age of this former country residence. The weather-worn structure was reconstructed as a residental building.

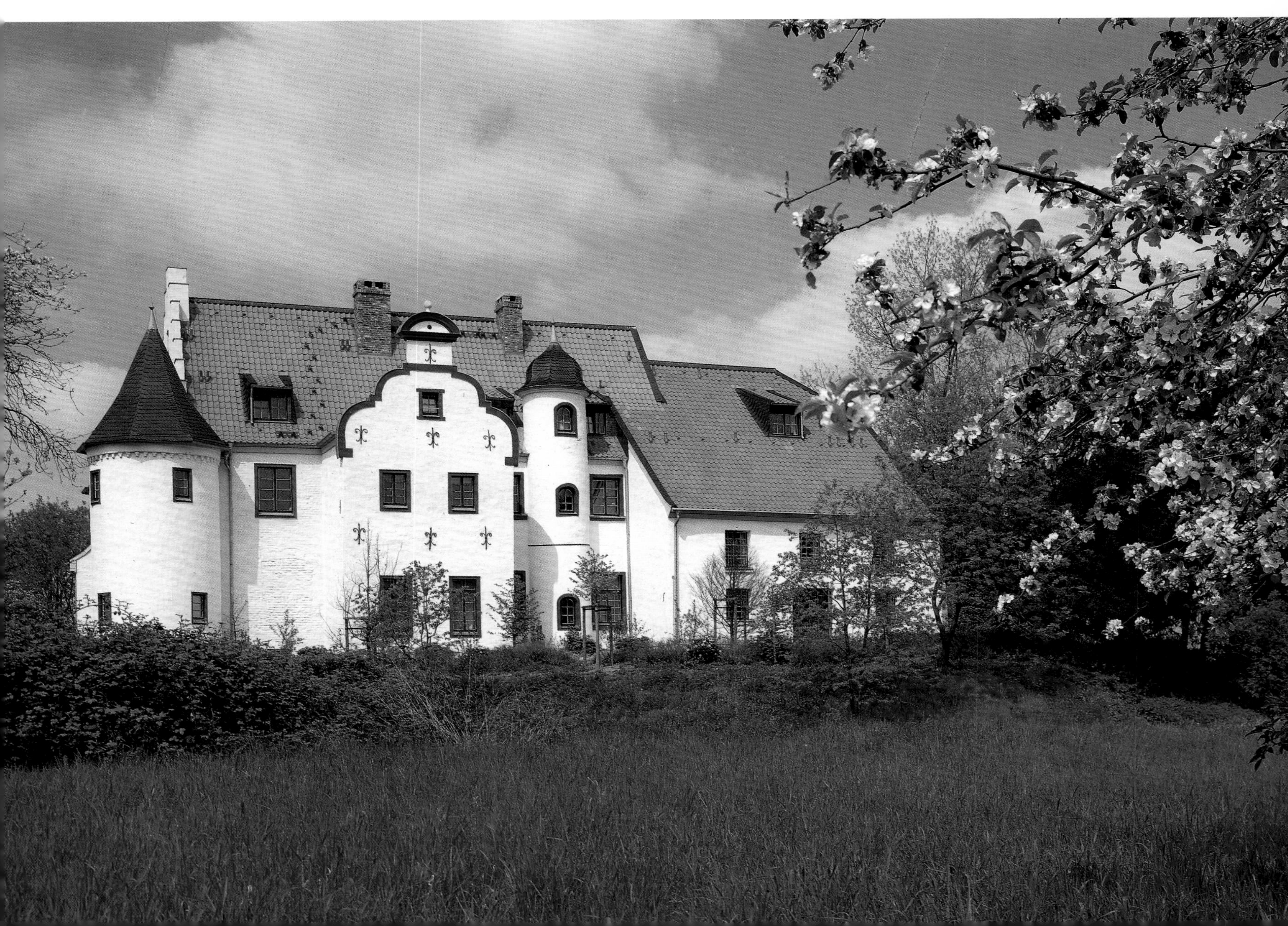

Die Hälfte des Krefelder Stadtgebietes ist unbebaute Landschaft. Reste der Überschwemmungsarme des Rheins, Niepkuhlen genannt, vereinen eine bunte Tier- und Pflanzenwelt.

Die Eiszeit stauchte Sand, Kies und Geröll zu einem flachen Hügel, dem Egelsberg. Auf dem Plateau steht die Mühle ideal im Wind, in deren Schatten Segelflugzeuge starten.

Half of the surface area of Krefeld consists of undeveloped countryside. Old flood canals of the Rhine, called "Niepkuhlen", host brightly coloured flora and fauna.

The ice age formed sand, pebbles and débris into a gentle hill, the Egelsberg. Its plateau is an ideal site for a mill, being exposed to the wind. Here gliders begin their flight in the shadow of the mill.

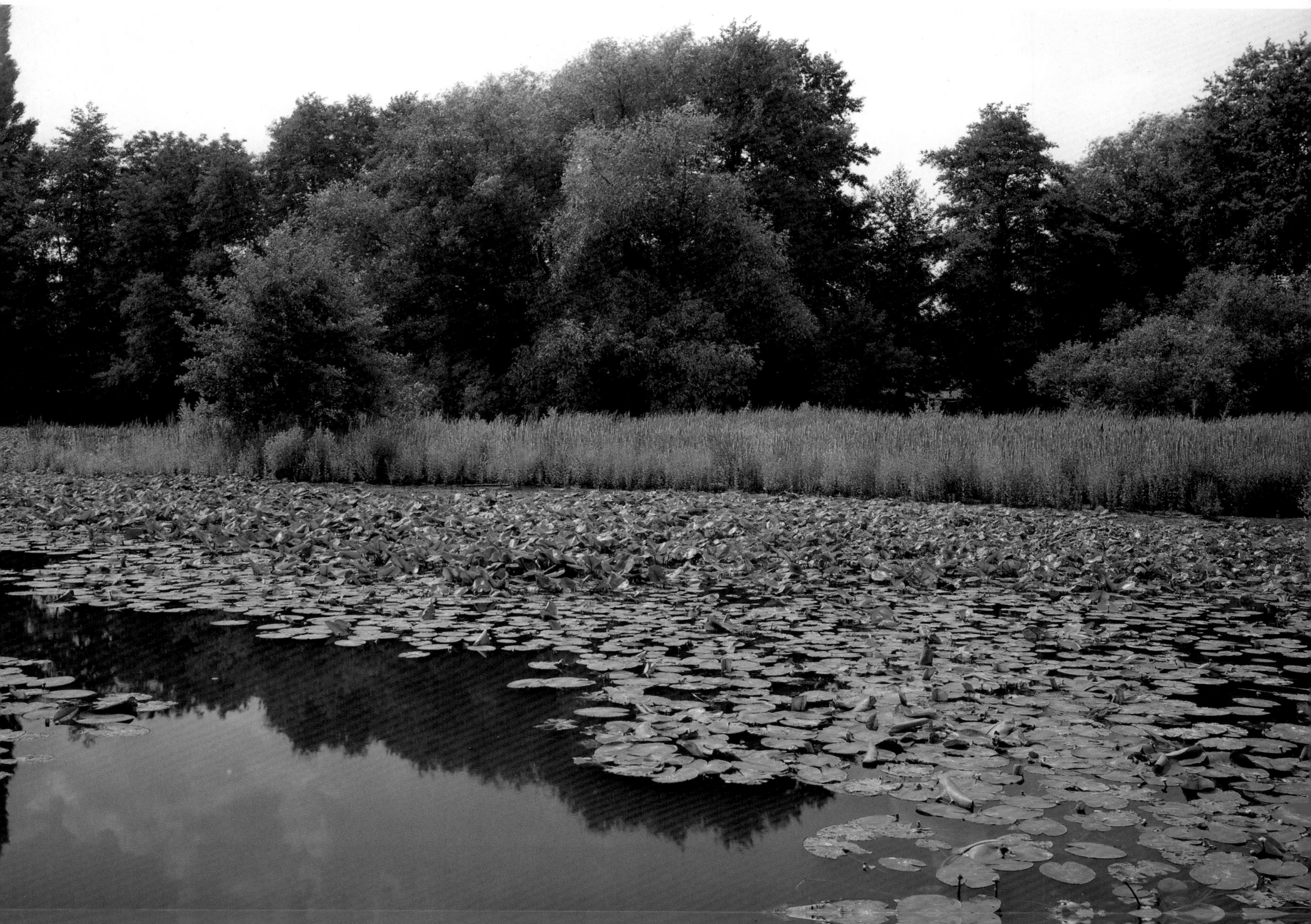

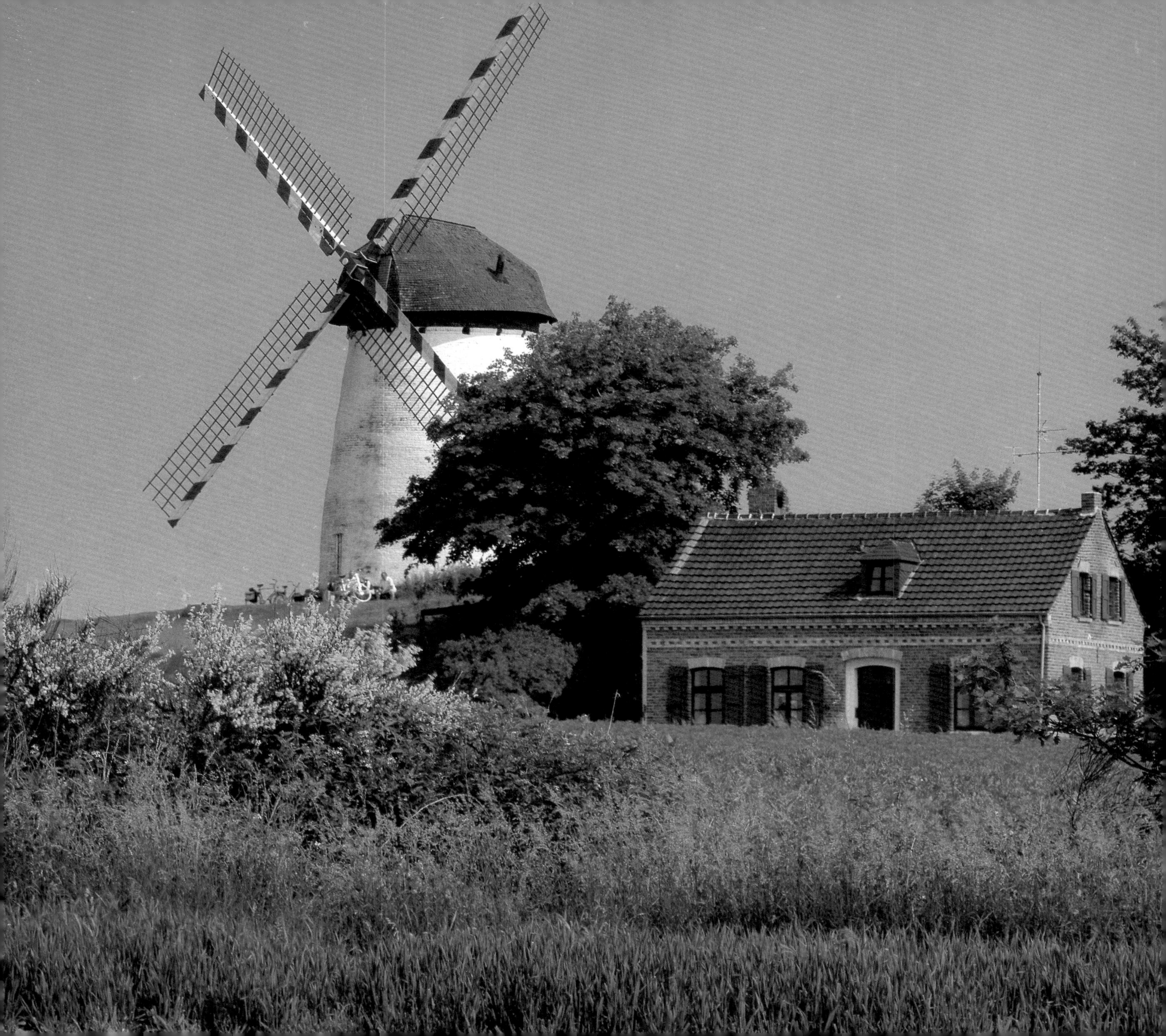

Auf den Bau eines Rhein-Maas-Kanals vertrauten die Erbauer der Krefelder Edelstahlwerke. Der Kanal kam nicht, aber Krefelder Edelstahl ist in aller Welt ein begehrtes Produkt.

The builders of the stainless steel works in Krefeld counted on the Rhine-Maas-Canal being built. The canal was not built, but Krefeld's stainless steel is wanted all over the world.

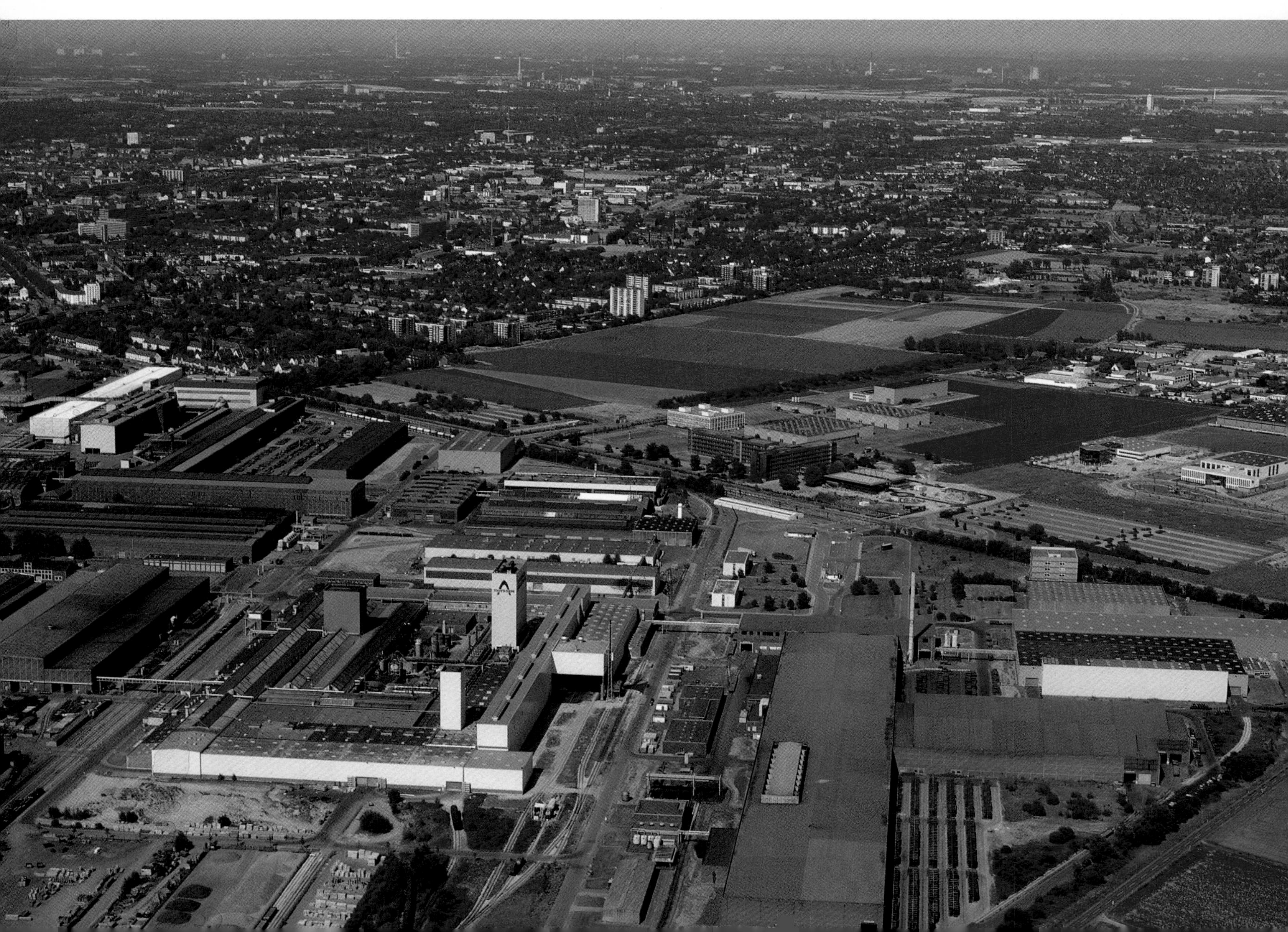

In Krefeld wird immer noch Seide gewebt, werden elegante Krawatten entworfen und genäht. Bier wird gebraut, und der Hochgeschwindigkeitszug ICE rollt aus Uerdinger Hallen.

Silk is still woven in Krefeld, elegant ties are designed and sewn, beer is brewed and the high speed train ICE rolls off the production line at Uerdingen.

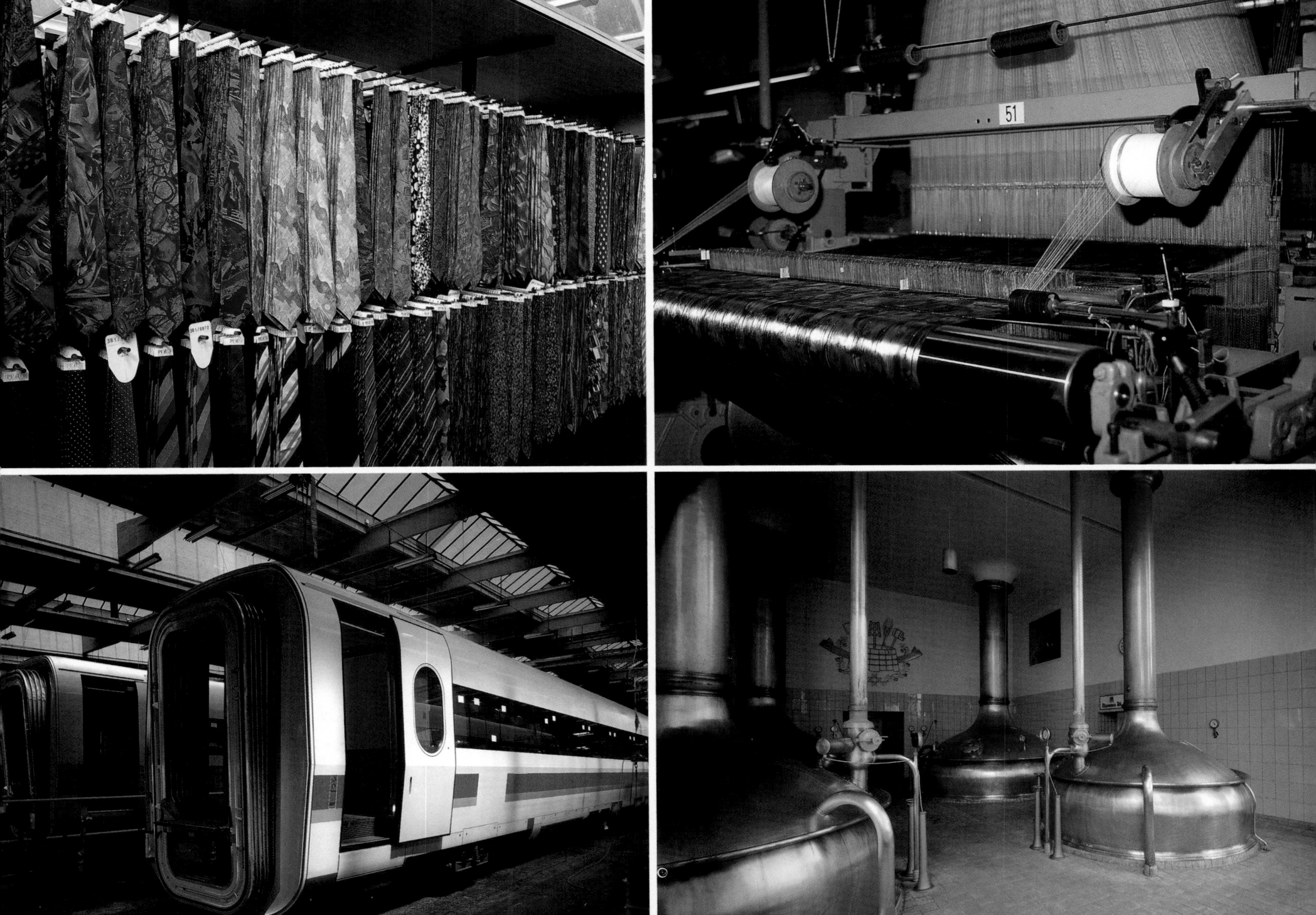

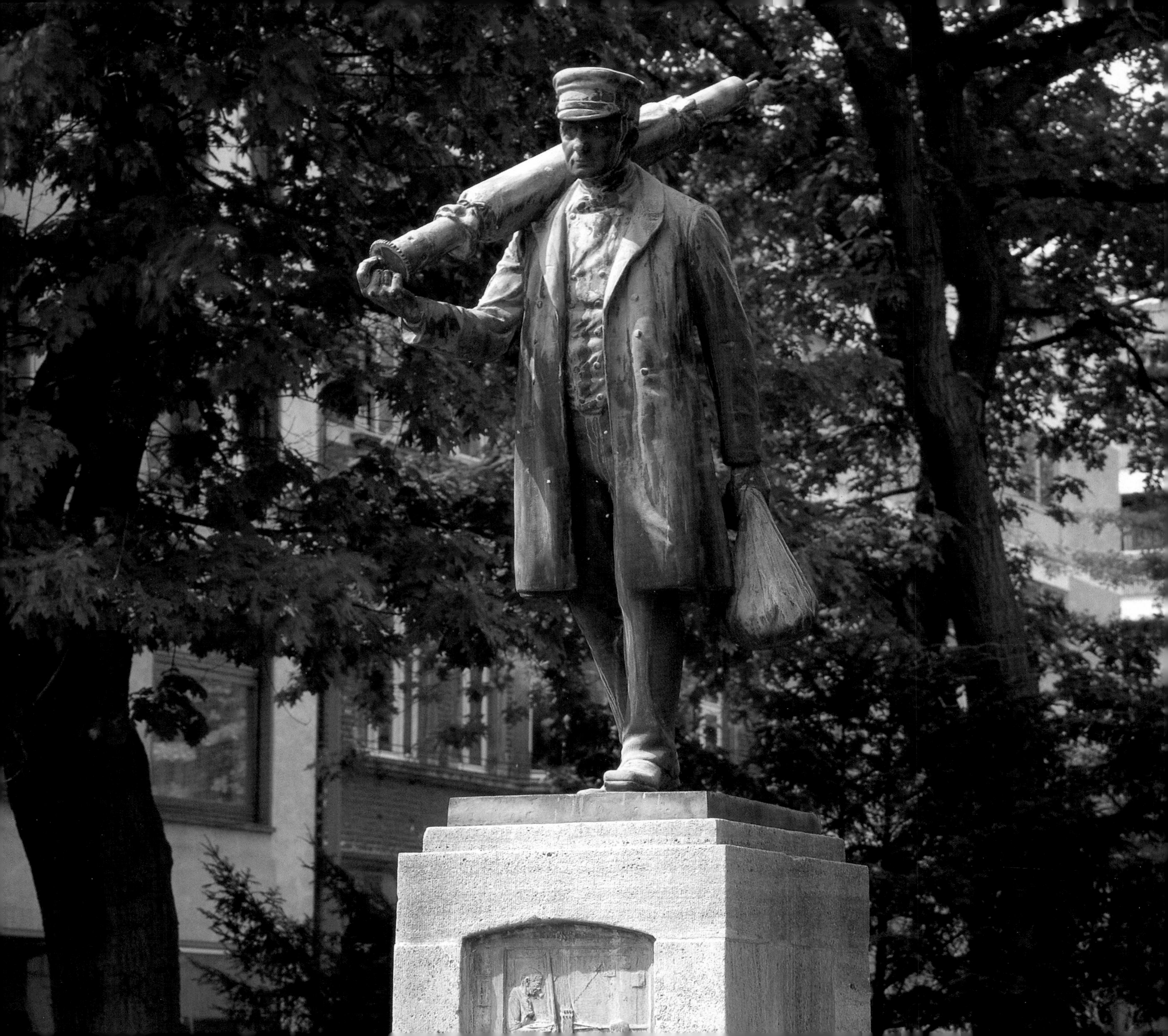

Meister Ponzelar/ Master Weaver

Im knielangen Überrock, darunter die Weste, an der Hand das Bündel mit den Spulen, auf der Schulter die Rolle mit Seidenstoff, dem Krefelder Weber setzte die Stadt dies Denkmal.

A knee-length topcoat over his vest, in his hand a bag of spools, on his shoulder a bolt of silk: this monument was dedicated by the city to the weavers of Krefeld.

BILDNACHWEIS / mention of sources used

HOLGER KLAES Seiten: Titelbild u. 10, Rücktitel u. 5, 6, 11, 12, 15, 16, 17, 18, 19, 20, 21, 22, 23, 24, 25, 26, 27, 28, 29, 30, 31, 32, 33, 35, 38, 39, 40, 42/43, 44, 45, 46, 47, 48, 49, 50, 51, 52, 53, 54, 55, 56, 57, 58, 59, 60, 62, 64, 65, 66, 67, 68, 69, 71 (4), 72

Horst Ziethen 34, 36, 61; Ruth Kaiser 8, 12, 63; Stadtverwaltung Krefeld 7, 9; Kaiser-Wilhelm-Museum, Krefeld 14; Laenderpress, Düsseldorf 37; Luftbild Martin Frank 70

Alter Stich auf Seite 4 / Stadtverwaltung Krefeld

Vorsatzseiten: Aktuelle Lageplankarte stellte die Stadt Krefeld (Vermessungs- u. Katasteramt) zur Verfügung.

Nachsatzseiten: Historische Karte stammt aus der Kartenaufnahme der Rheinlande 1803-1820 durch Tranchot und von Müffling und wurde vom Landesvermessungsamt NRW zur Verfügung gestellt.

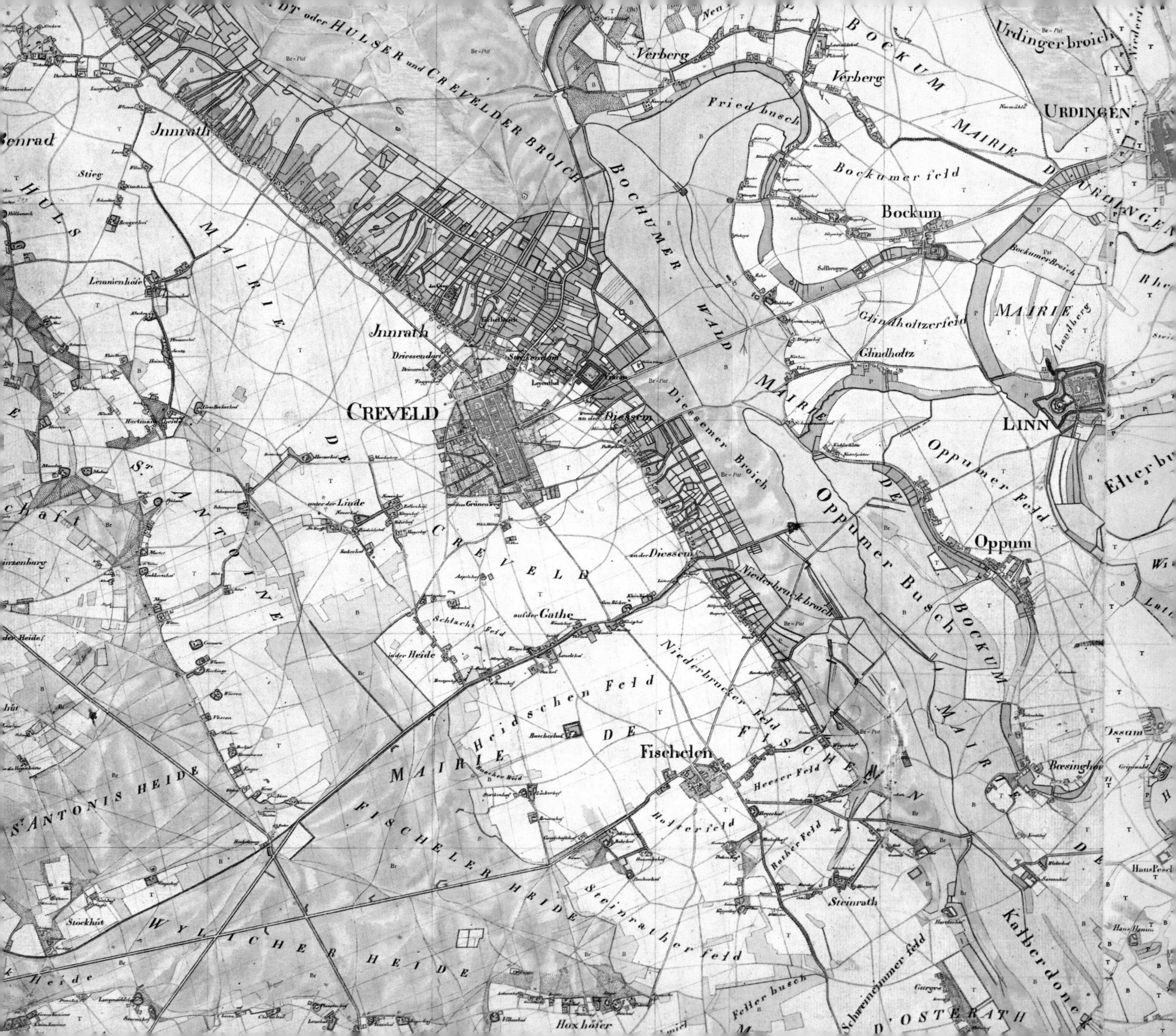

DT oder HULSER und CREVELDER BROICH
Verberg
BOCKUM
Urdinger broich
URDINGEN
Fried busch
MAIRIE
Bockumer feld
Bockum
Jnnrath
Stieg
HULS
MAIRIE
BOCHUMER
WALD
Lemmenhöfe
Glindholtzerfeld
Glindholtz
Bockumer Broich
MAIRIE
Landberg
Jnnrath
Driessendorf
CREVELD
Leyenthal
Diessem
Diessemer Broich
LINN
Oppumer Feld
Elterbu
DE
S.T ANTOINE
unter der Linde
CREVELD
an der Diessem
Oppumer Busch
Oppum
Niederbruckbroich
auf der Gathe
Schlacht feld
in der Heide
Niederbrucker Feld
BOCKUM
Heidschen Feld
Buscherhof
DE
Fischelen
FISCHELN
MAIRIE
Ossum
S.T ANTONIS HEIDE
MAIRIE
Heeser Feld
FISCHELER HEIDE
Holterfeld
Rother Feld
Steinrather feld
Steinrath
Kalberdonck
Stockhüt
WYLICHE HEIDE
Heide
Schweinenummer feld
Feller busch
Hoxhöfer
D'OSTERATH